VITREORETINAL SURGERY

VITREORETINAL SURGERY

Editors

Sandeep Saxena MS
Professor and Incharge Retina Service
Department of Ophthalmology
CSM Medical University
(Erstwhile King George's Medical University)
Lucknow, India

Carsten H Meyer MD
Professor and Head
Department of Ophthalmology
Pallas Klinik
Olten, Switzerland

Masahito Ohji MD
Professor and Chairman
Department of Ophthalmology
Shiga University of Medical Science
Shiga, Japan

Levent Akduman MD
Associate Professor
Department of Ophthalmology
Saint Louis University Eye Institute
Saint Louis University
Saint Louis, USA

Foreword

Maurice B Landers III MD

JAYPEE - HIGHLIGHTS
MEDICAL PUBLISHERS, INC.

Jaypee Brothers Medical Publishers (P) Ltd.

Headquarter

Jaypee Brothers Medical Publishers (P) Ltd
4838/24, Ansari Road, Daryaganj
New Delhi 110 002, India
Phone: +91-11-43574357
Fax: +91-11-43574314
Email: jaypee@jaypeebrothers.com

Overseas Offices

J.P. Medical Ltd.,
83 Victoria Street London
SW1H 0HW (UK)
Phone: +44-2031708910
Fax: +02-03-0086180
Email: info@jpmedpub.com

Jaypee-Highlights Medical Publishers Inc.
City of Knowledge, Bld. 237, Clayton
Panama City, Panama
Phone: 507-317-0160
Fax: +50-73-010499
Email: cservice@jphmedical.com

Website: www.jaypeebrothers.com
Website: www.jaypeedigital.com

Inquiries for bulk sales may be solicited at: jaypee@jaypeebrothers.com

Vitreoretinal Surgery

First Edition*:* **2012**

ISBN 978-93-5025-579-7

Printed at: Ajanta Offset & Packagings Ltd., New Delhi

Dedicated to

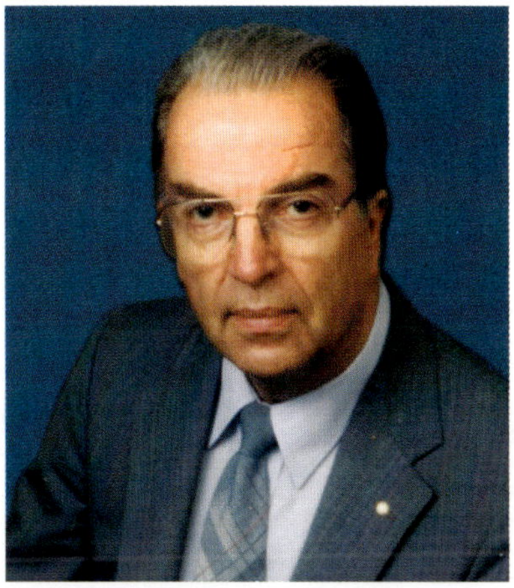

Late Prof Robert Machemer MD
(1933-2009)

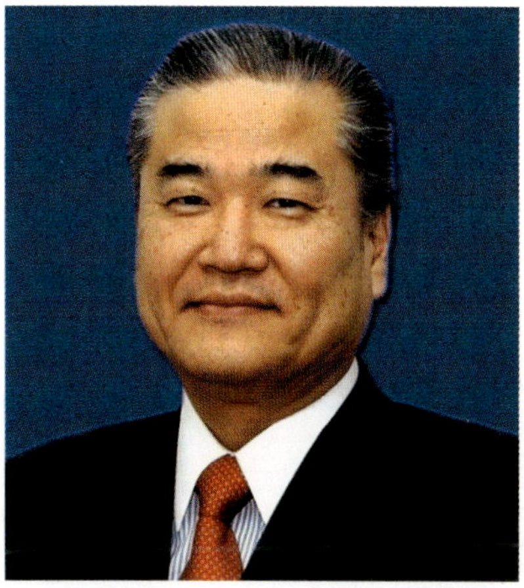

Late Prof Yasuo Tano MD
(1948-2009)

My parents Dr Rajesh C Saxena and Madhu Saxena, and to my family Sangeeta, Shreeya and Aishwarya

Sandeep

My loving wife Barbara and my children Paula and Philipp, who give my life support, happiness and dedication, for their unconditional love throughout successful as well as most challenging times

Carsten

My parents Isamu Ohji and Shigeko Ohji, and to my family Mifumi, Meiko, Hiroshi and Wako

Masahito

My parents Nebahat Akduman and Sabri Akduman, and to my family Isin, Yigit, Kaan and Koray

Levent

Contributors

Nakhleh E Abu-Yaghi MBBS
Assistant Professor
Department of Ophthalmology
The University of Jordan, Amman, Jordan

Levent Akduman MD
Associate Professor
Department of Ophthalmology
Saint Louis University Eye Institute
Saint Louis University, Saint Louis, USA

Jose Badal MD
Consultant
Hospital Moises Broggi, Barcelona, Spain

Sophie J Bakri MD
Associate Professor of Ophthalmology
Vitreoretinal Diseases and Surgery
Mayo Clinic, Rochester, USA

Susanne Binder MD
Professor and Head
Department of Ophthalmology
Krankenanstalt Rudolfstiftung, Vienna, and
Chair, Ludwig Boltzmann Institute for Retinology and Biomicroscopic Laser Surgery, Vienna, Austria

Kevin J Blinder MD
Professor of Clinical Ophthalmology and Visual Sciences
Washington University School of Medicine
The Retina Institute of St Louis, Saint Louis, USA

Ebru Nevin Cetin MD
Assistant Professor
Department of Ophthalmology
Pamukkale University, Denizli, Turkey

Steve Charles MD FACS FICS
Clinical Professor
University of Tennessee, Memphis, USA
Charles Retina Institute, Memphis, USA and
Adjunct Professor
Columbia College of Physicians and Surgeons, and
Chinese University of Hong Kong, Hong Kong

Lawrence P Chong MD
Consultant, VMR Institute
Huntington Beach, and
Clinical Professor of Ophthalmology
University of Southern California
Los Angeles, USA

Elaine de Paula Fiod Costa MD
Ophthalmologist
Department of Ophthalmology
Federal University of Sao Paulo, Sao Paulo, Brazil

Eduardo Dib MD
Ophthalmologist
Department of Ophthalmology
Federal University of Sao Paulo, Sao Paulo, Brazil

Andreas Ebneter MD
The Queen Elizabeth Hospital and
Department of Ophthalmology
Royal Adelaide Hospital, Adelaide, Australia

Dean Eliott MD
Professor
Associate Director, Retina Service
Massachusetts Eye and Ear Infirmary
Harvard Medical School, Boston, USA

Benjamin J Ernst MD
Vitreoretinal Fellow
Rocky Mountain Lions Eye Institute
University of Colorado
Aurora, USA

Lisa J Faia MD
Associated Retinal Consultants
William Beaumont Hospital
Royal Oak, USA

Michel Eid Farah MD
Professor
Department of Ophthalmology
Federal University of Sao Paulo
Sao Paulo, Brazil

Stephen S Feman MD MPH FACS
Walter and Sharon Ryan Davisson Professor
Department of Ophthalmology
Saint Louis University Eye Institute
Saint Louis University, Saint Louis, USA

Anne Fung MD
Vitreoretinal Consultant
Pacific Eye Associates
San Francisco, USA

Anna Gabrielian MD
Senior Vitreo-Retinal Surgery Fellow
Illinois Retina Associates
Rush University Medical Center, Chicago, USA

Jose Garcia-Arumi MD
Chairman and Professor
Universidad Autónoma de Barcelona
Instituto de Microcirugía Ocular (IMO), Barcelona, Spain

Alain Gaudric MD
Professor and Chairman
Service d'Ophtalmologie
Hôpital Lariboisière
Université Paris 7, Paris, France

Jagjit Singh Gilhotra M Med FRANZCO
The Queen Elizabeth Hospital
Department of Ophthalmology
Royal Adelaide Hospital and South Australian Institute of Ophthalmology, Adelaide, Australia

Lingam Gopal MS FRCS
Director Research
Medical Research Foundation
Sankara Nethralaya, Chennai, India

Kaan Gündüz MD
Professor
Department of Ophthalmology
Ankara University, Ankara, Turkey

Seenu M Hariprasad MD
Associate Professor and Director of Clinical Research
Chief, Vitreoretinal Service
Section of Ophthalmology and Visual Science
University of Chicago, Chicago, USA

Tarek S Hassan MD
Professor, Department of Ophthalmology
William Beaumont School of Medicine
Oakland University
Partner, Associated Retinal Consultants, Royal Oak, USA

Heinrich Heimann MD
Consultant Ophthalmic Surgeon
Royal Liverpool University Hospital
Liverpool, United Kingdom

Yasushi Ikuno MD
Associate Professor
Department of Ophthalmology
Osaka University Graduate School of Medicine
Osaka, Japan

Astha Jain MBBS
Department of Ophthalmology
CSM Medical University, Lucknow, India

Rajeev Jain MS
Save Sight Centre
New Delhi, India

Humeyra Karacal MD
Assistant Professor
Department of Ophthalmology and Visual Sciences
Washington University School of Medicine
St. Louis, USA

Pearse A Keane MRCOphth MSc
Moorfields Eye Hospital
London, United Kingdom

Ferenc Kuhn MD PhD
Associate Professor of Clinical Ophthalmology
University of Alabama at Birmingham
Associate Director of Clinical Research
Helen Keller Foundation for Research and Education
Birmingham, Alabama, USA and
Chief Vitreoretinal Surgeon, Milos Klinika
Belgrade, Serbia

Timothy YY Lai MD FRCSEd
Associate Professor
Department of Ophthalmology and Visual Sciences
The Chinese University of Hong Kong, Hong Kong

Wico W Lai MD FACS
Associate Professor
Eye Institute and the Research Center of Heart
Brain, Hormone and Healthy Aging
The University of Hong Kong, Pokfulam, Hong Kong

Paolo Lanzetta MD
Associate Professor
Department of Ophthalmology
University of Udine, Udine, Italy

Gary KY Lee MBBS MRCSEd
Hong Kong Eye Hospital, Hong Kong

Amy Lo PhD
Assistant Professor
Eye Institute and the Research Center of Heart, Brain,
Hormone and Healthy Aging
The University of Hong Kong, Pokfulam, Hong Kong

Mauricio Maia MD
Professor
Department of Ophthalmology
Federal University of Sao Paulo, Sao Paulo, Brazil

Ajit Babu Majji MD
Consultant
Smt. Kanuri Shantamma Centre for Vitreoretinal Diseases
LV Prasad Eye Institute, Hyderabad, India

Nicholas Marchase MD
Department of Ophthalmology
Callahan Eye Foundation Hospital
Birmingham, USA

Gloria Dal Mas MD
Department of Ophthalmology
University of Udine, Udine, Italy

Ranjana Mathur M Med FRCS (Ed) MS DNB
Senior Consultant
Vitreoretinal Service
Singapore National Eye Centre, Singapore

Colin A McCannel MD
Jules Stein Eye Institute
University of California, Los Angeles (UCLA)
Los Angeles, USA

Carsten H Meyer MD
Professor and Head
Department of Ophthalmology
Pallas Klinik, Olten, Switzerland

Dimple Modi MD MPH
Retina Fellow
Bascom Palmer Eye Institute
University of Miami, Miami, USA

Shaheeda Mohamed MBBS MRCSEd
Hong Kong Eye Hospital, Hong Kong

Milton Nunes de Moraes-Filho MD
Ophthalmologist
Department of Ophthalmology
Federal University of Sao Paulo, Sao Paulo, Brazil

Masahito Ohji MD
Professor and Chairman
Department of Ophthalmology
Shiga University of Medical Science, Shiga, Japan

Ozay Oz MD
Associate Professor
Sevgi Eye Center, Adana, Turkey

Claudine E Pang MRCS (Ed)
Singapore National Eye Center, Singapore

Eylem Yaman Pinarci MD
Instructor
Istanbul Medical and Research Center
Baskent University, Istanbul, Turkey

Kamalesh J Ramaiya MD
Vitreoretinal Surgeon
Eye Associates of New Mexico, Albuquerque, USA

Eduardo Buchele Rodrigues MD
Ophthalmologist
Department of Ophthalmology
Federal University of Sao Paulo, Sao Paulo, Brazil

Srinivas R Sadda MD
Associate Professor
Director, Medical Retina, Doheny Eye Institute
University of Southern California, Los Angeles, USA

Valentina Sarao MD
Department of Ophthalmology
University of Udine, Udine, Italy

Osamu Sawada MD
Associate Professor
Department of Ophthalmology
Shiga University of Medical Science
Shiga, Japan

Sandeep Saxena MS
Professor and Incharge
Retina Service
Department of Ophthalmology
CSM Medical University
(Erstwhile King George's Medical University)
Lucknow, India

Hermann D Schubert MD
Professor of Clinical Ophthalmology and Pathology
Edward S Harkness Eye Institute
New York-Presbyterian Hospital
Columbia University, New York, USA

Neha Sinha MBBS
Department of Ophthalmology
CSM Medical University
Lucknow, India

Ulrike Stolba MD
Associate Professor
Department of Ophthalmology and
L Boltzmann Institute of Retinology
Rudolf Foundation Clinic, Vienna, Austria

Ramin Tadayoni MD
Service d'Ophtalmologie
Hôpital Lariboisière
Université Paris 7, Paris, France

Ryan M Tarantola MD
Assistant Professor
Vitreoretinal Diseases
Department of Ophthalmology
Saint Louis University Eye Institute
Saint Louis University
Saint Louis, USA

Paul E Tornambe MD FACS
Retina Consultants, San Diego
Poway, USA

Michael T Trese MD
Clinical Professor of Ophthalmology
Oakland University William Beaumont School of Medicine
and
Chief Pediatric and Adult Vitreoretinal Surgery
William Beaumont Hospital, Royal Oak, USA

Daniele Veritti MD
Department of Ophthalmology
University of Udine, Udine, Italy

David Wong FRCS FRCOphth
Professor
Eye Institute and the Research Center of Heart, Brain,
Hormone and Healthy Aging
The University of Hong Kong, Pokfulam, Hong Kong

Edmund YM Wong M Med FRCS (Ed)
Senior Consultant
Singapore National Eye Center, Singapore

Ian Y Wong MRCS
Assistant Professor
Eye Institute and the Research Center of Heart
Brain, Hormone and Healthy Aging
The University of Hong Kong
Pokfulam, Hong Kong

David M Wu MD PhD
Doheny Eye Institute
Keck School of Medicine
University of Southern California, Los Angeles, USA

Widad Yusof MD FRCS
Eye Institute and the Research Center of Heart,
Brain, Hormone and Healthy Aging
The University of Hong Kong, Pokfulam, Hong Kong

Miguel Zapata MD
Associate Professor
Universidad Autonoma de Barcelona
Hospital Universitario Valle Hebron
Barcelona, Spain

Foreword

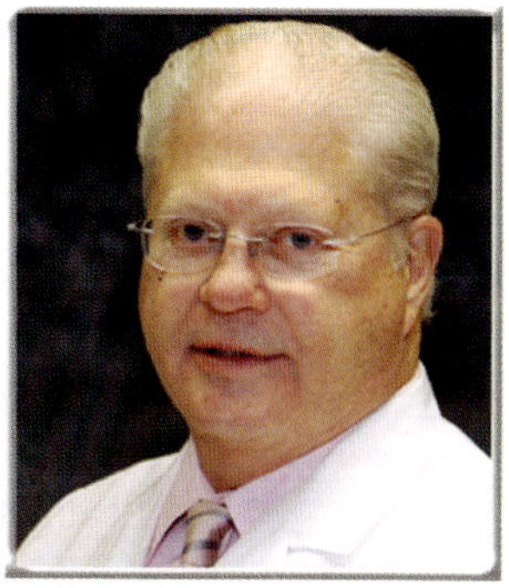

Dr Sandeep Saxena, along with Drs Carsten H Meyer, Masahito Ohji and Levent Akduman, has once again put together a remarkable book, this time covering the field of vitreoretinal surgery.

This book is destined to become a classic in the field. Clearly written by multiple international experts, the detailed reference lists following each chapter provide extensive background support for the text.

The illustrations are outstanding. Combining excellent schematic drawings, beautiful clinical photographs, fluorescein angiograms, and OCT images…the illustrations provide the reader, whether novice or expert, with a remarkably lucid journey through the complex world of vitreoretinal surgery.

The book is divided into eleven sections, initially covering Principles, Techiques and Instrumentation in Vitrectomy, and moving on through sections on the management of Retinal Detachment, Diabetic Retinopathy, Retinal Vascular Disorders and Inflammation, Macular Surgery, Trauma, Endophthalmitis, Pediatric Vitreoretinal Surgery, Viral Retinitis, and then several miscellaneous chapters, covering surgery for dislocated lenses, retinal detachments associated with optic disc pits, parasitic disease surgery, and retinal detachments associated with choroidal colobomas. The book concludes with a chapter on eye wall resections for ocular tumors.

This is an outstanding book. Experienced vitreoretinal surgeons will be pleased to have it in their library, young ophthalmologists, whether residents or fellows just starting out in the field, will find it an excellent guide book to start them on their lifelong journey into the field of vitreoretinal surgery.

Maurice B Landers III MD
Professor of Ophthalmology
Director, Vitreoretinal Service
Department of Ophthalmology
University of North Carolina
Chapel Hill, North Carolina, USA

Preface

The field of vitreoretinal diseases is technology driven. Because of the rapidity of the new developments, it is difficult for anyone to stay current in the latest advances in emerging technologies.

The best way to comprehend vitreoretinal surgery is to appreciate the underlying principles involved. With this deeper level of understanding, integration of surgical techniques and instrumentation becomes possible. Each unique source of information increases the value of the whole by more than just an additive amount; the increase in knowledge is a multiplicative function of the number of sources of information. Our ability to evaluate, perceive and think about vitreoretinal diseases is increased by the number of ways we can gain unique information. This is not merely obtaining more data; the information gained exists in an interlocking milieu.

As new surgical techniques, lasers and instruments are introduced; one must learn their intricacies for applying them to the treatment of vitreoretinal diseases. In turn, the adoption of new technology brings with it the need to learn new skills and develop new treatment algorithms. Advancing capabilities furthermore allows intervention for new indications.

As techniques, indications, and equipment evolve, better outcomes result but may also be accompanied by new sets of complications. Keeping up with these changes is vital. New technology and surgical approaches must be adapted to the specific socioeconomic conditions and disease presentations in different parts of the world.

'***Vitreoretinal Surgery***' provides a comprehensive text combined with integrated visual reference, in the form of colored figures. This book attempts to update the state-of-the-art vitreoretinal surgery in a lucid, authoritative and well-illustrated manner.

The value of this book lies in the quality and expertise of the text chapters contributors from across the globe. Contributors from Japan, Australia, Hong Kong, Singapore, India, Middle East, Turkey, Austria, Germany, France, Spain, Switzerland, United Kingdom, Italy, United States of America and Brazil provide a global perspective about the subject.

The book is intended for the experienced ophthalmologists, postgraduates as well as those in training. This pragmatic book provides an understanding of vitreoretinal surgery so important to the everyday practice.

There is something in this book for everyone.

Sandeep Saxena
Carsten H Meyer
Masahito Ohji
Levent Akduman

Contents

Section 2: Retinal Detachment

Section 3: Diabetic Retinopathy

Section 4: Other Retinal Vascular Disorders and Inflammation

Section 5: Macular Surgery

Section 6: Trauma

Section 7: Endophthalmitis

Section 8: Pediatric Vitreoretinal Surgery

Section 9: Surgical Techniques in Viral Retinitis

Section 10: Miscellaneous

Section 11: Oncology

SECTION 1

Principles, Techniques and Instrumentation in Vitrectomy

Wide-Angle Viewing Systems for Vitreoretinal Surgery

1

Lisa J Faia, Tarek S Hassan

Introduction

Wide-angle viewing systems are used for many intraocular procedures that involve vitrectomy and diagnostic inspection of the peripheral and posterior retina. A wide-angle system can be converted to a conventionally focused contact lens system when high magnification is required. Many complex surgeries, such as those with diabetic vitreous hemorrhages, tractional retinal detachments and proliferative vitreoretinopathy, can be more readily completed with the use of a wide-angle viewing system, particularly when there is significant pathology anterior to the equator. Panretinal endophotocoagulation, dissection of epiretinal and subretinal membranes, and gas-fluid exchange are all facilitated. The surgeon can concentrate on a focused area of the retina while still having a broad field of view. This is of particular importance during the peeling and dissection of membranes and the creation of a posterior vitreous detachment, as these maneuvers can exert significant and potentially dangerous, peripheral vitreoretinal traction that could lead to retinal breaks or detachment. These systems can be used with phakic, aphakic and pseudophakic patients and under various conditions, such as fluid, air, gas and silicone oil. The indirect systems can remain in focus with minimal adjustment when the index of refraction of the vitreous substitute is changed.

Wide-angle viewing systems offer a number of advantages over standard-view contact lens systems. They give a broader view of the pathology with better depth of field while displaying versatility, as they can be used with contact lenses, binocular indirect ophthalmoscopes, or no lenses at all. They provide the surgeon with a good surgical view under conditions other than fluid, such as with air, gas, or silicone oil. They also allow one to avoid the disadvantages seen with contact lens systems, such as corneal trauma, changes in intraocular pressure (IOP), poor view with lens or corneal opacities, or the need for multiple lenses. Disadvantages with wide-angle viewing systems include the need initially for more expensive equipment and the negotiation of a steeper learning curve in trying to obtain an optimally focused wide-field view. Contact lenses have traditionally been more readily available, less expensive, requiring of less maintenance, and not needing an associated re-inverting system.

Wide-angle viewing systems are either noncontact or contact in nature. Noncontact viewing systems are typically made of a series of lenses that are mechanically suspended above the surface of the eye. They allow the surgeon to manipulate the eye and still maintain good visualization while the eye is rotated during surgery. They provide good views in eyes with atypical corneal curvatures and opacities. The surgeon can operate without a skilled assistant as the lenses provide good depth of view in all fields of eye movement. They avoid the corneal trauma that can be seen with contact systems. Wide-field contact lens systems require a skilled assistant (for those that are hand held), can change IOP, do not allow much eye movement (as the image can be lost or distorted when the eye is rotated or the optical center of the lens is not matched with the moving eye), and can be difficult to use in eyes with corneal abnormalities. On the other hand, the wide-field contact lens systems can provide up to 150° field of view and do not have the disadvantages associated with noncontact systems, such as the learning curve needed to obtain and maintain focus, cost, adaptability to microscopes, and reduced optical resolution.[1]

Overview of Available Systems

Visualization of the posterior segment during vitreoretinal surgery can be accomplished via various contact and noncontact methods. Hand-held, plano-concave contact lenses neutralize the high convergence effect of the corneal curvature, which thereby permits the operating microscope to focus on the central vitreous and posterior retina with an approximately 20° view. For work on the equatorial retina, the surgeon may tilt this flat contact lens for a fairly highly magnified view, albeit with some slight aberration. Lenses may be used with sew-on retaining rings that stabilize them without an assistant; however, a series of special prismatic lenses may be required to view the periphery.[1] A biconcave lens increases the visual field to 35°. The Landers biconcave lens (Ocular Instruments, Bellevue, WA, USA) allows visualization of the fundus beyond the equator in gas-filled pseudophakic and phakic eyes.

All wide-angle systems generate an inverted fundus view and thus require a device to convert the image to a normal orientation for the surgeon. Indirect ophthalmoscopic viewing lenses, such as the Pan Funduscope (Rodenstock, Munich, Germany), were developed for panretinal photocoagulation and allow a wider, though inverted, view through the pupil. Such an inverted view is difficult and impractical for surgical viewing. The stereoscopic digital inverter (SDI, InterMed Sales Corporation, Miami, Florida, USA) is one of a class of devices that were developed to re-invert the image for use with wide-field lenses.[2] Currently available wide-angle viewing systems include:

1. The Volk re-inverting operating lens system (ROLS) [Volk miniature indirect contact lenses with both standard lenses and self-stabilizing lenses] (Volk Optical, Inc., Mentor, OH, USA).
2. The AVI inverter (Avi Greenblatt, New York, New York, USA) with miniature indirect contact lenses.
3. The Iris Medical contact wide-angle system (Iris Medical Instruments, Mountain View, CA, USA).
4. The BIOM (Binocular Indirect Ophthalmoscope)/SDI (Stereoscopic Diagonal Inverter) noncontact system with or without a miniature, indirect viewing contact lens[3] (Oculus, Inc., Lynnwood, WA, USA).
5. The EIBOS (Erected Image Binocular Ophthalmoscope) noncontact system (Möller-Wedel International GmbH, Wedel, Germany).

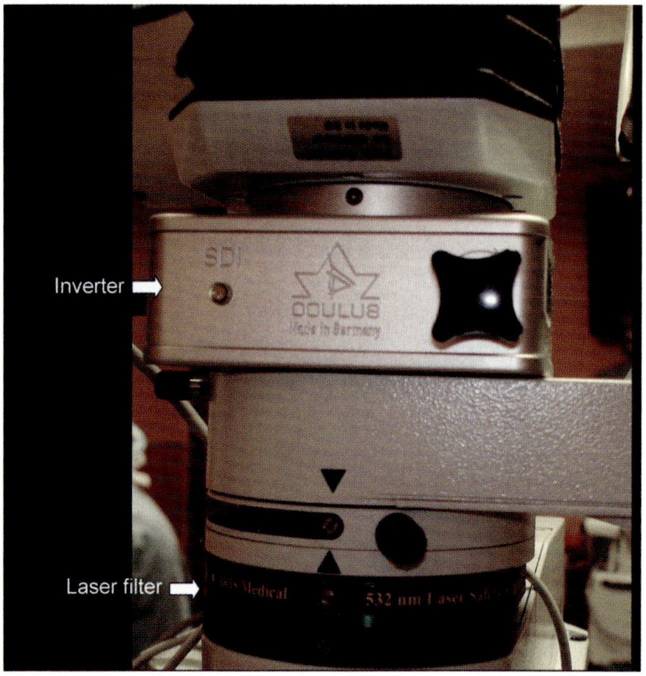

▲ **Figure 1.1**

SDI and laser filter. The SDI, along with the laser filter, is mounted into the stack of the microscope. They are not sterile but away from the eye and do not necessarily need to be draped

The SDI (Fig. 1.1) can be used with noncontact and contact lens because it is mounted in the stack of the scope. Other systems incorporate the ROLS or AVI image inverter with miniature indirect wide-angle contact lenses. The SDI can be changed automatically from an inverted image to non-inverted image with a foot pedal or assistant, where the ROLS and AVI require manual engagement. It is possible to use any inverter system with any objective lens.

The ROLS inverter by Volk uses a single-element image-erecting prism with four optical surfaces that are shared by the right and left eye systems. It is offered in a "Zeiss style", fitting Zeiss, Topcon, Moeller and Inam scopes that accept Zeiss accessories and a "Wild style", which fits only the Leica or Wild microscopes. A diode laser safety filter is built into the inverter (Fig. 1.1). The ROLS does not contact the eye and needs no sterilization. The AVI system sits in the stack of the microscope, is relatively compact (less than 1.5 inches thick and approximately one pound in weight), and is compatible with Wild, Zeiss and Moeller scopes. With the miniature indirect contact lens, the AVI system can offer 130° of peripheral viewing.

Comparison of Contact Lens Systems

Two traditionally used wide-angle contact lens systems include a floating plano-concave lens, supported by a sutured lens ring and a plano-concave irrigating hand-held contact lens.[4,5] A contact lens with one suture has also been described.[6] Sutureless and self-stabilizing lenses are attractive options for wide-angle viewing. Chalam et al.[7] described a standard 60-D plano-concave lens with the radius of curvature of 6.7 mm (less than the corneal curvature) modified with the addition of four footplates that facilitate lens stability and centration without the aid of an assistant. Viscoelastic material is placed between the lens and cornea, creating negative suction which keeps the lens firmly in place on the cornea. This lens allows one to circumvent one drawback of the sew-on lens ring, which is the potential bleeding from the suture placement that can track under the lens and then obscure the surgeon's view. Ikuno et al.[8] have recently introduced a sutureless contact lens system in which the lens is affixed with silicone bands. This system improves upon many of the drawbacks mentioned above, though rotation of globe is difficult due to the restriction caused by the silicone bands.

The MiniQuad lens (Volk Optical, Inc., Mentor, OH, USA) is a modified self-stabilizing contact lens. The posterior contact surface of the lens is extended with four footplates. The static field of view of the lens is 106°, while the dynamic view increases its field to 127°. The surgeon has unobstructed entry of the instruments through the sclerotomies. Scleral indentation, if required, can be done without interference of the footplates. Unfortunately, the lens may not be completely self-retaining in all situations and centration may require minimal assistance in some instances.[9]

Nakata et al.[10] have described features of the ClariVIT contact lens made of glass and polymethyl methacrylate without a plastic rim (Volk Optical, Inc., Mentor, OH, USA). The diameter is reduced to 16.2 mm (compared to the 18 mm diameter of the MiniQuad). A smaller diameter helps eliminate contact between surgical instruments and the wide-angle lens. The optical properties are otherwise identical to the standard wide-angle lens. Its field of view (127°) is the same as the MiniQuad and it allows for a good view through a small pupil even when the vitreous cavity is filled with gas.

The Volk wide-angle contact lenses can be sterilized with ethylene oxide gas at 130° F or disinfected with Sterrad, Steris, or glutaraldehyde. Sterilization of other contact lenses is traditionally done either by ethylene oxide gas or chemically by glutaraldehyde 2% or povidone iodine 5%. Sterilization via autoclaving is cost effective, fast and widely used. Unfortunately, autoclaving can irreparably damage most lenses. Shah et al.[11] described a wide-angle contact lens, which has two lens pieces contained together within a high temperature-resistant (150°C) plastic casing. The inferior lens has footplates and is made of acrylic and the superior lens is made of glass. This self-stabilizing wide-angle contact lens can be sterilized via autoclaving and is thus less costly and needs reduced time for sterilization. The field of view is 106° in the static view and 127° in the dynamic view. After use, its parts are detached, cleaned, put in a lens case and wrapped. The flash autoclave allows for immediate use when needed.

Comparison of Noncontact Wide-angle Systems

The BIOM (Fig. 1.2) is a noncontact device used for vitreous surgery under the operating microscope. It provides a field of view of typically up to 120°, and a dynamic view of up to 135°. It is adaptable to many microscopes and can be used with multiple wide-angle contact lenses. Its versatility allows it to be flipped in and out of use during surgery (Figs 1.3A and B). It is readily adaptable for use with various lighting systems, such as the bullet light pipe and peripheral chandelier devices, which produce wide-angle illumination that enhances the surgeon's view and allows for bimanual surgical techniques.

There are 2 models of the BIOM: A closed cone device and an open arm device that extends from a dove-tailed plate screwed onto the bottom of a microscope. There is a condensing lens on the top of the small indirect viewing tower on both models, as well as a smaller objective lens that is combined with the SDI in the stack on the microscope. The surgeon simply moves the indirect viewing tower in or out from under the microscope lens system to switch between

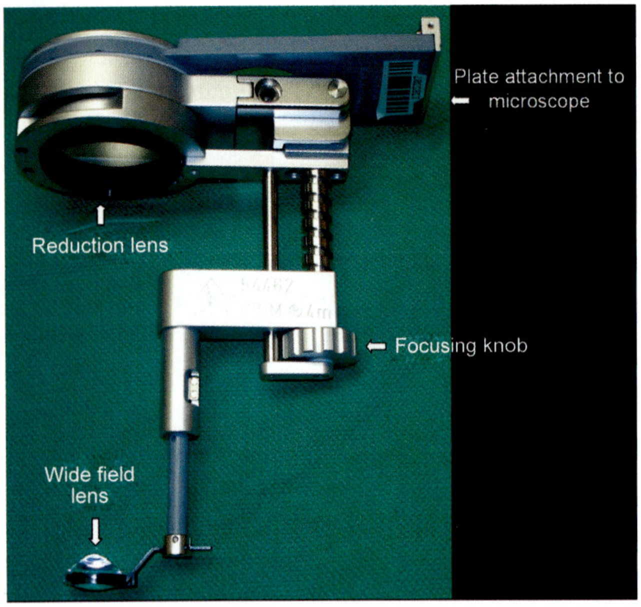

▲ **Figure 1.2**

BIOM. The BIOM, in addition to the plate used to anchor it onto the scope, also has a knurled knob for focusing, which may be adjusted via an assistant or automated pedal. The reduction lens and wide-angle lens come in disposable and nondisposable forms

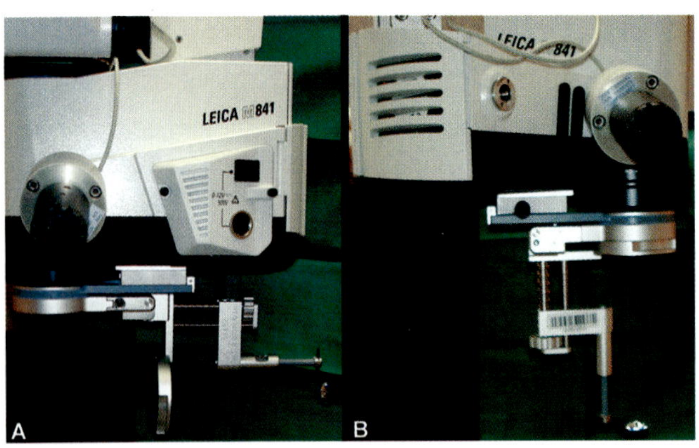

▲ **Figures 1.3A and B**

BIOM in different positions. (A) The BIOM is flipped up, allowing the use of the microscope with other lenses; (B) The BIOM and wide-angle lens are engaged

the BIOM wide-angle intraocular system and regular viewing. The surgeon then inverts the image by either using a foot pedal or assistant to activate the inverter. Gross focus is obtained by manipulating the microscope focus while fine focus is obtained by adjusting the knurled knob on the BIOM device (turning it counterclockwise allows the objective lens to elevate and focus down).

Sterilization can be accomplished via gas or autoclave. The lenses can be either sterilized with ethylene oxide or alkaline glutaraldehyde solution (e.g. Cidex). The SDI is incorporated into the scope and is not sterile. It has an internalized prismatic system with near-zero light escape to achieve maximal illumination and light intensity. The SDI inverts the indirect image from the BIOM to a conventional upright image. The interaction between the surgical scope and BIOM has the following variables, all of which can be manipulated to vary the image for the surgeon:

1. Power of the BIOM objective lens
2. Distance of the BIOM wide-field lens from the scope
3. Distance of the BIOM wide-field lens from the cornea.

The EIBOS noncontact lens system is similar to the combined BIOM/SDI system in function but has a one-piece design with the lenses and inverter housed in a single unit (Figs 1.4A and B). It thus cannot be used with varying wide-angle contact lenses. This one-piece design does not allow sterilization of the entire unit, so it must be draped with a sterile covering. The objective lens itself can be sterilized to prevent contamination of the surgical field. The entire unit is spring balanced as a safety feature so the objective lens does not contact the eye.

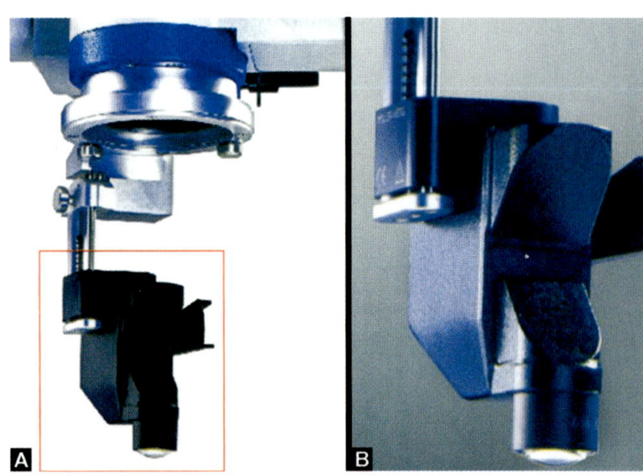

▲ **Figures 1.4A and B**

EIBOS. (A) The entire EIBOS unit is spring balanced and allows for a shorter microscope stack; (B) The EIBOS is a one-piece design with the lenses and inverter housed in a single unit

Focusing is done with a mounted sterile lever, which changes the internal lens distances without changing the distance of the lens from the patient's eye. The retinal image appears in the conventional orientation without the surgeon having to specifically manipulate an inverter. This combined system allows for a shorter scope stack, which thereby leads to better ergonomic management of the surgical field such as with the introduction and removal of instrumentation and devices around the eye.

Adjuncts to Viewing

Intermittent corneal wetting with balanced salt solution (BSS), viscoelastic, or hydroxypropyl methylcellulose solution diluted with BSS is required with noncontact viewing systems to maintain corneal clarity. Good endoillumination enhances the performance of wide-angle viewing systems, whether provided by a conventional light pipe, wide-angle endoilluminator, lighted instruments, single or multiport chandelier illumination systems, or a chandelier lighted infusion system. The microscope light is turned off when endoillumination is used. Slightly tilting the globe and using endoillumination in both a diffuse and tangential orientation maximizes the surgeon's view of the periphery. Magnification is achieved and manipulated by using the zoom function of the microscope and/or by lowering the microscope so the objective lens is closer to cornea. Having a clear visual axis with as large of a pupil as possible certainly enhances posterior segment visualization. Ideally, a pupil larger than 2.5 mm offers a near full view of the fundus. Iris hooks can enlarge the pupil but lensectomy, synechiolysis, penetrating keratoplasty, or keratoprosthesis may at times be needed to clear the visual axis.

Wide-angle viewing systems are used for many intraocular procedures and for effective inspection of the peripheral retina. They can be used with phakic, aphakic and pseudophakic eyes as well as under various viewing conditions in eyes filled with gas, fluid, or silicone oil. They offer a broad view of the patient's pathology while providing good depth perception. Both contact and noncontact systems are available. For contact lenses, there are suture and sutureless lenses available with dynamic views of 150°. Noncontact systems provide 135° of view but avoid several disadvantages of contact lens systems. Proper case selection and use of illumination and magnification are adjunctive maneuvers that aid in viewing with these systems and are as vital to obtaining an ideal surgical view as the specific wide-angle viewing system that is selected.

References

1. DeGregorio PG, Hammer ME, Grizzard WS. Wide-angle viewing systems for vitreoretinal surgeries. In: Peyman GA, Meffert SA, Conway MD, Chou F, Dunitz M (Eds). Vitreoretinal Surgical Techniques. Blackwell Science Inc.; 2001. pp. 99-106.
2. Spitznas M, Reiver J. A stereoscopic diagonal inverter (SDI) for wide-angle vitreous surgery. Graefes Ach Clin Exp Ophthalmol. 1987;225:9-12.
3. Spitznas M. A binocular indirect ophthalmoscope (BIOM) for wide-angle vitreous surgery. Graefes Ach Clin Exp Ophthalmol. 1987;225:13-5.
4. Tolentino FI, Freeman HM. A new lens for closed pars plana vitrectomy. Arch Ophthalmol. 1979;97:2197-8.
5. Parel JM, Machemer R. Steam-sterilizable fundus contact lenses. Arch Ophthalmol. 1981;99:151.
6. Lewis JM, Ohji M, Tano Y. A technique for contact lens fixation during vitreous surgery. Ophthalmic Surg Lasers. 1996;27:891-3.
7. Chalam KV, Patel CC, Shah VA. Newly designed self-retaining contact lens for vitreous surgery. Am J Ophthalmol. 2003;135:544-6.
8. Ikuno Y, Ohji M, Kusaka S, et al. Sutureless contact lens ring system during vitrectomy. Am J Ophthalmol. 2002; 133:847-8.
9. Shah VA, Chalam KV. Newly designed self-retaining prism contact lens for vitreous surgery. Retina. 2003;23:721-2.
10. Nakata K, Ohji M, Ikuno Y, et al. Wide-angle viewing lens for vitrectomy. Am J Ophthalmol. 2004;137:760-2.
11. Shah VA, Chalam KV. Autoclavable wide-angle contact lens for vitreous surgery. Am J Ophthalmol. 2004;137:359-60.

2 Illumination Considerations for Vitreous Surgery

Colin A McCannel

Introduction

Visualization of the posterior segment for vitreoretinal surgery requires a combination of an appropriate viewing system and sufficient light delivered into the vitreous cavity. There are conceptually two types of viewing systems, standard contact lenses and wide-angle viewing systems. Among wide-angle systems, there are contact and noncontact systems. However, the focus of this chapter will be illumination during vitrectomy surgery.

The light requirements differ between the viewing systems. The wider the angle of the viewing system, the more widespread the light delivery must be for optimal viewing. Additionally, the smaller the diameter of the fiber optic used, such as in small gauge vitrectomy, the more light may be required.

Illumination Strategies

▶ Endoillumination

Early in the evolution of vitrectomy surgery, visualization moved from the indirect ophthalmoscope or operating microscope mounted slit lamp to endoillumination using light delivered by fiber optic instruments. The most common source of endoillumination is the "light pipe". The light pipe allows maximal safety and efficiency in the delivery of light into the vitreous cavity. Most of the heat is left at the light source and the fiber optic allows efficient transfer of the light from the source to the vitreous cavity. Since the first use of endoillumination, many variations of endoillumination have evolved, most to facilitate bimanual surgery. Lighted instruments, including lighted forceps, scissors and picks as well as chandelier type illumination systems have enjoyed various levels of popularity.

Categorically, there are two endoillumination approaches, focal and diffuse light. Before the popularity of wide-angle viewing systems, focal light delivered by light pipes was perhaps the most common type of endoillumination in use. When operating with wide-angle viewing, the field needing illumination is far greater than can be accomplished with a standard light pipe. As a result, wide-angle viewing strategies have become more popular.

Focal illumination has the advantage of allowing excellent visualization of fine detail, including the semitransparent vitreous. Diffuse illumination allows a wide field to be visible at one time, but visualization of detail or the vitreous is far less optimal. The difference may be compared to spot lights versus flood lights as used in stage, cinema production and other circumstance, where the spot light is used to draw out detail whereas the flood light serves as a general overview illumination.

Light Pipes

Standard spread: The standard light pipe generally has a flat surface at the end of the fiber optic. Such a termination of the fiber optic results in a cone of light with a relatively small divergence angle. The spotlight-like illumination allows for detail by intensely illuminating a small area. This type of light pipe was commonly used before the advent and popularization of wide-angle viewing. The surgeon cannot enjoy the full benefits of wide-angle viewing with a small cone of light illuminating a portion of the fundus well, while leaving most of the field too dark.

Wide-angle spread: Wide-angle light pipes have rounded tips that result in a broader divergence angle spreading of light over and illuminating a wider field. Variations range from bullet-shaped tips to the more rounded, "cannonball" type, tips. The bullet-shaped tip delivers a relatively brighter illumination in the direction the tip is pointing with a continuous drop-off in brightness as the distance increases from the central bright portion of illumination. In contrast, a more rounded tip results in a more uniform light delivery in all directions. The "cannonball" light is such an example. While the obvious advantage of these light pipe tip designs is the wide field of diffuse illumination, there are also disadvantages. Some structures may be less easily visualized with the more diffuse light. Perhaps most notably vitreous is poorly seen with diffuse lighting.

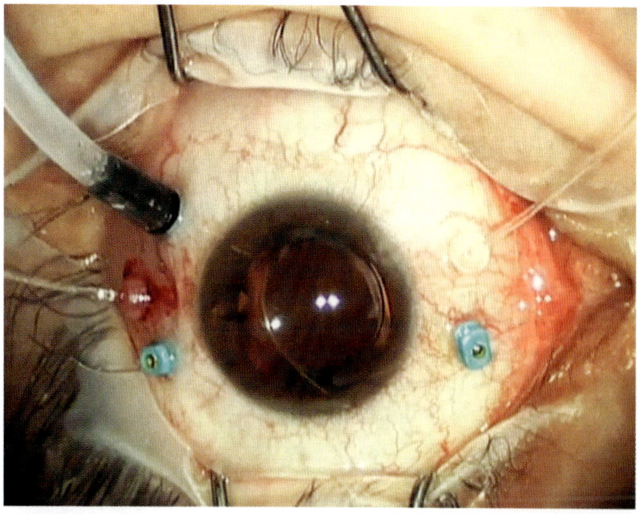

▲ **Figure 2.1**

Installed dual fiber chandelier. Appearance of the vitrectomy setup with a standard three port vitrectomy with dual port chandelier installed. The additional fiber optics add some complexity to the setup

Chandelier Illumination

Chandelier illumination systems are designed to allow the surgeon to perform true bimanual surgery, i.e. active instruments in each hand. Whether or not any given surgeon finds the additional complexity of the chandelier illumination system an acceptable trade-off likely depends on his or her reliance of bimanual surgical techniques. When bimanual techniques are not employed, the benefit over fiber optic illumination may be limited, though undoubtedly there are surgeons that routinely use chandelier systems. Some of the limitations of the chandelier systems include insufficient illumination in any one place while excellent overall illumination is achieved. In other words, at the point of surgical dissection, far away from the source point, the illumination may not always be adequate or as good as a nearby source point, i.e. a light pipe. Shadowing by instruments is a significant limitation of many chandelier systems. Concerns have been raised about the buildup of thermal energy at the light tip, which may cause damage to the local tissues.[1] Last not least, many surgeons find the additional complexity of having fiber optics connected to the eye undesirable (Fig. 2.1).

Chandelier systems can be principally divided into single and multi-source point systems. The single source point chandeliers are by far more common and most manufacturers have a version. Most single source point systems are inserted through pars plana via separate sclerotomies at the usual 2.5–4 mm posterior to the limbus, such as the Tornambe Torpedo®, or Awh chandelier.[2,3] Older such systems may require a fairly large sclerotomy, while more recent versions utilize small gauge technology, i.e. 25- or 27-gauge fibers.[2-4] Some manufacturers offer combination instrumentation, such as an illuminated infusion cannula. The advantage of such a system is the lack of additional sclerotomies or fibers emanating from the surgical field.

Among the multi-point source illumination systems, the "Multiport Illumination System" developed by Spitznas was perhaps the first such system.[5] Its great advantage is that the light comes from three point sources, one associated with each sclerotomy. Due to its bulky nature it never reached high levels of popularity. Today, there are dual fiber versions of multi-point source of illumination utilizing small gauge fibers and separate sclerotomies, such as the Eckardt twinlight.[6,7] The multi-point source systems have the great advantage of having less areas lacking illumination due to instrument shadows. However, the increased number of fibers emanating from the surgical field increases complexity and thus reduces desirability.

Illuminated Instruments

There is almost no instrument category that does not have an illuminated version, ranging from illuminated vitrectomy instruments,[8] forceps, scissors, picks,[9] flute needles,[8] to illuminated laser probes. The main commonality among these instruments is that there are significant trade-offs. Perhaps the most common surgeon complaints preventing these instruments from being used widely are that the light is never quite bright enough in the right place, yet there is a lot of glare because it is very bright. The 3-function tissue manipulator is a multifunction instrument that may be an exception to the lack of real world practicality. It combines light, aspiration and cautery in one instrument and has advocates for its use in the complex surgery of diabetic patients. Since the instrument can be rotated to get the light in nearly the perfect place, visualization is quite good with this illuminated instrument.

Microscope Mounted Slit Lamp

An alternative way of delivering light into the eye during vitrectomy is by means of a microscope mounted slit lamp. A description of this means of illumination dates back to the late 1960s when vitrectomy surgery was just starting.[10-13] Advocates of this approach continue to exist and describe excellent visualization. While slit lamp fundus illumination has been used most commonly with non-wide angle viewing, it can also be used in conjunction with a wide-angle fundus viewing lens.[14] Among its advantages are that the surgeon can perform bimanual surgery without specialized illuminated instruments, or chandelier type illumination systems. Furthermore, it allows for monoport vitrectomy or vitrectomy-less epiretinal membrane peeling with excellent vitreous and macular visualization. Disadvantages have not been formally reported, but may include the lack of surgeon familiarity and limited area of illumination. These may explain why the technique has never found widespread adoption.

The Light Source

Types of Light

Sources producing the light that is delivered into the eye by the fiber optics utilize a range of bulb technology. They are, in order of increasing light output, halogen (10–30 lumens/W), metal halide (65–115 lumens/W), xenon (277–355 lumens/W) and mercury vapor (up to 402 lumens/W).[15] The use of bulbs with brighter light was necessitated by the advent of small gauge vitrectomy surgery. The typical halogen light source sufficient for delivering bright endoillumination into the eye via 20 gauge fibers is insufficiently bright to do the same with smaller gauges. The cross-sectional surface area of 23- and 25-gauge fibers is 50% and 31% of 20-gauge fibers, respectively. For this reason, the light source has to be approximately twice or four times brighter for the same resultant intraocular illumination for 23- and 25-gauge, respectively. Even more light is required for 27- or 29-gauge fiber optics, with cross-sectional areas of 20% and 12% of 20-gauge fibers, respectively, such as used in some modern chandelier and multifunction instrument illumination systems.

The differing light bulb technologies additionally have differing light composition in terms of the wavelengths that make up the light. In general commercial or residential lighting this characteristic is referred to as color temperature. A light composed of more short wavelength light, i.e. blue light, has a cooler color temperature, i.e. higher Kelvin number, compared to one that has less component short wavelength light. Metal halide gas produces a more blue-white color, approximately 6500 Kelvin, while xenon gas produces a more natural 4500 Kelvin color temperature and halogen a light of approximately 1200 Kelvin. While the color temperature is important for visualization of retinal or epiretinal structures, the spectral composition is related to the risk of phototoxicity.

Light-induced Retinal and Retinal Pigment Epithelial Damage

A discussion of illumination during vitrectomy surgery is not complete without discussion of the potential for light-induced retinal and retinal pigment epithelial damage.[16-19] Experimental studies have also demonstrated light phototoxic effects on the retina and retinal pigment epithelium.[20-23] Reports of clinical retinal light toxicity have occurred since the early days of vitrectomy surgery and continue to do so.[17,20,21,24-29] Additionally, there have been at least 16 cases of suspected phototoxicity reported to the Federal Drug Administration in the United States implicating one manufacturers Xenon light source with a 420 nm cut-off filter.[30]

Types of Light Toxicity

Light energy can cause phototoxicity by either thermal or photochemical injury. Thermal injury is thought to set in when the tissue temperature is increased by 10° C or more resulting in denatured protein and similar thermal effects. This mechanism of injury underlies the retinal photocoagulation. Photochemical injury results in tissue damage without thermal effects.

Risk of Light Toxicity

There are three important factors that affect the risk of phototoxicity from light. These include the wavelength of the light (nanometers), the intensity of light exposure, or power level (watts per square millimeter) and the duration of exposure. The amount of energy contained in light depends on the wavelength. Shorter wavelength photons contain more energy compared to longer wavelength photons. Thus, at a given power level, shorter wavelength light is more damaging. The power delivered to a surface, such as the retina, is expressed as irradiance and is related to the brightness of the light. Furthermore the total energy exposure of a surface is measured in joules per square millimeter and calculated by multiplying the irradiance by exposure time.

The wavelength of light is dictated by the light source. Ham and colleagues reported the action spectrum and relative risk for retinal damage when the retina is exposed to various wavelengths of UV or blue light.[31] This work led to the creation of what is called the aphakic hazard curve (Fig. 2.2) often used in comparison with the spectral output of vitrectomy light sources. Essentially, their work showed that as the wavelength shortens the risk of phototoxicity increases at a given exposure.

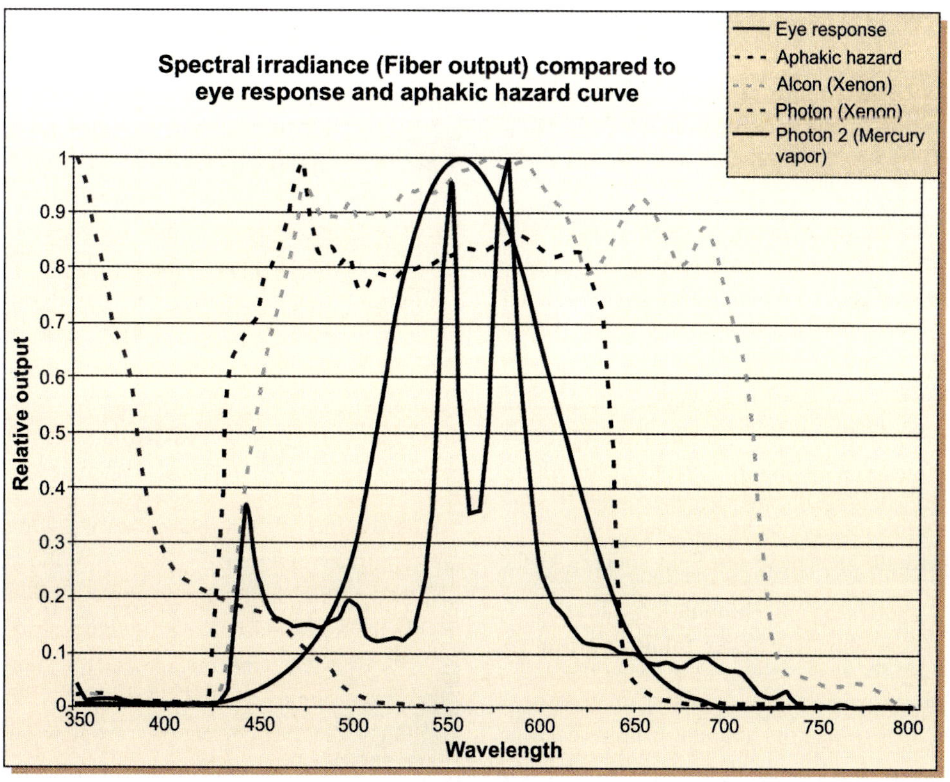

▲ Figure 2.2

Aphakic hazard curve, light response of eye, and various light sources. Spectral output curve of a two xenon light sources, Alcon xenon (interrupted light gray) and Photon (interrupted dark gray), and a mercury vapor light (Photon 2, solid gray curve), normal photopic spectral sensitivity curve (solid black curve), and spectral curve of phototoxic hazard in aphakic eyes (interrupted black line). The relative output of the Photon and Alcon xenon light is filtered by an integrated 420 nm filter, while the mercury vapor by a 435 nm filter. The output of the xenon light has a broad spectral composition, while mercury vapor bulb has two peaks at 550 nm and 580 nm

Light Toxicity Risk Reduction

The use of filters to eliminate some of the shorter wavelengths from the light delivered into the eye is a means to allow increased brightness and duration while minimizing the phototoxic effects. Some manufacturers allow dialing in different filters on the light source console by the surgeon in order to allow use of light with minimal short wavelength (blue, UV) to maximize safety and tolerability of the light by the retina. The disadvantage of these filters is that the light changes in color and many surgeons accustomed to white light may find the green or yellow light produced by eliminating the short wavelengths unfamiliar and uncomfortable to operate with. Kraushar et al.[32] reported that their studies of filtered monochromatic light devoid of short wavelength was insufficient for vitrectomy surgery. Since epiretinal membranes and vitreous are essentially colorless and best visualized with full spectrum light, this is not surprising. It must be kept in mind that these conclusions were based on light sources other than the modern high output xenon and mercury vapor bulbs were used, as additional brightness may overcome some of the disadvantages of colored light. Koch et al.[33] reported using filters that block the wavelengths below 420 nm reduced the amount of short wave length light by about one-third when used in a multiport chandelier type illumination system.

The intensity of retinal exposure is a factor of the brightness of the light (lumens) and the working distance. Modern xenon and mercury vapor light sources allow for tremendous brightness, i.e. amount of light delivered into the eye. Surgeons should be aware of the brightness and attempt to minimize the amount of retinal light exposure by utilizing the smallest amount of light needed to get the job done well. Inadvertent excessive light may be delivered into the eye following a bulb change in the light source. At the same intensity setting on the console, a new bulb will deliver more light than a bulb near the end of its useful life. Also, surgeons should be aware of the beam splitter characteristics of the operating microscope. Many operating microscopes have beam splitters that reduce the amount of light reaching the surgeon in favor of light being directed to an assistant scope or camera port for video recording. If the beam splitter devotes a low percentage of the light to the surgeon, a compensatory increase of intraocular light delivery can result in excellent visualization for the surgeon, but may lead to unsafe light levels in the eye. Furthermore, the surgeons should always be aware of the working distance. The light intensity varies exponentially with the working distance, i.e. at a constant light intensity setting, doubling the working distance reduces the retinal illumination by a factor of four. Meyer et al.[23] concluded that bright endoilluminators pose a significant risk of phototoxicity based on their work in owl and monkeys. Vander et al.[34] found no toxicity from a chandelier system, while an endoillumination probe easily produced phototoxic lesions in their experimental setting. The duration of exposure is also important. Longer exposure times at any intensity will increase the risk of phototoxicity. This is accentuated when the light at the retina is very intense (bright) and relatively small amounts of additional exposure rapidly lead to toxicity (Fig. 2.3).

Light Toxicity Predisposing Factors

Other factors that may predispose to phototoxicity include photosensitizing medications that the patient is taking[35,36] or dyes used during vitreoretinal surgery. Patients should be reviewed preoperatively as there are medications that are

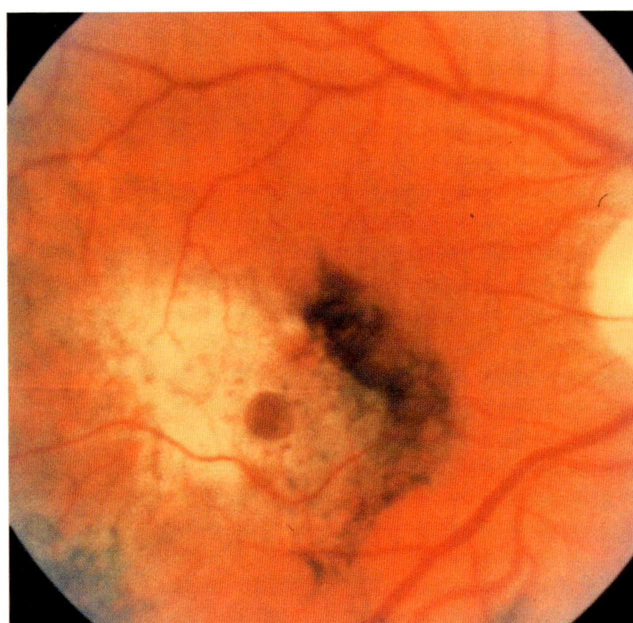

Figure 2.3

Case of phototoxicity. 72-year-old male underwent pars plana vitrectomy for epimacular membrane peel. Following surgery, he suffered progressive vision decline to the counting finger level, from 20/30 preoperatively. The surgeon described the procedure as completely uncomplicated and, reportedly, a halogen light source was used

TABLE 2.1: Selected photosensitizing medications that may increase risk of retinal phototoxicity during vitrectomy

Drug class	***Examples***
Antihistamines	Astemizole, Azatadine, Brompheniramine, Buclizine, Carbinoxamine, Cetirizine, Chlorpheniramine, Clemastine, Cyclizine, Cyproheptadine, Dexchlorpheniramine Dimenhydrinate, Diphenhydramine, Diphenylpyraline, Doxylamine, Hydroxyzine, Loratadine, Meclizine, Methapyrilene, Methdilazine, Orphenadrine, Pheniramine, Promethazine, Pyrilamine, Terfenadine, Trimeprazine, Tripelennamine, Triprolidine
Fluoroquinolones	Ciprofloxacin, Ofloxacin, Levofloxacin, Moxifloxacin, Lomefloxacin,* Sparfloxacin*
Oral estrogens and progestogens	Ethinyl estradiol, Medroxyprogesterone, Megestrol, Norethindrone, Norgestrel, Quinestrol, Chlorotrianisene, Diethylstilbestro,l Estradiol, Estrogens,Cconjugated estrogens, Esterified, Estropipate
Non-steroidal anti-inflammatory agents	Ibuprofen, Ketoprofen, Naproxen, Celecoxib
Phenothiazines*	Chlorpromazine, Fluphenazine, Perazine, Perphenazine, Thioridazine
Sulfonamides*	Acetazolamide, Sulfacytine, Sulfadiazine, Sulfadoxine, Sulfamethizole, Sulfamethoxazole, Sulfapyridine, Sulfasalazine, Sulfinpyrazone, Sulfisoxazole
Sulfonylureas*	Acetohexamide,* Chlorpropamide,* Glipizide,* Glyburide,* Tolazamide,* Tolbutamide*
Thiazide diuretics*	Furosemide,* Bumetanide,* Hydrochlorothiazide*
Tetracyclines*	Tetracycline,* Doxycycline,* Methacycline,* Minocycline,* Oxytetracycline,* Chlortetracycline,* Demeclocycline,* Declomycin,* Vibramycin*
Tricyclic antidepressents	Amitriptyline, Amoxapine, Clomipramine, Desipramine, Doxepin, Imipramine, Isocarboxazid, Maprotiline, Mirtazapine, Nortriptyline, Protriptyline, Sertaline, Trimipramine
HMG-CoA reductase inhibitors	Statins (atorvastatin, fluvastatin, lovastatin, pravastatin, simvastatin)
Antifungals	Terbinafine, Itraconazole, Voriconazole, Griseofulvin
Miscellaneous	Bithionol (antiparasitic),* Naladixic acid,* Amiodarone,* Verteporfin, Diltiazem, Dapsone, Isotretinoin (Accutane),* Etretinate (Tegison),* Tretinoin (Retin-A, Vitamin A Acid),* Dacarbazine*

*Thought to more likely to cause photosensitivity

known photosensitizers (Table 2.1). The magnitude of phototoxic risk to the retina during vitrectomy surgery, if any, attributable to these medications is not well understood. Dyes commonly used during vitrectomy include indocyanine green, infracyanine green, trypan blue and brilliant blue. Indocyanine green use has been reported to result in toxicity retinal or retinal pigment epithelial toxicity. It is possible that at least a portion of the toxicity is related to the light absorbing properties of the dye. Direct toxicity has, however, been reported. None the less, minimizing light intensity and maximizing working distance of the endoilluminator when using these dyes is probably advisable and likely reduces at least the phototoxic component of the dyes toxicity.

In summary, there have been many changes in delivery and utilization of light in the eye during vitrectomy surgery. Many of these changes have been possible through the development of high intensity light sources. The development of these light sources, in turn, were necessitated by the advent of small gauge vitrectomy instrumentation and resulted in a flurry of new instruments. Currently, the most important consideration with regard to endoillumination is for surgeon not to over utilize light, i.e. use light at too bright settings.

The newer light sources are extremely powerful and capable of inadvertently causing retinal phototoxicity and associated vision loss.

References

1. Shimada H, Nakashizuka H, Hattori T, et al. Thermal injury caused by chandelier fiber probe. Am J Ophthalmol. 2007;143:167-9.
2. Oshima Y, Awh CC, Tano Y. Self-retaining 27-gauge transconjunctival chandelier endoillumination for panoramic viewing during vitreous surgery. Am J Ophthalmol. 2007;143:166-7.
3. Oshima Y, Awh CC, Tano Y. A more convenient chandelier system utilizing a 29-gauge optical fiber housed within a retractable 27-gauge needle. Retina. 2008;28:1559-60.
4. Uemoto R, Nakasato S, Mizuki N. New technique for inserting 27-gauge twinlight chandelier illumination fibers into the eye using intravenous cannula. Retina. 2009;29:1040-2.
5. Koch FH, Pawlowski D, Spitznas M. A multiport illumination system for panoramic bimanual vitreous surgery. Graefes Arch Clin Exp Ophthalmol. 1991;229:425-9.
6. Eckardt C. Twin lights: a new chandelier illumination for bimanual surgery. Retina. 2003;23:893-4.
7. Eckardt C, Eckert T, Eckardt U. 27-gauge Twinlight chandelier illumination system for bimanual transconjunctival vitrectomy. Retina. 2008;28:518-9.
8. Fisher YL, Gross NE, Wang C. Inexpensive illuminated vitrectomy cutter. Retina. 2003;23:891.
9. Williams GA, Abrams GW, Mieler WF. Illuminated retinal picks for vitreous surgery. Arch Ophthalmol. 1989;107:1086.
10. McPherson SD, Jr. A modified Zeiss operating slit-lamp microscope. Trans Am Ophthalmol Soc. 1968;66:419-20.
11. Primbs GB. Slit-lamp biomicroscope for operating room use. Trans Sect Ophthalmol Am Acad Ophthalmol Otolaryngol. 1975;79:OP427.
12. Bonnet M. [Biomicroscopy of the fundus in retinal detachment surgery (author's transl)]. J Fr Ophtalmol. 1979;2:209-16.
13. Schirmer KE. Slit-lamp fundus microscopy without contact lens and with laser attachment. Arch Ophthalmol. 1981;99:155-7.
14. Ohji M, Tano Y. Vitreoretinal surgery with slit-lamp illumination combined with a wide-angle-viewing contact lens. Am J Ophthalmol. 2004;137:955-6.
15. Oshima Y, Chow DR, Awh CC, et al. Novel mercury vapor illuminator combined with a 27/29-gauge chandelier light fiber for vitreous surgery. Retina. 2008;28:171-3.
16. Glickman RD. Phototoxicity to the retina: mechanisms of damage. Int J Toxicol. 2002;21:473-90.
17. Fuller D, Machemer R, Knighton RW. Retinal damage produced by intraocular fiber optic light. Am J Ophthalmol. 1978;85:519-37.
18. Azzolini C, Brancato R, Venturi G, et al. Updating on intraoperative light-induced retinal injury. Int Ophthalmol. 1994;18:269-76.
19. Wu J, Seregard S, Algvere PV. Photochemical damage of the retina. Surv Ophthalmol. 2006;51:461-81.
20. Yanagi Y, Inoue Y, Jang WD, et al. A2e mediated phototoxic effects of endoilluminators. Br J Ophthalmol. 2006;90:229-32.
21. Yanagi Y, Iriyama A, Jang WD, et al. Evaluation of the safety of xenon/bandpass light in vitrectomy using the A2E-laden RPE model. Graefes Arch Clin Exp Ophthalmol. 2007;245:677-81.
22. Zilis JD, Machemer R. Light damage in detached retina. Am J Ophthalmol. 1991;111:47-50.
23. Meyers SM, Bonner RF. Retinal irradiance from vitrectomy endoilluminators. Am J Ophthalmol. 1982;94:26-9.
24. Kuhn F, Morris R, Massey M. Photic retinal injury from endoillumination during vitrectomy. Am J Ophthalmol. 1991;111:42-6.
25. Poliner LS, Tornambe PE. Retinal pigment epitheliopathy after macular hole surgery. Ophthalmology. 1992;99:1671-7.
26. Duker JS. Retinal pigment epitheliopathy after macular hole surgery. Ophthalmology. 1993;100:1604-5.
27. Michels M, Lewis H, Abrams GW, et al. Macular phototoxicity caused by fiberoptic endoillumination during pars plana vitrectomy. Am J Ophthalmol. 1992;114:287-96.
28. Michels M. Intraoperative retinal phototoxicity. Int Ophthalmol Clin.1995;35:157-72.
29. Andonegui Navarro J, Marcuerquiaga Arriaga J. [Xenon light induced phototoxic lesions]. Arch Soc Esp Oftalmol. 2000;75:117-20.
30. (MAUDE) Maufde. Manufacturer and user facility device experience.
31. Ham WT, Mueller HA, Ruffolo JJ, et al. Action spectrum for retinal injury from near-ultraviolet radiation in the aphakic monkey. Am J Ophthalmol. 1982;93:299-306.
32. Kraushar MF, Harris MJ, Morse PH. Monochromatic endoillumination for epimacular membrane surgery. Ophthalmic Surg. 1989;20:508-10.
33. Koch FH, Schmidt HP, Monks T, et al. The retinal irradiance and spectral properties of the multiport illumination system for vitreous surgery. Am J Ophthalmol. 1993;116:489-96.
34. Vander JF, Eagle RC, Brown GC, et al. Retinal tolerance of an implantable light source for use during vitrectomy surgery. Ophthalmic Surg. 1991;22:735-9.
35. Costagliola C, Menzione M, Chiosi F, et al. Retinal phototoxicity induced by hydrochlorothiazide after exposure to a UV tanning device. Photochem Photobiol. 2008;84:1294-7.
36. Mauget-Faysse M, Quaranta M, Francoz, et al. Incidental retinal phototoxicity associated with ingestion of photosensitizing drugs. Graefes Arch Clin Exp Ophthalmol. 2001;239:501-8.

3 Vitreoretinal Instrumentation

Steve Charles

Vitreoretinal instrumentation has evolved over a period of time to provide state-of-the-art pars plana vitrectomy (PPV) techniques.[1-4]

Surgical Fluidics

Surgical fluidics is a broad term that encompasses infusion and aspiration fluidics as well as the relationship between aspiration fluidics, and cutting parameters. Although aspiration fluidics has received the most attention, infusion fluidics are discussed first in this chapter because this subject requires special attention with the advent of 23/25/27-gauge vitrectomy.

▶ Infusion System Concepts

Since the inception of vitreoretinal surgery, surgeons have occasionally experienced excessively low intraocular pressure (IOP) during vitreoretinal surgery. New techniques and technologies have greatly improved surgical outcomes, but created special challenges with respect to the infusion system. A major cause of excessively low IOP during vitrectomy is inadvertent suprachoroidal infusion. Straight-in trocar-cannula trajectory to produce sclerotomies perpendicular to the sclera were used when 25-gauge, 0.5 mm sutureless vitrectomy was introduced. When 23-gauge, sutureless surgery was subsequently developed; oblique trocar-cannula entry was utilized in order to construct a scleral tunnel to reduce wound leakage from the larger, 0.75 mm wounds. Initially, surgeons used a two plane oblique approach; the initial trocar-cannula insertion segment was approximately 30° relative to the sclera and the second segment trajectory perpendicular to the sclera. Some surgeons even believed that a biplanar incision was constructed, although this is not the case because the wound was constructed before the change in trajectory. More recently, most surgeons using both 23- and 25-gauge systems have switched to oblique entry; often with very steep angles (5–10°). Although near tangential entry creates a long scleral tunnel, it increases the chances of infusing into the choroid because of the tangential trajectory, and because a 4 mm long cannula may not be able to traverse the long scleral tunnel and reach the vitreous cavity (Fig. 3.1). If the cannula is in the choroid early in the case, the choroid expands elastically allowing infusion without hypotony; later the choroid may limit infusion alerting the surgeon to the problem (Fig. 3.2). Unfortunately some surgeons incorrectly conclude that the hypotony was the primary problem and it subsequently caused a choroidal effusion. The evidence that acute choroidal effusion can occur from low IOP in cataract as well vitreoretinal surgery is not compelling.

The author always advised inspecting the infusion cannula with the operating microscope or indirect ophthalmoscope after insertion when using 20-gauge sutured infusion ports. Unfortunately, many of us have discontinued this practice since we began using 23/25/27-gauge sutureless vitrectomy; clearly we must not omit this crucial step. Using the naked eye and an external endoilluminator illumination do not provide sufficient magnification to make certain that the cannula has penetrated the choroid, and nonpigmented pars plana epithelium.

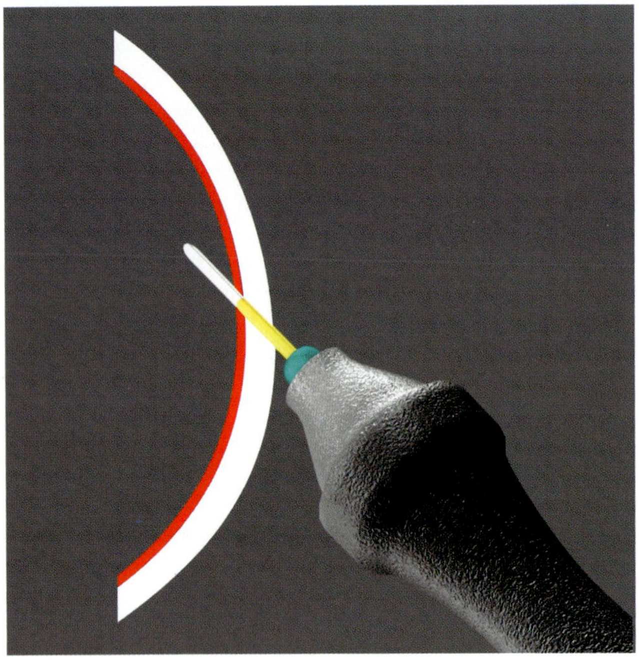

▲ Figure 3.1
Near-tangential trocar insertion

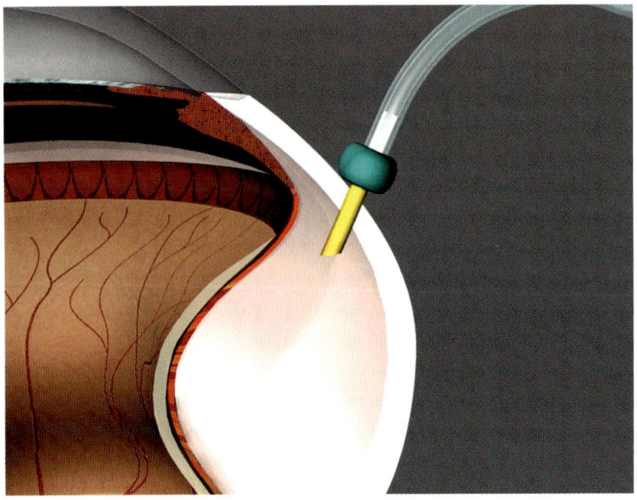

▲ Figure 3.2
Suprachoroidal infusion

Adhesively fastening the infusion cannula tubing and associated stopcock(s) and connectors to the drape is imperative to prevent traction on the infusion cannula, and the eye because inadvertent and unrecognized pulling on the tubing by the assistant or surgeon can easily pull the cannula partially out causing a suprachoroidal infusion (Fig. 3.3). Adhesively fastening the infusion cannula tubing to the drape with eye in the primary position, with a short tubing loop can result in a suprachoroidal infusion when the eye is rotated to view the periphery creating tension on the cannula and rotation of the tip into the choroid or partial pull out. Scleral depression is another opportunity to cause inadvertent suprachoroidal infusion by causing pressure on the cannula as the eye is rotated by the depressor. Placing the infusion cannula too close to the lower lid rather than just inferior to the horizontal meridian is a common cause of suprachoroidal infusion created when the eye is rotated down to visualize the inferior periphery.

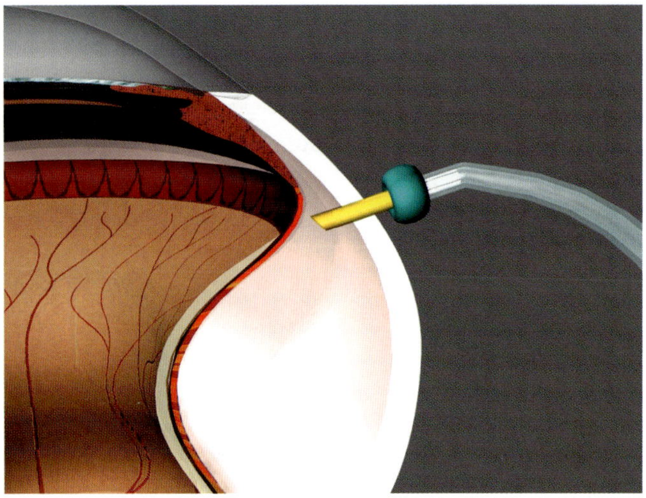

▲ Figure 3.3
Inadvertent angulation of the infusion cannula

Kinking of the more flexible silicone tubing terminal segment of the infusion cannula can be caused by the surgeon or assistant by accidentally pulling on the tubing. Kinking is exacerbated by using excessively low infusion pressure settings (10–25 mm Hg), which is insufficient to straighten out the tubing kink. The author has always used 45 mm Hg, except when operating on small children or patients with low systemic blood pressure, typically under general anesthesia. There is no evidence that infusion pressure of 35–45 mm Hg causes ischemic damage or impact visual outcomes. Simply stated, there are many disadvantages of using low infusion pressure, but no proven advantages.

Infusion Line Resistance

Many surgeons incorrectly believe that infusion pressure equals IOP; this in only true during no flow, no leak scenarios. With typical flow rates, there are significant frictional losses in the infusion system, typically 10–20 mm Hg. Although air pressure over infusion fluid (Alcon VGFI®) provides rapid, console-based control and digital readout in mm Hg not bottle height, it does not compensate for frictional losses occurring during flow. The Alcon Constellation® Vision System has an IOP compensation system, which measures achieved flow rates using known, precise infusion pressure during push priming to determine resistance in the infusion line and cannula. The infusion pressure is increased using digital feedback from real time infusion flow sensing to compensate for frictional losses in the infusion system. It is important to remember that no technology can completely overcome frictional losses in the line when excessively low pressure settings (10–25 mm Hg) are used, especially when combined with high vacuums and resultant outflow rates. Kinking as well as having a few bubbles in the infusion line increase resistance to flow and cause pressure drop, ultimately resulting in excessively low IOP. The IOP compensation system is most effective when used to slow the rate of IOP drop when using a 23- or especially 25-gauge infusion and a 20-gauge fragmenter to remove dense lens nuclear fragments. Occlusion break will result in ocular collapse if the surgeon does not respond quickly enough; the IOP compensation system gives the surgeon more time to reduce vacuum when an occlusion break is recognized. Scleral buckle pull up, pressure on eye during scleral depression, large angle eye rotation or excessive pressure on the fundus contact lens may cause vitreous, blood, residual silicone oil droplets or tissue to flow retrograde into the infusion cannula causing plugging thereby preventing infusion flow.

Regurgitation Issues

Using excessively low IOP settings (10–25 mm Hg) significantly increase the chances of regurgitation of air or perfluorooctane (PFO) bubbles when taking the foot off the foot pedal. Using 650 mm Hg vacuum is necessary and safe when using 25-gauge systems, but it allows gases that are always dissolved in the fluid to transition to gas bubbles. These bubbles ordinarily disappear into the vitreous cutter and aspiration system, but can regurgitate if excessively low IOP settings (10–25 mm Hg) are used.

▶ Aspiration Fluidics

Developing an understanding of aspiration fluidic systems is essential for the vitreoretinal as well as phaco surgeon. A pressure difference (trans-orifice pressure, delta P) across the port of a vitrectomy cutter, extrusion cannula, phaco probe, or irrigation/aspiration handpiece causes flow to occur through the port via connected tubing to the cassette. Various systems are used to create the pressure difference in the cassette; venturi and peristaltic pumps being the most common. Although venturi systems inherently produce a vacuum and peristaltic pumps produce a constant flow rate based on revolutions/minute, pressure and flow sensing can alter the behavior of venturi and peristaltic pumps to a limited extent emulating the other type of pump. Fluid flow mathematical relationships are identical to Ohm's law for electrical systems: E = IR (voltage = current X resistance); voltage is analogous to pressure difference (force) and current is analogous to flow. Venturi as well as peristaltic pumps are connected to vitreous cutters and phaco handpieces through lengthy segments (typically 84 inches) of relatively small bore, elastomeric tubing. Resistance to flow is proportional to the length of the tubing and to the fourth power of the internal diameter of tubing or handpiece lumen and port. Tubing expansion due to pressure increase and contraction due to applied vacuum or tubing elastomeric forces alters the shape of pressure/vaccum signals in the tubing. The signal from changes in viscosity, obstructed flow, or occlusion break is delayed by travel up the tubing to the console and any system fluidic response to the event must then travel back down the tubing to the port, adding further delay. In addition to tubing delays, time is required for sensors to detect change, electronics to process the signal, and valves controlling vacuum to modify vacuum levels in the cassette. Peristaltic pumps are significantly slower than venturi pumps; therefore, the ability of sensors in the console to alter vacuum level or change the flow rate of peristaltic pumps in response to rapid changes in resistance at the port is limited. Console-based flow control works best for quasi-steady state control; not large step changes in resistance at the port. Digital aspiration flow sensing which is incorporated in the Alcon Constellation® Vision System can be used to flow limit in vacuum control mode or provide proportional (linear) flow control.

Surgeon response time is approximately 400 milliseconds, while the most advanced vitreoretinal system available today reacts in about 25 milliseconds. If the surgeon recognizes movement of the retina toward the port, cognitive preprocessing is required before the frontal lobes; cerebellum and motor strip produce a neural response which must then travel down the spinal cord at about 1 m/sec finally producing muscle contraction in the hamstrings and anterior tibial compartment lifting the foot on the foot pedal treadle.

The author developed the term "port-based flow limiting" to describe various methods of limiting flow directly at the port, thereby avoiding the system, valve actuation, cassette capacitance, and bidirectional signal propagation delays inherent to console-based flow control.

Sudden elastic deformation of dense epiretinal membrane (ERM) or scar tissue through the cutter port produces fluid surge, which can result in iatrogenic retinal breaks. Fluid surge after dense ERM suddenly elastically deforms through the port and is directly analogous to occlusion break in phaco, just as minimizing pulsatile vitreoretinal traction is similar to anterior chamber stability in phaco.

The author developed the term "pulse flow" to describe the volume of fluid that travels through the port each time it opens and closes. Decreasing pulse flow produces less pulsatile vitreoretinal traction, thereby decreasing motion of detached retina as well as pulsatile forces on attached retina (Fig. 3.4). Greater pulse flow creates more distant effects, while low pulse flow limits effects the local region near the port; this is referred to as near field and far field effects. This is very similar to the well known observation that low frequency sounds travel through walls and great distances, while high frequency sounds are easily dissipated and do not propagate over significant distances.

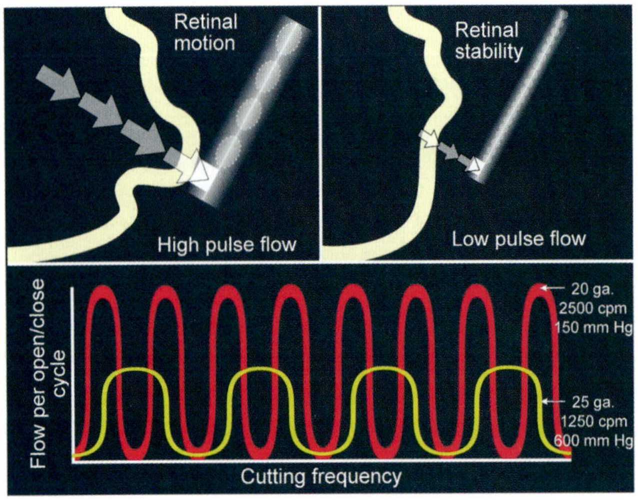

▲ **Figure 3.4**
Pulse flow effects

Higher cutting rates produce greater port-based flow limiting, thereby reducing pulsatile vitreoretinal traction. In addition, higher cutting rates reduce travel of collagen fibers before they are sheared which also reduces vitreoretinal traction. This is particularly important when surgeons make the too common mistake of withdrawing the cutter, while vacuum is applied which greatly increases vitreoretinal traction. The author believes that this dangerous habit originates from the precautions required when using early generation systems with slow response time fluidics and low cutting rates or more recently from using a phaco-like technique. In vitrectomy the objective is to cut vitreous in its original position by moving the port to the vitreous, while the objective in phaco is to mobilize lens material away from the capsule and to the port in the center of the capsular bag. Higher cutting rates do not produce higher cutting velocities or better cutting. It is thought that vitreous cutter's primary mechanism is shearing; a pair of square edges moving past each other, not inertial cutting dependent on high velocities. Some surgeons have suggested incorrectly that higher cutting rates are more efficient. Efficiency is defined as a greater ratio of vitreous to infusion fluid volumes and is entirely technique driven. If the port is embedded in vitreous, the technique is efficient; conversely, if the port is primarily removing infusion fluid, the technique is inefficient. The author terms the optimal technique "continuous engage and advance." If the cutter removes the same volume of fluid during each port open/close cycle as is the case with the Alcon UltraVit® driven by the Constellation® Vision System, higher cutting rates actually increase flow rates, while still reducing pulsatile vitreoretinal traction.

Smaller lumens produce port-based flow limiting because resistance to flow is proportional to the fourth power of the diameter. Advanced phaco probes produce high vacuum, low flow phaco by using smaller diameter ports (Alcon MicroFlare® and MicroTaper ABS®). Port-based flow limiting in phaco reduces surge and, therefore, capsular rupture rates after occlusion break as well as increase anterior chamber stability. Similarly, 25-gauge vitreous cutters (0.5 mm outside diameter) produce more port-based flow limiting than 23-gauge (0.75 mm outside diameter) and much more than 20-gauge (0.89 mm outside diameter).

The author developed dual actuation for vitreous cutters (Alcon InnoVit®) to eliminate the spring return mechanism used with single actuation systems, thereby facilitating higher cutting rates (Fig. 3.5). Alcon engineers more recently applied dual actuation to axial (guillotine) cutters as UltraVit®. Duty

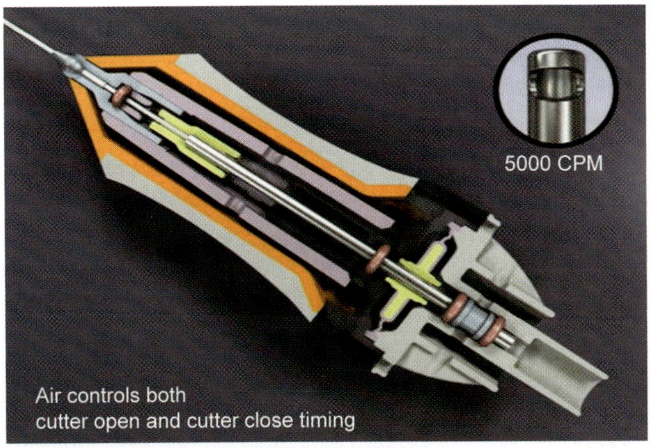

▲ **Figure 3.5**
Alcon Innovit® dual-actuation mechanism

cycle is defined as port open time divided by total time. Single actuation pneumatic cutters duty cycle is dependent on friction, spring rates, actuating pressure and cutting rate, but duty cycle control is not possible. Duty cycle control is another way of implementing port-based flow limiting. Alcon engineers developed a method of controlling duty cycle with dual actuation cutters by varying the open and close timing of twin actuation valves; this technology is implemented on the Alcon Constellation® Vision System. Biased open duty cycle result in less port-based flow limiting and higher flow rates, generally reserved for core vitrectomy. Biased closed duty cycle results in more port-based flow limiting and reduced flow rates, more suitable for peripheral vitreous shaving. As cutting rates move toward 5000 cuts/min the effect of duty cycle control is significantly reduced.

The author recommends using the highest possible cutting rates for all cases and almost all tasks. If the vitreous has been removed and a very dense segment of ERM or scar tissue has been separated from the retina, lower cutting rates can be used, if the highest vacuum level and biased open duty cycle proves insufficient to imbricate the tissue into the port. Dual linear control or 3D control should be avoided because they both utilize lower cutting rates, thereby increasing pulsatile vitreoretinal traction, travel of uncut vitreous through the port, and surge after sudden elastic deformation of dense tissue through the port.

Port-based flow limiting, unlike console-based flow control is instantaneous. Port-based flow limiting is safer for all tasks and all cases, and is best implemented by using the highest possible cutting rate and smaller lumens (23-gauge or preferably 25-gauge). Duty cycle control, enabled by dual actuation should be used in a biased closed mode, if less than maximum cutting rates are used; especially when performing peripheral vitreous shaving.

The Alcon Constellation Vision System

The Constellation is the culmination of over three decades of evolutionary development of vitreous cutters and fluidics, new and improved tools, xenon illumination sources, phaco technology, new laser technology, systems integration, efficiency systems, and advanced user interface design. The author is the principle architect of the Alcon Constellation® Vision System.

The vitreous infusion suction cutter (VISC) and roto-extractor were single port, large incision, so-called full function, slow speed, rotary, electric cutters with aspiration provided by a syringe operated by the assistant. The Berkeley Bioengineering Ocutome 800, developed by Conor O'Malley, MD and Ralph Heinz was the first three-port, 20-gauge (0.89 mm) system and had the first light weight, pneumatic probe and surgeon foot pedal to control on-off aspiration; a major advance. Berkeley Bioengineering subsequently was acquired by Coopervision and Coopervision was later acquired by Alcon Laboratories. The Coopervision Ocutome 8000 developed by Carl Wang, his engineering team, and the author had the first linear suction (now used on all vitrectomy and phaco machines), an integrated light source, and a connected fragmenter. The MidLabs MVS system developed by Carl Wang and the author had the first disposable pneumatic cutter; a crucial improvement over reusable cutters with low performance cutting. After the original MidLabs was acquired by Alcon Laboratories, the author started InnoVision and began development of the Ocular connection machine (OCM). The OCM had a dual actuation InnoVit® cutter with limited angle rotary cutting at 1500 cuts/min, linear diathermy, tool ID, an articulated arm with integrated tubing management, servo controlled IOP, a graphical user interface with soft keys, integrated xenon illuminator, integrated fragmenter, auto-gas mixing, auto fluid-air exchange (FAX) valving, and power scissors. The InnoVision OCM technology was never commercialized and was later acquired by Alcon laboratories and the author became a consultant for Alcon. Many of the OCM concepts were improved upon and incorporated into the Accurus®

system, which included an advanced graphical user interface with soft keys and global functions, vented gas forced infusion (VGFI), integrated fragmenter, silicone injector (VFC), and a halogen light source. 25-gauge and later 23-gauge tools were developed for the Accurus platform and are now in their third generation. The EyeLite® 532 nm diode pumped laser and later a xenon illumination source were developed to use with the Accurus system, but not integrated into the console or control interface.

The Constellation system incorporates new, improved implementations of all the concepts incorporated in the OCM as well as the Accurus and adds many new capabilities. The vitreous cutter is the pivotal component of any vitreoretinal surgery system; the Constellation UltraVit cutter utilizes dual pneumatic actuation (no spring return axial cutter) like the InnoVit® and currently operates at 5000 cuts/min. Because it is diaphragm driven, it eliminates the friction of the InnoVit piston, provides the familiar axial cutter format, and scales better to 23-, 25- and even 27-gauge form factors. The cutter is driven using a proprietary variable duty cycle technology dependent on the dual actuation system. Variable duty cycle control enables use of a biased closed approach to produce increased port-based flow limiting when working in close proximity to the retina; so-called vitreous shaving. Alternatively, port-based flow limiting can be decreased by using a biased open approach enabling greater flow rates when doing core vitrectomy. The aspiration system has a low latency response time to a foot pedal command for vacuum decrease or increase because of a new, triple proportional valve aspiration system and cassette design. Sensor-based, fast response, digital flow control and flow limiting facilitate working safely near the retinal surface. The aspiration system provides continuous linear (proportional) reflux as well as micro-reflux for all aspiration tools enabled by routing the infusion system through the vacuum cassette.

The Constellation utilizes a real-time operating system and distributed processor architecture to ensure reliability as well as 2X faster response time than the Accurus. It has a switched Ethernet architecture with 42 printed circuit boards, a Pentium CPU, five microprocessors, many FPGAs, and uses over 600,000 lines of code. The electronics have power backup for situations, such as the cord being pulled out or power failure in the operating room to facilitate rapid resumption of surgery.

Integrated pressurized infusion using a two chamber system is unique to the Constellation IOP compensation and is accomplished by sensing fluidic resistance in the infusion circuit during push priming by sensing flow and pressure. The infusion pressure is automatically increased as flow increases during surgery to control the IOP within +/– 2 mm Hg. IOP compensation will reduce sudden IOP decrease and resultant bleeding after dense ERM deformation through the cutter port. IOP compensation is especially valuable in high flow scenarios, such as removal of dislocated dense lens fragments using the fragmenter with 23- or 25-gauge infusion. The infusion system has automatic bottle out warning and enables changing the bottle with no interruption in fluid flow or bubbles.

The Constellation can be configured with one or two, dual-port xenon illumination sources to facilitate use of illuminated tools, chandeliers, and torpedoes. The all new xenon illuminator design is more efficient and produces 2X longer, 400 hour lamp life than the earlier Alcon HBI. The author typically uses 12–16% intensity settings because of the efficient xenon source and fiber coupling technology. The xenon optical system produces greater than 25 lumens using 23-gauge and 25-gauge fibers at 200 hours. Radio frequency identification (RFID) connectors on the illumination tools automatically adjust the initial xenon source intensity depending on specific tool characteristics; light throughput, typical working distance and divergence angle. This set-point is 8–10 lumens, which is the optimal light intensity for all tools in 20-, 23-, and 25-gauge. The surgeon can increase illumination, if needed, to the maximum FDA allowed output.

RFID in the tool connectors activates parameter and mode set-up, decreasing set-up time as well as workload and training requirements for the circulator. RFID also activates a new time saving; push prime system for the vitreous cutter and any connected extrusion tools. A sterile articulated arm incorporating a tubing management system enables priming and testing of all infusion, and aspiration components before the patient is anesthetized, prepped, and draped (Fig. 3.6), significantly decreasing set-up time and eliminating the need for a Mayo stand to support the tubing and surgical drape. Embedded wizards and digital instructional video facilitate faster set-up especially when using less experienced personnel.

The Constellation is usually configured with an embedded PurePoint 532 nm laser (Fig. 3.7). The PurePoint laser is a novel, advanced, thin-disc 532 nm solid state laser. The thin-disc laser engine reduces thermal lensing, which are localized changes in the index of refraction of the Nd Vanadate lasing medium as it heats up. The thin-disc design produces a more constant laser output especially with higher powers and firing

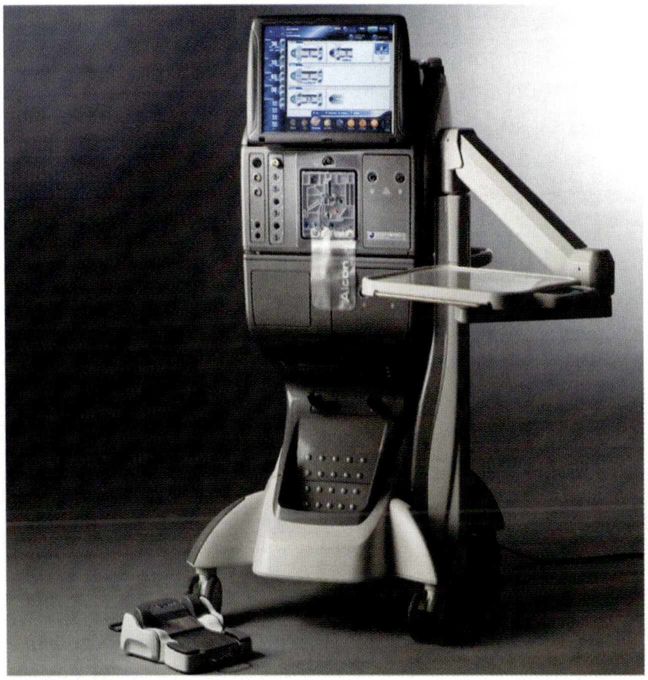

▲ **Figure 3.6**
Constellation® Vision System with articulated arm

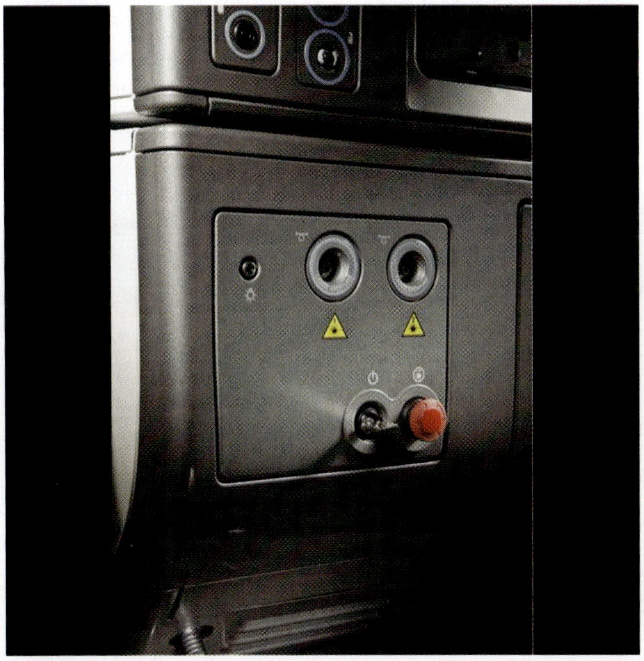

▲ **Figure 3.7**
PurePoint laser interface

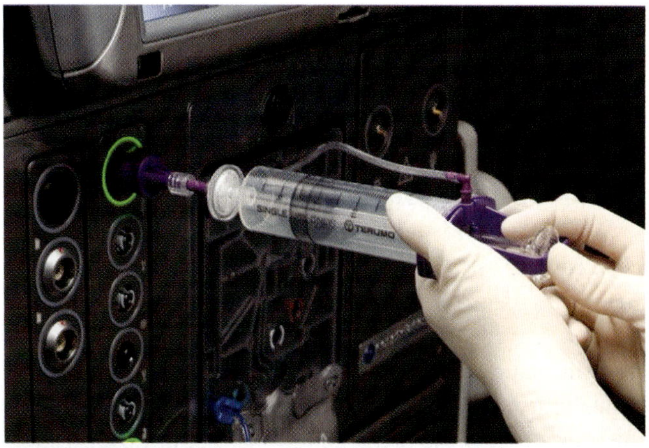

▲ **Figure 3.8**
Automated gas mixing

rates because of thermal stability. The lithium triborate frequency upconversion crystal (1064–532 nm), thermal electric cooler, and all optomechanical components are solder mounted in a fixed, mechanically and thermally stable position. A separate foot pedal controls laser power and standby/ready/standby control with voice verification eliminating dependence on the circulating nurse. The Constellation graphical user interface eliminates the need for a separate display and controls.

An Auto Infusion Valve replaces the stopcock used for FAX eliminating delay, while air travels through 84 inches of tubing and bubbles. The auto infusion valve can be controlled by the surgeon's foot pedal or the scrub tech using the Constellation sterile graphical user interface.

Auto gas syringe fill system enables filling the syringe from attached tanks of sulfur hexafluoride (SF_6) and octafluoropropane (C_3F_8), reduces gas wastage, ensures sterility, and eliminates the need for the circulator to assist the scrub tech (Fig. 3.8). A software applet calculates how much air to add to the gas to produce the surgeon's desired concentration of gas in air.

The VFC power silicone/perfluorocarbon liquid (PFCL) injector supports simultaneous aspiration and has RFID to automatically configure the Constellation mode.

Advanced phaco technology including Ozil torsional phaco is embedded in the Constellation to support both combined phacoemulsification-vitrectomy (phaco-vit) procedures as well as phaco only procedures. The Constellation, digital, fast, non-pulsatile flow control is superior to conventional peristaltic pump technology for phaco procedures.

The Constellation has proportional control of new, higher frequency, 1.5 MHz, sinusoidal diathermy system producing 10 watts maximum. Higher frequency diathermy produces a more focused lesion, possibly reducing retinal damage. Proportional control eliminates the need for the nurse or scrub technician to adjust the power and facilitates optimal intensity.

Power forceps with linear (proportional) control as well as power scissors with single-cut and multi-cut modes support disposable Alcon Grieshaber® disposable DSP ILM, and end-grasping forceps as well as vertical and curved scissors tips. Bimanual surgery is supported by single pedal linear control of power forceps to grasp and stabilize ERM during the initial segment of pedal travel, followed by control of the power scissors with further depression of the pedal.

Turnover time is greatly reduced because RFID on all tools initiates automated push-prime, testing and console set-up. The articulated arm system enables sterile setup and testing prior to or in parallel with surgery initiation. RFID and a barcode reader identify all consumables without RFID generate consumable use data for a wireless printer or LAN based connection. Surgical parameters and steps, laser log, and consumable use reports are generated automatically and printed on wireless printer for inventory control, cost accounting, billing, analysis, or incorporation into an operative note.

In summary, the Alcon Constellation® Vision System addresses all the needs of the vitreoretinal and cataract surgeon using the most advanced surgical and efficient technologies.

Management of Epiretinal Membranes

Membrane Peeling

Robert Machemer, MD, developed ERM peeling only 2 years after he developed PPV. He used a bent 23-gauge needle to peel macular puckers, which we now more correctly call epimacular membranes (EMMs). His technique, although effective, required a sharp needle tip adjacent to the retina surface. Conor O'Malley, MD, soon thereafter introduced the pic, a rounded tip instrument, safer for membrane peeling. The author developed forceps membrane peeling using end-grasping forceps and a pinch peeling technique because membranes slip off the needles and pics, and because forceps were still required to remove the membrane from the eye. A single-step, end-grasping forceps membrane peeling approach is safer and faster than initiating peeling with a blade, pic or membrane scraper and subsequently removing the ERM with forceps. End-grasping forceps are used with both blades on the anterior surface of the ERM; a safer approach than attempting to place one blade under the membrane risking retinal damage using a technique similar to peeling with needles, microvitreoretinal (MVR) blades or pics. Using pics or MVR blades requires finding or making an "edge." Finding the outer margin of an ERM can be difficult with thin, transparent, reflective membranes; retinal surface damage and retinal breaks can result from using this approach. Using an MVR blade is a potentially dangerous maneuver if the patient moves, or the visualization is not optimal. The author developed the MVR blade and was an early adopter of pics but has only used end-grasping forceps membrane peeling for more than three decades. An end-grasping forceps technique requires perfect alignment of the forceps blades at the tip which cannot be maintained with blades with long axial gripping surfaces particularly with multiple cleaning and sterilization cycles for reusable tools or, worse yet, reuse of disposable forceps. Smaller 23-gauge and 25-gauge forceps are more vulnerable to damage during cleaning and sterilization; the author uses disposable 25-gauge Alcon Grieshaber® DSP ILM forceps (Alcon, Ft. Worth, TX) for all ERMs, proliferative vitreoretinopathy (PVR) membranes, and internal limiting membrane (ILM) peeling without pics, MVR blades, membrane scrapers or staining (Fig. 3.9). The author developed 20-gauge conformal forceps so the blade tips would have the same radius of curvature as the retinal

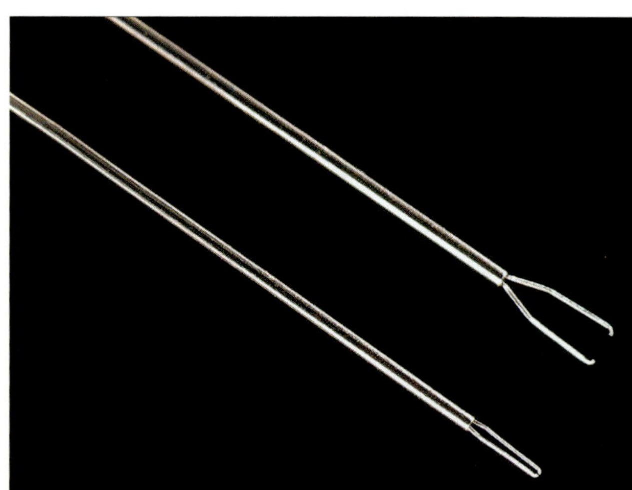

▲ **Figure 3.9**
Alcon 25-gauge ILM forceps

surface in contrast to the Eckardt forceps (Dutch Ophthalmic USA, Exeter, NH) that have sharp corners that tend to grasp retina. The 25-gauge DSP ILM forceps are small enough that radius of curvature is not a significant issue.

Yasuo Tano, MD, developed the diamond-dusted membrane scraper, which some surgeons have adopted. The author prefers the end-grasping forceps technique because it is less likely to damage the retinal surface, especially in smaller 23/25/27-gauge form factors that produce greater force per unit area.

Internal Limiting Membrane Peeling

Internal limiting membrane peeling was introduced for macular hole surgery and has been widely accepted; it is generally agreed that it improves closure rates. A few papers suggested that ILM produced worse visual outcome despite hole closure; the author strongly believes that reduced visual outcome is due to indocyanine green (ICG) toxicity, and not ILM peeling. The standard justification for ILM peeling is to remove "tangential traction." Successful ILM peeling guarantees removal of residual posterior vitreous cortex not contiguous with the detached vitreous and any ERM that might be present. The author believes that an additional and critical role for ILM peeling is increasing retinal compliance by approximately 50% so the inward directed surface tension force from a gas bubble can virtually immediately reapproximate the inner margins of the hole.

Anslem Kampnik, MD, has emphasized that ILM peeling in EMM surgery reduces membrane recurrence rates. The author been following his recommendations by peeling ILM in all EMM cases for several years, agree with his observation and believe that an additional benefit is elimination of residual striae, thereby producing better visual outcome and faster improvement.

Staining and Particulate Marking

Many surgeons still use ICG staining of the ILM, although its use is fortunately decreasing. The author has never used ICG because of concerns about the toxicity of the agent and vehicle, osmolarity, pH, and because it is simply unnecessary. One factor driving dangerous and unnecessary ICG use is using noncontact optical systems, such as the BIOM and EIBOS systems that decrease both axial and lateral resolution. Another factor driving use of staining is the use of chandelier or Tornambe Torpedo® illumination; eliminating the possibility of focal, specular and retroillumination essential for optimal visualization. An additional factor driving ICG use is using inadequate, often reusable forceps that are incapable of end-grasping. The only safe and effective stain is brilliant blue, now used by the author in all ILM staining situations.

Triamcinolone particulate marking, often incorrectly referred to as staining, is not specific to ILM or ERMs. The optimal use for triamcinolone is for visualizing the vitreous. Triamcinolone is more often required with a Tornambe Torpedo® (Alcon) or a chandelier illumination system that produces diffuse illumination making visualization of the vitreous, ILM and ERMs difficult. Triamcinolone is useful when learning vitrectomy and for identification of the posterior vitreous cortex anatomy in complex cases.

Scissors Segmentation and Delamination

The author developed scissors segmentation of ERMs more than three decades ago to address the issue of iatrogenic retinal tears caused when attempting to peel adherent ERMs, which are common in diabetic traction retinal detachment cases. Segmentation is used to reduce tangential force on the retina by separating ERM into "epicenters," better termed vascularized adherence sites. Segmentation is performed by placing one blade of the scissors under the ERM, between the retina and ERM, and the other blade above the ERM. Although this was initially performed with "vertical scissors," curved scissors are far superior for segmentation because blade width is much greater than blade thickness; vertical scissors require more space between the retina and ERM than curved scissors (Fig. 3.10). Segmentation is now primarily

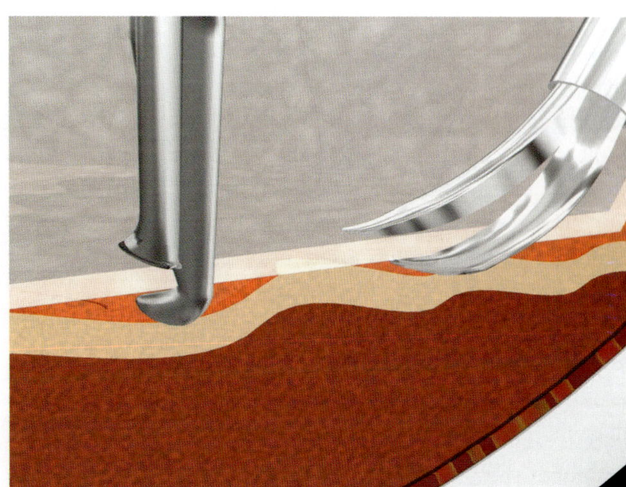

Figure 3.10
Curved versus vertical scissors

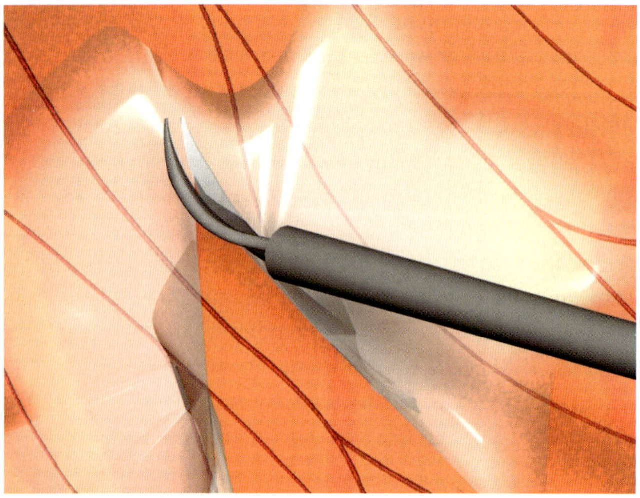

▲ Figure 3.11
Access segmentation

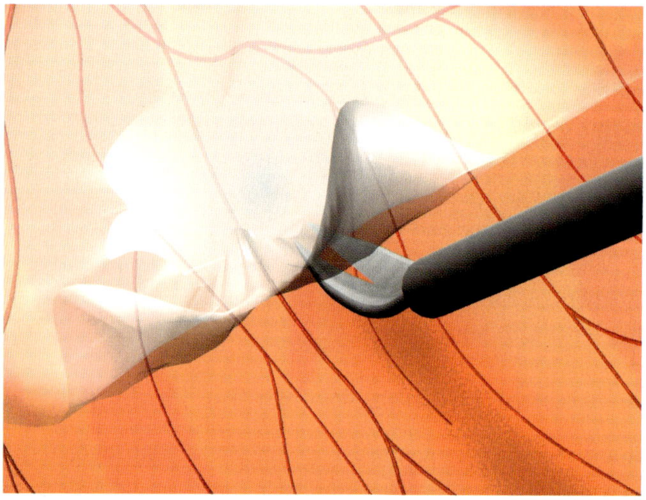

▲ Figure 3.12
ERM delamination

used for access segmentation to expose the delamination plane (Fig. 3.11). Using curved scissors for both segmentation and delamination expedites transitioning from access segmentation to delamination without tool exchange.

The author developed scissors delamination two years after developing segmentation to address the issue of residual ERM after segmentation. Residual ERMs in diabetic traction retinal detachment cases can result in small areas of chronic retinal elevation that ultimately cause atrophic retinal holes and late rhegmatogenous retinal detachments. In addition, bleeding from the cut edges provide a substrate for glial recurrence.

Scissors delamination is performed by inserting both scissors blades in the potential space between the ERM and the retina, and severing the attachment points. Simplistically, segmentation means to cut up the ERM and delamination means to cut it off. Initially, delamination was performed with "horizontal" scissors, actually 135º. For almost two decades, the author has used only curved scissors for conformal delamination. Curved scissors are preferred over "horizontal" because the curvature of the scissors matches the curvature of the retina, reducing the likelihood of impaling the retina with scissors tips. If the scissors are introduced under the ERM with the blades wide open and then closed, attachment points will be torn instead of sheared, which causes retinal breaks. When the scissors are introduced under the ERM with the blades closed and then opened, similar to the technique used for blunt dissection in general surgery, attachment points will be torn instead of sheared, creating retinal breaks. The optimal technique is to open the scissors just enough to engage an attachment point, cut, pull back slightly, move laterally to the next attachment point, advance slightly and cut again. It is not necessary to lift or stabilize the ERM using "bimanual surgery" when disposable scissors or reasonably new reusable scissors are used. Because ERMs are under tension and there is a pressure gradient across the retina, the membrane will scroll up and separate from the retina without lifting (Fig. 3.12).

Inside-out Versus Outside-in Technique

Robert Machemer, MD, used an outside-in technique for bent needle membrane peeling and many surgeons emulate this technique when using delamination. A better approach for end-grasping forceps membrane peeling, scissors segmentation as well as scissors delamination, is to initiate the dissection centrally and peel, segment or delaminate outward (Fig. 3.13). Inside-out dissection is safer because the retina is thicker and 100 times stronger centrally than in the periphery especially in ischemic patients and post-panretinal photocoagulation; the retina is redundant centrally in traction retinal detachment cases and the view is better centrally.

▶ Cutter Delamination

High cutting rate vitrectomy cutters can be used for segmentation and delamination of epiretinal tissue, decreasing but not

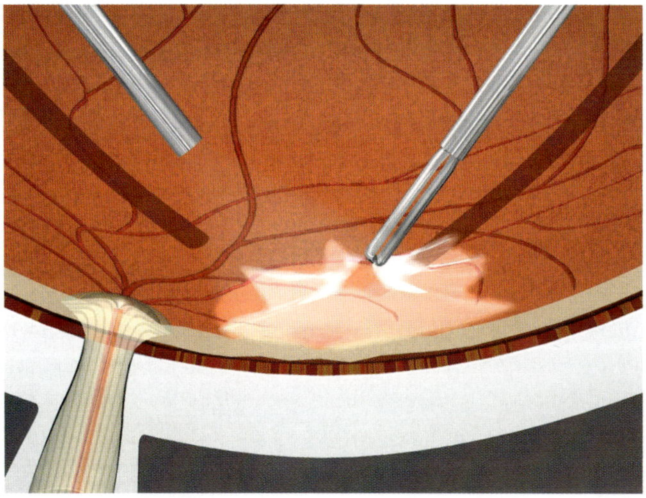

▲ **Figure 3.13**
Forceps membrane peeling

eliminating the need for scissors. Segmentation can be performed by placing the cutter directly over concave retina, port up between retinal attachment points where clearance from the retina is the highest, and removing the bridging posterior vitreous cortex and associated ERM. The author has described two techniques of cutter delamination—conformal cutter delamination and foldback cutter delamination. Conformal cutter delamination involves placing the cutter opening at the leading edge of the epiretinal tissue and modulating the angle of attack, so the cutter removes the epiretinal tissue without removing the underlying retina. Foldback delamination involves placing the cutter on surface of the epiretinal tissue, with the cutter port behind the leading edge of the ERM and allowing the epiretinal tissue to foldback into the cutter. This technique is only effective for flexible, less dense ERMs.

▶ En Bloc Dissection

En bloc dissection as initially described utilized an outside-in technique and advocated using the posterior vitreous cortex to lift the ERM. Putting traction on the posterior vitreous cortex results in peripheral retinal breaks, while the surgeon is focusing on the ERM dissection. En bloc is a poor term when applied to ERM dissection; it is only meaningful in cancer surgery when the concept is to minimize dispersion of cancer cells. A better way to think about this issue is to forget the outdated notion that the standard surgical algorithm is: first core vitrectomy, then create a posterior vitreous detachment (PVD) and finally dissect ERMs. If a PVD is not present in a diabetic traction retinal detachment case, then go directly to an inside-out delamination starting at or near the optic nerve head. It is not necessary to remove all ERM in one piece as suggested by the term en bloc; it is preferable to segment in several pieces, each of which will be contiguous with the posterior vitreous cortex. When most or all the ERM has been delaminated using an inside-out direction, creation of PVD will be accomplished as well or it will be irrelevant because there are no longer any posterior attachment points.

▶ Bimanual Surgery

Bimanual surgery is a misleading term; the point of bimanual surgery is to accomplish what the author calls forceps stabilization of ERM using forceps to offset the scissors push-out force. Scissors cut at a point that starts near the pivot point and moves toward the tip, creating undesirable push-out force. In contrast, a vitreous cutter cuts on a curved line which makes manufacturing much more difficult and requires vacuum for imbrications into the port, but eliminates push-out force. An unintended consequence of bimanual surgery is inadvertent lifting of the ERM causing iatrogenic retinal breaks. Making small delamination cuts with disposable scissors almost closed, obviates the need to lift the ERM and visualize the attachment points. Bimanual surgery requires the use of either illuminated tools, which are not available in 23-gauge or 25-gauge, or a chandelier or Torpedo which produces diffuse illumination making visualization of vitreous, ILM and transparent membranes more difficult.

Exchanges and Subretinal Fluid Drainage

▶ Surface Tension Management and Exchanges

Air, various inert gases (SF_6, C_3F_8), silicone oil, and PFCLs are utilized primarily because they are immiscible in water [balanced salt solution (BSS), retina, vitreous]. This immiscibility is best referred to as interfacial surface tension. Surface tension is a physical property of liquids that depends on intermolecular attraction forces within the liquid itself. Whereas deep in a liquid all molecules are attracted to neighboring molecules in all directions, on the surface of a liquid, molecules are only attracted to those in the plane of the surface and underneath it, but not above the surface. This causes surface liquid molecules to form a "film" of closely packed molecules. The energy required to break this film is termed surface tension. Different liquids will have different surface tensions, which depend on the chemical characteristics of their molecules and their intermolecular attraction forces. Liquids with high electrostatic intermolecular attraction forces, such as water (surface tension of 73 dynes/cm), have higher surface tension than nonpolar liquids, such as silicone oil (surface tension of 20 dynes/cm). PFCLs have intermediate surface tension properties (50 dynes/cm). When two immiscible liquid phases interact, the particular tension at the interphase is called interfacial tension. The surface tension or interfacial tension values of clinical significance for vitreous surgery are: water/air (or gas) = 73 dynes/cm, silicone oil/water = 40 dynes/cm, and PFO/water = 50 dynes/cm. As mentioned above, vitreous, retina, BSS, and aqueous humor behave as water.

Surface tension management of rhegmatogenous retinal detachments is based on creating a "liquid surface" interface at the level of a retinal hole (or holes). This interface, by virtue of its surface tension, creates a virtual film over the hole that prevents passage of fluid through the hole and restores the transretinal pressure gradient. This enables the retinal pigment epithelium (RPE) cells to absorb the subretinal fluid (SRF), or the surgeon to intraoperatively remove the fluid without reaccumulation. The term "tamponade" is meaningless from a physics perspective. It is derived from French, and means "to plug" not "to press." The interfacial tension of an air or gas bubble "seals" the hole even when it is not in contact with the RPE.

Density (specific gravity) determines if a substance will sink or float and the force it will produce at the retinal contact surface. Air, gases and silicone oil are less dense than saline or vitreous and migrate opposite to the gravity vector, and rise inside the eye. PFCLs are almost twice as dense as saline or vitreous and, therefore, sink to the lowest part of the eye.

Air, SF_6 and C_3F_8 have identical intraoperative properties, although they are different with respect to bubble expansion and duration in the eye. Gases, such as C_3F_8, produce greater duration in the eye because the gaseous diffusion rate of these larger molecules is much slower than nitrogen in the blood. Abrams showed that an empirical iso-expansive mixture of each inert gas with air could be determined so that complete intraocular filling could be used without increased postoperative pressure. The iso-expansive concentration is approximately 25% for SF_6 and 18% for C_3F_8. Nitrous oxide anesthesia should not be used with air or mixtures of any of the inert gases, as it can cause rapid intraoperative expansion of a pre-existing bubble or marked postoperative shrinkage of the bubble. All patients should wear a warning bracelet until the bubble is noticed by the anesthesia personnel in case the patient undergoes emergency, nonophthalmic surgery.

Interfacial Tension Agents

Exchange techniques are utilized in vitreoretinal surgery to inject or remove interfacial tension agents; air and longer acting gases, PFCLs, and silicone oil after the vitreous has been removed. Although these substances are often called tamponade agents, this is a poor term. Using correct terms from physics and chemistry promotes better understanding of surgical concepts. For example; some surgeons inject gas after EMM surgery thinking it will press on and eliminate retinal folds, which is simply not the case. Interfacial tension is not related to viscosity or density. Air and air-gas mixtures produce greater interfacial tension (70 nM/M) than silicone oil (40–45 nM/M) or PFO (50 nM/M). The silicone-PFO interface produces only 5–7 nM/M interfacial tension, explaining why these substances become mixtures overtime. Density determines where the bubble goes; interfacial tension determines what it does. Many surgeons have said that you cannot use PFO with 25-gauge surgery because it is too viscous, which is incorrect; PFO is less viscous than BSS, although it has almost twice the density demonstrating that density and viscosity are not related. PFO has similar interfacial tension to silicone oil, although oil has over 1,000 times greater viscosity. Most surgeons use FAX coupled with internal drainage of SRF (IDS) to attach the retina, treat the retinal breaks with endophotocoagulation, and then perform air-silicone exchange (ASX) for PVR cases. They are often surprised when some or the entire inferior retina is detached on the first postoperative day; this is because the interfacial tension of air is greater than that of silicone oil and the force of residual traction is greater than the interfacial tension of oil. Emulsification is related to many factors, but the most significant parameter is interfacial tension (which is not related to viscosity) explaining why the emulsification rate of 1,000 cs oil is same as 5,000 cs oil. Factors in silicone oil emulsification include steep bubble radius due to an incomplete fill and use of viscoelastics, postoperative bleeding or inflammation, all of which decrease interfacial tension, much like a detergent. Nystagmus is another factor in emulsification because it increases the shear rate, in essence spinning off small bubbles.

There are many ways to plan for the use of interfacial tension agents: does the agent float (air, gas and silicone oil) or sink (PFO); does the agent absorb overtime (air, gas) or remain in place (PFO, oil); can the patient see through the bubble (silicone oil) or not (air, gas, PFO), and can the substance be left in the eye for long-term (oil) or only medium-term (gas, PFO).

Nomenclature

Logical terminology is essential in a procedural context. English language convention is that word order is relevant; FAX means replace fluid with air. Often surgeons incorrectly call this gas-fluid exchange which actually means remove gas and replace it with fluid. The preferred naming convention is to use IDS for internal drainage of subretinal fluid, FAX for fluid-air exchange, AGX for air-gas exchange, ASX for air-silicone exchange, PGX for PFO-gas exchange, PSX for PFO-silicone exchange, etc.

Drainage of Subretinal Fluid

Total FAX (Fig. 3.14) and near total IDS is utilized by most vitreoretinal surgeons when repairing retinal detachments using vitrectomy. The author invented IDS over three decades ago; the concept is to drain SRF through pre-existing or iatrogenic retinal breaks or a drainage retinotomy rather than through the sclera, choroid, and RPE, risking bleeding and retinal incarceration. Unlike the use of cryopexy during scleral buckling while the retina is still detached, vitrectomy using IDS and FAX permits post-reattachment retinopexy, which in turn enables precise location of the endolaser without overtreatment, and treating both the retina and RPE which results in stronger adherence. In addition, internal drainage when coupled with FAX enables assessment of residual vitreoretinal traction, a maneuver the author refers to as the reattachment experiment. Assessment of residual vitreoretinal traction can determine the need for interface vitrectomy, additional forceps peeling of ERMs, scissors segmentation/delamination, or retinectomy, all performed "under" air.

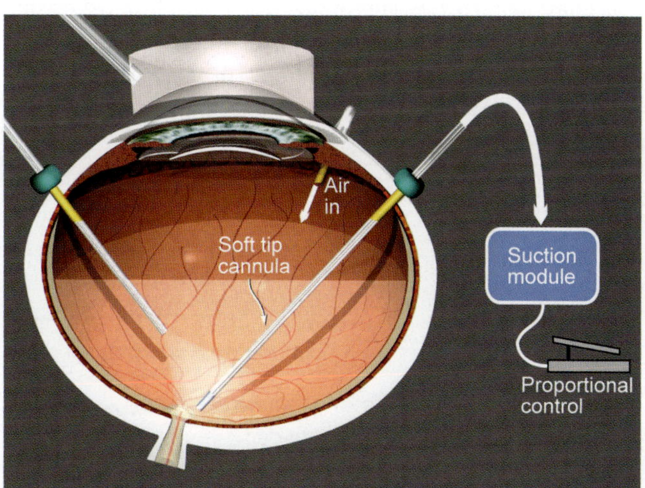

▲ **Figure 3.14**
Fluid-air exchange

The author performed the first IDS using the vitreous cutter, which is still a useful technique in some cases. Soon thereafter the author developed the flute needle; a nontapered, end-opening, blunt cannula with a port on the handle to control fluid egress with the surgeon's fingertip (hence the term flute, like the musical instrument). This cannula was also used to remove free blood products using a technique called "vacuum cleaning" similar to cleaning the bottom of a swimming pool. Many surgeons called this "passive egress" which is incorrect; IOP can produce a substantial pressure difference across the port relative to atmospheric pressure which is no safer than so-called active suction. Conor O'Malley soon thereafter suggested that fluid egress would be better controlled by using the console and footpedal, a technique he called "extrusion." The author immediately adopted extrusion because it prevented inadvertent motion of the tip when covering/uncovering the port on the handle and enabled more precise vacuum control as well as foot pedal controlled reflux.

Sandy Grizzard and Harry Flynn independently developed various flexible or soft-tip cannulas which are preferable to rigid cannulas for all applications. Soft-tip cannulas are less likely to damage the retina, optic nerve, RPE, or choroid due to patient movement or positioning errors caused by suboptimal visualization. Soft-tip cannulas should be inserted through the retina break or drainage retinotomy to a position just above the RPE to reduce the likelihood of retinal incarceration in the port. Small diameter, especially 25G, soft-tip cannulas are very flexible and will flex to conform to the RPE surface when inserted through a retinal break or retinotomy. 25-gauge soft-tip cannulas always provide sufficient flow rates when used with proportional (linear) vacuum with a preset maximum of 600–650 mm Hg.

Internal drainage of SRF should be initiated before starting FAX to prevent SRF from being displaced posteriorly by the buoyancy of the air. Internal drainage can be performed through a pre-existing retinal break or mid-peripheral drainage retinotomy well away from the macula and vascular arcades. Internal drainage should be continued during FAX to prevent posterior displacement of SRF; the view is often transiently lost until bubbles coalesce necessitating very stable positioning of the soft-tip cannula. Removal of the flap from flap tears not only eliminates traction, but it also reduces the likelihood of retinal incarceration in the soft-tip cannula.

Drainage Retinotomy

Although the author developed IDS as well as retinectomy, drainage retinotomies were infrequently used by the author for many years. More recently, small drainage retinotomies have been utilized safely and effectively when the tear could not be adequately visualized or adequately reached with the soft-tip cannula. The retinotomy should be made posteriorly, away from retinal vessels, but outside the temporal arcades. The soft-tip cannula can then be used to drain all the SRF through the retinotomy.

Total intraoperative reattachment eliminates postoperative questions concerning leakage through the tear or effectiveness of the RPE pump. In addition, retinopexy performed after reattachment allows for more precise localization, less risk of RPE migration, and permits treatment of the retina as well as the RPE ensuring better adherence. The guesswork method of using a small expanding bubble without completion of SRF drainage leaves many questions unanswered at the time of vitrectomy and consequently lowers the success rate.

Intraocular Lens Fogging During Fluid-Air Exchange

Fogging is not specific to silicone IOLs, although they have a greater thermal mass than polymethylmethacrylate or acrylic IOLs and have a higher posterior capsular opacification rate than acrylic IOLs. Fogging occurs when a YAG laser capsulotomy has been performed, and the cataract or vitreous surgeon removes the anterior vitreous cortex enabling the warm air bubble to come into contact with the relatively cooler IOL, resulting in condensation. PFO reattachment technique is ideal when fogging of the intraocular lens (IOL) occurs. When fogging occurs, the air should be replaced with infusion fluid and the retina attached with PFO followed by endophotocoagulation around all retinal breaks, and finally by placing the soft-tip cannula in the optic nerve cup to perform a PGX. Often a few drops of PFO will be retained if fogging occurs during the PGX, but these can be removed at a later time, if necessary. Alternatively, ASX could be performed; condensation will disappear when oil reaches the posterior surface of the IOL and IDS followed by endophotocoagulation to all breaks can then be completed under oil.

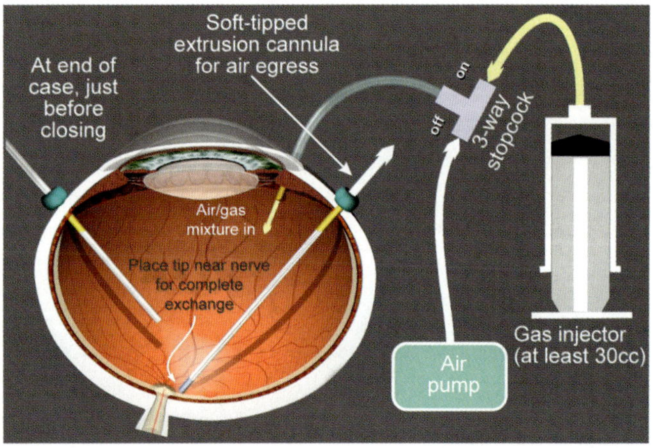

▲ Figure 3.15
Air-gas exchange

Air-Gas Exchange

Air-gas exchange is performed after IDS, combined with FAX is used to attach the retina and endophotocoagulation has been completed around all retinal breaks (Fig. 3.15). It is essential to use an iso-expansive gas concentration as developed by Gary Abrams to prevent high IOP or undersize bubbles. SF_6 should be mixed with air to achieve a 25% concentration; 18% is appropriate for C_3F_8. It is dangerous to estimate the volume of the air bubble in the vitreous cavity and inject a higher gas concentration. This inaccurate method solves no problems and can result in very high IOP and central retinal artery occlusion or inadequate postoperative bubble size. Some surgeons use partial FAX and higher gas concentrations which are inaccurate and prone to high IOP or inadequate bubbles. The air-gas concentration should be carefully determined, many errors have occurred by confusing cubic centimeters with percent; a potential disaster if a different size syringe is used than that used when the percent calculation was done.

Liquid Perfluorocarbon

Liquid PFC (PFO or perfluorodecalin,) can be used to remove SRF in cases without PVR or giant breaks. There are pros and cons of using PFO compared to IDS, although the

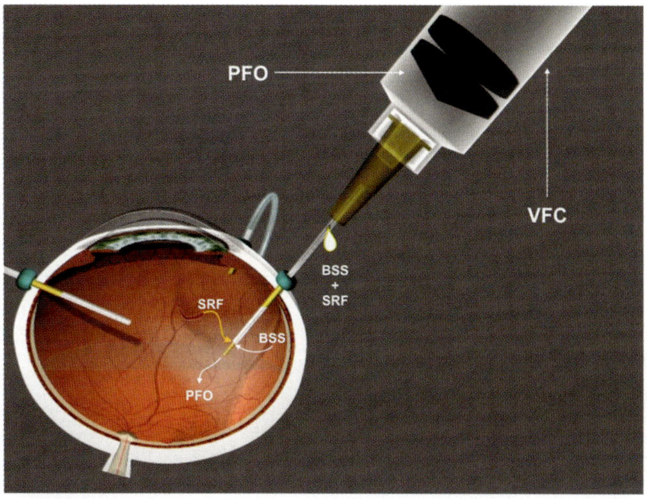

▲ **Figure 3.16**
PFO injection

techniques can be combined. PFO should be injected slowly, near the retinal surface, away from retinal breaks; preferably into the optic nerve cup or nasally to prevent damage to the macula. The MedOne 25-gauge dual-bore PFO injection cannula permits fluid egress as the PFO is injected to maintain a normal IOP (Fig. 3.16). The cannula must be retracted as the PFO level rises to avoid loss of PFO through the fluid egress port.

Perfluorooctane is best injected by using the Alcon VFC connected to the MedOne dual-bore cannula. The maximum infusion pressure should be set at 45 mm Hg and the surgeon should continuously visualize the fundus during the VFC injection of PFO. The VFC at 10 psi can also be used to inject tissue plasminogen activator into the subretinal space in cases of massive subretinal hemorrhage.

Subretinal fluid as well as infusion fluid, floats anteriorly when PFO is injected into the vitreous cavity which often results in SRF being displaced anterior to the most anterior retinal break unless a giant retinal break is present. Anterior displacement of SRF can be managed by extending a retinal break to the ora with scissors or the vitreous cutter, making a very small drainage retinotomy right at the ora, or by inserting a soft-tip cannula through a retinal break and carefully removing the SRF without removing PFO.

Removal of the PFO should be made carefully under air infusion, to prevent any layer of BSS that may be above the PFO to enter the subretinal space. Sometimes, a small amount of SRF can become trapped in a toroidal configuration anterior to the retinal tear and may be difficult to perceive until the PFO is removed, and the surgeon notices the presence of posterior SRF. To achieve complete removal of PFO and SRF, the removal of PFO should begin anteriorly trying to remove any amount of infusion fluid, liquid vitreous and SRF above the PFO meniscus. The tip of the soft-tip cannula should slowly be moved to the location of the retinal tear and aspiration should be continued until the PFO-air meniscus is clearly observed. If any SRF above the PFO is present, the surgeon can remove it at this time immediately above the PFO meniscus through the retinal tear. This is critical in giant retinal tear cases to prevent slippage.

▶ Medium Term Perfluorooctane

The author has used medium term PFO off label to repair selected inferior retinal detachments and giant retinal breaks since PFO became available. The technique allows the patient to stand, sit, fly, and even work and drive if there is good vision in the other eye. The technique involves completing the vitrectomy and removing peripheral traction for 360° followed by attaching the retina with PFO, and then endophotocoagulation surrounding all retinal breaks and suspicious areas. A total PFO fill is utilized and air turned on after total PFO fill, a very thin air bubble at the pars plana prevents PFO loss while removing the cannulas. Using 4 mg of subconjunctival Decadron and frequent topical Durezol reduces the foreign body reaction that can occur with PFO left in the eye for 14–16 days until the laser treatment areas are pigmented.

▶ Giant Retinal Breaks

David Wong emphasizes that a full fill with PFO with the infusion fluid turned off prevents posterior slippage of the giant break. Exchange of PFO for air to enable AGX or ASX must be done precisely to prevent slippage; the soft-tip cannula for PFO removal must be positioned above the PFO-fluid interface, just below the air-fluid interface at all times so that all BSS (containing SRF) is removed before any PFO. The cannula must be slowly advanced posteriorly as the exchange is done.

▶ Air-Silicone Exchange

Air-silicone exchange is preferable to fluid-silicone exchange because air helps keep silicone out of the anterior chamber. If silicone oil gains entry to the anterior chamber, it can be removed by injecting Viscoat through a phaco-like sideport

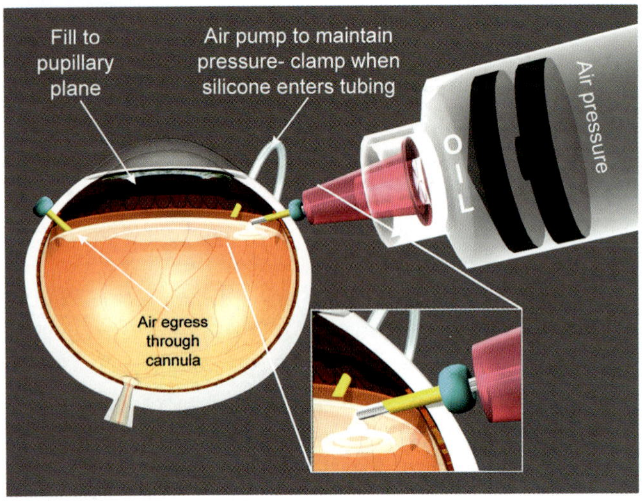

▲ **Figure 3.17**

Air-silicone exchange

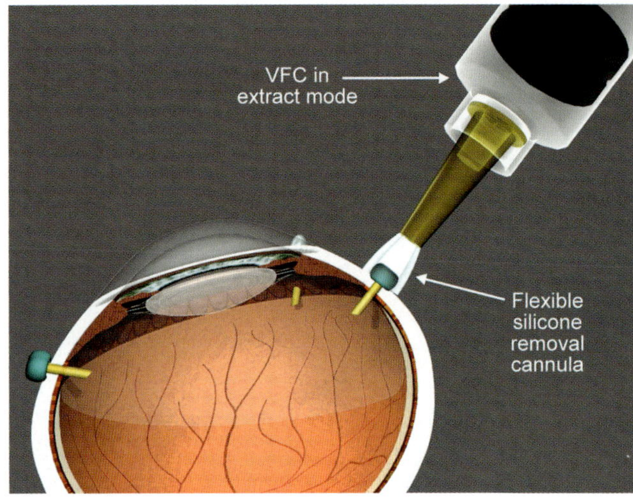

▲ **Figure 3.18**

Silicone removal

incision and leaving it in place. The author uses 25-gauge, transconjunctival vitrectomy in all cases and performs ASX by injecting 1,000 cs oil through one 25-gauge cannula with an Alcon 25-gauge metal silicone oil injection cannula while allowing air to escape through the other open cannula (Fig. 3.17). The air infusion cannula line is clamped when oil refluxes up the infusion tubing and the oil injection is continued, carefully monitoring the IOP until all the air comes out of the open cannula in phakic or IOL eyes. Silicone oil is filled up to the pupillary plane in aphakic eyes. Air egress is made possible in phakic eyes and IOL eyes by positioning the eye and patient's head so the open cannula is at the highest point, although an air bubble can be removed by extrusion with the soft-tip cannula if care is taken to keep the tip out of the oil. Pushing air back into the console air pump is inappropriate because it risks contamination of the console, over-pressurization of the eye and incomplete filling with oil. Injection of oil using the infusion port and tubing is not a good technique because of the high resistance of the tubing and cannula; the short, thin wall silicone injection cannula is preferred approach.

▶ Silicone Removal

Silicone oil should not be removed unless the retina is 100% attached, all retinal breaks are surrounded by confluent laser and, preferably, three rows of 360° laser have been applied. It is not necessary to remove oil in older patients especially if an IOL is present and silicone does not enter the anterior chamber. The author uses 25-gauge, three-port technique to remove silicone oil by placing an Alcon silicone oil extraction cannula over the outside of the nasal cannula hub (Fig. 3.18); aspiration is provided by the Alcon Constellation VFC. The infusion maintains the IOP, and the temporal cannula is left open to allow additional egress of small silicone bubbles. Complete silicone oil removal is facilitated by positioning the eye and patient's head so the cannula used for extraction is at the highest point. Repeated fluid-air-fluid exchanges may be needed to displace any silicone oil that may be adherent to the zonules. This technique allows complete removal of all silicone oil through the 25-gauge cannulas.

▶ Silicone Reoperations

The author has reoperated all silicone cases for EMMs or PVR redetachment without removing the oil for over 25 years. In recent years, the author developed another method which works well with 25-gauge silicone reoperations, a two-port, sequential, inject oil and remove SRF method using the Alcon 25-gauge silicone oil injection cannula. End-grasping Alcon 25-gauge DSP ILM forceps are used for ERM peeling "under" oil and the cutter is used for retinectomy, if needed, as well as removal of residual vitreous traction and SRF. Forceps membrane peeling, scissors segmentation/delamination, retinectomy, laser, etc. are effective "under" silicone. Silicone is injected sequentially with the VFC to replace silicone as needed. The suction (vacuum) is used at the highest setting (600–650 mm Hg) and scissors segmentation/

delamination, forceps membrane peeling, retinectomy, subretinal surgery, and endophotocoagulation work in the usual manner.

Interface Vitrectomy

The author developed a concept known as interface vitrectomy, which is based on performing a variety of techniques with air, PFO, or silicone oil in the eye. Vitrectomy, forceps membrane peeling, scissors segmentation/delamination, diathermy, and retinectomy all work well with these agents in the eye. The term "interface" emphasizes that the vitreous cutter must be placed outside the air, PFO or silicone oil bubble. Air and silicone oil float in infusion fluid, but PFO sinks; it is crucial to understand that there is always a fluid layer at the retinal surface, the retina is over 90% water as well as immiscible in air, PFO or oil. The author introduced the concept of endophotocoagulation "under" air over three decades ago and Stanley Chang introduced membrane peeling "under" PFO for PVR cases many years ago as well. Interface vitrectomy prevents an increase of SRF during traction removal, allows realistic assessment of remaining traction, confines bleeding to the interface, and stabilizes the retina. Air stabilizes the retina by spring dampening, silicone oil by viscous dampening, and PFO by inertial (F = MA) and gravitational (high specific gravity) effect. The author uses 25-gauge vitrectomy for these cases and is very careful to avoid applying vacuum while the port is in silicone oil. Moderate amounts of subretinal silicone can be removed in conjunction with retinectomy and ERM removal without plugging the vitreous cutter by using 600–650 mm Hg vacuum.

Prior to the development of FAX by the author, fluid was withdrawn through a single needle which was then used to inject gas into the collapsed eye after turning a stopcock. Air-gas exchange is usually best performed at the end of the case, after FAX and retinopexy. Similarly, most surgeons perform FAX and retinopexy before ASX. Some surgeons recommend fluid-silicone exchange and omit the FAX step. The fluid-silicone exchange approach can make visualization as well as complete reattachment for retinopexy more difficult.

Fluid PFCL exchange is preferred to FAX before PFCL placement in retinal detachment, PVR, and giant break cases. Perfluorocarbon-gas or PFCL-silicone exchange is usually performed after laser retinopexy.

▶ Vitrectomy Under Air

Certain portions of the vitreous surgery procedure can be completed after FAX. At times, continuous severe bleeding cannot be controlled with combined extrusion and bipolar diathermy or endophotocoagulation. If internal FAX is performed in such an instance, the bubble will confine the blood to a small space so that overall visualization is improved and diathermy or endophotocoagulation of the vessel can be completed. The air-vitreous interface is quite visible which facilitates removal of residual vitreous by placing the cutter port barely into the vitreous.

The air-vitreous interface facilitates visualization of residual vitreous after an exchange is performed. The author often places the vitreous cutter port just posterior to the air-vitreous interface and performs additional vitrectomy under air. This can be done with PFO and silicone oil as well, which is termed "interface vitrectomy".

Forceps membrane peeling, scissors segmentation and delamination, subretinal surgery, retinectomy, laser endophotocoagulation, and foreign body removal can all be performed under air, if it is not an aphakic eye with striate keratopathy. Fogging of intraocular lenses, if a YAG capsulotomy has been performed, is a serious limitation of this method.

▶ Postoperative Positioning

Postoperative positioning requirements will depend on the location of the tears being treated, and lens status. A phakic patient can develop a gas cataract from contact of the gas to the posterior lens surface. While this cataract can be transitory, once it persists for longer than 48 hours, it may become permanent. The first requirement is that the location of the treated tear is at the highest-most position in the eye to allow contact with the gas. Once the laser retinopexy becomes pigmented, further head positioning is not required to keep the retina attached. Once this occurs on a pseudophakic patient, strict head positioning can be relieved. If the patient is phakic, some degree of forward head tilt depending on the remaining size of the bubble is usually required to keep the gas away from the posterior lens surface.

Making an analogy to a "cast on a broken arm" can enhance patient acceptance. Phrases like "put the bubble on the trouble" and "longer duration bubbles result in higher success rates" help the patient gain understanding. Numerous pillows facilitate comfortable positioning. A comparison can be made to sleeping with crossed arms on a school desk and a table at home used with a pillow for padding. Wingback chairs and sofas are similar to the car, bus or airplane seating position and can be used to explain the required position. Some surgeons recommend expensive special chairs or support systems, which the author believes to be unnecessary; these devices require immobility, which increases muscle cramping, psychological stress and deep venous thrombosis.

The reduced atmospheric pressures intrinsic to air travel or rapid ground travel to higher altitudes dictate marked caution when a bubble is present. Bubble expansion from air travel causes a severe increase in IOP and can cause vascular occlusion. Air travel is best prohibited while an air/gas bubble is present, although clinically it has been observed that a bubble less than 10% of ocular volume can be tolerated. Ground travel should be used to prevent this severe problem. Patients should be cautioned to avoid rapid ground travel from low to high altitudes.

An understanding of physics, fluidics, and how tools and vitreoretinal systems work is essential to logical, efficient, effective vitreoretinal surgery. In this era of incredible advances in biotechnology, the surgeon must not de-emphasize understanding their surgical systems, tools and techniques.

References

1. Charles S. An engineering approach to vitreoretinal surgery. Retina. 2004;24:435-44.
2. Chang S, McCuen B, Charles S. New techniques for hemostasis during diabetic vitrectomy. Retina. 2003;23:120-2.
3. Charles S. Techniques and tools for dissection of epiretinal membranes. Graefes Arch Clin Exp Ophthalmol. 2003;241:347-52.
4. Charles S, Calzada J, Wood B. Vitreous Microsurgery, 4th edition. Baltimore, Maryland: Lippincott, Williams and Wilkins; 2006.

20-Gauge Pars Plana Vitrectomy

4

Andreas Ebneter, Rajeev Jain, Jagjit Singh Gilhotra

Introduction and Brief History

The invention of vitrectomy has been closely associated with the name Robert Machemer. Born and educated in Germany, he joined the Bascom Palmer Eye Institute as a research fellow in the mid 1960 and was appointed on a faculty position only few months later. Initially, Machemer was involved in the study of retinal detachments but his interest was soon drawn towards the vitreous cavity. In those days, vitreous surgery involved the use of forceps and scissors and access was gained through lens extraction in an open sky approach. The main problems of this technique were irritation of the iris and damage to the corneal endothelium. Machemer was convinced that these complications could be reduced by the use of appropriate small instruments, thus causing less trauma to the iris and the anterior segment structures. The first instrument he and his colleagues developed consisted of a drill enclosed in a 17-gauge cylinder with an additional side opening. To make removal of vitreous more effective, suction was added. This instrument was used in an open sky approach. The first trials in human subjects were encouraging and postoperative irritation was significantly reduced.[1]

The next phase of the development aimed at avoiding access through the anterior chamber and lens removal. Based on his experience with inducing experimental retinal detachments in monkeys, Machemer intuitively knew that a pars plana approach would be promising. Collapse of the eye was avoided by adding a continuous infusion into the vitreous cavity. On April 20, 1970, the first closed vitrectomy was performed on a human eye. Machemer writes about this case "This man had been blind for years; he had vision of counting fingers at 2 feet, slight cataract and his vitreous was opaque. We were very lucky to select a patient with a condition that we know today to be easiest to treat, just hemorrhage. We were also lucky that we did not have any complication. One can imagine the enthusiasm that we had when the first operation was a full success and the patient could see 20/50."

During further refinement, the drill was substituted by a distally closed second tube, which was precisely fitted in the outer one. The inner tube was turning and cut the vitreous when it was aspired through the lateral hole at the moment where the two holes coincided. Despite remarkably fast progress in the early stages of the development of pars plana vitrectomy, it took more than 10 years and several attempts with different companies to produce the first commercially available vitrectomy system. Carefully selected surgeons were subsequently trained in special courses. The first pathologies treated were vitreous hemorrhages, membranes in proliferative diabetic retinopathy and retinal detachments resulting from vitreous traction.

For illumination, the coaxial light of the operating microscope shining though the pupil was used initially but visibility was not sufficient in patients with small pupils or complex retinal pathologies. A fiber optic lighting system was subsequently developed. While initially cutting, aspiration and infusion were all in the same instrument, Connor O'Malley introduced the concept of several ports at the expense of bimanual work.[2] The new approach with separation of functions and several access ports turned out to be very successful and the new technique was quickly adopted by the vitreoretinal community.

In 1996, Chen[3] described a technique for creating a self-sealing pars plana sclerotomy. This involved an initial scleral incision based 6 mm posterior to the limbus and creating a scleral flap that was theoretically self-sealing. Kwok et al.[4] described a variation of this method by rotating the orientation of the scleral tunnel by 90°, resulting in a tunnel parallel to and 3–4 mm behind the corneoscleral limbus. They used a 20-gauge round body hypodermic needle rather than a microvitreoretinal blade.

De Juan and Hickingbotham[5] devised and introduced a range of 25-guage instruments in 1990 for use through conventional sclerotomies. However, it was only in 2002, with the advent of the microcannulae array, that the 25-gauge transconjunctival sutureless vitrectomy system was introduced by Fujii et al.[6] This was followed by the introduction of a 23-gauge system by Eckardt[7] in 2005. Since then various surgeons have used sutureless technique for almost all the vitreoretinal procedures.[8]

Indications for 20-Gauge Vitrectomy

20-gauge vitrectomy historically is the gold standard for the treatment of vitreoretinal disorders. However, the advent of small gauge instrumentation was well received and the evolution quick. Today, most cases can be performed using 23- or 25-gauge instrumentation with success rates comparable to 20-gauge instrumentation.[9] Nevertheless, despite the many advantages of the small gauge techniques, 20-gauge vitrectomy is still the only surgical technique to allow appropriate treatment of the entire spectrum of vitreoretinal disorders and is for some pathologies the only suitable modality.

20-gauge vitrectomy is preferable in cases where meticulous shaving of the anterior and posterior vitreous base is key to success or where a wide range of instruments is necessary. Typical examples include advanced proliferative vitreoretinopathy (PVR), subretinal fibrosis or choroidal neovascular membranes, scar tissue, removal of intraocular foreign bodies or dislocated nuclear matter. However, the outcome ultimately depends in many cases on the experience and proficiency of the surgeon with the platform he chooses and universal recommendations are difficult to establish.

Indications for Posterior Segment Vitrectomy

1. Diagnostic:
   a. Diagnosis of infectious endophthalmitis (bacterial/parasitic/fungal)
   b. Intraocular tumors like lymphoma/reticulum cell sarcoma
   c. Amyloidosis
2. Therapeutic:
   a. Nonresolving vitreous opacities: vitreous hemorrhage, vitreous debris/floaters, vitreous membranes, asteroid hyalosis, etc.
   b. Rhegmatogenous retinal detachment (RRD): primary rhegmatogenous detachment, recurrent retinal detachment, proliferative vitreoretinopathy (PVR) changes, giant retinal tears, posterior breaks, colobomatous detachments, detachments with associated choroidal detachments.
   c. Tractional retinal detachments (TRD): especially when the macula is involved or threatened like in diabetic eye disease, healed vasculitis including Eales' disease, retinal vein occlusions, sickle cell disease, retinopathy of prematurity, etc.
   d. Combined rhegmatogenous and tractional retinal detachment.
   e. Posterior subluxations/dislocations: natural lens, intraocular lens, capsular tension ring, nucleus/cortex drop during phacoemulsification.
   f. Vitreo-macular tractions (VMTS) or Vitreopapillary tractions
   g. Epiretinal membranes (ERM)
   h. Macular holes
   i. Trauma: retained intraocular foreign body, nonresolving vitreous hemorrhage, vitreous incarceration in the wound.
   j. Miscellaneous: radial keratotomy, macular transpositions, intraocular cysticercosis, malignant glaucoma, etc.

Advantages of 20-Gauge Vitrectomy

Rigid instruments: The rigidity of the instruments results in excellent maneuverability of the globe. This is important to achieve close shaving of the vitreous base. Bending of instruments makes manipulation of the globe more difficult, particularly in complex cases.

Wide range of instruments: Particularly helpful for some tasks are curved instruments. These are not available or to a lesser extent for 23- or 25- gauge platforms. The design is limited by the size of the ports because curved instruments physically can not be inserted through a narrow, rigid straight port.

Water-tight sutures: Suturing results in reliable closure of the sclerotomies. As a consequence, hypotony is less frequent.[10-12] On the other hand, high intraocular post-operative pressures are more likely to occur after suturing.[13] The risk of endophthalmitis tends to be lower after 20-gauge vitrectomy, although in the latest studies, the difference does not appear to be statistically significant.[14-19]

Higher flow rates: The larger internal diameter results in faster removal of the vitreous. However, the gain in time is, at least partially, lost during the suturing of the sclerotomies and sclera. The literature on procedure times is not univocal.

Reduced risk of jamming: Jamming means entrapment of thick hemorrhage and condensed peripheral vitreous between the port and the instrument by repeated movement. This phenomenon has been described for 23- and 25-guage platforms during removal of vitreous hemorrhages.[20-22] It may result in peripheral retinal breaks or oral dialysis.

Cheaper: Many of the 20-gauge instruments are reusable whereas disposable instruments are common for 23- and 25-gauge vitrectomy. This makes 20-gauge vitrectomy in general cheaper.

Disadvantages of 20-Gauge Vitrectomy

Need for sutures: For water-tight closure the entry ports need to be sutured. Suturing of at least two tissue levels is necessary, namely sclera and conjunctiva. Some surgeons also suture Tenon's capsule as a separate layer. Although, in our experience this is not necessary. The need for sutures may increase surgery times and potentially cause suture-related complications like granulomatas.

Postoperative pain and discomfort: Due to the larger tissue trauma patients suffer from more pain postoperatively.[23,24] Patients may benefit from additional local anesthetic agents (e.g. Sub-Tenon) given at the end of the procedure if the surgery was done under general anesthetic.

Long visual recovery: Again owing to the surgical trauma, it takes longer for the more inflamed eyes to recover after surgery and reach the level of their full visual potential.[25,26]

Surgically induced astigmatism: 20-gauge vitrectomy results in significantly more surgically induced astigmatism.[27-30] This may be relevant in procedures primarily aiming at improving macular function and visual acuity.

Basic Concepts

Vitrectomy Machines

Many different vitrectomy machines are available in the market. A common characteristic of all modern products is that they contain a Venturi pump to provide a vacuum controlled aspiration system. A vacuum controlled aspiration system is operated by setting a desired vacuum level. The flow rate is not controlled and information on flow not directly available. The advantages are quick response times and good fluidic performance while aspirating air. Therefore, this is the preferred system for vitrectomies. Most machines have additional pumps to offer another modality with flow control.

In a Venturi pump, compressed gas at high pressure is directed past an orifice on the side wall of the tube. This creates a vacuum at the side orifice exploiting the Venturi effect (Fig. 4.1). Peristaltic, scroll or vane pumps are used

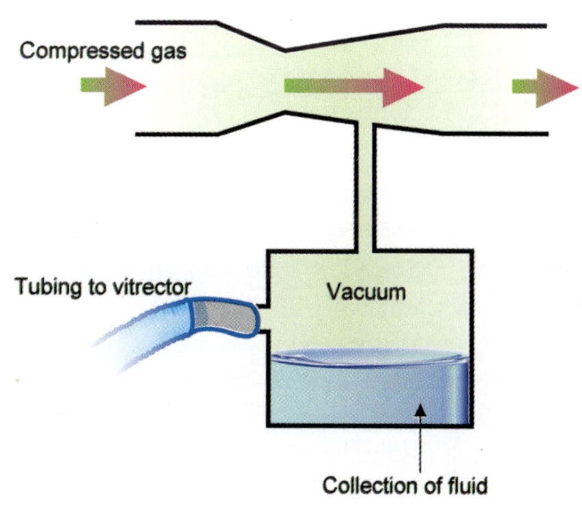

▲ Figure 4.1

Venturi pump. Compressed gas flows through a tube with locally decreasing diameter, which causes increased flow velocity. A vacuum results at the side orifice located in the tube section with increasing diameter for flow controlled aspiration systems. Disadvantages are the slow response times, undesired occlusion break responses and the vacuum cannot be linearly decreased during tip occlusion.

For the outcome probably more important than the performance differences between the different models and brands is, that the surgeon is very familiar with the machine he uses, including setting it up and trouble-shooting. He should be able to utilize the full potential of the machine by appropriately applying the available functions. For many models, the use of the foot pedal can be programmed according to the individual needs and preferences of the surgeon.

Types of Cutters

An ideal cutter produces a minimum of traction and allows fast removal of tissue. Obstruction and surge should be avoided for smooth cutting. At the beginning of the vitrectomy era cutting rates of 400–500 cuts per minute (cpm) were used. However, slow cutting rates have disadvantages, mainly exertion of traction to surrounding tissues and over time the trend has been to increase cut rates for smoother cutting to allow closer work to the retina. Today, cut rates of 1500 cpm are considered to be standard. High-speed vitrectomies have cutting rates of 2500 cpm. High-speed vitrectomies create less transorifice pressure variation, which results in decreased surgically induced movements of the retina and iatrogenic traction. This concept is called aperture limited flow. The lower flow rates of high-speed tend to be compensated by the use of higher vacuum settings.

The first available, nondisposable vitreous cutters were driven by an electric motor. The inner tube of the vitrector was continuously rotating and cutting the vitreous at the port. A major drawback of this design was the high weight of the vitrector. High instrument weight leads to fatigue of the surgeon. Another problem with the rotary design is, that vitreous can be winded up and cause significant traction to the retina. Nondisposable axial cutters eliminated the winding problem but were still subject to wear resulting in poor cutting. The first disposable cutters were axial, pneumatic devices. The pneumatic design allows a dramatic reduction of weight. The production cost of pneumatic vitrectors is lower, which makes single-use affordable. Wear-induced cutting difficulties become obsolete.

An advantage of the rotatory design is that the port is closer to the tip of the vitrector and the duty cycle is constant. The term "duty cycle" describes the time ratio between open and closed port. The necessary slowing down and the inversion of the movement direction of the blade in pneumatic axial cutters entails the longer distance between instrument tip and port opening, causes a variable cutting velocity at the port and is the reason for the decrease of the duty cycle with increasing cutting rates. Other factors determining the duty cycle in the axial design are the actuation pressure pulse and the spring constant. The significance of the duty cycle on flow will be discussed in the following section of this chapter. Dual pneumatic actuation in modern cutters homogenizes the cutting velocity and the duty cycle becomes almost constant and independent from the cut rate.

Fluid Dynamics and Cutter Parameters

For cutting to happen at the port of the vitrector, tissue needs to be aspirated through the port opening into the outer vitrector tube lumen. The piece of tissue in the lumen is then chopped by the blade and evacuated through the inner lumen of the cutter. The driving force for the displacement of tissue into the cutter is the transorifice pressure (TOP), which is the pressure gradient between the intraocular pressure and the pressure in the vitrector lumen. These two pressures can be varied independently by choosing the infusion pressure, which affects the intraocular pressure and the vacuum respectively, which varies the pressure in the lumen at the tip of the vitrector. Although these two parameters are arbitrarily adjustable, they are not the only determinants of the effective transorifice pressure. It is essential to remember, that the infusion pressure, which is displayed by the vitrectomy machine interface, in most situations does not equal the intraocular pressure. Likewise, the vacuum pressure most commonly does not represent the intraluminal pressure of the vitrector. The reason being the pressure dissipation caused by the fluidic resistance to flow in the system according to Ohm's law (P=RxI; where P = pressure, R = resistance, I = flow). The only situation where the infusion pressure matches the intraocular pressure and the intraluminal pressure of the vitrector corresponds to the vacuum generated at the machine level is when there is no flow. The higher the flow, the higher are the differences. No flow occurs, when the port is closed by the cutting blade or obstructed by a tissue fragment. As a consequence, the machine settings may alter between different procedures. It makes sense to distinguish between high-flow and low-flow maneuvers.

During low-flow maneuvers pressure dissipation is minimal. Examples are peeling, endophotocoagulation or the use of scissors. In these circumstances the infusion pressure in theory should be adapted to the stage of the vitrectomy.

30–40 mm Hg for the core vitrectomy and lower (20–25 mm Hg) in the periphery to reduce the risk of traction-induced iatrogenic retinal breaks. However, in reality most surgeons set the infusion pressure during low-flow maneuvers at 25–30 mm Hg and do not vary it. Some surgeons even advocate the use of higher infusion pressures of approximately 45 mm Hg assuming a normal diastolic blood pressure to avoid a soft eye.[31] If the intraocular pressure is chosen higher, there is a risk of compromised blood flow resulting in retinal ischemia.

Phacofragmentation is a high-flow maneuver which under all circumstances requires a higher infusion pressures of 50–60 mm Hg. Too low an infusion pressure results in a soft eye which can lead to retinal, choroidal and iris bleeding as well as miosis. Additionally, excessive deformation of a soft eye induced by instrument manipulations causes corneal astigmatism with resulting compromised view.

Variation of the infusion pressure can be achieved in two different ways. Traditionally, the infusion pressure was set by choosing the appropriate bottle height with gravity being the driving force. Gas-forced infusion is a more accurate method, which provides an exact display readout. In this more modern approach, the infusion bottle is air-pressurized by the vitrectomy machine. The response time to a vacuum-induced drop in pressure is identical for the two methods. Gas-forced infusion systems can be controlled much faster and more accurate than the height of the infusion bottle. In a venting gas-forced infusion system the air pressure in the bottle can be dropped quickly to atmosphere levels by venting the space in the infusion bottle.

As mentioned above, most vitrectomy machines use a Venturi pump to create the vacuum for the vitrectomy. The suction force is directly controlled by the surgeon via the foot pedal. The term "linear suction" means that the foot pedal position is proportional to the suction force. The fluidic resistance on the vitrector side of the system depends on the diameter of the tool lumen, the length of the fluid channel, the viscosity of the fluid and the duty cycle. The port opening is in general larger than the inner diameter of vitrector and hence does not affect the resistance. The vitrector lumen is an important determinant and fluidic resistance and increases proportionally to the fourth power of the diameter. The vacuum settings in 25-gauge vitrectomy are about four times higher (600 mm Hg) than for 20-gauge vitrectomy (150 mm Hg). Resistance also increases proportional to the length of the fluid channel. Shortening of the tubing system thus helps to reduce the resistance. This is especially helpful when highly viscous substances like silicone oil need to be removed from the eye. The viscosity of the vitreous is also somewhat higher than for balanced salt solution (BSS). In reality, the fluid removed during the vitrectomy is a mixture of BSS and cut vitreous and the resulting viscosity is therefore dependant on the proportion of these two components. Nuclear fragments, epiretinal membranes and scar tissue need to be deformed while transported through the cutter which requires additional suction force.

The resistance on the infusion side of the system is determined by the length and the diameter of the tubing and the viscosity of the BSS. These parameters do not change during the procedure and the resistance on the infusion side remains hence constant.

The relationship between cutting rate and flow depends on the substance that is removed. For pure BSS the flow decreases with higher cutting rates due to a reduced duty cycle. This is called port-based flow limitation. For vitreous, there is a parabolic relationship with highest performance at medium range cutting rates and decreased flow for both low and high cutting speeds. At low-speed, the low vitreous flow rate is due to flow obstruction. At high-speed, the flow is hampered by the decreased duty cycle, resulting again in port-based flow limitation.[32]

Surgical Technique

Preparation of the Patient

Adequate positioning and preparation of the patient greatly influences the subsequent surgical procedure, the patient's comfort and the postoperative outcome. It is worthwhile to spend the time necessary to carefully position and drape the patient. The patient should lay flat on his back with the head resting in a headrest. Attention should be paid that the patient be as far back and close to the surgeon as possible and the pupillary plane be horizontal. This allows the surgeon to sit in a comfortable upright position and avoids pooling of fluid in the nasal corner of the lid aperture.

The eyelashes and the periorbital region are then thoroughly cleaned with povidone-iodine 10% solution.[33] The solution should be applied in a centrifugal manner. Moving from the peripheral to central site should be avoided as this carries the risk of contamination. Make sure that lid margin and eyelashes are appropriately exposed during the cleaning procedure as they provide an ideal environment for bacteria that can potentially cause postoperative intraocular infections. Also, it is crucial that povidone-iodine solution gets on the conjunctiva and disseminates to reach the fornices. Alternatively, the conjunctival cul-de-sac is rinsed with povidone-iodine 5%.[34] The time for the povidone-iodine solution to act should be 3–5 minutes to allow optimal antiseptic effect.[35] The periorbital area is then dried using sterile cotton gauze. Again, special attention should be attributed to the eyelashes. They need to be very dry to make sure that the drape will stick to them and prevent the eyelashes from coming forward on to the operation site where they could get in contact with and contaminate surgical instruments.

After appropriate drying a drape is placed on the patient's face. Various types of drapes are available and choice depends on availability and preference of the surgeon. Make sure that the underlying skin is not under tension and full eyelid mobility is possible. Starting over the nose, the transparent sticky tape part of the drape needs to be carefully tucked into the nasal palpebral fissure, then continuing towards temporal. It is then incised horizontally at about 1/3 the distance between lower and upper lid using forceps and big scissors. Relaxing incisions can be made if necessary. The lid speculum is then positioned. The eye should now be nicely exposed and all eyelashes covered by tape. The eye is rinsed immediately before the start of the surgical procedure to clean conjunctiva and cornea from povidone-iodine.

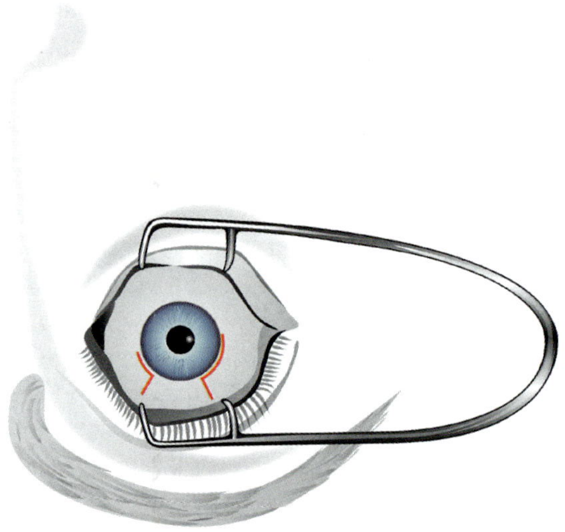

▲ **Figure 4.2**

Conjunctival flaps. The extent of the temporal flap should be about 60°, centered at the lateral rectus muscle. The superonasal flap measures 30°

Incision of Conjunctiva

As a general principle, as little conjunctiva should be incised as possible to reduce the amount of postoperative scaring. A 360° conjunctival perimetry is necessary only for buckle surgery.

For a standard 20-gauge vitrectomy without encircling band two conjunctival flaps are created. The temporal one should be 60° in extent, centered at the lateral rectus. The incision consists of a radial cut and a perilimbal cut 1–2 mm from the limbus. Alternatively, some surgeons cut directly at the limbus. This results in a triangular conjunctival flap. The superonasal flap should be about 30° in extent, also triangular and respecting the same principles as the temporal one (Fig. 4.2). Ensure the Tenon's layer has been dissected to expose bare sclera. After creation of the flaps the exposed vessels are coagulated using external diathermy.

Some surgeon aiming at even less invasiveness and conjunctival scarring use three radial slits only over the sclerotomies to access the subconjunctival space and the sclera. Blunt forceps (e.g. Moorfields) in one hand are used to grasp the conjunctiva and create a fold parallel to the limbus. Scissors held radial, perpendicular to the conjunctival fold, are then pressed on the bulbus to cut conjunctiva and episclera/Tenon's layer (Fig. 4.3). It is crucial to make sure that the cuts incorporate the whole thickness of the Tenon's layer. A similar approach with instruments rotated 90° can be used to create incisions orientated parallel to the limbus (Fig. 4.4).

For a 360° conjunctival perimetry the conjunctiva is incised as close to the limbus as possible. Two opposite radial cuts are used to avoid tear during the procedure. These radial cuts should be placed on oblique meridians to avoid damage to the extraocular muscles and spare the quadrant in which the lock of any bands is going to be (Fig. 4.5). The aim is to avoid conjunctival wounds overlying implant material to reduce the risk of poor wound healing, postoperative exposure and infection.

Sclerotomies and Infusion Cannula

The first sclerotomy to be placed is the infusion sclerotomy in the inferotemporal quadrant. 4.0 mm from the limbus in phakic eyes and 3.0 mm from the limbus in aphakic/pseudophakic eyes or 3.5 mm for all situations. The use of calipers is recommended to measure the distances. Placement of sclerotomies in the horizontal meridian should be avoided

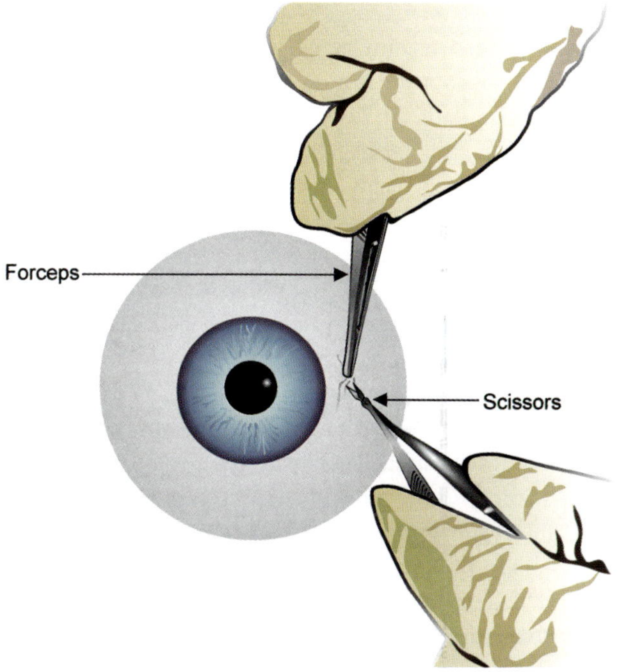

▲ Figure 4.3

Incision of the conjunctiva to obtain a radial out. The forceps grasp the conjunctiva and underlying episclera/Tenon's layer to create a fold orientated parallel to the limbus. The scissors held perpendicular to the fold cut down onto the sclera. A radial cut results

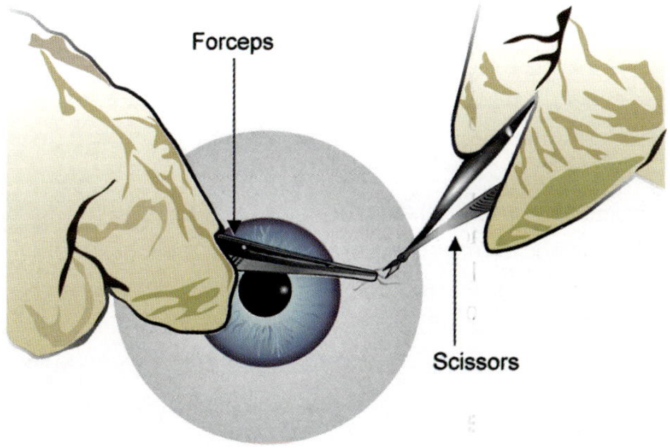

▲ Figure 4.4

Incision of the conjunctiva to obtain a cut orientated parallel to the limbus. The forceps grasp the conjunctiva and underlying episclera/Tenon's layer to create a fold orientated perpendicular to the limbus. The scissors held perpendicular to the fold cut down onto the sclera. A cut parallel to the limus results

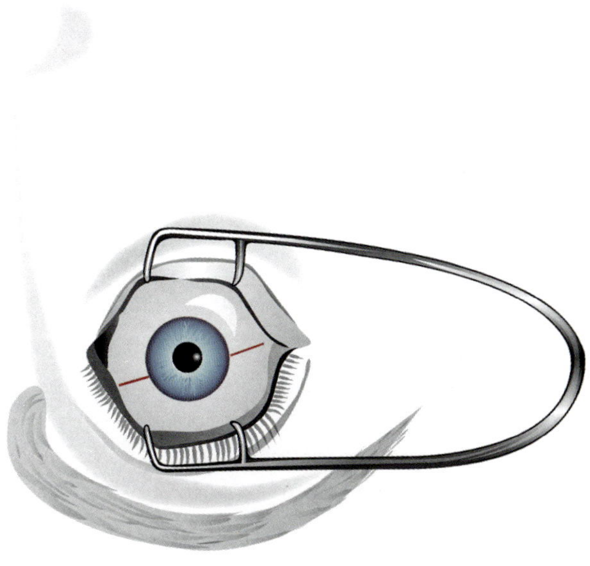

▲ Figure 4.5

Peritomy for scleral buckling procedure. The conjunctiva is incised for 360° at the limbus. Two radial relaxing incisions are placed on oblique meridians to avoid damage to the extraocular muscles

because damage to the long ciliary arteries and nerves could occur. Avoid positioning of the infusion too inferior as this leads to restriction of eye movements during the surgical procedure. The infusion cannula needs to be sutured to avoid disinsertion during surgery. We recommend the use of 7/0 vicryl, which at the end of the procedure is used for the sclerotomy wound closure. Alternatively, a Dacron suture can be used but needs to be replaced by 7/0 vicryl for closure of the sclerotomy. A suture with two radial bites and a diagonal loop is placed where the sclerotomy is going to be created. Pointing towards the center of the eye, a microvitreoretinal blade is then inserted between the radial bites to create a 20-gauge hole through sclera and choroid. In theory, a limbus-parallel orientation of the blade is preferable, in accordance with the orientation of the scleral fibers. Furthermore, inadvertent radial enlargement of the sclerotomy is less likely. In addition, if the wound needs to be enlarged to accommodate removal of an intraocular foreign body, it is safer to orientate it parallel to the limbus. However, a radial orientation is also acceptable. A smart combination of sclerotomies orientated parallel and radial to the limbus facilitates suturing of the sclerotomies at the end of the procedure (Fig. 4.6).

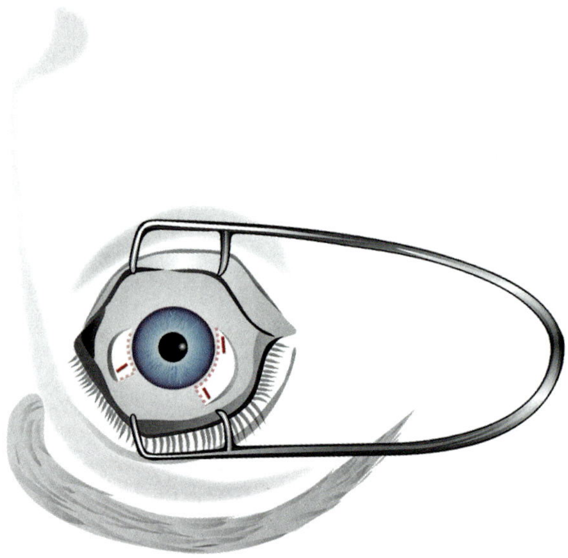

▲ **Figure 4.6**

Combination of sclerotomies of limbus parallel and radial orientation for easier suturing. The right eye is shown as an example for a right-handed surgeon. Radial orientation of the superotemporal incision makes suturing of this sclerotomy easier. Backhand stitching is not necessary in this example

A standard 4 mm infusion cannula is now inserted through the sclerotomy. Before the infusion is turned on, correct position of the infusion cannula and full penetration of the choroid must be checked. This is done by visualizing the tip of the cannula, shining light from the side with the endoilluminator. Once the surgeon is convinced that the position of the cannula is correct, the infusion can be turned on and then off to repressurize the globe if necessary.

Once correct positioning is confirmed and the globe has been toned, the infusion cannula must be tied down. Two throws are followed by a slip knot. It is important to tie the infusion cannula down firmly to prevent tilting of the port which can cause complications such as damage to the lens or iatrogenic retinal tears. The infusion line is now taped on to the drape, creating a loop in such manner that the infusion cannula is orientated perpendicularly to the entry site plane, tip pointing towards the center of the eye. The loop of the infusion line should not be too long to avoid that it impedes the rotating-in of the indirect viewing system. During this rotation process the assistant needs to be careful not to catch the infusion line with the lens of the independent viewing system (IVS) and rip off the infusion cannula.

Finally, the two superior sclerotomies for the instrumentation are created in the same fashion as described above apart from the suture which is not necessary for the instrumentation sites. The two superior sclerotomies should be placed about 150° apart, one in the superonasal and one in the superotemporal quadrant. Sclerotomies placed too close together or too far apart reduce the maneuverability and stability of the globe during surgery.

Different causes can result in a situation where the tip of the infusion cannula cannot be seen. Non-penetration due to subchoroidal hemorrhage or thickened choroid, dense vitreous hemorrhage or opaque optic media. In these situations, if the media are clear, the cannula is removed. A MVR blade is inserted again under direct visual control. Once full penetration of the wall structures is ascertained by visualization of the blade tip, a longer 6 mm infusion cannula is inserted. The tip can now be visualized in situations with thickened wall structures. Sometimes even after inserting the 6 mm cannula the tip itself is not visible but its position can be localized because protrusion of the overlaying choroid can be seen. In these cases the choroid can be punctured from inside with a MVR blade (inserted from the superonasal sclerotomy in aphakic and pseudophakic eyes and through the superotemporal sclerotomy in phakic eyes) to make the tip of cannula appear in the vitreous cavity. However, in situations with obstructed view from opaque media or vitreous blood, visual confirmation of the tip position is not possible and the infusion must be turned on in a blind manner, in general after placement of a 6 mm cannula.

▶ Machine Settings

As a general rule, the infusion should only be running when the sclerotomies are occupied by instruments. This is to avoid vitreous from becoming incarcerated in the sclerotomies. Incarceration of vitreous carries the risk of causing unwanted traction to the retina, which in turn can result in iatrogenic retinal breaks. Furthermore, detached retina could be dragged along causing even more extensive retinal damage. However, rigorous implementation of this principle is not always possible, especially during later stages of the procedure. And it must be pointed out, that the risk of retinal complications are minimal if the retina is flat and once the vitreous has been thoroughly removed around the sclerotomies.

As previously described, several parameters determine the flow from and towards the vitrectomy machine. However, only infusion pressure, vacuum and cut rate can be varied by the surgeon. Relevant flow-determining parameters given by the design and dimensions of the instruments are the duty cycle and the internal shaft inner surface area. The type of cutting mechanism (pneumatic or electric) and the blade movement (axial or partial rotational) are not flow limiting factors.

Infusion Height/Pressure

A standard setting for the infusion pressure is 25–30 mm Hg, assuming a situation with normal flow and normal diastolic blood pressure. This pressure level needs to be increased to up to 60 mm Hg during high-flow steps of the procedure (e.g. phacofragmentation, induction of PVD) to compensate for increased pressure dissipation in the afferent tubing. Care must be taken to observe the blood vessels if retinal blood flow is compromised for any reason. The ultimate target is always to assure a sufficient retinal circulation. Winking of veins can often be seen and is perfectly fine. Winking of the arteries during low-flow maneuvers only occurs if the intraocular pressure is higher than 50 mm Hg and should be avoided at any time.

Vacuum

The vacuum is the other parameter that can be varied to influence the transorifice pressure and flow in the machine-eye circuit. In general, lower vacuum settings allow a smoother but also slower cutting process. The actual vacuum is controlled by the foot pedal. Under standard conditions, the vacuum is capped at 150 mm Hg for 20-gauge vitrectomy.

Cutting Rate

1500 cpm is considered the standard cutting rate today and seems appropriate for most cases. It allows gentle removal of vitreous with appropriate flow in a reasonable amount of time. However, high cut rates are not desirable in all conditions. For tissue of high density, lower cut rates give better performance because more tissue deformation at the port is necessary to result in cutting of appropriate size tissue blocks. The disadvantage of slow cut rate is the increased risk of fluid surge and pulse pressure variation at the port. In dual-linear vitrectomy machines the cutting speed and aspiration can be controlled in real-time via the foot pedal and adapted to the needs.

▶ Use of the Light Pipe

If possible, insert the light pipe first into the eye. This will retroilluminate the other superior sclerotomy which makes insertion of the second instrument easier. The light source should be directed on to the area where one is working with the vitrector or another instrument, or behind it to work with retroillumination. If possible, direct the light source away from the macula to avoid light toxicity. The light pipe should only be inserted as far as necessary to minimize obstruction of the view by the light source. Furthermore, the overall view is better if the light source is further away from the retina. If the light pipe is directed at the vitrector, it may cause scatter and glare. However, it is crucial to always be aware of the position of the tip of the light pipe in the eye, which should always be in view. It is too easy to forget about it while concentrating on the working instrument and unintentionally cause iatrogenic damage. The surgeon should adopt a habit to pull the light pipe out of the eye or lift it up slightly when changing instruments.

The light pipe can also be useful for shaving of vitreous that has become incarcerated in a sclerotomy. For this purpose, it is best held on the sclera from outside to transilluminate the vitreous. The vitreous is demonstrated nicely in this manner. Similarly, the light pipe can be used as an indenting instrument when the base is shaved, illuminating the vitreous also by transillumination.

▶ Vitrectomy

The first step in removal of the vitreous is usually a core vitrectomy. The vitrector should be moved slowly and gently. Let the vitreous come to the port instead of chasing it around. The port should always be visible for the surgeon when doing the vitrectomy. Afterwards the vitreous is removed on the same side as the instrument entry. Crossing of the midline should be avoided anterior to the equator in phakic eyes to avoid lens touches (Fig. 4.7). In aphakic or pseudophakic eyes crossing the midline is possible.

The vitreous is attached at its base, close to the ora serrata. Therefore this is a safe place to hold the vitrector with minimal risk of tissue structures jumping unanticipated in the port. If the retina is detached from large areas and very mobile, heavy liquids may be necessary to stabilize it and safely remove the vitreous. The heavy liquids are therefore sometimes called the third hand of the surgeon. Thereafter the vitreous is removed from the most difficult site of the eye, most commonly the area of a RRD.

The amount of vitreous to be removed depends on the pathology present. Also bear in mind that a posterior vitreous detachment needs to be induced in most pathologies. This is easier with some vitreous left to hold on to for induction of

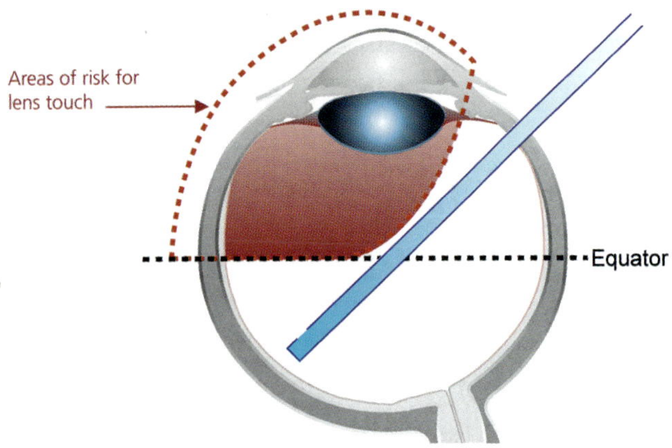

▲ **Figure 4.7**

Crossing of midline in phakic eyes. Crossing of the midline in phakic eyes should be avoided because of increased risk of lens touch

a PVD. Just as an analogy: trying to pull the hair of a bald man (equivalent to most of the vitreous removed) is more difficult than pulling it in a man with a full head of hair.

Use of Plugs

Plugs are used for two main reasons: Firstly and probably most importantly, to avoid incarceration of loose retina in the sclerotomies and secondly, to avoid preoperative hypotony.

The risk of incarceration of retina is greatest in eyes with extensive superior rhegmatogenous retinal detachments. In patients with shallow RD or detachments far away from the sclerotomies the risk is much less prevalent. One must note that plugs can disinsert, resulting in the risk of vitreous incarceration. Thus, it is important to remove all vitreous around the sclerotomies to avoid vitreous from incarcerating. Furthermore, it is advisable to use some heavy liquid to stabilize very bullous detachments or drain SRF to shallow the RD. In addition, turn the infusion off when removing instruments out of the eye.

Preoperative hypotony is unlikely to occur if the bottle height is chosen adequately (e.g. high enough to favor influx of fluid into the eye over outflow through the sclerotomies) and the sclerotomies are as small and tight as possible. When all these considerations are put into practice meticulously, plugs are hardly ever needed, unless for extensive detachments located near the sclerotomies.

Closing of Sclerotomies and Conjunctiva

The technique most commonly used to close the sclerotomies is by a figure-of-eight using a 7-0 Vicryl suture. The edge of the sclerotomy is grasped with a fine toothed forceps (e.g. colibri or 0, 12) to pass the suture in half thickness of the sclera. To create a figure-of-eight, the first pass is done at one end of the sclerotomy. A second pass follows at the other end of the sclerotomy. It is best to use a 2-1-1 knot to tie the suture off. In sclerotomies that have enlarged during surgery or in thinned sclera, two independent sutures may be necessary. This is preferable to a double-X figure-of-eight. Closure of the conjunctiva is crucial to avoid many possible complications after both vitrectomies and scleral buckle surgeries and should be done carefully. Closure using a layered approach with separate suturing of Tenon's and conjunctiva or closure of the conjunctiva alone is possible. The advantage of a layered approach is that tension is removed from the conjunctiva which is particularly useful in brittle or very thin conjunctiva. If Tenon's is sutured, the anterior edge of it is attached to both edges of the muscle insertions by two sutures in each quadrant. Vicryl 7-0 is suitable to suture Tenon's capsule. Alternatively, 6-0 plain gut sutures can be used.

In case of a 360° peritomy, the initial step of conjunctival closure consists of bringing the two opposite edges created by the relaxing incision together at the limbus. Care must be taken to adequately identify these conjunctival edges before suturing. The Vicryl 7-0 suture is first passed through one edge of conjunctiva, then through the corneoscleral tissue right at the limbus and finally through the remaining conjunctival corner. In this manner, the position of the suture is clearly defined and postoperative displacement of the conjunctival closure site is avoided. The preferred knot is again a 2-1-1 sequence. The relaxing incision is then sutured from the limbus back in the direction of the fornix using interrupted or running sutures. The edges of the conjunctiva should always be everted to avoid formation of conjunctival cysts. Closure of the conjunctiva in the opposite position is done in similar fashion (Fig. 4.8). Alternatively, a 360° running suture can be used to close a 360° peritomy. The advantage being, that hooding of the conjunctiva on to the cornea, although occurring only rarely, is avoided.

Small radial conjunctival incisions in minimally invasive vitrectomies are closed using interrupted sutures, preferably with buried knots to maximize the patient's postoperative comfort.

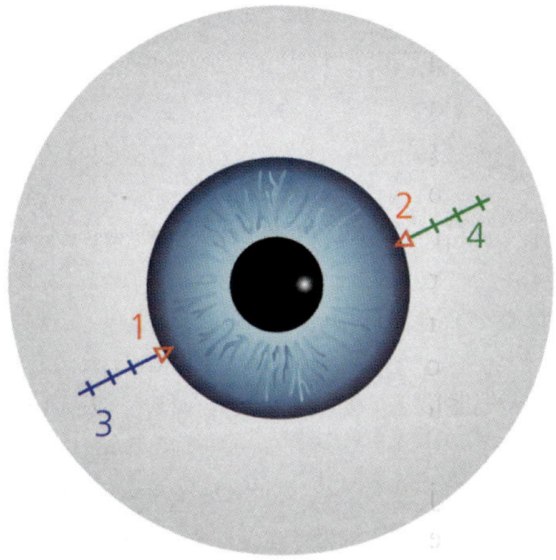

▲ **Figure 4.8**

Conjunctival closure of a 360° peritomy. The corners of the relaxing incisions are sutured in anatomically correct position to the corneoscleral tissue (1 and 2). The conjunctiva of the two relaxing incisions is then sutured from the limbus towards the fornix using interrupted or running sutures (3 and 4)

Tamponading Agents

The most common tamponading agents are silicone oil and inert gases. Their mode of action is in two ways. First, due to their high surface tension they adhere to the edges of holes in the retina and therefore prevent fluid from getting in the subretinal space. Second, they press the retina against the retinal pigment epithelium in the convex areas of the bubble.

The gases need to be used at non-expansile concentrations; otherwise they will expand by diffusion of nitrogen from the circulation and cause a rises of intraocular pressure. The tamponading gases are mixed with ambient air, which contains 80% nitrogen. For SF_6 the non-expansible concentration is 20–25% and for C_3F_8 12–16%. The gas bubble slowly disappears by diffusion into the circulation-lungs-ambient within 2–8 weeks respectively.

The alternative modality is the use of silicone oil. It is permanent, does not expand, the contact area is smaller and it comes in different viscosities. However, it has lower surface tension than gas. The likelihood of emulsification is lower for the high viscosity oils. However, because the handling is more laborious and the advantage appears to be limited in practice, high viscosity oil is used uncommonly. Heavy silicone oils are now also available for limited indication where one needs long-term tamponade on the inferior retina or in situations where the patient cannot posture.[36] In addition one can leave heavy liquids in the eye as a tamponading agent for up to 2 weeks.[37-40]

Complications

Intraoperative Complications

Iatrogenic Breaks and Retinal Incarceration

Intraoperative iatrogenic retinal breaks occur in about 5–10%,[41,42] depending on the complexity of the case. Treatment consists of retinopexy (cryo or laser) and tamponade. Entry site breaks result from the insertion of instruments or vitreous incarceration. The risk of entry site breaks can be reduced by meticulous removal of vitreous around the entry site at an early stage of the vitrectomy and the use of plugs if appropriate. Retinal damage can also result from unintended direct touch with intraocular instruments. Furthermore from cutter bites or from traction exerted while peeling membranes. The risk of tractional damage is reduced by using high-speed cutting when near the retina.

Bleeding

Different vessels can be responsible for intraoperative intravitreal bleeds. Bleeding from retinal vessels tends to be extensive. Hemorrhages of variable severity result from retinal neovascularization. Relevant intraoperative bleeding should be avoided as much as possible by coagulating the afferent vessels to structures that need to be cut or removed during the procedure. Minor bleedings can be controlled in the majority of cases by raising the infusion pressure. In case of severe bleedings, the corresponding vessel needs to be coagulated by endothermy. Careful direct compression of a vessel can be helpful as well.

Choroidal Hemorrhage

Choroidal hemorrhages are rare.[43] If they are only small and controlled, the procedure can be finished and the eye closed. However, if the extent is significant, continuation of the case is not recommended. All lowering of the intraocular pressures should be avoided by keeping the instruments in the eye at all times and elevating the infusion pressure to 60 mm Hg. The eye needs to be filled with silicone oil by infusing it through the three-way tap.[44]

Lens Touch

Lens touch increases the risk of postoperative cataract formation. It usually still allows one to complete the vitreoretinal procedure. Routine cataract surgery can be performed but attention should be paid to breaches of the posterior capsule (see below).

Postoperative Complications

The most common postoperative complication after vitrectomy is cataract progression. Nuclear sclerosis is accelerated and often posterior subcapsular opacification may develop. The cataract is remedied by routine cataract surgery. However, attention should be paid to some peculiarities in vitrectomized eyes. Compromized zonules and capsular weakness are more common. The anterior chamber is unusually deep due to lack of support from the vitreous. Lowering infusion pressure is required in many cases. Pupillary dilatation can be poor. Considering all these eventualities, gentle surgery is advised with careful attention to meticulous hydroprocedures to avoid any zonular or capsular stress.[45] In case of zonular weakness a capsular tension ring should be inserted prior to phacoemulsification or following nucleus removal.

Hypotony and serous choroidal effusions occur sometimes and can be associated with leaking sclerotomies. Treatment consists of resuturing which implies repeated use of the operating theater. Primary careful suturing pays off to avoid this. Extensive choroidal effusions are proinflammatory and can cause marked intraocular inflammation. Intensive topical steroid treatment is advised.

Vitreous hemorrhages can occur intraoperatively and persist or arise postoperatively. If mild, they generally clear spontaneously. Severe forms require surgical reintervention.

Endophthalmitis is a serious complication which occurs in 0.04–0.07% of patients.[46,47] Treatment is similar to post cataract surgery endophthalmitis except in cases where the vitreous cavity is filled with gas or another tamponading agent. In these cases the doses of intravitreal medications need to be adjusted.

Specific retinal complications are retinal detachment, epiretinal membranes and proliferative vitreoretinopathy. These usually require further surgery.

Future or Emerging Trends

Small Gauge, Sutureless

In recent years the development of 25-gauge and 23-gauge vitrectomy has been remarkable and most cases can now be performed with comparable success rates using these latter techniques. The main advantages of these transconjunctival sutureless techniques are increased patient comfort, possibly decreased operative times, improved postoperative astigmatism and reduced conjunctival scarring.

Sutureless 20-Gauge Vitrectomy

Recently, several attempts have been undertaken to develop access techniques that would allow to perform sutureless vitrectomies using the standard 20-gauge instruments. Gotzaridis[48] created a self-sealing tunnel incision using a microvitreoretinal blade after conjunctival diathermy. Postoperative hypotony occurred in 3.5% of patients at day 1 and was normalized 3 days later. Aguni et al.[49] achieved similar results in a small series of short duration vitrectomies. Lafeta and Claes[50] and Kim et al.[51] used an approach based on a cannulated system which allows use of standard 20-gauge instruments. Up to 38% of sclerotomies needed to be sutured with a single transconjunctival-scleral suture. Series to date are too small to draw a final conclusion. But the possible higher sclerotomy suturing rate relative to smaller-gauge approaches is the drawback of this method.

Simple Vitrectomy or Combination with Buckling Procedure

For macular disorders and pathologies involving only the vitreous body, simple vitrectomy is the appropriate treatment option. Typical examples are vitreous hemorrhages, macular holes, epiretinal membranes, simple retinal detachments, rarely vitreous floaters or uveitic disorders. However, when the pathology involves a tractional component to the peripheral retina, a combined procedure consisting of a vitrectomy and a buckling procedure may be necessary. Examples are certain rhegmatogenous retinal detachments, advanced cases of PVR or proliferative diabetic retinopathies comprising a peripheral retinal detachment. It is not possible to setup simple guidelines regarding the choice of the appropriate procedure and each case needs to be evaluated individually. Treatment choices may also vary between different surgeons. For many conditions, an evidence-based choice is not possible due to the absence of appropriate studies. The decisions are largely based on the surgeon's experience; however principles and goals of surgery are the same.

Acknowledgment

The authors would like to thank Quoc Nguyen from the Adelaide Health Service Graphic Design team for the illustrations in this chapter.

References

1. Machemer R. The development of pars plana vitrectomy: a personal account. Graefes Arch Clin Exp Ophthalmol. 1995;233:453-68.
2. O'Malley C, Heintz RM. Vitrectomy via the pars plana—a new instrument system. Trans Pac Coast Otoophthalmological Soc annu meet. 1972;53:121-37.
3. Chen JC. Sutureless pars plana vitrectomy through self-sealing sclerotomies. Arch Ophthalmol. 1996;114:1273-5.
4. Kwok AK, Tham CC, Lam DS, et al. Modified sutureless sclerotomies in pars plana vitrectomy. Am J Ophthalmol. 1999;127:731-3.
5. de Juan EJ, Hickingbotham D. Refinements in microinstrumentation for vitreous surgery. Am J Ophthalmol. 1990;109:218-20.
6. Fujii GY, De Juan E, Humayun MS, et al. A new 25-gauge instrument system for transconjunctival sutureless vitrectomy surgery. Ophthalmology. 2002;109:1807-12.
7. Eckardt C. Transconjunctival sutureless 23-gauge vitrectomy. Retina. 2005;25:208-11.
8. Warrier SK, Jain R, Gilhotra JS, et al. Sutureless vitrectomy. Indian J Ophthalmol. 2008;56:453-8.
9. Spirn MJ. Comparison of 25-, 23- and 20-gauge vitrectomy. Curr Opin Ophthalmol. 2009;20:195-9
10. Gupta OP, Weichel ED, Regillo CD, et al. Postoperative complications associated with 25-gauge pars plana vitrectomy. Ophthalmic Surg Lasers Imaging. 2007;38:270-5.
11. Schadlu R, Shah GK. Early postoperative intraocular pressure after 23-gauge sutureless small-incision pars plana vitrectomy. Retina. 2009;29:1043-4.
12. Shaikh S, Ho S, Richmond PP, et al. Untoward outcomes in 25-gauge versus 20-gauge vitreoretinal surgery. Retina. 2007;27:1048-53.
13. Misra A, Ho-Yen G, Burton RL. 23-gauge sutureless vitrectomy and 20-gauge vitrectomy: a case series comparison. Eye. 2009;23:1187-91.
14. Chen JK, Khurana RN, Nguyen QD, et al. The incidence of endophthalmitis following transconjunctival sutureless 25- vs 20-gauge vitrectomy. Eye. 2009;23:780-4.
15. Hu AY, Bourges JL, Shah SP, et al. Endophthalmitis after pars plana vitrectomy a 20- and 25-gauge comparison. Ophthalmology. 2009;116:1360-5.
16. Kunimoto DY, Kaiser RS. Incidence of endophthalmitis after 20- and 25-gauge vitrectomy. Ophthalmology. 2007;114:2133-7.
17. Mason JO, Yunker JJ, Vail RS, et al. Incidence of endophthalmitis following 20-gauge and 25-gauge vitrectomy. Retina. 2008;28:1352-4.
18. Scott IU, Flynn HW, Dev S, et al. Endophthalmitis after 25-gauge and 20-gauge pars plana vitrectomy: incidence and outcomes. Retina. 2008;28:138-42.
19. Shimada H, Nakashizuka H, Hattori T, et al. Incidence of endophthalmitis after 20- and 25-gauge vitrectomy causes and prevention. Ophthalmology. 2008;115:2215-20.
20. Nagpal M, Wartikar S, Nagpal K. Comparison of clinical outcomes and wound dynamics of sclerotomy ports of 20-, 25-, and 23-gauge vitrectomy. Retina. 2009;29:225-31.
21. Nam DH, Ku M, Sohn HJ, et al. Jamming of 23-gauge instruments in the microcannula during vitrectomy for severe vitreous haemorrhage. Acta Ophthalmol; 2009.
22. Shinoda H, Nakajima T, Shinoda K, et al. Jamming of 25-gauge instruments in the cannula during vitrectomy for vitreous haemorrhage. Acta Ophthalmol. 2008;86:160-4.
23. Kellner L, Wimpissinger B, Stolba U, et al. 25-gauge vs 20-gauge system for pars plana vitrectomy: a prospective randomised clinical trial. Br J Ophthalmol. 2007;91:945-8.
24. Wimpissinger B, Kellner L, Brannath W, et al. 23-Gauge versus 20-gauge system for pars plana vitrectomy: a prospective randomised clinical trial. Br J Ophthalmol. 2008;92:1483-7.
25. Inoue Y, Kadonosono K, Yamakawa T, et al. Surgically-induced inflammation with 20-, 23-, and 25-gauge vitrectomy systems: an experimental study. Retina. 2009;29:477-80.
26. Lakhanpal RR, Humayun MS, de Juan E, et al. Outcomes of 140 consecutive cases of 25-gauge transconjunctival surgery for posterior segment disease. Ophthalmology. 2005;112:817-24.
27. Galway G, Drury B, Cronin BG, et al. A comparison of induced astigmatism in 20- vs 25-gauge vitrectomy procedures. Eye. 2010;24:315-7.
28. Kim YK, Hyon JY, Woo SJ, et al. Surgically induced astigmatism after 23-gauge transconjunctival sutureless vitrectomy. Eye. 2010;24:799-804.
29. Okamoto F, Okamoto C, Sakata N, et al. Changes in corneal topography after 25-gauge transconjunctival sutureless vitrectomy versus after 20-gauge standard vitrectomy. Ophthalmology. 2007;114:2138-41.
30. Yanyali A, Celik E, Horozoglu F, et al. Corneal topographic changes after transconjunctival (25-gauge) sutureless vitrectomy. Am J Ophthalmol. 2005;140:939-41.
31. Charles S, Calzada J, Wood B. Vitreous Microsurgery, 4th edition. Philadelphia: Lippincott Williams and Wilkins; 2006.
32. Magalhaes O, Chong L, DeBoer C, et al. Vitreous dynamics: vitreous flow analysis in 20-, 23-, and 25-gauge cutters. Retina. 2008;28:236-41.
33. Gordon-Bennett P, Karas A, Flanagan D, et al. A survey of measures used for the prevention of postoperative endophthalmitis after cataract surgery in the United Kingdom. Eye. 2008;22:620-7.
34. Mino de Kaspar H, Chang RT, Singh K, et al. Prospective randomized comparison of 2 different methods of 5% povidone-iodine applications for anterior segment intraocular surgery. Arch Ophthalmol. 2005;123:161-5.
35. Ferguson AW, Scott JA, McGavigan J, et al. Comparison of 5% povidone-iodine solution against 1% povidone-iodine solution in preoperative cataract surgery antisepsis: a prospective randomised double blind study. Br J Ophthalmol. 2003;87:163-7.
36. Heimann H, Stappler T, Wong D. Heavy tamponade 1: a review of indications, use, and complications. Eye. 2008;22:1342-59.

37. Bryan JS, Friedman SM, Mames RN, et al. Experimental vitreous replacement with perfluorotri-n-propylamine. Arch Ophthalmol. 1994;112:1098-102.
38. Chang S, Sparrow JR, Iwamoto T, et al. Experimental studies of tolerance to intravitreal perfluoro-n-octane liquid. Retina. 1991;11:367-74.
39. Flores-Aguilar M, Munguia D, Loeb E, et al. Intraocular tolerance of perfluorooctylbromide (perflubron). Retina. 1995;15:3-13.
40. Velikay M, Wedrich A, Stolba U, et al. Experimental long-term vitreous replacement with purified and nonpurified perfluorodecalin. Am J Ophthalmol. 1993;116:565-70.
41. Carter JB, Michels RG, Glaser BM, et al. Iatrogenic retinal breaks complicating pars plana vitrectomy. Ophthalmology. 1990;97:848-53.
42. Sjaarda RN, Glaser BM, Thompson JT, et al. Distribution of iatrogenic retinal breaks in macular hole surgery. Ophthalmology. 1995;102:1387-92.
43. Sharma T, Virdi DS, Parikh S, et al. A case-control study of suprachoroidal hemorrhage during pars plana vitrectomy. Ophthalmic Surg Lasers. 1997;28:640-4.
44. Williamson TH. Vitroretinal Surgery. New York: Springer; 2008.
45. Sharma N, Pal N, Azad RV, Vajpayee RB. Phacoemulsification in eyes following vitreoretinal surgery. In: Vajpayee RB, Sharma N, Pandey SK, Titiyal JS (Eds). Phacoemulsification Surgery. Kent: Anshan; 2006. pp. 343-7.
46. Cohen SM, Flynn HW, Murray TG, et al. Endophthalmitis after pars plana vitrectomy. The Postvitrectomy Endophthalmitis Study Group. Ophthalmology. 1995;102:705-12.
47. Eifrig CW, Scott IU, Flynn HW, et al. Endophthalmitis after pars plana vitrectomy: Incidence, causative organisms, and visual acuity outcomes. Am J Ophthalmol. 2004;138:799-802.
48. Gotzaridis EV. Three-port 20-gauge transconjunctival pars plana vitrectomy. Retina. 2007;27:382-4.
49. Aguni JS, Meyer CH, Rodrigues EB. Transconjunctival 20-gauge vitrectomy: a pilot study. Ophthalmologica. 2009;223:12-6.
50. Lafeta AP, Claes C. Twenty-gauge transconjunctival sutureless vitrectomy trocar system. Retina. 2007;27:1136-41.
51. Kim JE, Shah SN, Choi DL, et al. Transconjunctival 20-gauge pars plana vitrectomy using a single entry cannulated sutureless system. Retina. 2009;29:1294-8.

5 23-Gauge Pars Plana Vitrectomy

Gary KY Lee, Timothy YY Lai

Introduction

The application of 23-gauge pars plana vitrectomy for vitreoretinal procedures was first reported by Singh et al.[1] in 1996. The instrument was a portable electronic system designed for simple office-based procedures such as vitreous biopsy. Due to the limited array of instrumentations available for surgical procedures, the system did not gain widespread acceptance within the vitreoretinal community. It was not until nearly a decade later, when the first fully integrated 23-gauge system with complete instrumentarium was developed by Eckardt in collaboration with the Dutch Ophthalmic Research Center (DORC, Zuidland, the Netherlands). This new system was designed to overcome the excessive flexibility of instruments associated with the earlier developed 25-gauge pars plana transconjunctival vitrectomy system which might cause difficulty in maneuvering the globe during surgery.

Since the publication of the first report on the safety and efficacy of 23-gauge vitrectomy by Eckardt in 2005,[2] the 23-gauge vitrectomy system has rapidly gained popularity with expanding clinical applications in various vitreoretinal conditions. Apart from the initial 23-gauge pars plana vitrectomy system by DORC, newly improved 23-gauge pars plana vitrectomy systems are also commercially available from most major vitreoretinal surgical instrument manufacturers such as Alcon Laboratories (Fort Worth, TX, USA), Synergetics (St Charles, MO, USA), Oertli (Berneck, Switzerland), and Geuder (Heidelberg, Germany) (Fig. 5.1). With the increasing availability and better designed instruments, 23-gauge system has become one of the preferred vitrectomy systems in the vitreoretinal community in recent years. According to the 2009 Preferences and Trends (PAT) Survey conducted by the American Society of Retina Specialists (ASRS), close to 80% of respondents commonly utilize the small gauge vitrectomy systems.

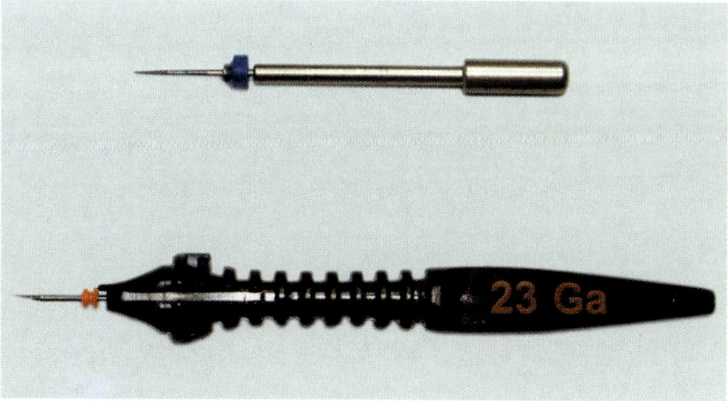

▲ **Figure 5.1**

23-Gauge vitrectomy trocar systems by DORC (top) and Alcon (bottom)

Operative Techniques

▶ Anesthesia

As with conventional 20-gauge pars plana vitrectomy, 23-gauge pars plana vitrectomy can be performed under general anesthesia or retrobulbar anesthesia. In case of using the retrobulbar anesthesia, proper techniques should be taken to avoid subconjunctival accumulation of the local anesthetic agent. Any ballooning of bulbar conjunctiva would render subsequent insertions of the transconjunctival cannulas more difficult to perform and might potentially increase the risk of postoperative wound leakage due to poor wound construction.

Two-step Sclerotomy Technique

The original method of inserting the transconjunctival microcannulas was described by Eckardt.[2,3] This method involves a two-step technique with the use of a specially designed pressure plate and a 23-gauge stiletto blade for entering into the vitreous cavity. The first step involves displacing the conjunctiva over the intended sclerotomy site with a forceps or cotton applicator. This displacement of the conjunctiva over the scleral incision allows coverage of the sclerotomy by intact conjunctiva at the end of the operation and thereby decreases the chance of wound leakage and potential entry of micro-organisms. After displacing the conjunctiva, a pressure plate can be applied firmly on the displaced conjunctiva against the sclera (Fig. 5.2A). The edge of the pressure plate should be placed at the corneoscleral limbus. At this position, the central opening of the plate is located 3.5 mm posterior to the limbus. Apart from acting as a tool for measurement, the pressure plate also prevents slipping of the displaced conjunctiva over the sclerotomy site and allows the surgeon to rotate the globe during the insertions of the cannulas. Moreover, flattening the sclera during the incision with the stiletto blade would increase the length of the scleral wound and enhance the self-sealing effect.

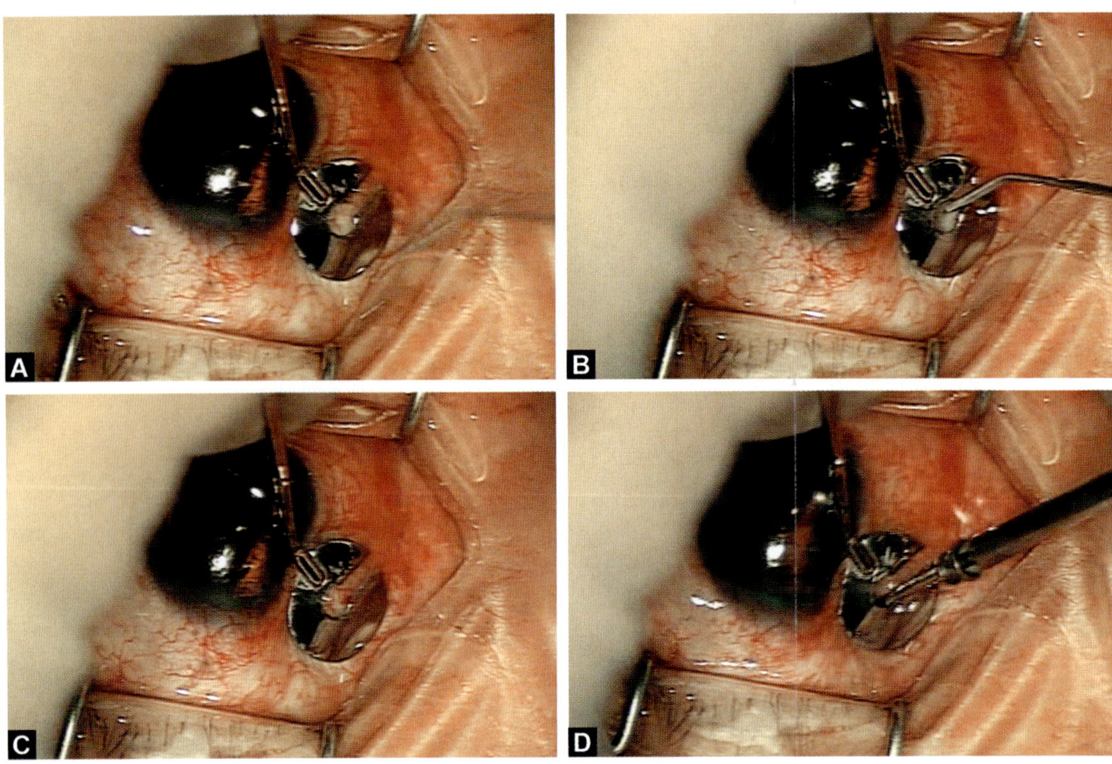

Figures 5.2A to D

Steps for insertion of the 23-gauge vitrectomy microcannulas using the two-step technique. (A) Using a pressure plate, the conjunctiva over the intended sclerotomy site is displaced and pressed firmly against the sclera; (B) The transconjunctival scleral tunnel incision is performed using a 45°-angled-stiletto blade through the central opening of the pressure plate at an angle of 30°; (C) The pressure plate is kept in place against the sclera after creation of the scleral tunnel so that the conjunctival opening is still in line with the tunnel; (D) The microcannula is inserted into the scleral tunnel through the conjunctival opening using a blunt trocar inserter. The direction of insertion is shifted from the initial tangential path to a more perpendicular course towards the center of the globe

With the pressure plate held firmly in place, a 45° angled-stiletto blade is used to create a 30° oblique scleral tunnel (Fig. 5.2B). The scleral tunnel should be made parallel to the corneoscleral limbus in order to ensure that the full length of the wound is in equal distance from the limbus and within the pars plana. During the passage of the stiletto blade, the surgeon may experience some rotation of the globe in the direction of the incision. This can be avoided by using a new sharp blade and by stabilizing the globe with the pressure plate. Some surgeons advocate an anteroposterior scleral tunnel with the blade aiming towards the posterior pole. It is thought that this technique would allow splitting rather than cutting of the concentrically arrange scleral fibers, allowing faster postoperative wound healing. However, this benefit is offset by the potential risk of retinal damage if the internal opening is created too close to the ora serrata.

The pressure plate should be kept in place after withdrawal of the blade (Fig. 5.2C). With the DORC system, the microcannula is inserted through the conjunctival incision into the scleral tunnel with a blunt inserter. During the insertion of the microcannula, the direction of insertion should be shifted from the original tangential path to a more perpendicular direction towards the center of the globe (Fig. 5.2D). This maneuver helps exert the necessary pressure on the globe to minimize any rotational movements. The pressure plate can be slowly withdrawn before the complete insertion of the trocar. During removal of the trocar, the microcannula should be held in place with forceps to avoid dislodgement. The microcannula is then left in place and plugged. Normally, the first microcannula is inserted at the inferotemporal quadrant for the infusion line. Two more microcannulas are then placed at the superotemporal and superonasal quadrants for the microsurgical instruments. In case of combined phacovitrectomy, the microcannulas should be inserted before the phacoemulsification procedures as this allows better control of vitreous pressure during phacoemulsification.

▶ Single-step Sclerotomy Technique

The main limitation of the previously described two-step sclerotomy technique is the difficulty in identifying and tracing the original conjunctival incision after the first stiletto cut. This might cause problems during insertion of the blunt inserter and result in double-incision through the conjunctiva. To tackle this limitation, manufacturers have introduced one-step trocar or cannula systems. With the one-step technique, the blunt inserter is replaced with a sharp needle trocar for the creation of the conjunctival incision and scleral tunnel without the use of a stiletto blade. Similar to the two-step system, a scleral tunnel at a 30° angle parallel to the limbus is created after the conjunctiva is displaced. Compared with the stiletto blade, the needle trocar has a slightly greater tissue resistance during incision and this might occasionally result in a more significant globe rotation. However, newly designed needle trocar systems have greatly enhanced the blade design and the increased sharpness has allowed less resistance during wound construction with a more water tight wound (Figs 5.3A to F).

▶ Vitrectomy

Techniques of vitrectomy using the 23-gauge system are similar to the conventional 20-gauge system due to the similar stiffness of the instruments. Nevertheless, forceful insertion and manipulation of instruments can lead to bending within the metal cannula and later difficulty during removal of instruments. Careful handling of instruments is important to prevent this complication. Dislodgement of microcannula during vitrectomy is another potential problem for 23-gauge system. It is usually related to incomplete insertion of the microcannula at the start of the operation. With the help of a blunt inserter, the dislodged microcannula can usually be reinserted smoothly into the original sclerotomy. Gentle and slow removal of microsurgical instruments through the lumen of the cannula will also be useful in preventing dislodgement of the microcannula. Since no suture is used to hold the infusion line, dislodgement of the infusion line may sometimes occur and can lead to sudden hypotony and collapse of the globe. Extra caution is therefore needed when securing the connection of the infusion line before starting vitrectomy.

▶ Removal of Microcannulas

Removal of the microcannulas should be started by lowering the intraocular pressure to about 20 mm Hg. The two superior cannulas for the surgical instruments should be plugged before removal and the infusion cannula is removed last. The microcannulas are held by forceps and withdrawn along the direction of the scleral tunnel (Figs 5.4A to F). A cotton wool applicator is used to press on the conjunctiva and rotate back the conjunctiva over the sclerotomy immediately after removing the microcannulas (Figs 5.4B and D). Sustained pressure for 30–60 seconds is generally adequate to allow self-opposition of the sclerotomy wounds and to stop any bleeding from the wound area. Globe pressure and the

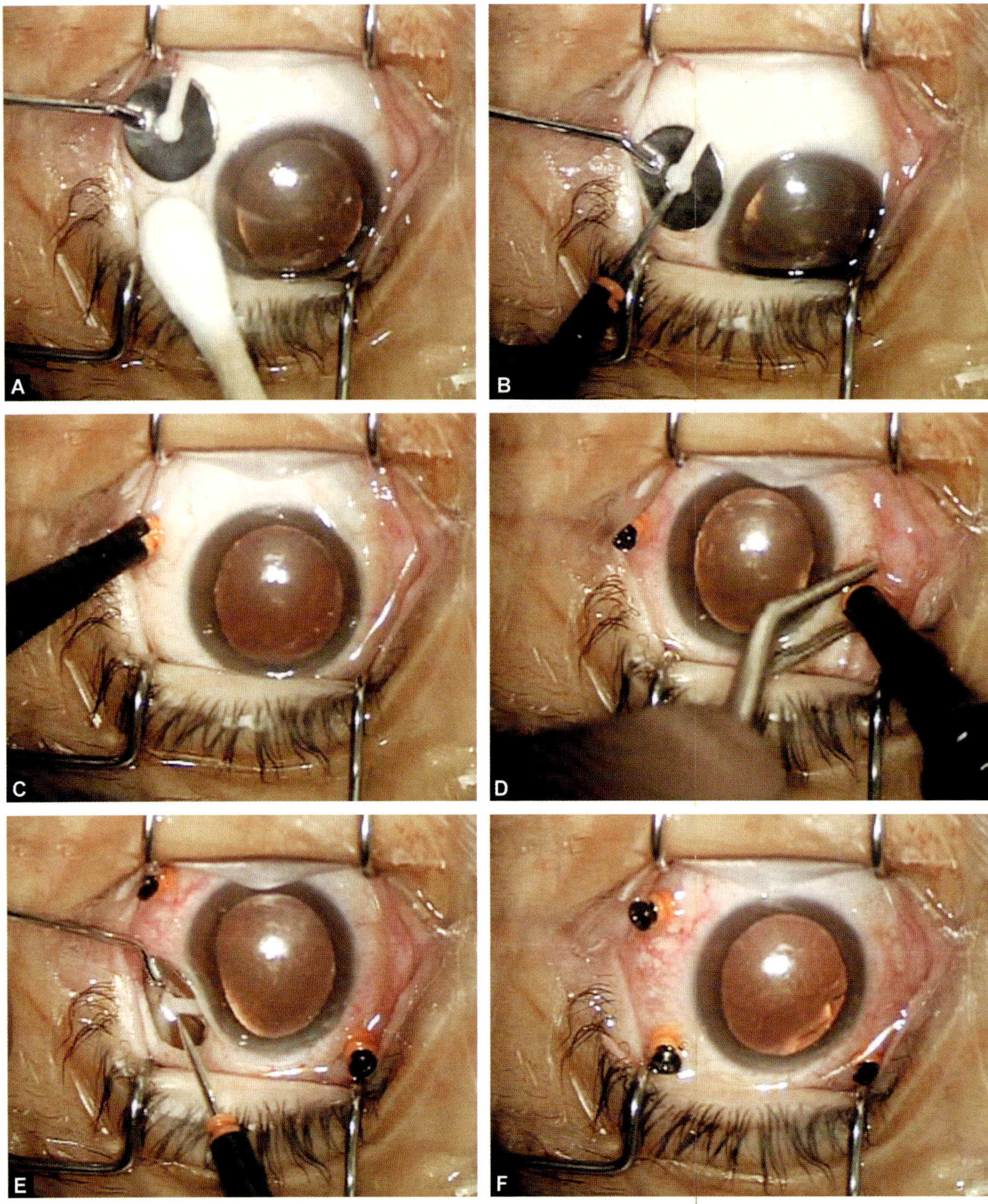

▲ **Figures 5.3A to F**

Steps for insertion of the 23-gauge vitrectomy microcannulas using the one-step technique. (A) The conjunctiva is displaced over the intended sclerotomy site and pressed firmly against the sclera using the pressure plate; (B and C) A sharp trocar needle is used for the transconjunctival scleral tunnel incision through the central opening of the pressure plate at an angle of 30°; (D) A forceps can be used to provide a counterforce and to hold the cannula in place while the needle is being withdrawn; (E) A third transconjunctival sclerotomy is being created by the sharp needle at a 30° angle; (F) All three sclerotomy microcannulas with plugs in place

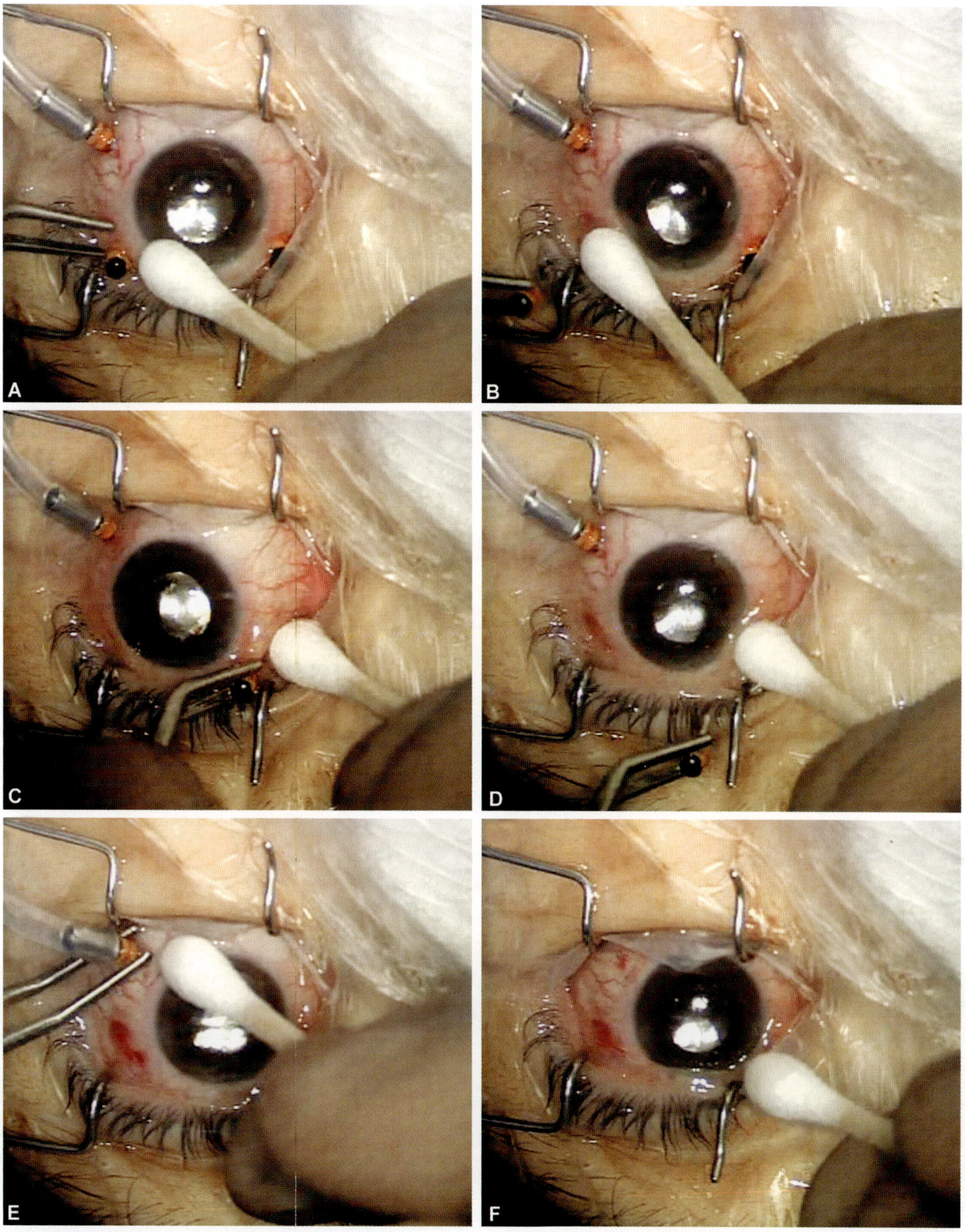

▲ **Figures 5.4A to F**

Steps for removal of the 23-gauge vitrectomy microcannulas. (A) The microcannula is grasped with a forceps and removed along the path of the scleral tunnel; (B) A cotton wool applicator is applied on the wound after removal of the microcannula to oppose the scleral wound edges and to stop any bleeding; (C and D) The procedure is repeated for removal of the superonasal microcannula; (E) After stopping the infusion of balanced salt solution or the gas infusion is clamped, the microcannula with the infusion line is removed last; (F) All three microcannulas removed external opening of the scleral tunnels should be checked carefully. In case of persistent leakage from the sclerotomy and overt hypotony, the scleral wound should be sutured and the globe reinflated with air, gas or balanced salt solution as required.

Indications of 23-Gauge Vitrectomy

There has been a continuous expansion in the clinical indications for 23-gauge vitrectomy system. With the increase in the spectrum of various 23-gauge instruments and improved surgical technique, the indications for 23-gauge system are now almost identical to the conventional 20-gauge system (Table 5.1).

The 23-gauge vitrectomy system offers a clear advantage over the conventional 20-gauge system in surgically less complicated conditions, such as for removal of vitreous hemorrhage followed by endolaser panretinal photocoagulation. Macular pathologies, including macular hole, epiretinal membrane and vitreomacular traction syndrome, are also amongst the most suitable indications for 23-gauge surgery. In general, most studies have demonstrated good success rate in using 23-gauge vitrectomy for macular hole and epiretinal membrane peeling.[4,5] 23-gauge vitrectomy has also been successfully applied in the treatment of retinal detachment and the primary anatomical success rate appeared to be comparable with conventional 20-gauge pars plana vitrectomy.[6] Moreover, 23-gauge vitrectomy is also feasible in complex retinal detachment surgery with silicone oil tamponade for retinal detachments associated with proliferative vitreoretinopathy, diabetic tractional retinal detachment and giant retinal tear.[7] Removal of silicone oil of low viscosity is also possible with 23-gauge system by expelling the oil passively through the microcannula under the hydrostatic pressure from the infusion line. In cases with high viscosity silicone oil, such passive removal would be excessively time-consuming and impractical. In this instance, one sclerotomy can be enlarged to 20-gauge in order to accommodate the use of conventional 20-gauge instruments.

TABLE 5.1: Indications of 23-gauge vitrectomy

- Macular conditions:
  - Epiretinal membrane
  - Macular hole (idiopathic or secondary)
  - Vitreomacular traction syndrome
  - Myopic foveoschisis
- Vitreous hemorrhage
- Vitreous biopsy
- Primary rhegmatogenous retinal detachment
- Proliferative diabetic retinopathy with or without tractional retinal detachment
- Removal of silicone oil (low viscosity)

Contraindications of 23-Gauge Vitrectomy

Conditions that involve ultrasonic endofragmentation of retained lens fragments are amongst the few contraindications of 23-gauge vitrectomy. At the time of writing, a 23-gauge phacofragmatome is still not yet commercially available. The design of the microcannulas also prohibits the passage of various angled tools. For conditions that require the use of such special instruments, 23-gauge vitrectomy may not be the preferable choice. Nonetheless, some 23-gauge instruments with retractable and bendable materials are now available and these instruments can facilitate intraoperative procedures by allowing improved accessibility.

Advantages of 23-Gauge Vitrectomy

One of the most obvious advantages of using 23-gauge vitrectomy is the shortening of operation time during creation and closure of sclerotomies. The wound opening and closure time was significantly shorter for the 23-gauge system when compared with the conventional 20-gauge system. In addition to shortening the operation time, patients who had 23-gauge pars plana vitrectomy also had significantly less pain postoperatively compared with the 20-gauge system.[8] The increased level of patients' comfort can be attributable to the absence of suture and conjunctival peritomy, thereby allowing a faster wound healing and less inflammatory reaction (Figs 5.5A and B). The smaller wound sizes in 23-gauge surgery also allow a shorter recovery time and minimize postoperative discomfort.

Reoperations in patients who have previously underwent multiple conventional 20-gauge vitrectomies can be

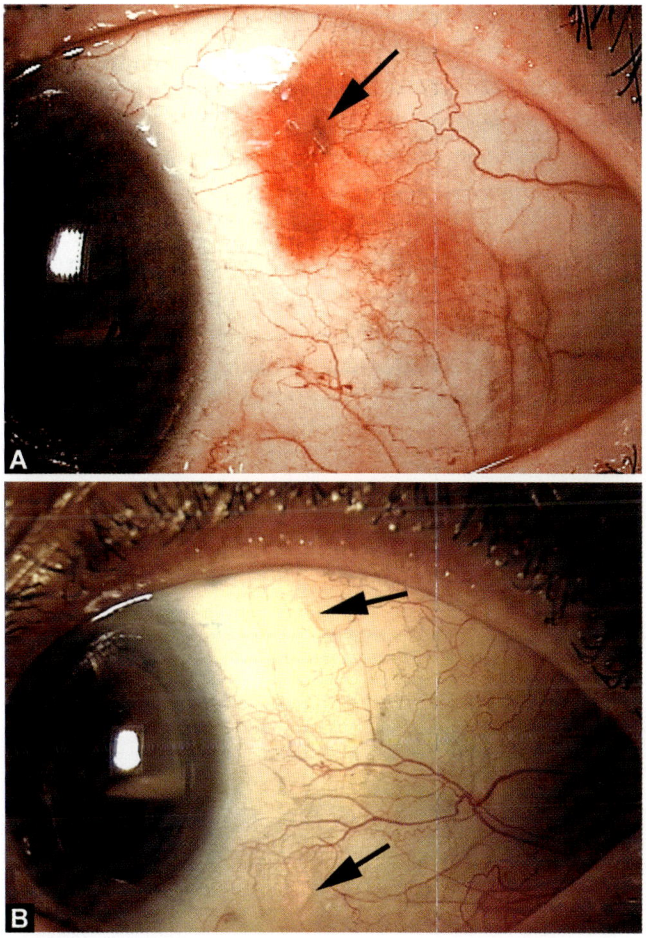

▲ **Figures 5.5A and B**

Postoperative slit-lamp photographs of a patient after 23-gauge transconjunctival vitrectomy.(A) At day 1 postoperation, there was mild subconjunctival hemorrhage associated with a well-sealed sclerotomy wound (arrow). No leakage was seen at the sclerotomy site; (B) At week 1 postoperation, the sclerotomies (arrows) were barely visible under the conjunctiva

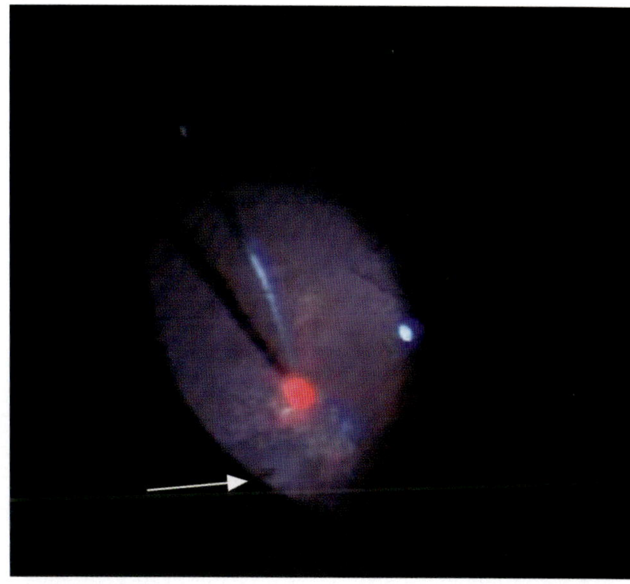

▲ **Figure 5.6**

Intraoperative photograph of 23-gauge endolaser photocoagulation for treating a peripheral retinal break (arrow)

challenging not only due to extensive conjunctival scarring, but also because of the difficulty in finding a new site for sclerotomy. The sutureless transconjunctival approach of 23-gauge surgery enables the surgeon to preserve the mobility of conjunctiva even after repeated operations. This is especially important in glaucoma patients who may later require filtering surgery. The smaller diameter of the scleral wound in 23-gauge vitrectomy also leaves more fresh sites for future sclerotomies. Compared with conventional 20-gauge vitrectomy, there is less surgically induced astigmatism following 23-gauge vitrectomy.[9] This allows for faster stabilization of postoperative refraction and faster visual rehabilitation of the patients.

The cutting port of a 23-gauge vitreous cutter is located closer to the tip when compared with a conventional 20-gauge cutter. This feature enables the surgeon to cut the vitreous closer to the retina more efficiently. The smaller caliber of the cutting probe also enables access into narrower tissue plane. Together with the newer vitrectomy machines with cut rate up to 5000 cuts per minute (cpm), dissection of tractional membranes is made much easier with a 23-gauge probe and the need for microscissors is greatly reduced.

Compared with 25-gauge system, 23-gauge instruments are much stiffer and less flexible. Maneuvering of surgical instruments and control of globe movements are much more efficient with 23-gauge instruments. This is especially important when performing endolaser and accessing the peripheral retina (Fig. 5.6). The closer resemblance to the conventional 20-gauge system also shortens the learning process for changing from 20-gauge to 23-gauge system. Reusable 23-gauge microsurgical instruments are also more durable and easier to clean than 25-gauge instruments.

In pediatric patients, postoperative inflammation after intraocular surgery is known to be more severe compared with their adult counterparts. The smaller wound size of

23-gauge vitrectomy system can help to minimize surgical trauma and decrease the postoperative reaction in this age group. The faster wound healing also allows an early rehabilitation for the developing visual system.

Disadvantages of 23-Gauge Vitrectomy

Eckardt noted in his original series of 23-gauge vitrectomy that the vitreous cutter was "somewhat slower" for extensive vitrectomy when compared with using conventional 20-gauge system.[2] This slower cutting is due to the limitation in flow rate by the smaller lumen of the 23-gauge cutter. A simple vitrectomy using a 23-gauge system may need up to 30% more time than using a 20-gauge system. The decrease in aspiration efficiency is also obvious when using a 23-gauge silicone tipped flute needle for removal of nonclotting blood in the vitreous cavity and during fluid-gas exchange. The cutting performance of some newer 23-gauge cutters has been improved by the thin-wall design that increases the lumen diameter. When vitrectomy is performed under a high-flow rate, the difference in cutting efficiency between 23-guage and 20-guage is now minimal.

In conventional 20-gauge vitrectomy, examination and assessment of the peripheral retina by scleral indentation is facilitated by opening the conjunctiva and exposing the anterior sclera. In 23-gague vitrectomy, due to the intact conjunctiva, scleral indentation might be less efficient and more difficult to perform. This limitation in scleral indentation is especially obvious over the nasal anterior retina and near the equator. Moreover, scleral indentation should be performed more cautiously due to potential easier dislodgement of the infusion line. Another difficulty with 23-gauge vitrectomy might develop during fluid-air exchange. Due to the potential space between the lumen of the cannula and the microsurgical instrument, bubbles might foam up due to air leak around the instrument and this can obscure the surgical view (Fig. 5.7). This can be prevented by avoiding the use of excessive viscous material to lubricate the ocular surface during the surgery.

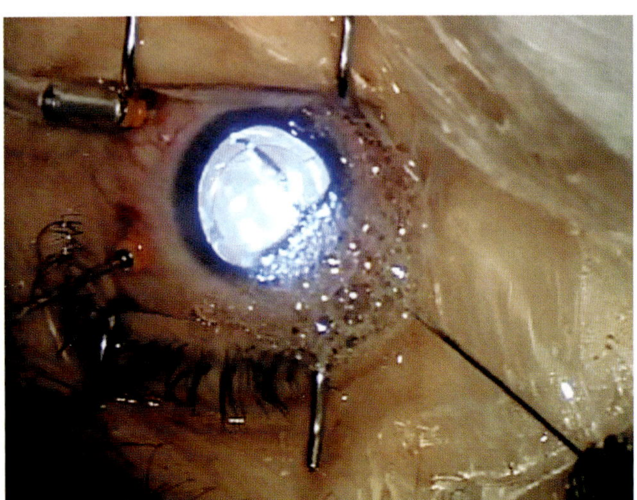

▲ Figure 5.7
Intraoperative photograph of bubble foaming due to air leak around the microsurgical instrument within the microcannula

Complications of 23-Gauge Vitrectomy

▶ Subconjunctival Hemorrhage

Subconjunctival hemorrhage is usually the consequence of damaging the conjunctival or episcleral vessels during insertion or removal of the microcannula. Apart from the cosmetic concern, inspection of the sclerotomy for leakage at the end of the operation can be made difficult by the overlying blood. In patients taking aspirin or anticoagulants, withholding the medications before the operation might help to decrease the risk of this complication.

▶ Wound Leak and Hypotony

Postoperative hypotony due to leakage from sclerotomies, though not common, may sometimes result in choroidal detachment and warrant reoperation for suturing of the scleral wound. Such sclerotomy leakage is most commonly related to poor techniques during wound construction and removal of the microcannulas. A leaking sclerotomy can be detected by observing the formation of a subconjunctival bleb over the sclerotomy site. It is imperative for the surgeon to examine for any leakage at the end of the operation and to close any leaking sclerotomy with suture. The incidences of postoperative hypotony have been estimated to be 11.3% at 2 hours and 3.8% at 1 day.[10] It has been shown that up to 11% of cases which had 23-guage pars plana vitrectomy required intraoperative suture placement for leaking sclerotomies.[10] Risk factors of leaking sclerotomies include prior vitrectomy, young patients, high myopia and vitreous base dissection.

Endophthalmitis

In a large retrospective case series, the incidence of endophthalmitis after 25-gauge vitrectomy has been shown to be 12 times higher than conventional 20-gauge vitrectomy.[11] The sutureless nature of the scleral wound poses a definite risk for this devastating complication. However, subsequent series using 25- and 23-gauge transconjunctival vitrectomy have shown that there were no obvious increased incidence of endophthalmitis compared with 20-gauge vitrectomy.[12,13] Wound leakage and postoperative hypotony should be avoided in order to minimize the chance of bacterial entry and hence the risk of endophthalmitis.

Conclusion

The safety and efficacy of 23-gauge transconjunctival sutureless vitrectomy in the management of various vitreoretinal conditions have been demonstrated in multiple studies in recent years. Unlike its 25-gauge counterpart, the 23-gauge vitrectomy system has the benefits of allowing microincisional sutureless procedures while working with instruments with greater stiffness and higher flow dynamics similar to the conventional 20-gauge system. With the increasing availability of different 23-gauge instruments, 23-gauge vitrectomy system has a good potential to replace 20-gauge system as the standard of vitreoretinal surgery.

References

1. Singh S, Josephberg RJ, Zaidman GW. Office-based diagnostic pars plana vitrectomy. Invest Ophthalmol Vis Sci. 1996;37:402.
2. Eckardt C. Transconjunctival sutureless 23-gauge vitrectomy. Retina. 2005;25:208-11.
3. Eckardt C. Transconjunctival 23-gauge vitrectomy. In: Rizzo S, Patelli F, Chow DR (Eds). Essential in Ophthalmology: Vitreoretinal Surgery. Berlin Heidelberg: Springer-Verlag; 2009. pp. 38-9.
4. Konstantinidis L, Berguiga M, Beknazar E, et al. Anatomic and functional outcome after 23-gauge vitrectomy, peeling, and intravitreal triamcinolone for idiopathic macular epiretinal membrane. Retina. 2009;29:1119-27.
5. Kusuhara S, Ooto S, Kimura D, et al. Outcomes of 23- and 25-gauge transconjunctival sutureless vitrectomies for idiopathic macular holes. Br J Ophthalmol. 2008;92:1261-4.
6. Tsang CW, Cheung BT, Lam RF, et al. Primary 23-gauge transconjunctival sutureless vitrectomy for rhegmatogenous retinal detachment. Retina. 2008;28:1075-81.
7. Oliveira LB, Reis PA. Silicone oil tamponade in 23-gauge transconjunctival sutureless vitrectomy. Retina. 2007;27:1054-8.
8. Wimpissinge B, Kellner L, Brannath, et al. 23-gauge versus 20-gauge system for pars planar vitrectomy: a prospective randomized clinical trial. Br J Ophthalmol. 2008;92:1483-7.
9. Park DH, Shin JP, Kim SY. Surgically induced astigmatism in combined phacoemulsification and vitrectomy; 23-gauge transconjunctival sutureless vitrectomy versus 20-gauge standard vitrectomy. Graefes Arch Clin Exp Ophthalmol. 2009;10:1331-7.
10. Woo SJ, Park KH, Hwang JM, et al. Risk factors associated with sclerotomy leakage and postoperative hypotony after 23-gauge transconjunctival sutureless vitrectomy. Retina. 2009;29:456-63.
11. Kunimoto DY, Kaiser RS. Wills Eye Retina Service. Incidence of endophthalmitis after 20- and 25-gauge vitrectomy. Ophthalmology. 2007;114:2133-7.
12. Hu AY, Bourges JL, Shah SP, et al. Endophthalmitis after pars plana vitrectomy a 20- and 25-gauge comparison. Ophthalmology. 2009;116:1360-5.
13. Parolini B, Romanelli F, Prigione G, et al. Incidence of endophthalmitis in a large series of 23-gauge and 20-gauge transconjunctival pars plana vitrectomy. Graefes Arch Clin Exp Ophthalmol. 2009;247:895-8.

6

The Use of Silicone Oil in Vitreoretinal Surgery

Lawrence P Chong

Introduction

Silicone oil is used as an intraocular tamponade in the pars plana vitrectomy repair of retinal detachment. Rarely, it is also instilled into eyes with chronic hypotony to maintain a minimal pressure for visual function. Silicone oil tamponade has a number of advantages over gas tamponade. Unlike gas tamponades, silicone oil is not absorbed so the injected volume never decreases. This allows prolonged tamponade and improved tamponade of inferior retinal breaks without positioning. Patients can see through the silicone oil (although there is a hyperopic refractive shift). Silicone oil does not expand so air travel or return to higher elevations is permitted.

Disadvantages of silicone oil include the need to surgically remove the oil as an additional procedure. Oil migrating into the anterior chamber can damage the corneal endothelium[1] or cause glaucoma. Oil escaping the eye through sclerotomies can accumulate in the periorbit. Like all long acting tamponades, oil can induce cataract formation. Infectious endophthalmitis in a silicone oil filled eye presents with a clear media unlike typical endophthalmitis. The key symptom is pain and the key finding is white necrotic retina.[2]

Silicone oils (polymerized siloxane with organic side chains) are silicon analogues of carbon-based organic compounds, and can form long and complex molecules based on silicon rather than carbon. Chains are formed of alternating silicon-oxygen atoms (…Si-O-Si-O-Si..) or siloxane, rather than carbon atoms (…C-C-C-C…). Other species attach to the tetravalent silicon atoms, not to the divalent oxygen atoms which are fully committed to forming the siloxane chain. Two methyl groups are attached to each silicon atom in polydimethylsiloxane which is used clinically (Fig. 6.1). The polydimethylsiloxane are crystal clear optically and have an index of refraction that ranges from 1.375 to 1.4035. The molecular weight per unit of polydimethylsiloxane is 74. There are approximately 200 molecules in an average chain giving a molecular weight of approximately 15,000. As the viscosity of the silicone oil increases, the average chain length increases, the specific gravity increases and therefore the total molecular weight increases. A viscosity between 0.65 and 60,000 centistokes (corresponding to specific gravities between 0.761 and 0.973) can be obtained from readily available stock fluids or from their combination. One can breakdown the molecular weight of silicone oil combinations by gel penetration chromatography. These gel chromatograms

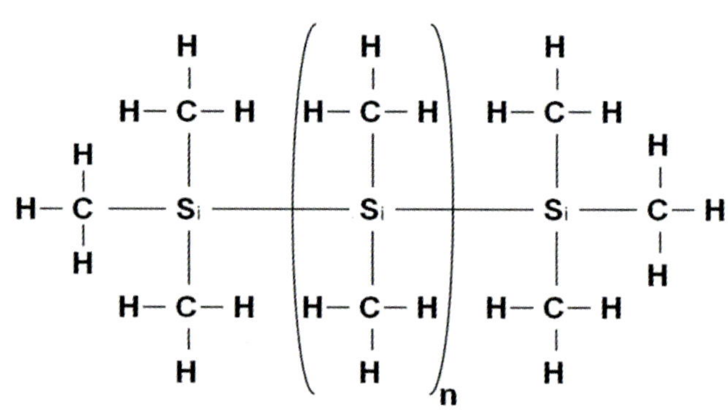

▲ **Figure 6.1**

Chemical structure of polydimethylsiloxane

give the distribution of the various molecular weights. High molecular weight and single peak concentrations are the most ideal. Various catalysts are used in the preparation of silicone oil and these are considered industry trade secrets. Contamination by catalysts was a problem in the early years.

Liquid silicone is nonwettable and moisture repellent. It is impermeable to solutes but permits the diffusion of gases and water vapor. The physical characteristics of liquid silicone with viscosities greater than 50 centistoke are heat stable so heat sterilization is possible.[3]

Liquid silicone was first injected into the vitreous cavity of rabbits by Stone who reported that silicone fluids of various viscosities were well tolerated.[4] Silicone oil was first used for intraocular tamponade by Paul Cibis for direct injection into nonvitrectomized eyes.[5] It was used extensively in the United States until about 1970 when published reports of toxicity diminished its popularity.[6] However, its use continued in Europe with the work of Scott [7-10] and Leaver.[11]

A randomized controlled clinical trial comparing silicone oil to gas for the vitrectomy repair of complex retinal detachments showed the equivalency of SF_6 gas versus oil for anatomic and visual outcomes, but oil-filled eyes had less hypotony.[12] As a result of this study and subsequent Food and Drug Administration approval silicone use regained popularity in the United States.

Presently, silicone oil can be obtained in two different viscosities: 1000 and 5000 centistoke. Higher viscosity oil was introduced because it was believed to cause less emulsification. Oil emulsification promotes migration of oil into the anterior chamber, which causes injury to the corneal endothelium or glaucoma. However, emulsifying agents in the vitreous cavity such as lipoproteins may be more important factors in causing emulsification returning 1000 centistoke oil to popularity. Heavier than water oils are discussed in another chapter in this book.

Silicone oil can be instilled into an air filled eye after the retina is attached by simultaneous air-fluid exchange. This is most easily achieved with a silicone oil pump. Although 1000 centistoke oil can be manually pushed through a large bore needle (18-gauge) with a syringe, this requires significant effort and time. The added step of air-fluid exchange can be avoided by proceeding to direct silicone oil-fluid exchange but this requires a silicone oil pump. As fluid is removed from the subretinal space through a retinal opening with a cannula, oil is simultaneously instilled with a pump. Silicone oil-perfluorocarbon liquid exchange can also be performed, but there is a risk of admixture of the two liquids which makes complete removal of the mixture difficult or impossible.[13] This phenomenon may be unique to perfluoro-n-octane and is not seen with perfluorodecalin.

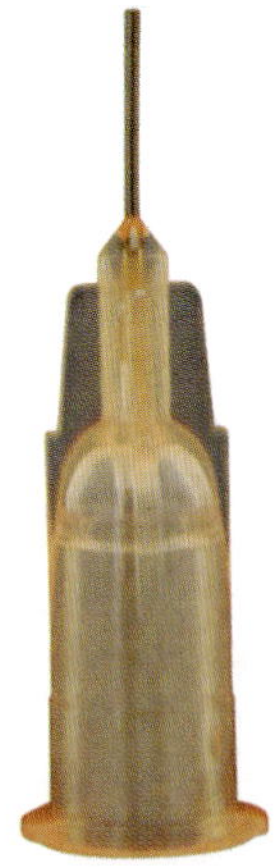

▶ **Figure 6.2**

Oil can be instilled through a thin wall needle which fits through a 23-gauge transconjunctival cannula

Oil can be instilled by pump through a 23-gauge transconjunctival cannula using a thin walled needle (MedOne Surgical, Inc. Sarasota FL, USA) (Fig. 6.2). One thousand centistokes oil can be passively removed through two open 23- or 25-gauge cannulas.[14] Five thousand centistokes oil can also be removed by pump using modified tubing which fits over the 23-gauge transconjunctival cannula (Fig. 6.3).[15] Both of these techniques are slower than making a separate sclerotomy opening large enough to accommodate an 18-gauge cannula for oil removal. It is prohibitively slow to infuse oil through 25-gauge transconjunctival cannula.

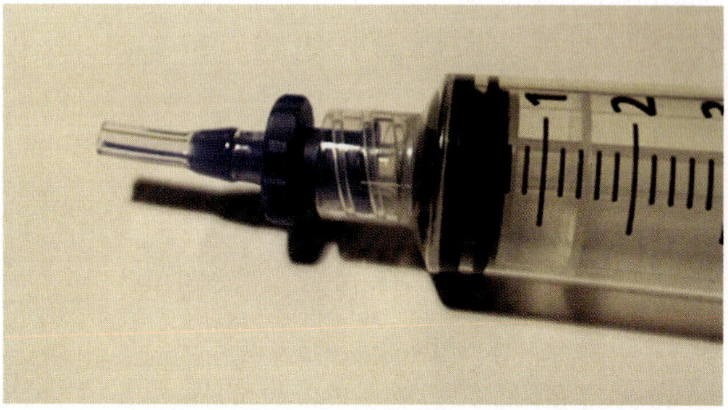

▲ **Figure 6.3**

Modified tubing from either the 25-gauge Alcon infusion line or the aspiration line can be used to connect the 25-gauge cannula to the viscous fluid injection/extraction syringe. The tubing is the correct diameter to snugly fit over the entire cannula

When oil is used after vitrectomy with sutureless transconjunctival vitrectomy systems, the sclerotomy sites must be sutured closed after the cannulas are removed. Otherwise, oil will eventually leak from these sites causing periorbital complications.

Ando demonstrated that an inferior peripheral iridectomy prevents pupillary block by the silicone oil in aphakic eyes and the consequent migration of oil into the anterior chamber.[16] Therefore, an inferior peripheral iridectomy is mandatory in all aphakic eyes. The inferior peripheral iridectomy is made with the vitreous cutter before the air-fluid exchange or oil-fluid exchange. There is no need for an inferior peripheral iridectomy in phakic eyes or pseudophakic eyes with intact capsules. However, care must be taken not to overpressurize the eye with oil which can then break through the zonules into the anterior chamber. Once this occurs, it is usually impossible to keep oil from eventually migrating through the broken zonules into the anterior chamber. Oil can be removed from the anterior chamber by making two paracentesis sites 180° apart at the limbus. A viscoelastic is instilled through one site displacing the oil bubble which exits through the second paracentesis site. However, this absence of oil from the anterior chamber is usually temporary. When the eye is pseudophakic and has a posterior capsule opening, the surgeon will have to judge if the capsular opening is small enough to prevent oil from migrating through or whether the opening is too large and an inferior peripheral iridectomy is needed.

Author's technique for the instillation of oil after 20-gauge vitrectomy in an air-filled eye is as follows. First suture one of the superior sclerotomies closed. Then enlarge the second superior sclerotomy to accommodate the oil infusion cannula. Author either vents the inferotemporal cannula to atmosphere or reduce the air infusion to zero. In this way as oil fills the eye, the air escapes through the inferotemporal cannula. Midway through the fill, author inserts a 30-gauge needle through the pars plana, until it is visible behind the lens. Author uses this needle to vent air from inside the eye. The 30-gauge needle is attached to a 3 ml syringe without the plunger. Author uses this as a handle. As the silicone oil fills the eye and approaches the lens, the meniscus of the oil bubble first touches the lens and then sweeps across the posterior surface of the lens. The air bubble gets smaller and escapes through the 30-gauge needle. This observation is most important, because if it is not seen, then the oil fill is incomplete. The fill is complete once the air bubble disappears from view. After adjusting the eye pressure to around 20 mm, author then removes the oil infusion cannula and suture the sclerotomy closed.

Author uses the same technique for the instillation of oil after 25- or 23-gauge vitrectomy with the following modification. After removing both superior cannulas, author sutures one of the superior sclerotomies closed. Author enlarges the second superior sclerotomy to accommodate the oil infusion cannula. Author then disconnects the infusion line from the third cannula. Author injects oil into the eye until he sees oil visible in the outer lumen of the remaining cannula. This indicates that oil is at the level of the pars plana. He then inserts the 30-gauge needle to remove the remaining air.

In an aphakic eye author uses the same technique as described above, but fills with oil into the anterior chamber. Author equilibrates the eye with the outside atmospheric pressure before closing the sclerotomy. This leaves the eye with a low pressure, but in all cases by the next morning the oil has migrated posteriorly.

When oil is used in place of gas for uncomplicated retinal detachments, the oil is removed after retinopexy is deemed complete. Usually this is 2–4 weeks. When oil is used for complex retinal detachments, the oil is removed when the cellular process of proliferative vitreoretinopathy (PVR) is deemed complete. Usually this is at 6 months. In penetrating ocular injury complicated by retinal detachment and PVR, the PVR process can be quite prolonged and oil is removed after a year.

The use of silicone oil is particularly advantageous in penetrating ocular injury with posterior segment involvement.[17] It allows prolonged tamponade that keeps retina attached longer which downregulates PVR. It allows visibility to the posterior segment in the postoperative period which allows the surgeon to monitor PVR and plan for timely vitrectomy revision based on recurrence of PVR membrane and detachment. It reduces bleeding from the penetration site.

Another strong indication for the use of silicone oil is the repair of retinal detachment caused by viral retinitis.[18-20] In these cases, the vitreous is usually not detached and is impossible to detach from the underlying necrotic retina. Silicone oil is usually left indefinitely in these cases. Ganciclovir implants last much longer in silicone oil-filled eye.[21]

Oil should be used with caution after vitrectomy for diabetic retinal detachment. The entrapment of blood, protein and growth factors in the preretinal space promotes fibrous reproliferation.[22,23] The same occurs after relaxing retinotomy. Meticulous hemostasis should be performed before oil instillation.

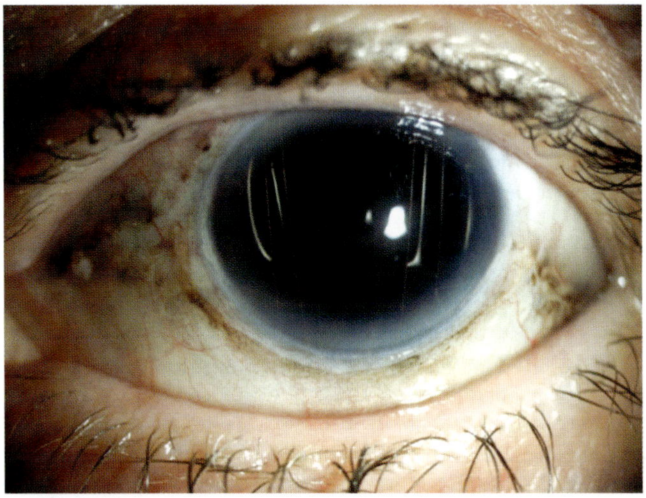

▲ **Figure 6.4**

Iris retention sutures preventing oil from migrating into the anterior chamber of aphakic eye with inadequate iris (Dr Ronald C Gentile)

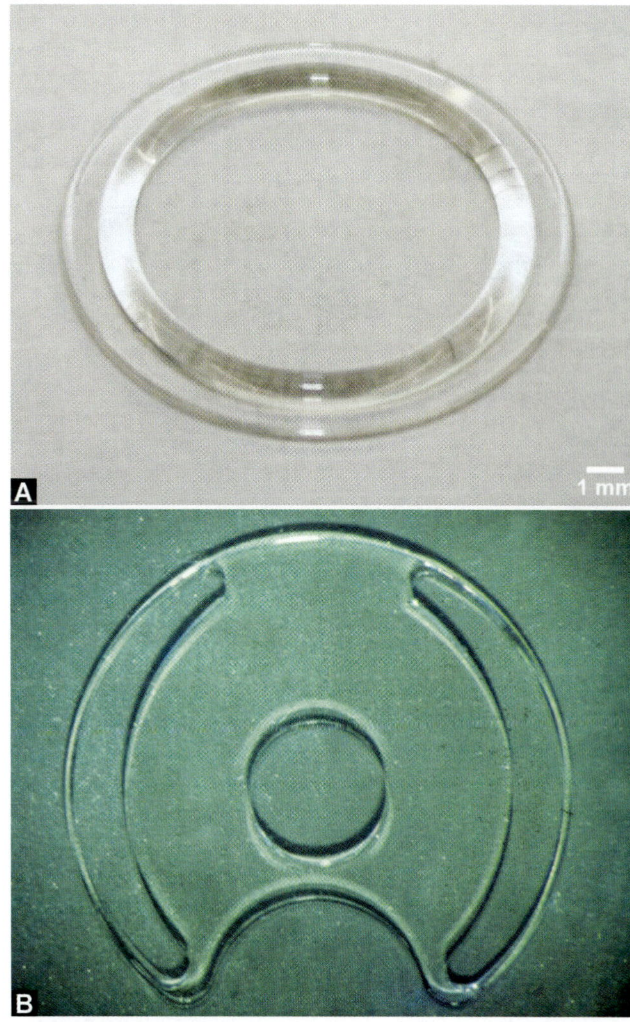

▲ **Figures 6.5A and B**

(A) Current model of silicone diaphragm; (B) Original polymethyl-methacrylate diaphragm [Source: (A) Acri Tec, Hennigsdorf, Germany; (B) Prof Gabriele Thumann]

It is almost impossible to keep oil out of the anterior chamber in aphakic eyes without sufficient iris or pressure. In these cases, iris retention sutures[24] (Fig. 6.4) or an iris diaphragm[25,26] (Figs 6.5A and B) can be employed.

Silicone oil may be used to treat chronic hypotony.[27,28] However, even after infusing enough oil eye to close the central retinal artery 50% of the time, the intraocular pressure the next day usually is in the single digits. Because of the difficulties of keeping oil out of the anterior chamber in aphakic eyes, a reasonable alternative is the periodic injection of cohesive viscoelastics in these eyes.[29]

Oil has also been used as a tamponade in macular hole repair,[30-33] retinal detachments associated with myopic macular degeneration and staphyloma[34] and retinal detachments associated with myopic macular holes.[35]

The use of silicone oil in pseudophakic eyes with silicone lenses is problematic when there is an opening in the posterior capsule. The oil droplets which adhere to the surface of the intraocular lens (IOL) may be impossible to remove requiring a lens exchange.[36-38] Therefore, a nonsilicone IOL is recommended if there is likelihood that oil may be instilled into the eye or if oil is present in the eye.[39] In the future it may be possible to remove these oil droplets using a fluorinated alkane.[40,41]

Silicone oil tamponade should be removed if possible from the eye. The silicone oil study demonstrated an improvement of vision, but a risk of recurrent retinal detachment after removing silicone oil.[42] This risk may be mitigated by 360° laser treatment to the retinal periphery.[43] Even after oil removal, small oil bubbles may continue to emerge from iris crypts and other locations.[44]

References

1. Foulks GN, Hatchell DL, Proia AD, et al. Histopathology of silicone oil keratopathy in humans. Cornea. 1991;10:29-37.
2. Chong LP, de Juan E , McCuen BW, et al. Endophthalmitis in a silicone oil-filled eye. Am J Ophthalmol. 1986;102:660-1.

3. Armaly MF. Ocular tolerance to silicones. Arch Ophthalmol. 1962;68:390-5.
4. Stone W. Alloplasty in surgery of the eye. N Engl J Med. 1958;258:486-90.
5. Cibis PA, Becker B, Okun E, et al. The use of liquid silicone oil in retinal detachment surgery. Arch Ophthalmol. 1962;68:590-9.
6. Mukai N, Lee PF, Schepens CL. Intravitreous injection of silicone: an experimental study. Ann Ophthalmol. 1972;4:273-87.
7. Scott JD. Treatment of the detached immobile retina. Trans Ophthalmol Soc UK. 1972;92:351-7.
8. Scott JD. The treatment of massive vitreous retraction. Trans Ophthalmol Soc UK. 1973;93:417-23.
9. Scott JD. Macular holes and retinal detachment. Trans Ophthalmol Soc UK. 1974;94:319-24.
10. Scott JD. A rationale for the use of liquid silicone. Trans Ophthalmol Soc UK. 1977;99:235-41.
11. Grey RHB, Leaver PK. Result of silicone oil injection in massive preretinal retraction. Trans Ophthalmol Soc UK. 1977;97:238-41.
12. Vitrectomy with silicone oil or sulfur hexafluoride gas in eyes with severe proliferative vitreoretinopathy: results of a randomized clinical trial. Silicone Study Report 1. Arch Ophthalmol. 1997;110:770-9.
13. Veckeneer MA, de Voogd S, Lindstedt EW, et al. An epidemic of sticky silicone oil at the Rotterdam Eye Hospital. Patient review and chemical analyses. Graefes Archive Clin Exp Ophthalmol. 2008;246:917-22.
14. Patwardhan SD, Azad R, Shad V, et al. The safety and efficacy of passive removal of silicone oil with a 23 gauge transconjunctival sutureless system. Retina. 2010;30:1237-41.
15. Song AM, Shen D, Ke Z, et al. A new approach for active removal of 5,000 centistokes silicone oil through 23-gauge cannula. Retina. 2010;30:1302-7.
16. Beekhuis WH, Ando F, Zivojnovic R, et al. Basal iridectomy at 6 o'clock in the aphakic eye treated with silicone oil: prevention of keratopathy and secondary glaucoma. Br J Ophthalmol. 1983;71:197-200.
17. Lemmen KD, Heimann K. Early vitrectomy with primary silicone oil injection in very severely injured eyes. Klinische Monatsblatter fur Augenheilkunde. 1988;193:594-601.
18. Freeman WR, Quiceno JL, Crapotta JA, et al. Surgical repair of rhegmatogenous retinal detachment in immunosuppressed patients with cytomegalovirus retinitis. Ophthalmology. 1992;99:466-74.
19. Kuppermann BD, Flores-Aguilar M, Quiceno JI, et al. A masked prospective evaluation of outcome parameters for cytomegalovirus-related retinal detachment surgery in patients with acquired immune deficiency syndrome. Ophthalmology. 1994;101:46-55.
20. Jabs DA, Enger C, Haller J, et al. Retinal detachments in patients with cytomegalovirus retinitis. Arch Ophthalmol. 1991;1098:794-9.
21. Perkins SL, Yang CH, Ashton PA, et al. Pharmacokinetics of the ganciclovir implant in the silicone-filled eye. Retina. 2001;21:10-4.
22. Heimann K, Dahl B, Dimopoulos S, et al. Pars plana vitrectomy and silicone oil injection in proliferative diabetic retinopathy. Graefes Arch Clin Exp Ophthalmol. 1989;227:152-6.
23. Asaria RH, Kon CH, Bunce C, et al. Silicone oil concentrates fibrogenic growth factors in the retro-oil fluid. Br J Ophthalmol. 2004;88:1439-42.
24. Gentile RC, Eliott D. Silicone oil rentention sutures in aphakic eyes with iris loss. Arch Ophthalmol. 2010;128:1596-9.
25. Keller GK, Dahlke C, Kuckelhorn R, et al. Experience with the artificial iris diaphragm in hypotonic eyes. (German) Ophthalmologe. 2003;100:203-8.
26. Thumann G, Kirchof B, Bartz-Schimdt KU, et al. The artificial iris diaphragm for vitreoretinal silicone oil surgery. Retina. 1997;17:330-7.
27. Morse LS, McCuen BW. The use of silicone oil in uveitis and hypotony. Retina. 1991;11:399-404.
28. Kapur R, Birnbaum AD, Goldstein DA, et al. Treating uveitis-associated hypotony with pars plana vitrectomy and silicone oil injection. Retina. 2010;30:140-5.
29. Tosi GM, Schiff W, Barile G, et al. Management of severe hypotony with intravitreal injection of viscoelastic. Amer J Ophthalmol. 2005;140:952-4.
30. Goldbaum MH, McCuen BW, Hanneken AM, et al. Silicone oil tamponade to seal macular holes without position restrictions. Ophthalmology. 1998;105:2140-7.
31. Pertile G, Claes C. Silicone oil vs gas for the treatment of full-thickness macular hole. Bulletin de la Societe Belge d Ophtalmologie. 1999;274:31-6.
32. Karia N, Laidlaw A, West J, et al. Macular hole surgery using silicone oil tamponade. Br J Ophthalmol. 2001;85:1320-3.
33. Lai JC, Stinnett SS, McCuen BW. Comparison of silicone oil versus gas tamponade in the treatment of idiopathic full-thickness macular hole. Ophthalmology. 2003;110:1170-4.
34. Scholda C, Egger SF. Silicone oil tamponade in eyes with posterior staphyloma and retinal detachment caused by macular hole. Acta Ophthalmologica Scandinavica. 1998;76:704-6.
35. Wolfensberger TJ, Gonvers M. Long-term follow-up of retinal detachment due to macular hole in myopic eyes treated by temporary silicone oil tamponade and laser photocoagulation. Ophthalmology. 1999;106:1786-91.
36. Senn P, Schmid MK, Schipper I, et al. Interaction between silicone oil and silicone intraocular lenses: an in vitro study. Ophthalmic Surg Lasers. 1997;28:776-9.
37. Dick B, Stoffeins B, Pavlovic S, et al. Interaction of silicone oil with various intraocular lenses. A light and scanning electron microscop study. Klin Monbl Augenheilkd. 1997;211:192-206.
38. Apple DJ, Issacs RT, Kent DG, et al. Silicone oil adhesion to intraocular lenses: an experimental study comparing various biomaterial. J Cataract Refract Surg. 1997;23:536-44.

39. Oner FH, Saatchi OA, Sarioglu S, et al. Interaction of intraocular lenses with various concentration of silicone oil: an experimental study. Ophthalmologica. 2003;217:124-8.
40. Liang Y, Kociok N, Leszczuk M, et al. A cleaning solution for silicone intraocular lenses: "sticky silicone oil." Br J Ophthalmol. 2008;92:1522-7.
41. Stappler T, Williams R, Wong D. F4H5: a novel substance for the removal of silicone oil from intraocular lenses. Br J Ophthalmol. 2010;94:364-7.
42. Hutton WL, Azen SP, Blumenkranz MS, et al. The effect of silicone oil removal: silicone study report 5. Arch Ophthalmol. 1994;112:778-85.
43. Falkner-Radler CL, Graf A, Binder S. Outcome after silicone oil removal and simultaneous 360 endolaser treatment. Acta Ophthalmol. 2010;89:e46-51.
44. Bifrare YD, Wolfensberger TJ. Re-emergence of hidden residual intraocular silicone oil bubble after previous silicone oil removal. Klin Montbl Augenheilkd. 2006;223:450-2.

7 Long-term Intraocular Tamponade with Silicone Oil

Wico W Lai, Widad Yusof, Amy Lo, Ian Y Wong, David Wong

Introduction

Silicone oil was first introduced by Cibis[1,2] to treat retinal detachment in humans in the 1960s prior to the introduction of pars plana vitrectomy.[3] Almost from the beginning, there have been serious concerns regarding possible silicone toxicity. Apart from complications such as cataract formation, glaucoma and poor visual outcome,[4] there were observed histological changes.[5-7] These concerns led many surgeons to discontinue using silicone oil altogether. This was particularly the case in the USA and even in Europe where only a few surgeons would continue to use silicone oil as an intraoperative tool. Scott[8] and others persisted to use silicone oil, initially without and subsequently combined with vitrectomy. They were spurred on by the ability to achieve a significantly higher success rate in complex retinal detachments especially those with proliferative vitreoretinopathy (which was referred to as massive preretinal proliferation). With the advent of pars plana vitrectomy[3] in the 1970s and the continued surgical refinement by Scott,[8] Zivojnovic,[9,10] Gabel,[11] Kampik,[11] Leaver,[12] McLeod,[12] Gonvers,[13] Heimann,[14] Lucke,[15] Foerster,[15] Laqua[15] and others, silicone oil eventually became an internal tamponade agent of choice for complex retinal detachment in many European countries by the 1980s. The further refinement of microvitreoretinal surgical instrumentations and techniques[16,17] greatly increased the success rate of retinal reattachment.

Although the use of silicone oil gained popularity in Europe, long-acting gases was used as primary intraocular tamponades in the United States.[18,19] This divergence in the choice of tamponade agent inevitably led to a series of randomized control studies, the Silicone Study,[20-27] comparing the efficacy and safety of silicone oil versus that of long-acting gases for the treatment of rhegmatogenous retinal detachment (RRD) with proliferative vitreoretinopathy (PVR). A classification system for PVR was also developed[28] which was subsequently updated[29] and in a modern guise is still currently in clinical use, especially for clinical trials and audits of surgical outcome.

The Silicone Study[20-27]

- *Background:* The treatment of retinal detachment complicated by PVR was controversial. Pars plana vitrectomy with temporary tamponade provided by intraocular gas were successful in reattaching the retina in some patients while not in others (redetached).

  Prolonged tamponade with liquid silicone were thought to result in improved anatomical success, but has the disadvantage of silicone-related complications, particularly glaucoma and keratopathy.
- *Aim:* To compare effectiveness of intraocular silicone oil with that of an intraocular long-acting gas [initially sulfur hexafluoride (SF_6), later perfluoropropane (C_3F_8)] for the management of retinal detachment complicated by proliferative vitreoretinopathy (PVR), using vitrectomy and associated techniques.

  To evaluate the ocular complications that result from the use of silicone oil and gas.
- *Methods:* Randomized, multicenter surgical trial. Eligibility criteria included but were not limited to PVR

TABLE 7.1: Silicone study classification system for proliferative vitreoretinopathy[29]

Grade	Clinical signs
A	Vitreous haze, vitreous pigment clumps
B	Inner retinal wrinkling, rolled edge of retinal breaks
CP P1: 1 Quadrants (1–3 clock hours) P2: 2 Quadrants (4–6 clock hours) P3: 3 Quadrants (7–9 clock hours) P4: 4 Quadrants (10–12 clock hours)	Starfolds and/or diffuse contraction (See below on contraction type) in posterior retina and/or subretinal membrane in posterior retina
CA A1: 1 Quadrants (1–3 clock hours) A2: 2 Quadrants (4–6 clock hours) A3: 3 Quadrants (7–9 clock hours) A4: 4 Quadrants (10–12 clock hours)	Circumferential and/or perpendicular and/or anterior traction in anterior retina

of Grade C 3 or greater according to the Retina Society Classification (Tables 7.1 and 7.2) and visual acuity of light perception or better.

All study patients underwent vitrectomy and were randomized intraoperatively (after air/fluid exchange) either to silicone oil or to gas.

Two groups of eyes were entered into the study: eyes that had not had a prior vitrectomy (group 1) and those that had undergone previous vitrectomy outside the study (group 2).

- *Main outcome measures:* Visual acuity of 5/200 or greater. Macular reattachment for 6 months following the final surgical procedure.
- *Cohort:* Recruitment began on September 1, 1985 and was completed on June 30, 1991. One hundred and fifty one eyes were randomized to receive either SF_6 gas or silicone oil (113 in group 1 and 38 in group 2). Four hundred and four eyes were randomized to receive either C_3F_8 gas or silicone oil (232 and 172 in groups 1 and 2, respectively). There are 11 reports of findings for this study.

TABLE 7.2: Silicone study classification of contraction type in proliferative vitreoretinopathy[22,29]

Type number	Contraction type	Location of PVR	Clinical signs
1	Focal	Posterior	Starfold
2	Diffuse	Posterior	Confluent irregular retinal folds in posterior retina; remainder of retina drawn posterior; optic disc may not be visible
3	Subretinal	Posterior	"Napkin ring" around disc, or "clothesline" elevation of retina
4	Circumferential	Anterior	Irregular retinal folds in the anterior; series of radial folds more posteriorly; peripheral retina within vitreous base stretched inward
5	Perpendicular	Anterior	Smooth circumferential fold of retina at insertion of posterior hyaloid
6	Anterior	Anterior	Circumferential fold of retina at insertion of posterior hyaloid pulled forward; trough of peripheral retina anteriorly; ciliary process stretched with possible hypotony; iris retracted

- *Findings:*

  Anatomic and vision outcome comparing group 1 versus group 2: Anatomic and vision results and prevalence of complications suggest that the differences in outcomes between groups 1 and 2 were not as great as previously believed.

  IOP abnormalities: Chronic hypotony was more prevalent in C_3F_8 gas eyes than in silicone oil eyes, more prevalent in eyes with anatomical failure and correlated with poor postoperative vision, corneal opacity and retinal detachment.

  The presence of diffuse contraction of the retina anterior to the equator should alert the vitrectomy surgeon that the eye is likely to be hypotonous postoperatively.

  Retinotomy: Eyes undergoing vitreous surgery for the first time for the treatment of PVR can be treated successfully in most instances by conventional techniques without the need for relaxing retinotomy.

  Retinotomy may be required more frequently in patients undergoing repeat vitreous surgery for PVR. Silicone oil and C_3F_8 gas appeared to be equally effective tamponade modalities.

  In eyes undergoing retinotomy that have not been previously vitrectomized, silicone oil may initially increase the likelihood of visual success and may decrease the likelihood of hypotony at 6 months; however, long-term observations at 24 months suggested a trend toward worsening in silicone oil-filled eyes and improvement in gas-filled eyes.

  Outcomes after silicone oil removal: Eyes with attached retinas at the time of oil removal generally showed improvement in visual acuity at the last follow-up examination. There was an increased risk of recurrent retinal detachment at the last follow-up examination in the oil-removed eyes.

  Corneal abnormalities: The postoperative incidence rates of corneal abnormalities are equivalent between oil and gas.

  Postoperative macular pucker: The occurrence of macular pucker following successful surgery for retinal detachments complicated by severe PVR was not influenced by the choice of intraocular tamponade.

  Prognosis using the silicone study classification system: Identification of the anteroposterior extent of the PVR was prognostic of visual acuity and hypotony at 24 months.

  Comparison of outcome in anterior versus posterior PVR: Eyes with anterior PVR and clinically significant posterior PVR changes had a better visual prognosis if silicone oil rather than C_3F_8 gas was used.

  Long-term outcome: National Eye Institute funded an extension of the Silicone Study.

  During 6 years of follow-up, attachment of the macula was maintained for all eyes.

  No significant differences in the rates of complete retinal attachment, visual acuity greater than 5/200 or glaucoma were found between treatment groups. Gas-treated eyes had more hypotony.

  Success in the first operation for PVR is paramount in obtaining better visual results.

  If anatomically and visually successful at 3 years, there is an excellent chance that the results will be maintained over the long term.

Chemical Properties of Silicone Oil

Silicone is a siloxane of repeated units. It is chemically relatively inert. Silicone oil is a polymer with a backbone of $[R2\text{-}Si\text{-}O]_n$ where R2 are 2 methyl groups, having a common siloxane (-Si-O-) repeating unit as their backbone. Thus, one should use the name polydimethylsiloxane (PDMS). The more general term silicone can be used to describe all organosiloxane materials, including silicone fluids ("silicone oil") and silicone elastomers ("silicone rubber"). Although in ophthalmology authors often use the terms silicone oil, PDMS certainly has some of the properties of being hydrophobic, liquid and clear. However, it is not technically "oil" as well as hydrocarbon.

Depending on the length and molecular weight of the polymer, the viscosity differs and can be adjusted. In addition, different side groups on the Si atom of -Si-O- repeating units and different end terminals of the polymer chain can be synthesized, yielding silicone oils with various chemical and physical properties. For example, two methyl ($-CH_3-$) side groups can be attached to the Si atom, giving the dimethylsiloxane repeating units, which is the most common silicone oil with a lighter-than-water property. Or, different side groups can be attached to the same Si atom. For example, methyl and trifluoropropyl side groups are used to yield the trifluoropropylmethylsiloxane polymer, giving rise to fluorosilicone oils with the heavier-than-water property. Moreover, different monopolymers can be mixed in various ratios, yielding copolymers.

Polydimethylsiloxane has a specific gravity of about 0.97. It is immiscible with water and forms an interface with it. Note that the specific gravity remains the same irrespective of the shear viscosity. It makes sense, as the shear viscosity is simply dependent on the molecular weight. This in turn depends on the number of repeated units (siloxane monomers). Therefore in terms of density or specific gravity, large and small molecules should be the same. Similarly, the interfacial tension of silicone oil against water is the same irrespective of the viscosity. Again, this stands to reason at the oil-water interface, what is presented is the same molecular structure irrespective of how large or small is the siloxane polymer.

During the synthesis of silicone oils, a number of undesirable impurities may be present. These include unpolymerized residual monomers, low molecular weight oligomeric chains, cyclical forms and siloxane with hydroxy instead of methyl end groups. There could also be polymerization byproducts or catalytic impurities that may be toxic. The first silicone oils used were not intended for medical use. In addition to impurities, the oils were really a mixture of molecules of different molecular weights. The lower molecular weights have lower viscosity and the higher molecular weight molecules have higher viscosity. They were in fact blends, such that when mixed, the final product had a viscosity close to the specified viscosity (which in general tended to either 1,000 or 5,000). In general, it is thought that the presence of low molecular weight component that is important in emulsification silicone oil with MilliPascals (mPas) of 5,000 or more were found less likely to emulsify.[30]

Physical Properties of Silicone Oil

The effectiveness of an endotamponade depends on its ability to displace aqueous from the surface of the retina.[31] This ability is influenced by its specific gravity, buoyancy and interfacial surface tension, but principally by buoyancy.

▶ Specific Gravity

The specific gravity (SG) of a vitreous substitute will determine if it will sink or float in aqueous and will also determine the shape of an intraocular bubble.[31] The specific gravity of PDMS (0.97) is slightly lower than that of aqueous (1.00) and hence it floats in the vitreous cavity. The higher the specific gravity, the better it will contact with the retina.

Physical Properties of Tamponade

Silicone oil	***Viscosity (mPas) (25°C)***	***Specific gravity (25°C)***	***Refractive index (25°C)***
PDMS			
Siluron 1000	1000	0.97	1.404
Siluron 2000	2000–2400	0.97	1.404
Siluron 5000	5000	0.97	1.404
Fluorinated silicone/ Perfluorocarbon (PFCL)			
Perfluorodecalin (C10F18)	5.10	1.917	1.313
Perfluorophenanthrene ('Vitreon', C14F24)	8.03	2.03	
Perfluoro-octane (PFO)	1.4	1.78	1.27
Perfluorodecalin (PFD)	5.53	1.92	1.31
Fluoromethylcyclo-hexane (FMCH)	1.56	1.79	1.27
PDMS with high molecular weight additives			
Densiron 68	1349	1.06	1.387
Oxane HD	3800	1.02	1.4
HWS 46-3000	2903	1.118	1.366
PDMS with semi-fluorinated alkanes, alkenes			
F6H8	3.44	1.35	1.343
Perfluorohexylethan (O62)	0.75	1.62	1.29
Low-viscosity oligomer (OL62LV)	90	1.6	1.33
High-viscosity oli-gomer (OL62HV)	1750	1.6	1.33
Ethylsiloxane			
Ethylsiloxane with colloidal silica			

▶ Buoyancy

Buoyancy acting on a body inside a fluid is the upward force acting on the body exerted by a fluid. This upward force is opposed by the downward force of gravity that is the weight of the oil bubble. At equilibrium, buoyancy is equal in magnitude to the weight of fluid displaced by that body.

In the context of the eye, the body is the bubble of tamponade. The fluid is vitreous fluid. For example, if 1 ml of silicone oil is injected, then the buoyancy acting on the silicone oil bubble is equivalent to the weight of 1 ml of water, which is 1 gram. This as we noted previously is the upward force. The download force acting on the silicone oil bubble is 0.97 gram (that being the weight of 1 ml of silicone oil). The upward force is therefore higher than the download force. Therefore, the bubble of silicone oil floats. This floatation force however, is very small (1–0.97 g = 0.03 g). Similarly, 1 ml of air (or any gas for that matter) weighs about 0.001 g. The floatation force is therefore large being the difference between buoyancy and weight (1–0.001 g– 0.999 g). Likewise, PFCL and the so-called heavy silicone oils (e.g. Densiron-68 or Oxane HD) have specific gravities greater than 1. The floatation force is negative. In other words, these liquids sink and are sometimes referred to as "heavier-than-water" tamponades.

The histological changes observed previously on the retina by heavy liquids were thought to be due to their pressure or mechanical effects.[32,33] A recent study using a model eye chamber to examine the pressure effects of heavy tamponade agents have shown that the pressure increase due to these agents were minimal and was less than the diurnal fluctuations in the intraocular pressure.[34] We concluded from these studies that the histological changes are unlikely to be due to pure pressure effect. We speculated that the histological changes might be the result of the exclusion of water from the vitreoretinal interface. Winter et al.[35] measured using optical coherence tomography (OCT) in the laboratory the thickness of the film of aqueous between an oil bubble and the retina. The film of water is so thin that ionic exchange might be affected. The authors concluded that the exclusion of aqueous, which was important in the for the functioning of Muller cell potassium siphoning pump, could lead to the accumulation of excessive potassium ion and this in turn could give rise to hyperpolarization and excitotoxicity. Whether this is responsible for the histological changes is speculative.

Buoyancy dictates the floatation force. With large floatation force acting on air (and gas) bubbles, they take on the shape of a sphere with a relatively flat bottom (in geometry, this is referred to as a spherical cap). Whereas, with silicone oil the floatation force is small. It maintains a near spherical shape. For any given volume of gas used, the shape of air (or gas) bubble is very important. Apart from a small volume that goes to form the meniscus, the bulk of the volume contributes to the tamponade effect by making direct contact with the retina. In the case of silicone oil, the tamponade effect is much less for any given volume because of the spherical shape.

Based on the interfacial tensions alone, one would expect that air to form more rounded bubble compared to silicone oil (air has much higher interfacial tensions against water). However, the reverse is the case. The reason is that air and gas bubbles have far higher floatation forces compared to oil. That is the reason why the shape (and therefore the efficiency) of tamponade bubbles is determined principally by buoyancy and less by the interfacial tension with water.

It is important to appreciate that when a tamponade agent is used in an eye, there are in fact three phases in contact with each other. They are namely, oil against water, water against retina and retina against oil. The retina is hydrophilic.[36] In eye model studies, we have shown in the past that silicone oil virtually makes little or no contact with the retina until it is near 100% fill. In contrast, a very small bubble of air (or gas) could tamponade up to 90° of arc within the eye. This physical property of gaseous tamponade is exploited in the surgical procedure of pneumatic retinopexy. When a small bubble of C_3F_8 is injected (0.3 ml for example), it can be observed that the gas bubble remains fairly rounded in shape and do not offer much tamponade effect. When a gas bubble is small, the main determinant of its shape is the interfacial tension. Over the next few days, the bubble expands and as the volume gets larger, buoyancy becomes more important in governing the shape of the bubble and it takes on the shape of the spherical cap. Despite the small volume, up to 3–6 clock hours of the retina can be supported.

Along the same lines, it needs to be understood that in the case of silicone oil, a slight underfill would leave many clock hours of the retina unsupported. When using silicone oil, the most important consideration is to achieve 100% fill.[1]

Another important distinction between the behavior of gas and silicone oil is their ability to fit into the nooks and crannies or the recesses of the eye. This is important when scleral buckling is used. If a buckle was not correctly placed and a retinal break was to fall on the slope of an indent, the oil would not make contact or seal that break. On the same principle, the results of model eye chamber studies suggested that if an encircling element was used, by changing the shape of the eye cavity, the tamponade to the posterior pole might be enhanced.[36,37]

Table 7.3: Interfacial tension against water (mN/m) at (25°C) for various substances

Various substances	*Interfacial tension against water (mN/m)(25°C)*
Gas or air	80
Silicone oil	35
Perfluorcarbon liquids	40–45

Interfacial Tension or Surface Tension

Interfacial tension arises from the attractive van de Waal's forces between molecules at the interface, e.g. surface of a bubble of oil or air (Table 7.3). For a given bubble, the surface energy naturally wants to attain the smallest surface area for any given volume. This is achieved in the shape of a sphere. For the bubble to change it spherical shape, the surface energy has to be overcome. A bubble with a high surface has less tendency to deform or disperse into small bubbles. It is also less likely to go through small apertures. These are exactly the properties that we are seeking in tamponade agents. Gas has the highest interfacial tension when compared with that of silicone oil. It is also pertinent to understand that hydrogels and sodium hyaluronate as viscoelastic material are water-based. As such they do not form an interface with water and have no interfacial tension. Therefore, they technically do not act as tamponades. They are however, cohesive and therefore tend to stay as a single body. This property is exploited in vitreoretinal and cataract surgery. They can displace and separate tissue. Sodium hyaluronate can for example be used to open closed funnels associated long-standing retinal detachment or PVR in trauma. Hyaluronate being buoyancy neutral does have less tendency to go through retinal breaks in these immobile and stiff retinal detachments.

Viscosity

Viscosity is a measure of the resistance of a fluid to deformity by either shear stress (shear viscosity-tangential force, e.g. flow of silicone oil through injection cannula) or tensile stress (extensional viscosity-perpendicular force and away, e.g. pulling apart and forming separate bubbles-emulsification). A higher energy is needed to disperse a large and highly viscous (extensional viscosity) fluid bubble into small droplets (emulsification). Viscosity is expressed in centistokes (cs; 1cs = $10^{-6}m^2/s$), or more often these days as mPas. Silicone oil is usually classified clinically, based on its shear viscosity.

Generally, silicone oil with higher viscosity (e.g. 5,000 cs), is less likely to emulsify over time. Emulsified silicone oil may pass into the anterior segment blocking the trabecular meshwork as well as inducing inflammation by attracting neutrophils.[38]

Silicone oils are viscoelastic. When a force is applied, such as when it is mechanically stirred, silicone oil tends to behave as though it is less viscous. This phenomenon is called shear thinning. The shear viscosity decreases with increasing shear strain (applied force). The addition of high molecular weight polymer increased the extensional viscosity and in turn, increase the emulsification resistance.[39] Another advantage of adding the high molecular weight is that the oil becomes more viscoelastic such that it is easier to inject and aspirate. This has been demonstrated *in vitro* experiments using the viscous fluid injection at different pressures that authors normally use for vitrectomy. For the same shear viscosities, oils with the higher molecular weight components are consistently and significantly faster to inject.[40]

Refractive Indices

When injected in phakic eyes, silicone oil produces a hyperopic shift. Effectively, the oil reduces the converging power of the eye. The refractive index of PDMS is 1.40 and therefore close to that of the normal crystalline lens. When placed in the vitreous cavity, the oil conforms to the contour of the posterior lens surface and therefore effectively reduces the refractive power of the crystalline lens. A similar explanation applies for the hyperopic shift induced by silicone oil in pseudophakic eyes. Some intraocular lenses are designed so that all the refractive power is in the anterior surface. They are suitable for use in eyes filled with silicone oil as the normal hypermetropic shift would not occur. In aphakic eyes, as a result of buoyancy, the oil herniates through the pupil and forms a convex anterior surface. This effectively increases the overall refractive power of the eye and renders it less hypermetropic.[41]

Clinical Indications

Silicone oil used in retinal surgeries were first reported by Cibis in the early 1960s.[1] They used silicone oil (including heavier than water silicone oil, specific gravity 1.24) in patients with retinal detachment considered not treatable during that time. Their patients include those with "rolled-over retina", "massive vitreous hemorrhage" and "advanced retinal atrophy and multiple breaks". Although this procedure had resulted in retinal reattachment in some patients, improved visualization of ocular fundus and visual acuity, they acknowledged that it did not result in permanent attachment of the retina. Despite the drawbacks, the properties of silicone oil in clinical use were well documented: it is clear, relatively inert; it floats and have the tendency to emulsify in some cases. Early surgeons injected silicone oil without performing vitrectomy. They created room or capacity for the silicone oil by drainage of subretinal fluid only. The oil fill was therefore being incomplete. The early surgical outcomes were less favorable. Several reports of complications of silicone oil as intraocular tamponade also made its earlier use unpopular.[4-7]

It is not until the early 80s that its usage for long-term tamponade becomes more widespread, after the development of pars plana vitrectomy and refinement of other surgical techniques.[12,42-60] Its use is now critical to ensure good outcome in certain cases of vitreoretinal disease, including giant retinal tears.[61]

General

Generally the need to travel by air and anticipated difficulty in postoperative positioning (children, mentally challenged persons or those with physical disabilities) and the need for early visual rehabilitation due to poor vision in the fellow eye were acceptable justification for the use of silicone oil instead of gas. Silicone oil is transparent. Despite the changes in refraction, the use of this tamponade gives relatively satisfactory early rehabilitation. Surgery in patients with poor vision would be more practical with silicone oil as this allows better navigational vision in the immediate postoperative period. The main disadvantage of silicone oil is that a second surgery is needed to remove it.

Retinal Detachment with Severe Proliferative Vitreoretinopathy

The Silicone Study[20-27] was a prospective, randomized, multicentered clinical trial that began in 1985 and compared the visual and anatomical outcomes of using silicone versus long-acting gases (SF_6 or C_3F_8) in the treatment of RRD associated with advanced (at least grade C3, full thickness retinal folds in 3 or more quadrants) PVR. These two groups of patients were further randomized into those who had not undergone previous vitrectomy versus those that had had previous vitrectomy and gas tamponade. The following is a summary of the major results of the Silicone Study:

Silicone Study Report 1

Silicone oil was significantly superior to SF_6 in postoperative visual acuity and retinal reattachment. The incidences of hypotony and keratopathy were more frequent in the SF_6 group than in the silicone oil group.[22]

Silicone Study Report 2

C_3F_8 was found to be more effective than SF_6 and was equally effective as silicone oil in producing retinal reattachment, improving postoperative visual acuity and in resulting in lower incidence of complications.[24]

Silicone Study Report 3

Subgroup analysis was performed to examine the differences in outcomes between eyes that had not undergone prior vitrectomy (group 1) and eyes that had undergone at least one unsuccessful vitrectomy with gas tamponade (group 2) prior to entry into the study. The report found no difference between the two groups in the retinal reattachment rate and in achieving ambulatory vision. For both groups, those eyes that required multiple surgeries were less likely to achieve ambulatory vision. There was no difference in the incidence of hypotony between the two groups, but eyes in group 2 were more likely to develop keratopathy than those in group 1.[25]

Silicone Study Report 5

This study examined eyes that had undergone vitrectomy and relaxing retinotomy. The study showed that relaxing retinotomy was performed two times more likely in eyes that had undergone previous vitrectomy than those that had not. Both C_3F_8 and silicone oil appeared to be effective. In eyes that had not undergone a prior vitrectomy, those that did not undergo a relaxing retinotomy had better visual outcome and less incidence of hypotony. Overall, in those who had undergone prior vitrectomy and relaxing retinotomy, there was no difference in the final visual outcome compared with those that did not undergo a relaxing retinotomy. Subgroup analysis showed that those eyes that underwent a relaxing retinotomy and received silicone oil tamponade had worst visual and anatomical outcomes compared with those that did not undergo a relaxing retinotomy.[26]

Giant Retinal Tear

Silicone oil has been used as a long-term tamponding agent in the treatment of retinal detachment due to giant retinal tears (GRT).[61-63] In addition, it has been used as an intraocular tool to unfold a GRT and reattach the retina. Prior to the availability of silicone oil, air and gas had been used. This involved patients being operated in the prone with the surgeon often lying supine beneath the patient. The air bubble would therefore float upwards and unfold the GRT. Clearly, the patient had to be tied to the operating table which must have the ability of turning the upside down with the patient strapped firmly. It can be appreciated that performing surgery and fundoscopy could not be easy. Similarly, providing anesthesia and monitoring for an upside-down patient were also challenging. Silicone oil made the surgery much easier.

In GRT, the posterior flap is described as being "independently mobile". The mobility arises from the fact that the vitreous is no longer attached to the posterior edge of the retinal tear. As with any tear, the vitreous attachment is to the operculum, which in the case of the GRT is the anterior flap. If the extent of the tear was greater than 90° circumferentially, the posterior edge of the tear will have a tendency to slip posteriorly. With the onset of PVR, the edge of the tear can become rolled, which later develop into a fixed fold.

What silicone oil does is to enable the two ends of the retina to go "out to length". The surface energy of the tear enables the bubble to stay as a single bubble. As the injected bubble gets larger, the two ends of the retina tears become more widely separated. That means that any sagging of the posterior edge of the tear will be effectively pulled anteriorly. Therefore, even with the patient in the supine position, silicone oil is able to reattach the GRT. This however, is possible for tears up to 180° only. Clearly, if the break was much larger, then even if the two ends of the tear were returned to their respective anatomical positions, there could still be some sagging of the retina in between. In these situations, the retinal edge needed to be physically pulled anteriorly using a flute needle. The skill demanded of surgeons who often operated using indirect ophthalmoscopy was very high. The introduction of PFCL dramatically changed the way surgery for GRT was performed.[64,65] In combination with silicone oil, the anatomical results were much improved.[47] Some surgeons prefer direct PFCL-silicone oil exchange in order to avoid the complication of slippage.[66]

Whilst it is possible to repair GRTs with gas and obtain good anatomical results, the indication for silicone oil is not confined to treating cases associated established PVR. In GRT, the success rate using gas was around 70% with one operation. The surgical series using silicone oil from Leaver et al.[62] were close to 100% and although there are no randomized controlled trials for gas versus oil in GRT, most surgeons in US and virtually all surgeons in the UK will use primary silicone oil tamponade. The extent of the tear is such that much retinal pigment epithelial cells will find their way into the vitreous cavity. These cases are at high risk of developing PVR and the indication for use of silicone oil in these instances is in anticipation of the exaggerated wound healing response of PVR.

Severe Proliferative Diabetic Retinopathy

To date, there is no prospective randomized control trial comparing silicone oil with long acting gas in the treatment of eyes with complicated proliferative diabetic retinopathy (PDR). However, it has the potential of reducing postoperative vitreous hemorrhage, allows a more rapid visual recovery and reduces the need for face-down posturing.[67-70] Furthermore, the fundus is better visualized during the immediate postoperative period. Silicone oil may prevent the movement of vasoproliferative substances from the posterior pole to the anterior segment or prevent the diffusion of oxygen in the opposite direction, thus suppressing the development of anterior segment neovascularization.[71,72] This could be beneficial in diabetic patients needing vitrectomy in the presence of severe neovascularization of the anterior segment.[73,74] Equally postoperatively, any residual blood from the surgery or any recurrent hemorrhages will be confined by the silicone oil to the preretinal space, and in this situation, is likely to get organized into reproliferative membranes.

Macular Hole

The use of silicone oil in macular hole surgery is mainly indicated in patients with difficulty in posturing in the postoperative period, in those who need to travel by air and in those who are monocular. In addition, silicone oil has been used in cases where attempts using gas tamponades had failed. In a multicenter nonrandomized study, Goldbaum reported 80% of all macular holes and 86% of holes that were not treated previously were closed with a single silicone oil tamponade of the vitreous cavity.[75] In a subsequent study comparing C_3F_8 gas versus silicone oil tamponade, C_3F_8 was found to be more effective than silicone oil in achieving initial closure of macular holes.[76] Pertile and Claes compared SF_6 with silicone oil in a series of 54 macular holes treated with vitrectomy and ILM peel. They had high success rates of

94.7% and 97.1% using SF_6 and silicone oil respectively, but patients treated with silicone oil had significantly better visual results.[77] Stalmans reported using silicone oil for primary stage 2, 3 and 4 holes using infracyanine green and silicone oil and excellent anatomical closure rate (94%) and visual outcome (more than half saw 20/50 or better).[78]

The trend for macular hole surgery is to differentiate those that are smaller and require shorter tamponade and perhaps no posture from those that are larger and perhaps more chronic and less likely to close. In terms of surgery, the current trend is to use safer dyes with specific affinity to the ILM and to remove them. Early OCT studies show that macular holes often quite quickly close in the postoperative period (in terms of a few days). The justification for the use of silicone oil because it provides longer tamponade or that it obviates the need for posture will be increasingly untenable.

▶ Pathologic Myopia

Retinal detachment associated with macular holes may occur in eyes with pathologic myopia, especially in those eyes with posterior staphyloma.[79] Pars plana vitrectomy with intraocular silicone oil tamponade has been used in the treatment of this condition and has shown variable degrees of success.[80-82]

▶ Cytomegalovirus Retinitis

Silicone oil is commonly used in the setting of rhegmatogenous retinal detachment associated with cytomegalovirus (CMV) retinitis in immunologically compromised patients.[83-88] In CMV retinitis, widespread retinal necrosis develops and recurrence of the condition is common despite treatment. Pars plana vitrectomy, silicone oil tamponade and the use of the ganciclovir intraocular implant has been shown to achieve long-term stabilization of the atrophic retina, preservation or improvement of vision and extended control of the CMV retinitis.[89]

▶ Complicated Pediatric Retinal Detachment

The main indications for the use of silicone oil in the pediatric population are trauma, retinopathy of prematurity and myopia.[90] Silicone oil instillation has advantages over gas endotamponade since it is very difficult for children to keep the children in a prone position after the procedure. The outcomes, however, are generally poor.

Ferone[91] evaluated the efficacy of silicone oil as an intraocular tamponade for complicated retinal detachments in the pediatric population and showed that the results were generally disappointing due to the low rate of sustained retinal reattachment, poor vision after the surgery and high complication rates including corneal opacification and hypotony. The sequential use of conventional silicone oil and Densiron-68, a heavier than water silicone oil, may be a strategy in reducing the number of reoperations. Our case series shows that despite multiple surgical procedures, favorable visual outcome can be achieved.[92]

▶ Trauma

Pars plana vitrectomy allows severely traumatized eye to be repaired successfully. Silicone oil usage as endotemponade in vitrectomy for penetrating injury is beneficial because it minimizes intraoperative and postoperative hemorrhage which is a risk factor for PVR.[93] It maintains retinal attachment and prevents hypotony.

A series of severe ocular trauma managed with primary pars plana vitrectomy and silicone oil was reported by Spiegel et al.[94] In this retrospective study, pars plana vitrectomy and silicone oil filling were performed in 13 eyes as the primary surgical repair. The indications were laceration of the retina larger than 4 disc diameters, primary retinal detachment larger than two quadrants and/or persistent intrasurgical hemorrhage. All patients underwent surgery within 24 hours. Eleven eyes achieved a visual acuity ranging from 20/25–20/200. Silicone oil was removed in 11 of 13 eyes after 5.8 +/– 4.6 months. Recurrent proliferative vitreoretinopathy developed in two eyes.

In patients who failed initial vitrectomy, a repeat procedure with oil as a long-term tamponade may be tried to improve visual and anatomical outcome.[95,96] Antozky et al.[89] reported 42 cases of complicated retinal detachment following trauma after failed primary vitrectomy. At 6 months follow-up anatomic retinal reattachment was achieved in 50%. Many patients who had visual acuities of 5/200 or better at 6 months experienced a progressive decrease in visual acuity over 3 years, primarily because of recurrent retinal detachments and corneal edema. A final visual acuity of 5/200 or better was obtained in only five of the 42 eyes (12%) at the last follow-up examination. Generally, the prognoses of these eyes are poor even with oil.

Surgical Techniques in the Use of Silicone Oil

The surgical technique employed in vitreoretinal surgery varies from one surgeon to another and is subjected to personal preference. The maneuvers to achieve an endpoint are very much dependent on what is available and the retinal pathology presented at hand. However, the general surgical principle with regard to the use of silicone oil for internal tamponade is the same. The main consideration is related to the physical properties of silicone oil itself, which influence its behavior when it is used intraoperatively.

The tendency of silicone oil to be infused subretinally is much higher compared to gas due to its lower surface tension. This will occur in cases with large break and unrelieved retinal traction. Surface tension of silicone oil with different viscosity in clinical use has been found to be almost the same, giving them almost similar tamponading effects. The tendency to remain as one globule is advantageous as it does not obstruct view, ensuring a good fill and makes it easier to remove or ensuring a complete removal after the aim of tamponade is achieved.

The viscosity of silicone oil currently available for clinical use ranges from 1,000 cs–5,700 cs. A study on outcomes of complex retinal detachment repair using 1,000 cs versus 5,000 cs silicone oil did not show any difference in terms of anatomic and visual acuity outcomes, complication rates, retinal reattachment and ambulatory vision.[95] Higher viscosity oil is much more difficult to infuse or extrude and takes longer time; a larger wound is needed to accommodate a larger cannula at higher infusion pressure and thus may not be suitable for 23-gauge or 25-gauge system. However, a recent study has shown that active removal of Densiron-68, a heavier than water silicone oil, with a 23-gauge short cannula was feasible, simple and safe.[97] A combination of forces, such as the interfacial tension between the cannula and the oil, as well as the phenomenon of tubeless siphoning, made it feasible and reduces the risk of iatrogenic damage.[98]

For safety reasons, plastic syringe is preferred to glass. The flow of fluid in a tube is proportional to the fourth power of its radius and inversely proportional to the length of the tube (Poiseuille's Law). Thus, to reduce the resistance during injection, infusion line or cannula needs to be short and with the largest diameter permissible.

Infusion of Silicone Oil

Air-Silicone Oil Exchange

Silicone oil is injected after vitreous cavity has been replaced by air, the retina is flattened and retinal breaks have been sealed by laser or cryotherapy.

Injection of silicone oil is done through either of the two superior sclerotomies. It is important to ensure that the vitreous cavity is cleared from fluid or blood component to reduce the chance of oil emulsification later. The subretinal space should be as dry as possible to avoid underfilling, especially in cases with inferior break(s). To ensure that the air is replaced totally, the eye is tilted such that the infusion port is at its highest point to allow residual air to escape. Alternatively, a flute needle or a vitrectomy cutter can be used.

Slippage may occur during air-fluid exchange. A posterior retinotomy may be created and the subretinal fluid drained via this retinotomy. However, complete evacuation of the subretinal fluid may be difficult. If silicone oil is injected with residual subretinal fluid present, the vitreous cavity may be underfilled with silicone oil. Some advocate the use of an air-perfluorocarbon liquid (PFCL) exchange prior to silicone oil injection, but this also does not guarantee complete evacuation of the subretinal fluid. During the infusion of PFCL, subretinal fluid is displaced by the PFCL anteriorly and during the subsequent infusion of silicone oil, the anteriorly-displaced subretinal fluid is then pushed posteriorly by the silicone oil, giving rise to slippage. To overcome this problem, a total fill of vitreous cavity with PFCL up to the three-way tap before silicone oil injection is performed.[99] For details of the procedure, refer to the next section on perfluorocarbon liquid-silicone oil exchange.

The status of the lens has influence on the technique or maneuvers or additional procedures to be employed. Generally, it is easier to ensure total filling in phakic eyes compared to pseudophakic eyes, as the air will be displaced to the sides and escape through the ports without effort. In aphakic eyes, pseudophakic eyes with posterior capsular tear, sulcus fixated lens or in eyes with anterior chamber lens, an inferior peripheral iridotomy (Ando's inferior iridotomy)[16,100] is needed to prevent pupillary block glaucoma. For heavier than water silicone oil, a superior peripheral iridotomy should be done instead. The iridotomy is usually done with the vitrectomy cutter before silicone oil infusion. In creating an iridotomy, one technique is by applying suction under the posterior surface of the iris (as peripheral as possible and with low cut rate) where the iridotomy is intended; this creates a dimple on the iris surface, thus ensuring the correct location after which the cutter is activated to create an opening of adequate size. This is a more control way of creating an iridotomy compared to activating the cutter from the start blindly behind the iris. However, in the presence of peripheral capsular remnant or fibrosis, this may be difficult to be done without first removing it by cutting.

The adequacy of fill at the end of infusion is judged by: all air bubble has been expelled from the cavity, silicone oil begins to drain into the infusion cannula and the eye pressure is within normal limits digitally when the ports are closed. The eye must not be overfilled. Normally increase in intraocular pressure is compensated by increase in aqueous outflow and with the egress of aqueous, the intraocular pressure decreases. However, if the vitreous cavity is overfilled with silicone oil, the egression of aqueous will give rise to a shallow anterior chamber and intractable glaucoma that can only be effectively managed by removal of some silicone oil from the vitreous cavity. Similarly, applying and tightening encircling bands around the eye after the eye has been filled with silicone oil is another means of causing raised intraocular pressure postoperatively.

In pseudophakic eyes, extra care must be given, as there is the tendency for the oil to go into the anterior chamber in eyes with previous capsulotomy or zonular dehiscence. If silicone oil passes to the anterior chamber, viscoelastic material can be injected into the anterior chamber. However, it must be noted that subsequent anterior chamber washout of the viscoelastic often results in balance salt solution tracking posteriorly to the vitreous cavity and results in an subtotal of silicone oil.

The infusion pressure needs to be adjusted at the end of infusion so that the oil remains at the level of the iris plane. Injection of acetylcholine in such cases into the anterior chamber before the silicone oil is infused may constrict the pupil and helps to retain the silicone oil posteriorly. In cases where combined cataract surgery is performed, anterior segment wound closure must be secured to prevent sudden collapse of the anterior chamber, displacement of the silicone oil into it and prolapse of the iris. A facedown posture should be adopted immediately after silicone oil infusion. This might be difficult in the immediate recovery period when general anesthesia was used. In this instance, the patient should be postured with the head tilted to one side or the other.

Perfluorocarbon Liquid-Silicone Oil Exchange

Perfluorocarbon liquid is commonly used today during surgery for retinal detachment to aid subretinal fluid drainage, or to stabilize the retina during complex retinal procedures. PFCL can be exchanged with air first before silicone oil injection, as described above. However, there is always the possibility of slippage if this is done in cases where a large retinotomy was made to relieve traction or in cases of GRT. Slippage is the displacement of fluid under the retina posteriorly caused by the incoming air bubble during the exchange. This is due to the presence of residual subretinal fluid (SRF) anterior to the PFCL. This may lead to collection of subretinal fluid posteriorly, posterior displacement of the retinotomy edge, leaving a larger area of retinal pigment epithelium exposed. The latter may in turn, increase the risk of PVR and the development to retinal folds.

Slippage is less likely to occur in the case of GRT by using PFCL-silicone oil exchange. To accomplish this, the vitreous cavity is filled completely with PFCL and allowing it to overflow (overfill) into the infusion tubing until the level of three-way-tap before exchange (either air or oil) is done (Figs 7.1 to 7.3).[101] In the case of GRT, any SRF will be displaced by the PFCL anteriorly and expelled via one of the sclerotomies. A direct PFCL-silicone oil exchange can be performed. Silicone is infused through the 3-way-tap. In a 20-gauge system, passive aspiration using a flute need is all that is necessary. The interface between oil and PFCL is clearly seen. The tip of the fluting needle needs to be below that of the oil. In a 23-gauge system, active aspiration may be needed as the 23-gauge fluting needle offers considerable resistance such that it is important to ensure that the tip of the needle is below the silicone oil-PFCL interface and within the PFCL bubble. The infusion port should be clamped at the beginning to prevent the influx of balanced salt solution, which may enter the retinal break and causes slippage.

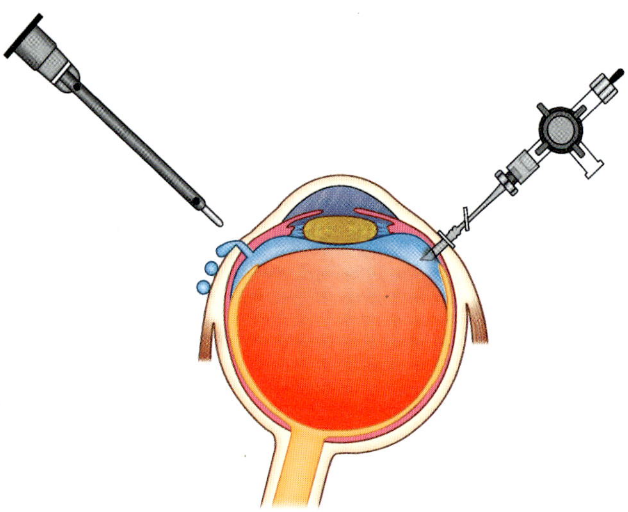

▲ **Figure 7.1**

Schematic diagram showing BSS infusion ensured that the fill of PFCL can only be up to the sclerotomies. Once the PFCL injection cannula was removed, the infusion of BSS would displace any PFCL above the sclerotomies out of the eye cavity

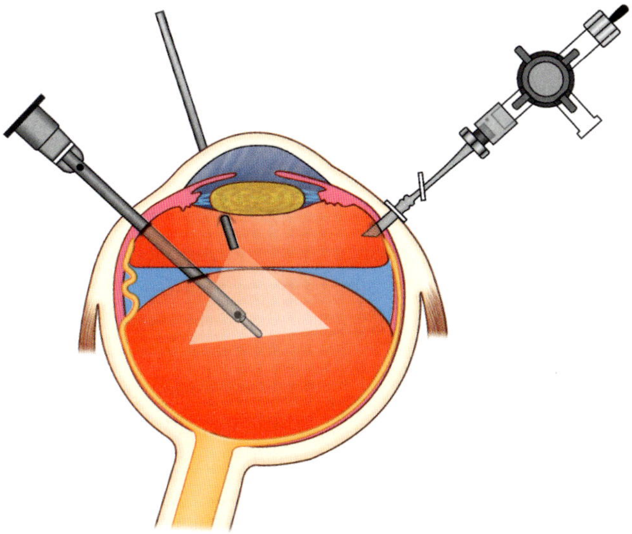

▲ Figure 7.2

Schematic diagram showing there may have a film of aqueous between the PFCL and silicone oil that can lead to slippage of the retina

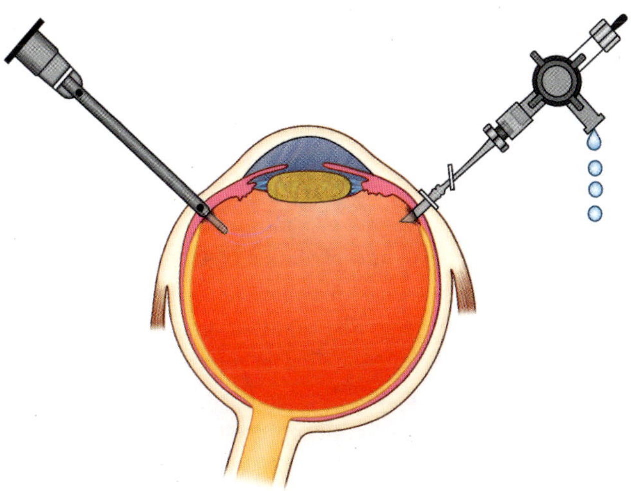

▲ Figure 7.3

Schematic diagram showing that by turning off the infusion of BSS and by filling the vitreous cavity totally with PFCL including the cannula, authors ensured that there was no aqueous in the system, thus eliminating slippage as a possible complication

Note: It may be advisable to leave one of the sclerotomy ports opened and in the uppermost position, so that any aqueous can be displaced out of the eye by the perfluorocarbon

The reason behind the lesser likelihood of slippage with PFCL-silicone exchange is because PFCL and silicone oil are both hydrophobic. The two liquids prefer to be in contact with each other and excludes aqueous from its interface. Once in contact, the two liquids effectively form a single bubble. The bubble will have a combined specific gravity greater than 1.0 and therefore aqueous stays on top of this bubble and effectively does not get displaced posteriorly to result in slippage. To accomplish this, during silicone oil injection, a flute needle should be passed from the silicone oil into the PFCL in order to make the two liquids join as a single bubble. The eye should be rotated so that any aqueous displaced anteriorly can be expelled. With further addition of the silicone oil, the conjoined bubble of PFCL and silicone oil becomes lighter as more of the PFCL gets removed. The evacuation of the last drop of PFCL is made easier by the contrast in refractive index.

Fluid-Silicone Oil Exchange

This is a direct exchange of fluid in the eye with silicone oil. Since oil floats over balanced salt solution and will push any subretinal fluid to the macula, a posterior drainage retinotomy needs to be created. An extrusion needle must be placed in the fluid phase in the vitreous cavity and through the retinal break or posterior retinotomy. This technique is technically difficult and probably the least done. A high pressure is needed to inject silicone oil into the eye. If passive aspiration was used to evacuate preretinal vitreous fluid or subretinal fluid, working with such high pressures could be daunting. The tip of the drainage or flute needle would often be very close to the retina. Towards the end, the retina could be accidentally aspirated into the needle because of the high pressures employed. If the tip of the draining needle was not at all times below the incoming bubble of oil, it could be partially blocked by the highly viscous silicone oil. That means high pressure would be necessary to drain the aqueous. The whole procedure would not be easily controlled. Fortunately, the new generation of vitrectomy machines allow for simultaneous injection of silicone oil under high pressure with the active aspiration (or linear extrusion under low pressure). Active aspiration meant that the oil could be injected whilst keeping the intraocular pressure at normal level. Nonetheless, the surgeon needs to be careful not to block up the drainage needle with oil and to palpate the globe periodically to get a feel of the intraocular pressure. It would be foolish to be too reliant on machines monitoring the intraocular pressure.

Removal of Silicone Oil

Silicone oil should be removed once the objective of tamponade is achieved to avoid or minimize its potential complications. In the Silicone Study, silicone oil removal was allowed after a minimum of 8 weeks following surgery.[102] Some suggested removal should be done within the first 6 months of surgery when conventional silicone oil is used.[103] It is advisable to have silicone oil removed earlier in cases with heavy silicone oil, that is, no longer than 3 months.[104] Various methods of silicone oil removal have been described.[98,105-119] The type of silicone oil and its viscosity, lens status and whether or not additional procedures are to be carried out, will influence the method used.

Generally, a minimum of two ports are employed; one for infusion of balanced salt solution and the other is for silicone oil aspiration. Many surgeons prefer a three port approach such that a triple-air-fluid exchange, a thorough internal search and if necessary supplementary laser photocoagulation can be carried out at the same time. Removal of silicone oil can be done passively by allowing oil to egress through a sclerotomy or by active aspiration using automated pump, or manually. Passive aspiration is slow, inefficient and may be dangerous. With passive aspiration one must remember that the pressure gradient is only that between the intraocular pressure and the atmospheric pressure. When the infusion bottle was raised to its maximum height, the pressure gradient would still be only about 110 cm H_2O or 80 mm Hg. This pressure gradient is low when trying to aspirate silicone oil especially if it was 5,000 mPas. With active aspiration, suction of up to 600 mm Hg could be achieved. A suction of 600 mm Hg refers to the pressure below atmospheric. The pressure gradient would therefore be 600 mm Hg plus the intraocular pressure. As flow is linearly dependent on the pressure gradient, it seems illogical not to employ suction and just use "passive" aspiration. The chief determinant of flow rate however is not so much the pressure gradient. It is the radius of the cannula used for the aspiration. Poiseuille's law reminds that flow is proportional to the fourth power of the radius. The speed of oil extraction using a 20-gauge cannula is very much faster than using a 23-gauge cannula. Two other factors are worth mentioning. The flow of course is inversely proportional to the length. Therefore, ideally the length should be kept to a minimum. Practically, this means that silicone oil cannot be removed using "linear extrusion". That is, oil cannot be aspirated via a length of tubing to a vacuum generated at the vitrectomy machine. The suction needs to be generated as close to the eye as possible. In other words, we should always use a pneumatically driven syringe or even simply a manual syringe with a short cannula attached to it. Lastly, the viscosity of the oil matters. Poiseuille's law applies to Newtonian fluids. Silicone oil is slightly viscoelastic. That means that 5,000 mPas does not take 5 times as long as 1,000 mPas. Furthermore, by adding high molecular weight polydimethlysiloxane to normal silicone oil, the extensional viscosity of the oil can be increased. This makes it easier to aspirate or inject than conventional silicone oil with similar shear viscosity. A group of authors has shown that it is possible to make silicone oils that are easier to inject (and to aspirate)[40] and yet more resistant to emulsify *in vitro.*[39]

In combined phacoemulsification and uncomplicated silicone oil removal, a posterior capsulotomy is made that is large enough to accommodate aspiration cannula that goes through the phacoemulsification wound. By comparison, fashion a continuous circular capsulorhexis in the posterior capsule requires more skill than in the anterior capsule. The floatation of the oil can cause the posterior capsule to bulge anteriorly. Because the capsular bag is empty, the posterior capsule is lax; there is more of a tendency for the rhexis to extend to the equator. By the judicious use of an appropriate amount of viscoelastic, performing the rhexis could be made easier to perform. After the capsulorhexis, a needle could be introduced through to the posterior chamber. Surprisingly, there is often little or no evidence of any anterior cortical vitreous behind the lens. The oil often herniates through the capsulorhexis. The infusion line is normally placed at the pars plana. It could also be sited in the anterior chamber via a corneal paracentesis. After the removal of oil, the intraocular lens could be placed in the bag. If however, there was any doubt about the integrity of the capsulorhexis, sulcus fixated intraocular lens could also be considered. If the eye was aphakic, sutured intraocular lens implant or iris claw lenses could be placed. The only caveat with all the additional maneuvers, great care must be taken in maintaining the intraocular pressure. With the presence of a large corneal wound and an absence of vitreous, there is nothing to prevent the collapse of the eye and protect it from the real risk of massive intraocular hemorrhage.

Implications of Silicone Oil Removal

Removal of silicone oil is associated with the potential risk of retinal redetachment. The rate of retinal redetachment after removal of silicone oil has improved in recent years. This might be attributable to the improvement in surgical management.[120] Reported retrospective series on redetachment rate after silicone oil removal can be as high as 30%.[121-129] The risk of redetachment is very difficult to quantify for each patient. The rate of redetachment is higher in eyes with PVR[120] or in eyes with risks of developing PVR.[121] Li et al.[128] reported the rate of redetachment by causes of initial detachment as PVR grade C (9.5%), PVR grade D (25%), trauma without intraocular foreign body (27.3%), with intraocular foreign body (33.3%), GRT (37.5%) and proliferative diabetic retinopathy with tractional retinal detachment (33.3%). In a recent retrospective series for eyes with retinal detachment with grade C PVR treated with silicone oil, the redetachment rate was found to be 18.36% after silicone oil removal.[127] Increased number of previous unsuccessful retinal detachment surgeries and longer axial lengths were associated with higher failure rates. Most redetachment occur within 6 months after silicone oil removal.[120,122,124,130] Prophylactic 360° laser[131] or the use of encircling band[123,125] may reduce the rate of retinal redetachment after silicone oil removal.

It is extremely difficult or impossible to ensure the eye is free of emulsified oil at the end of the procedure. Patients may complain of floaters due to the presence of residual oil droplets. Some may advocate air-fluid exchange at the end of oil removal to remove residual droplets. However, a study has shown that there was no difference in the incidence of floaters seen after silicone oil removal with passive drainage alone versus passive drainage combined with air-fluid exchange.[108]

In patients who were found to have glaucoma refractory to medical therapy, presumably due to oil emulsification, removal of silicone oil normalized the intraocular pressure (with or without antiglaucoma therapy) in the majority of cases (75%).[132] Twenty-five percent of eyes had persistent raised intraocular pressures despite of silicone oil removal. These could be due to neovascularization or chronic inflammation with increasing anterior synechiae formation. The majority of patients who developed glaucoma after silicone oil removal have open anterior chamber angles. Emulsification of silicone oil may play a role in the development of glaucoma. Whether the emulsified oil droplets led to blockage or damage of the trabecular meshwork is not known. Even in patients with no clinically observable droplets, there might be small droplets of the size of 1–3 µm which can only been "seen" as flare rather than cells. Moisseiev et al.[133] found removal of the emulsified oil did not affect the intraocular pressure in 91% of glaucomatous eyes in their series. Patients with medically uncontrolled glaucoma persisting after silicone oil removal may benefit from trans-scleral-cyclo-photocoagulation. Though variable, cyclo destructive treatment could achieve pressure reduction but often more than one treatment session might be required.[134]

The change in visual acuity after silicone oil removal is very difficult to predict for each patient because the interplay of multiple factors before (etiology of detachment, duration, number of previous surgeries, etc.) and during oil removal (perfusion, complications, additional procedures, etc.). Studies looking specifically at visual acuity change after oil removal are not many. Some 50–60% of patients had some improvement of their vision after removal of oil.[135-137]

Complications of Silicone Oil

General

Complications related to the use of silicone oil use can occur intraoperatively, during the postoperative period, or after its removal.

Silicone oil should be removed once the purpose of tamponade has been achieved. This is to minimize its long-term complication. Although silicone oils used in vitreoretinal surgery were generally considered as inert and nontoxic, it had been shown that intraocular silicone oil could damage the normal tissue structures and function if it was retained in eyeballs too long.[138]

Generally, silicone oil is removed between 6 weeks to 6 months following surgery if the retina remains attached and no intraocular pressure rise or other oil-related complications occur. However, in eyes with very poor ultimate anatomical or visual prognosis, it may be preferable to leave the oil in the eye. Lastly, removal of oil is be contraindicated if the eye has chronic hypotony.

Specific

Glaucoma: Glaucoma associated with intraocular silicone oil may be attributable to oil overfilling, pupillary block, blockage of trabecular meshwork by emulsified silicone oil and oil-related inflammation or trabeculitis or exacerbation of pre-existing glaucoma.[139,140]

Oil overfilling may be suspected when the intraocular pressure is high in the immediate postoperative period with shallowing of the anterior chamber and absence of an inferior silicone oil meniscus over aqueous in the posterior segment. Partial removal of the oil is necessary. This can be avoided by making sure the intraocular pressure is normal or slightly low and the silicone oil remains posterior to the lens-iris diaphragm after injection into the vitreous cavity.

Pupillary block glaucoma usually occurs during the early postoperative period, though it can occur at any time postoperatively.[16,141-143] It is more common in aphakic eyes due to close proximity of anterior surface of oil to the pupillary margin. It is less common in pseudophakic eye. An inferior peripheral iridotomy is usually done in these eyes prior to oil injection to avoid this complication. However, closure of the iridotomy by blood, fibrin or residual lens capsule can occur postoperatively, leading to aqueous misdirection, shallowing of the anterior chamber and intraocular pressure rise.

Cataract: Most clinical studies associate long-term silicone oil tamponade with cataract formation.[18,19,139,144,145] The proposed mechanisms are impaired metabolic exchange across the posterior lens capsule and/or direct toxicity of the silicone oil. A histologic study has identified increased posterior migration of lens epithelium and deposition of collagen contributing to cataract formation in oil-filled eye.[146]

If the silicone oil is *in situ*, then a combined phacoemulsification, posterior chamber intraocular lens implantation and silicone oil removal can be performed. The rate of posterior capsule opacification is 100%. There is a strong motivation to perform preoperative posterior capsulotomy. If the silicone oil has already been removed, Nd:YAG laser capsulotomy can be performed.

Keratopathy: Eyes with prolonged silicone oil tamponade invariably develop corneal abnormalities in the form of diffuse bullous keratopathy or band keratopathy. Silicone oil in the anterior chamber can often be missed by the novice vitreoretinal surgeon. If silicone oil completely fills the anterior chamber and no meniscus or fluid level can be seen, the casual observer can be deceived into thinking that the anterior chamber is fluid filled. In silicone oil-filled eyes, surgeons should always have a high index of suspicion of the anterior chamber being filled with silicone oil. Confirmatory signs of a silicone oil-filled anterior chamber includes the absence of flare in the anterior chamber, mid-dilated pupil and a shimmering reflex on the iris crypts. If in doubt, fluorescein sodium can be applied and the absence of flare in the anterior chamber would confirm the presence of a silicone oil-filled anterior chamber. Paradoxically, bubble of silicone oil seldom gives rise to keratopathy even when they are fairly large in size. This is probably due to the relative minimal contact between the silicone oil and the corneal endothelium. With the increased use of combined phacoemulsification, posterior chamber intraocular lens implantation, pars plana vitrectomy and silicone oil injection, silicone oil-induced keratopathy has become a rare complication. The exception occurs when the eye is hypotonic. In these phthisical eyes, even if they were pseudophakic and the posterior capsule seemed to be intact, a silicone oil-filled anterior chamber and subsequent keratopathy would be inevitable.

Band keratopathy is more common in younger patient, while bullous keratopathy is seen more in the older patient. In eyes with severe PVR, the independent risks for keratopathy are aphakic, pseudophakic, preoperative iris neovascularization, postoperative aqueous flare and in eyes with repeated surgery. The incidence of corneal abnormalities in the silicone study at 24 months was 27%. However, this did not differ significantly between the use of silicone oil or C_3F_8 gas.[147] Cornea touch by silicone oil was found to be a contributor, but not as an independent factor for the development of keratopathy.

While it is difficult to control the above factors in the prevention of keratopathy, minimizing the possible effects of silicone oil on corneal endothelium need to be emphasized. The management strategies include ensuring a patent inferior iridectomy, ensuring no silicone oil in the anterior chamber at the end of surgery and early removal of silicone oil if it has come in contact with corneal endothelium. Prolonged silicone-corneal endothelium contact will result in endothelial damage.[140,148] Histopathology of corneal button obtained after penetrating keratoplasty for silicone oil associated keratopathy has shown marked endothelial cell loss and degeneration.[149] While the cornea remains clear when the anterior chamber is filled with oil, corneal edema or opacification develops soon after removal of oil when aqueous fills the anterior chamber; this is a reflection of endothelial dysfunction.

In the blind eye with silicone oil-induced keratopathy, the calcium plaques can ulcerate and cause pain to the patient. These calcified plaques can be successfully removed by superficial keratectomy. It is also possible to employ photo keratectomy. These treatments are very worthwhile as it brings relief to these patients who often suffer from chronic pain. Band keratopathy may also benefit form chelation. Severe keratopathy needs keratoplasty if vision is to be improved. This maybe done before, during or after silicone oil has been removed from the eye. Graft failure rate after penetrating keratoplasty is higher when the silicone is retained in the eye (67%) compared to those removed before or during keratoplasty (25%).[150] The risk of transplant failure is significantly lower in eyes that do not undergo additional surgery.[151]

Recurrent retinal detachment: In the silicone study, rate of recurrent detachment does not appear to be related to the type of intraocular tamponade used. Early or late postoperative period redetachment occurs in half of the patients treated for retinal detachment complicated by severe PVR with either silicone oil or C_3F_8 gas.[24] Early redetachment is most likely due to unrelieved retinal traction, while reproliferation is the cause for late redetachment.[124,125] The risk of retinal redetachment decreases steeply with increasing time after silicone oil removal; 3–5 months after oil removal, retinal redetachment becomes unlikely.[49]

To minimize redetachment after silicone oil removal, meticulous membrane removal to relieve traction is important during the initial surgery and the use of pharmacologic strategies against reproliferation should be considered. Some authors have suggested the use of 360° laser before or during silicone oil removal to the effect of reducing the chance or redetachment.[128,152] A recent article suggests increasing number of previous surgeries and longer axial length are poor prognostic factors for anatomic success after silicone oil removal[127] in addition to aphakia.[128] Application of 360° laser retinopexy may be considered in these cases.

Hypotony: Hypotony, as defined by intraocular pressure of 5 mm Hg or less, is a late complication of complicated retinal detachment surgery. In the silicone study for severe PVR, hypotony occurs in 18% of silicone oil filled eye versus 31% of C_3F_8 at 36 months[153] and 3% versus 15% at 6 years.[20]

The reason for hypotony development is multifactorial and is not fully understood. Reduction of aqueous production due to damage to ciliary processes during repeated surgery might be the main cause. The continued anterior proliferation with traction on ciliary processes[38,51,153,154] and/or cilio-choroidal detachment[155] also results in aqueous hypo secretion and increase outflow. Increased uveoscleral outflow through large retinotomies especially if more than 180°[126] might be a contributing factor as well.

Treatment of postoperative hypotony is difficult. At the early postoperative period, a repeat surgery to relieve anterior proliferation and traction on the anterior retina and ciliary processes may be considered beneficial.[156,157] Subconjunctival injection of long-acting steroids may help in normalization of intraocular pressure in these eyes. However, there is no current effective treatment for eyes with established hypotony.

In silicone oil-filled eye, the possibility of inducing or potentiating hypotony or causing phthisis after removal of oil needs to be considered. In eyes with chronic hypotony or already at risk of developing hypotony, the silicone oil is best left *in situ*. Ultimately, the risks and benefits of silicone oil removal need to be discussed with the patient, depending on the condition of the affected eye and his fellow eye.

Silicone Oil Emulsification

Silicone oil emulsification is an inherent problem especially if its use is prolonged. This can lead to glaucoma and keratopathy. Often it is not possible to remove the emulsified oil totally; patients may develop visual disturbances or persistent intraocular pressure rise because of the emulsified silicone oil. Migration of emulsified silicone oil into the subretinal space may lead to retinal redetachment.

The tendency for silicone oil to emulsify is dependent on its viscosity and surface tension.[31] Clinically used silicone oil is usually classified by its viscosity. Generally, the higher viscosity oil has lower tendency to emulsify.[158] The problem with the use of higher viscosity silicone oils is that it is relatively more difficult to inject or remove them and it requires a large sclerotomy for removal. With the advent of 25-gauge and 23-gauge vitrectomy systems, lower viscosity silicone oils need to be used but without the added problem of easier emulsification. Recent *in vitro* studies have shown new low viscosity silicone oils have a reduced emulsification similar to that of 5,000 cs silicone oil by the addition of small amounts of very-long-chain silicone molecules to 1,000 cs silicone oil.[159]

Silicone oil emulsification can occur within a few days but more common after several months.[8,11] It is postulated that the combination of saccadic eye movement, shear between the silicone oil and aqueous liquids or intraocular fluids and reduction of interfacial tension by absorption of active component in the intraocular fluids contributed to the oil-emulsification process. Thus, adequate drying of posterior segment from fluid or blood or blood products and complete filling of the posterior segment may minimize silicone oil emulsification.

Recently, the addition of low concentrations of very high molecular weight polymers of the same chemistry as the bulk silicone oil has been shown to increase the emulsification resistance of tamponade agents while maintaining ease of injection and removal.[39] These materials have the potential to reduce the adverse clinical responses of current silicone oil tamponade agents.

Refractive Changes

Silicone oil in the vitreous cavity induced a myopic shift in aphakic eyes and a hypermetropic shift in phakic eyes. This tended to render phakic high myopes and aphakes closer to emmetropia. The resultant refraction was dependent on the shape of the silicone oil bubble inside the eye and influenced by the posture of the patient. In phakic patients the ability to accommodate was markedly reduced.[41]

Others

Using proper technique and addressing intraocular pathology adequately can avoid placing silicone oil in the wrong anatomical space. Suprachoroidal infusion of oil is avoidable by ensuring complete infusion cannula penetration into the vitreous cavity during injection. Particular attention should be given in cases with thickened choroid: in hypotonous eyes (e.g. due to chronic retinal detachment), inflamed eye (e.g. postoperative, uveitis or trauma) and in the eye with choroidal effusion or hemorrhage (e.g. trauma cases). Silicone oil can gain access to the subretinal space through persistent open break due to unrelieved traction. All traction, which prevents retinal flattening under air, must be relieved before injection of silicone oil is carried out. Postoperative subretinal migration of silicone oil may occur as well through of new large break in the presence of PVR and persistent traction.

In aphakic eyes and phakic or pseudophakic eyes with zonular dehiscence and pseudophakic eyes with posterior capsule defect, anterior migration of silicone oil can occur at the end of silicone oil infusion. Infusion pressure must be controlled towards the end of infusion to prevent anterior migration. In addition, the pupil may be constricted prior to silicone oil injection. In aphakic eye, anteriorly migrated oil may be displaced posteriorly by injecting viscoelastic in the anterior chamber and later replacing it with balance-salt solution. Alternatively, the patient can be instructed to maintain a facedown position. In phakic or pseudophakic eyes, it is best to remove the silicone oil and repeat the injection. It is important to ensure a patent inferior iridotomy is present in these cases. Postoperative closure of iridotomy due to blood or fibrin can lead to forward movement of silicone oil into the anterior chamber. In eyes that have previously done well, late anterior chamber migration of silicone oil may signify recurrent retinal detachment; silicone oil being noncompressible will be displaced anteriorly. The other reason is reduction of ocular volume due to development of chronic hypotony.

The use of heavier than water silicone oil improves tamponade of the inferior retina. There are two heavier than water silicone oil currently available. They are Oxane HD[160] (Silicone oil 5,700 cs-RMN3 mixture: viscosity 3,300 cs, density 1.02 g/cm^3) and Densiron-68[99,161-165] (Silicone oil 3,000 cs-F6H8 mixture: viscosity 1,400 cs, density 1.06 g/cm^3). Rizzo et al.[165] has reported on the use of heavy oil based on F_4H_6.

The use of heavy silicone oil is controversial.[40] PVR has a propensity for the inferior retina. There has been many attempts to find a heavier than water tamponade. These are used to treat complicated detachment of the inferior retina[99,160-163,166] or for managing persistent macula hole[164,165] or in patients who are unable to posture. For conventional silicone oil, removal of oil only requires anterior segment viewing system. Heavy oil sinks, thus require posterior segment viewing system and active extrusion by high vacuum relatively close to the retina using automated pump system. The use of heavier than water tamponade agent in patient with high risk of PVR may result in a shift of PVR development to the superior retina.

Heavier than water, silicone oil is associated with similar complications as conventional silicone oil. These include cataract formation, emulsification and glaucoma. The use of Densiron-68 may be associated with higher early postoperative intraocular pressure compared to conventional silicone oil.[167] Li et al.[99] reported complications such as posterior capsule opacification (25.9%), cataract (25%), intraocular inflammation (22.2%), emulsification (18.5%) and raised intraocular pressure (18.5%) in their series with the use of Densiron-68. Wickham et al.[166] did not observe an advantage following the use of Oxane HD in the treatment of inferior retinal detachments. Furthermore, it was difficult to remove and was associated with a higher incidence of complications. Ang et al.[168] reported postoperative complications in 77.8% of patients in their series with the use of Oxane HD, including emulsification (33.3%), epiretinal membrane (27.8%) and posterior capsular opacifications (22.2%). The interim report of the HSO study was inconclusive.

References

1. Cibis PA, Becker B, Okun E, et al. The use of liquid silicone in retinal detachment surgery. Arch Ophthalmol. 1962;68:590-9.
2. Cibis PA. Recent methods in the surgical treatment of retinal detachment: intravitreal procedures. Trans Ophthalmol Soc UK. 1965;85:111-27.
3. Machemer R, Buettner H, Norton EW, et al. Vitrectomy: a pars plana approach. Trans Am Acad Ophthalmol Otolaryngol. 1971;75:813-20.
4. Watzke RC. Silicone retinopiesis for retinal detachment. A long-term clinical evaluation. Arch Ophthalmol. 1967;77:185-96.
5. Jalkh AE, McMeel JW, Kozlowski IM, et al. Silicone oil retinopathy. Arch Ophthalmol. 1986;104:178-9.
6. Sugar HS, Okamura ID. Ocular findings six years after intravitreal silicone injection. Arch Ophthalmol. 1976;94:612-5.
7. Cockerham WD, Schepens CL, Freeman HM. Silicone injection in retinal detachment. Arch Ophthalmol. 1970; 83:704-12.
8. Scott JD. Treatment of massive vitreous retraction. Trans Ophthalmol Soc UK. 1975;95:429-32.
9. Zivojnovic R, Mertens DA, Baarsma GS. Fluid silicon in detachment for surgery (author's transl). Klin Monbl Augenheilkd. 1981;179:17-22.
10. Zivojnovic R, Mertens DA, Peperkamp E. Liquid silicone in amotio surgery (II). Report on 280 cases - further development of the technic. Klin Monbl Augenheilkd. 1982;181:444-52.
11. Gabel VP, Kampik A, Gabel C, et al. Silicone oil with high specific gravity for intraocular use. Br J Ophthalmol. 1987;71:262-7.
12. Leaver PK, McLeod D. Rationale and techniques of closed vitrectomy. Trans Ophthalmol Soc UK. 1977;97:242-7.
13. Gonvers M. Pars plana vitrectomy. Rev Med Suisse Romande. 1980;100:515-9.
14. Heimann K. Pars-plana-vitrectomy in the treatment of injuries with intraocular foreign bodies. Bull Soc Belge Ophtalmol. 1981;193:13-24.
15. Lucke KH, Foerster MH, Laqua H. Long-term results of vitrectomy and silicone oil in 500 cases of complicated retinal detachments. Am J Ophthalmol. 1987;104:624-33.
16. Ando F. Intraocular hypertension resulting from pupillary block by silicone oil. Am J Ophthalmol. 1985,99:87-8.
17. Machemer R, McCuen BW, de Juan E. Relaxing retinotomies and retinectomies. Am J Ophthalmol. 1986;102:7-12.
18. Chang S, Lincoff HA, Coleman DJ, et al. Perfluorocarbon gases in vitreous surgery. Ophthalmology. 1985;92:651-6.
19. Lincoff H, Coleman J, Kreissig I, et al. The perfluorocarbon gases in the treatment of retinal detachment. Ophthalmology. 1983;90:546-51.
20. Abrams GW, Azen SP, McCuen BW, et al. Vitrectomy with silicone oil or long-acting gas in eyes with severe proliferative vitreoretinopathy: results of additional and long-term follow-up. Silicone Study report 11. Arch Ophthalmol. 1997;115:335-44.
21. Azen SP, Boone DC, Barlow W, et al. Methods, statistical features, and baseline results of a standardized, multicentered ophthalmologic surgical trial: the Silicone Study. Control Clin Trials. 1991;12:438-55.
22. Silicone Study Group. Proliferative vitreoretinopathy. The Silicone Study Group. Am J Ophthalmol. 1985;99:593-5.
23. Silicone Study Group. Vitrectomy with silicone oil or sulfur hexafluoride gas in eyes with severe proliferative vitreoretinopathy: results of a randomized clinical trial. Silicone Study Report 1. Arch Ophthalmol. 1992;110:770-9.
24. Silicone Study Group. Vitrectomy with silicone oil or perfluoropropane gas in eyes with severe proliferative vitreoretinopathy: results of a randomized clinical trial. Silicone Study Report 2. Arch Ophthalmol. 1992;110:780-92.
25. McCuen BW, Azen SP, Stern W, et al. Vitrectomy with silicone oil or perfluoropropane gas in eyes with severe proliferative vitreoretinopathy. Silicone Study Report 3. Retin 1993;13:279-84.
26. Blumenkranz MS, Azen SP, Aaberg T, et al. Relaxing retinotomy with silicone oil or long-acting gas in eyes with severe proliferative vitreoretinopathy. Silicone Study Report 5. The Silicone Study Group. Am J Ophthalmol. 1993;116: 557-64.
27. Diddie KR, Azen SP, Freeman HM, et al. Anterior proliferative vitreoretinopathy in the silicone study. Silicone Study Report Number 10. Ophthalmology. 1996;103:1092-9.
28. Retina Society Terminology Committee. The classification of retinal detachment with proliferative vitreoretinopathy. Ophthalmology. 1983;90:121-5.
29. Machemer R, Aaberg TM, Freeman HM, et al. An updated classification of retinal detachment with proliferative vitreoretinopathy. Am J Ophthalmol. 1991;112:159-65.
30. Heidenkummer HP, Kampik A, Thierfelder S. Emulsification of silicone oils with specific physicochemical characteristics. Graefes Arch Clin Exp Ophthalmol. 1991;229:88-94.
31. Joussen AM, Wong D. The concept of heavy tamponades-chances and limitations. Graefes Arch Clin Exp Ophthalmol. 2008;246:1217-24.
32. Eckardt C, Nicolai U. Clinical and histologic findings after several weeks of intraocular tamponade with perfluorodecalin. Ophthalmologe. 1993;90:443-7.
33. Velikay M, Wedrich A, Stolba U, et al. Experimental long-term vitreous replacement with purified and nonpurified perfluorodecalin. Am J Ophthalmol. 1993;116:565-70.
34. Wong D, Williams R, Stappler T, et al. What pressure is exerted on the retina by heavy tamponade agents? Graefes Arch Clin Exp Ophthalmol. 2005;243:474-7.
35. Winter M, Eberhardt W, Scholz C, et al. Failure of potassium siphoning by Muller cells: a new hypothesis of perfluorocarbon liquid-induced retinopathy. Invest Ophthalmol Vis Sci. 2000;41:256-61.
36. Fawcett IM, Williams RL, Wong D. Contact angles of substances used for internal tamponade in retinal detachment surgery. Graefes Arch Clin Exp Ophthalmol. 1994;232:438-44.

37. Williams R, Wong D. The influence of explants on the physical efficiency of tamponade agents. Graefes Arch Clin Exp Ophthalmol. 1999;237:870-4.
38. Hiscott P, Magee RM, Colthurst M, et al. Clinicopathological correlation of epiretinal membranes and posterior lens opacification following perfluorohexyloctane tamponade. Br J Ophthalmol. 2001;85:179-83.
39. Williams RL, Day M, Garvey MJ, et al. Increasing the extensional viscosity of silicone oil reduces the tendency for emulsification. Retina. 2010;30:300-4.
40. Williams RL, Day MJ, Garvey MJ, et al. Injectability of silicone oil-based tamponade agents. Br J Ophthalmol. 2011;95:273-6.
41. Smith RC, Smith GT, Wong D. Refractive changes in silicone filled eyes. Eye. 1990;4 (Pt 1):230-4.
42. Machemer R. Vitrectomy in the management of severe diabetic retinopathies. Klin Monbl Augenheilkd. 1973;162:199-205.
43. Machemer R. Subtotal vitrectomy through the pars plana. Trans Am Acad Ophthalmol Otolaryngol. 1973;77:OP198-201.
44. Machemer R. A new concept for vitreous surgery. 7. Two instrument techniques in pars plana vitrectomy. Arch Ophthalmol. 1974;92:407-12.
45. Machemer R. Advances in vitrectomy through the pars-plana (author's transl). Klin Monbl Augenheilkd. 1974;164:572-9.
46. Machemer R. Vitrectomy in diabetic retinopathy: removal of preretinal proliferations. Trans Sect Ophthalmol Am Acad Ophthalmol Otolaryngol. 1975;79:OP394-5.
47. Machemer R, Allen AW. Retinal tears 180 degrees and greater. Management with vitrectomy and intravitreal gas. Arch Ophthalmol. 1976;94:1340-6.
48. Machemer R, Buettner H, Parel JM. Vitrectomy, a pars plana approach. Instrumentation. Mod Probl Ophthalmol. 1972;10:172-7.
49. Machemer R, Norton EW. Vitrectomy, a pars plana approach. II. Clinical experience. Mod Probl Ophthalmol. 1972;10:178-85.
50. Machemer R, Norton EW. Vitrectomy. 2. Complications and results. Ber Zusammenkunft Dtsch Ophthalmol Ges. 1972;71:428-33.
51. Machemer R, Parel JM, Norton EW. Vitrectomy: a pars plana approach. Technical improvements and further results. Trans Am Acad Ophthalmol Otolaryngol. 1972;76:462-6.
52. Mandelcorn M, Machemer R. Vitrectomy in the treatment os severe diabetic retinopathy, with follow-up. Mod Probl Ophthalmol. 1975;15:226.
53. Benson WE, Machemer R. Severe perforating injuries treated with pars plana vitrectomy. Am J Ophthalmol. 1976;81:728-32.
54. Mandelcorn MS, Blankenship G, Machemer R. Pars plana vitrectomy for the management of sever diabetic retinopathy. Am J Ophthalmol. 1976;81:561-70.
55. Machemer R. Pars plana vitrectomy. Summary. Trans Sect Ophthalmol Am Acad Ophthalmol Otolaryngol. 1976;81(3 Pt 1):431.
56. Machemer R. Pars plana vitrectomy. Removal of preretinal membranes. Trans Sect Ophthalmol Am Acad Ophthalmol Otolaryngol. 1976;81(3 Pt 1):420-5.
57. Buettner H, Machemer R. Histopathologic findings in human eyes after pars plana vitrectomy and lensectomy. Arch Ophthalmol. 1977;95(11):2029-33.
58. Treister G, Machemer R. Results of vitrectomy for rare proliferative and hemorrhagic diseases. Am J Ophthalmol. 1977;84:394-412.
59. Benson WE, Blankenship GW, Machemer R. Pars plana lens removal with vitrectomy. Am J Ophthalmol. 1977;84:150-2.
60. Abrams GW, Topping T, Machemer R. An improved method for practice vitrectomy. Arch Ophthalmol. 1978;96:521-5.
61. Wilson-Holt N, Leaver PK. Extended criteria for vitrectomy and fluid/silicone oil exchange. Eye. 1990;4:850-4.
62. Leaver PK, Lean JS. Management of giant retinal tears using vitrectomy and silicone oil/fluid exchange. A preliminary report. Trans Ophthalmol Soc UK. 1981;101:189-91.
63. Leaver PK, Billington BM. Vitrectomy and fluid/silicone-oil exchange for giant retinal tears: 5 years follow-up. Graefes Arch Clin Exp Ophthalmol. 1989;227:323-7.
64. Chang S. Low viscosity liquid fluorochemicals in vitreous surgery. Am J Ophthalmol. 1987;103:38-43.
65. Glaser BM, Carter JB, Kuppermann BD, et al. Perfluoro-octane in the treatment of giant retinal tears with proliferative vitreoretinopathy. Ophthalmology. 1991;98:1613-21.
66. Mathis A, Pagot V, Gazagne C, et al. Giant retinal tears. Surgical techniques and results using perfluorodecalin and silicone oil tamponade. Retina. 1992;12(3 Suppl):S7-10.
67. Brourman ND, Blumenkranz MS, Cox MS, et al. Silicone oil for the treatment of severe proliferative diabetic retinopathy. Ophthalmology. 1989;96:759-64.
68. McLeod D. Silicone-oil injection during closed microsurgery for diabetic retinal detachment. Graefes Arch Clin Exp Ophthalmol. 1986;224:55-9.
69. McLeod D. Microsurgical management of neovascularisation secondary to posterior segment ischaemia. Eye. 1991;5:252-9.
70. Oldendoerp J, Spitznas M. Factors influencing the results of vitreous surgery in diabetic retinopathy. I. Iris rubeosis and/or active neovascularization at the fundus. Graefes Arch Clin Exp Ophthalmol. 1989;227:1-8.
71. de Juan E, Hardy M, Hatchell DL, et al. The effect of intraocular silicone oil on anterior chamber oxygen pressure in cats. Arch Ophthalmol. 1986;104(7):1063-4.
72. Wilson CA, Berkowitz BA, McCuen BW, et al. Measurement of preretinal oxygen tension in the vitrectomized human eye using fluorine-19 magnetic resonance spectroscopy. Arch Ophthalmol. 1992;110:1098-100.
73. Castellarin A, Grigorian R, Bhagat N, et al. Vitrectomy with silicone oil infusion in severe diabetic retinopathy. Br J Ophthalmol. 2003;87:318-21.
74. McCuen BW, Rinkoff JS. Silicone oil for progressive anterior ocular neovascularization after failed diabetic vitrectomy. Arch Ophthalmol. 1989;107:677-82.

75. Goldbaum MH, McCuen BW, Hanneken AM, et al. Silicone oil tamponade to seal macular holes without position restrictions. Ophthalmology. 1998;105:2140-7.
76. Lai JC, Stinnett SS, McCuen BW. Comparison of silicone oil versus gas tamponade in the treatment of idiopathic full-thickness macular hole. Ophthalmology. 2003;110:1170-4.
77. Pertile G, Claes C. Silicone oil vs gas for the treatment of full-thickness macular hole. Bull Soc Belge Ophthalmol 1999;274:31-6.
78. Van De Moere A, Stalmans P. Anatomical and visual outcome of macular hole surgery with infracyanine green-assisted peeling of the internal limiting membrane, endodrainage, and silicone oil tamponade. Am J Ophthalmol. 2003;136:879-87.
79. Akiba J, Konno S, Yoshida A. Retinal detachment associated with a macular hole in severely myopic eyes. Am J Ophthalmol. 1999;128:654-5.
80. Gonvers M, Machemer R. A new approach to treating retinal detachment with macular hole. Am J Ophthalmol. 1982;94:468-72.
81. Haut J, Van Effenterre G, Flamand M. Treatment of macular hole retinal detachment with silicone oil, with or without argon laser photocoagulation. Ophthalmologica. 1983;187:25-8.
82. Wolfensberger TJ, Gonvers M. Long-term follow-up of retinal detachment due to macular hole in myopic eyes treated by temporary silicone oil tamponade and laser photocoagulation. Ophthalmology. 1999;106:1786-91.
83. Davis JL, Serfass MS, Lai MY, et al. Silicone oil in repair of retinal detachments caused by necrotizing retinitis in HIV infection. Arch Ophthalmol. 1995;113:1401-9.
84. Dugel PU, Liggett PE, Lee MB, et al. Repair of retinal detachment caused by cytomegalovirus retinitis in patients with the acquired immunodeficiency syndrome. Am J Ophthalmol. 1991;112:235-42.
85. Freeman WR, Henderly DE, Wan WL, et al. Prevalence, pathophysiology, and treatment of rhegmatogenous retinal detachment in treated cytomegalovirus retinitis. Am J Ophthalmol. 1987;103:527-36.
86. Freeman WR, Quiceno JI, Crapotta JA, et al. Surgical repair of rhegmatogenous retinal detachment in immunosuppressed patients with cytomegalovirus retinitis. Ophthalmology. 1992;99:466-74.
87. Garcia RF, Flores-Aguilar M, Quiceno JI, et al. Results of rhegmatogenous retinal detachment repair in cytomegalovirus retinitis with and without scleral buckling. Ophthalmology. 1995;102:236-45.
88. Lucke K, Reinking U, el-Hifnawi E, et al. Acute retinal necrosis. Klin Monbl Augenheilkd. 1988;193:602-7.
89. Martidis A, Danis RP, Ciulla TA. Treating cytomegalovirus retinitis-related retinal detachment by combining silicone oil tamponade and ganciclovir implant. Ophthalmic Surg Lasers. 2002;33:135-9.
90. Meier P. [Retinal detachment in children, differential diagnosis and current therapy]. Klin Monbl Augenheilkd. 2008;225:779-90.
91. Ferrone PJ, McCuen BW, de Juan E, et al. The efficacy of silicone oil for complicated retinal detachments in the pediatric population. Arch Ophthalmol. 1994;112:773-7.
92. Wong D, Cazabon S, Ali H, et al. Can the sequential use of conventional silicone oil and heavy oil be a strategy for the management of proliferative vitreoretinopathy? Ann Acad Med Singapore. 2006;35:181-4.
93. Girard P, Mimoun G, Karpouzas I, et al. Clinical risk factors for proliferative vitreoretinopathy after retinal detachment surgery. Retina. 1994;14:417-24.
94. Spiegel D, Nasemann J, Nawrocki J, et al. Severe ocular trauma managed with primary pars plana vitrectomy and silicone oil. Retina. 1997;17:275-85.
95. Antoszyk AN, McCuen BW, de Juan E, et al. Silicone oil injection after failed primary vitreous surgery in severe ocular trauma. Am J Ophthalmol. 1989;107:537-43.
96. Skorpik C, Menapace R, Gnad HD, et al. Silicone oil implantation in penetrating injuries complicated by PVR. Results from 1982 to 1986. Retina. 1989;9:8-14.
97. Romano MR, Groenwald C, Das R, et al. Removal of Densiron-68 with a 23-gauge transconjunctival vitrectomy system. Eye. 2009;23:715-7.
98. Stappler T, Williams R, Gibran SK, et al. A guide to the removal of heavy silicone oil. Br J Ophthalmol. 2008;92:844-7.
99. Li W, Zheng J, Zheng Q, et al. Clinical complications of Densiron 68 intraocular tamponade for complicated retinal detachment. Eye. 2010;24:21-8.
100. Beekhuis WH, Ando F, Zivojnovic R, et al. Basal iridectomy at 6 o'clock in the aphakic eye treated with silicone oil: prevention of keratopathy and secondary glaucoma. Br J Ophthalmol. 1987;71:197-200.
101. Li KK, Wong D. Avoiding retinal slippage during macular translocation surgery with 360° retinotomy. Graefes Arch Clin Exp Ophthalmol. 2008;246:649-51.
102. Hutton WL, Azen SP, Blumenkranz MS, et al. The effects of silicone oil removal. Silicone Study Report 6. Arch Ophthalmol. 1994;112:778-85.
103. Jiang Y, Li X. The best timing of silicone oil removal. Zhonghua Yan Ke Za Zhi. 1997;33:39-41.
104. Sandner D, Herbrig E, Engelmann K. High-density silicone oil (Densiron) as a primary intraocular tamponade: 12-month follow-up. Graefes Arch Clin Exp Ophthalmol. 2007;245:1097-105.
105. Avci R. Cataract surgery and transpupillary silicone oil removal through a single scleral tunnel incision under topical anesthesia; sutureless surgery. Int Ophthalmol. 2001;24:337-41.
106. Boscia F, Recchimurzo N, Cardascia N, et al. Phacoemulsification with transpupillary silicone oil removal and lens implantation through a corneal incision using topical anesthesia. J Cataract Refract Surg. 2003;29:1113-9.
107. Clark C, Habib MS, Steel DH. Combined phacoemulsification and transpupillary removal of heavy silicone oil. J Cataract Refract Surg. 2008;34:1640-3.
108. Dabil H, Akduman L, Olk RJ, et al. Comparison of silicone oil removal with passive drainage alone versus passive drainage combined with air-fluid exchange. Retina. 2002;22:597-601.

109. Dada VK, Talwar D, Sharma N, et al. Phacoemulsification combined with silicone oil removal through a posterior capsulorhexis. J Cataract Refract Surg. 2001;27:1243-7.
110. Fletcher ME, Peyman GA. A simplified technique for the removal of liquid silicone from vitrectomized eyes. Retina. 1985;5:168-71.
111. Frau E, Lautier-Frau M, Labetoulle M, et al. Phacoemulsification combined with silicone oil removal through the posterior capsulorhexis tear. Retina. 2002;22:158-62.
112. Herbert EN, Williamson TH. Combined removal of silicone oil plus internal search (ROSO-plus) following retinal detachment surgery. Eye. 2007;21:925-9.
113. Jonas JB, Hugger P, Sauder G. Topical anesthesia for transpupillary silicone oil removal combined with cataract surgery. J Cataract Refract Surg. 2005;31:1781-2.
114. Kapran Z, Acar. Removal of silicone oil with 25-gauge transconjunctival sutureless vitrectomy system. Retina. 2007;27:1059-64.
115. Kapran Z, Acar N, Unver YB, et al. Passive removal of silicone oil with a 25-gauge sutureless system. Jpn J Ophthalmol. 2008;52:63-6.
116. Korobelnik JF, Alietta A, Hannouche D, et al. Value of posterior capsulorrhexis during combined phacoemulsification and silicone oil removal. J Fr Ophtalmol. 1998;21:649-53.
117. Larkin GB, Flaxel CJ, Leaver PK. Phacoemulsification and silicone oil removal through a single corneal incision. Ophthalmology. 1998;105:2023-7.
118. Michel G, Meyer L, Naoun KO. Active drainage combined with air-fluid exchange for silicone oil removal: advantages and long-term follow-up. J Fr Ophtalmol. 2008;31:777-80.
119. Yildirim R, Aras C, Ozdamar A, et al. Silicone oil removal using a self-sealing corneal incision under topical anesthesia. Ophthalmic Surg Lasers. 1999;30:24-6.
120. Bassat IB, Desatnik H, Alhalel A, et al. Reduced rate of retinal detachment following silicone oil removal. Retina. 2000;20:597-603.
121. Abu El-Asrar AM, Al-Bishi SM, Kangave D. Outcome of temporary silicone oil tamponade in complex rhegmatogenous retinal detachment. Eur J Ophthalmol. 2003;13:474-81.
122. Falkner CI, Binder S, Kruger A. Outcome after silicone oil removal. Br J Ophthalmol. 2001;85:1324-7.
123. Goezinne F, EC LAH, Berendschot TT, et al. Low redetachment rate due to encircling scleral buckle in giant retinal tears treated with vitrectomy and silicone oil. Retina. 2008;28:485-92.
124. Jonas JB, Budde WM, Knorr HL. Timing of retinal redetachment after removal of intraocular silicone oil tamponade. Am J Ophthalmol. 1999;128:628-31.
125. Jonas JB, Knorr HL, Rank RM, et al. Retinal redetachment after removal of intraocular silicone oil tamponade. Br J Ophthalmol. 2001;85:1203-7.
126. La Heij EC, Hendrikse F, Kessels AG. Results and complications of temporary silicone oil tamponade in patients with complicated retinal detachments. Retina. 2001;21:107-14.
127. Lam RF, Cheung BT, Yuen CY, et al. Retinal redetachment after silicone oil removal in proliferative vitreoretinopathy: a prognostic factor analysis. Am J Ophthalmol. 2008;145:527-33.
128. Li H, Zhu X, Jiang D. Risk factors of retinal redetachment after expected silicone oil removal. Yan Ke Xue Bao. 2005;21:92-4.
129. Unlu N, Kocaoglan H, Acar MA, et al. Outcome of complex retinal detachment surgery after silicone oil removal. Int Ophthalmol. 2004;25:33-6.
130. Jonas JB, Budde WM, Panda-Jonas S. Cataract surgery combined with transpupillary silicone oil removal through planned posterior capsulotomy. Ophthalmology. 1998;105: 1234-7
131. Tufail A, Schwartz SD, Gregor ZJ. Prophylactic argon laser retinopexy prior to removal of silicone oil: a pilot study. Eye. 1997;11:328-30.
132. Nowack C, Lucke K, Laqua H. Removal of silicone oil in treatment of so-called emulsification glaucoma. Ophthalmologe. 1992;89:462-4.
133. Moisseiev J, Barak A, Manaim T, et al. Removal of silicone oil in the management of glaucoma in eyes with emulsified silicone. Retina. 1993;13:290-5.
134. Kumar A, Dada T, Singh RP, et al. Diode laser trans-scleral cyclophotocoagulation for glaucoma following silicone oil removal. Clin Experiment Ophthalmol. 2001;29:220-4.
135. Eckardt C, Behrendt S, Zwick A. Results of silicone oil removal from eyes treated with retinectomies. Ger J Ophthalmol. 1992;1:2-6.
136. Flaxel CJ, Mitchell SM, Aylward GW. Visual outcome after silicone oil removal and recurrent retinal detachment repair. Eye. 2000;14:834-8.
137. Scholda C, Egger S, Lakits A, et al. Silicone oil removal: results, risks and complications. Acta Ophthalmol Scand. 1997;75:695-9.
138. Zhong XF, Li YP, Lin JX, et al. Histopathological and ultrastructural characteristics of oil-associated complications in silicone oil-filled human eyes. Zhonghua Yan Ke Za Zhi. 2005;41:31-6.
139. Federman JL, Schubert HD. Complications associated with the use of silicone oil in 150 eyes after retina-vitreous surgery. Ophthalmology. 1988;95:870-6.
140. Gao RL, Neubauer L, Tang S, et al. Silicone oil in the anterior chamber. Graefes Arch Clin Exp Ophthalmol. 1989;227:106-9.
141. Burk LL, Shields MB, Proia AD, et al. Intraocular pressure following intravitreal silicone oil injection. Ophthalmic Surg. 1988;19:565-9.
142. Lucke K, Strobel B, Foerster M, et al. Secondary glaucoma after silicone oil surgery. Klin Monbl Augenheilkd. 1990;196: 205-9.
143. Zborowski-Gutman L, Treister G, Naveh N, et al. Acute glaucoma following vitrectomy and silicone oil injection. Br J Ophthalmol. 1987;71:903-6.
144. Haut J, Ullern M, Chermet M, et al. Complications of intraocular injections of silicone combined with vitrectomy. Ophthalmologica. 1980;180:29-35.
145. Okun E. Intravitreal surgery utilizing liquid silicone. A long term followup. Trans Pac Coast Otoophthalmol Soc Annu Meet. 1968;49:141-59.

146. Spraul CW, Jakobczyk-Zmija MJ, Aigner T, et al. Posterior fibrous pseudometaplasia of lens epithelial cells in phacic eyes filled with silicone oil. Graefes Arch Clin Exp Ophthalmol. 2002;240:829-34.
147. Abrams GW, Azen SP, Barr CC, et al. The incidence of corneal abnormalities in the Silicone Study. Silicone Study Report 7. Arch Ophthalmol. 1995;113:764-9.
148. Sternberg P, Hatchell DL, Foulks GN,et al. The effect of silicone oil on the cornea. Arch Ophthalmol. 1985;103:90-4.
149. Sekundo W, Hesse L, Schmidt J, et al. Histopathology of 8 corneal buttons after penetrating keratoplasty in silicone oil-associated keratopathy. Klin Monbl Augenheilkd. 2001;218:424-8.
150. Noorily SW, Foulks GN, McCuen BW. Results of penetrating keratoplasty associated with silicone oil retinal tamponade. Ophthalmology. 1991;98:1186-9.
151. Roters S, Hamzei P, Szurman P, et al. Combined penetrating keratoplasty and vitreoretinal surgery with silicone oil: a 1-year follow-up. Graefes Arch Clin Exp Ophthalmol. 2003;241: 24-33.
152. Laidlaw DA, Karia N, Bunce C, et al. Is prophylactic 360-degree laser retinopexy protective? Risk factors for retinal redetachment after removal of silicone oil. Ophthalmology. 2002;109:153-8.
153. Barr CC, Lai MY, Lean JS, et al. Postoperative intraocular pressure abnormalities in the Silicone Study. Silicone Study Report 4. Ophthalmology. 1993;100:1629-35.
154. McCuen BW, 2nd, Landers MB, 3rd, Machemer R. The use of silicone oil following failed vitrectomy for retinal detachment with advanced proliferative vitreoretinopathy. Ophthalmology. 1985;92:1029-34.
155. Minamoto A, Nakano KE, Tanimoto S, et al. Ultrasound biomicroscopy in the diagnosis of persistent hypotony after vitrectomy. Am J Ophthalmol. 1997;123:711-3.
156. Lewis H, Verdaguer JI. Surgical treatment for chronic hypotony and anterior proliferative vitreoretinopathy. Am J Ophthalmol. 1996;122:228-35.
157. Zarbin MA, Michels RG, Green WR. Dissection of epiciliary tissue to treat chronic hypotony after surgery for retinal detachment with proliferative vitreoretinopathy. Retina. 1991;11:208-13.
158. Heidenkummer HP, Kampik A, Thierfelder S. Experimental evaluation of in vitro stability of purified polydimethylsiloxanes (silicone oil) in viscosity ranges from 1000 to 5000 centistokes. Retina. 1992;12(3 Suppl):S28-32.
159. Caramoy A, Schroder S, Fauser S, et al. In vitro emulsification assessment of new silicone oils. Br J Ophthalmol. 2010;94: 509-12.
160. Meng Q, Zhang S, Cheng H, et al. Long-term outcomes of Oxane Hd as intraocular tamponade in the treatment of complicated retinal detachment. Graefes Arch Clin Exp Ophthalmol. 2010;248:1091-6.
161. Li W, Zheng Q, Wang X, et al. Clinical results of Densiron 68 intraocular tamponade for complicated retinal detachment. Ophthalmologica. 2010;224:354-60.
162. Auriol S, Pagot-Mathis V, Mahieu L, et al. Efficacy and safety of heavy silicone oil Densiron 68 in the treatment of complicated retinal detachment with large inferior retinectomy. Graefes Arch Clin Exp Ophthalmol. 2008;246:1383-9.
163. Herbrig E, Sandner D, Engelmann K. Anatomical and functional results of endotamponade with heavy silicone oil - Densiron 68 - in complicated retinal detachment. Ophthalmic Res. 2007;39:198-206.
164. Lappas A, Foerster AM, Kirchhof B. Use of heavy silicone oil (Densiron-68) in the treatment of persistent macular holes. Acta Ophthalmol. 2009;87:866-70.
165. Rizzo S, Genovesi-Ebert F, Vento A, et al. Heavy silicone oil (Densiron-68) for the treatment of persistent macular holes. Densiron-68 endotamponade for persistent macular holes. Graefes Arch Clin Exp Ophthalmol. 2009;247:1471-6.
166. Wickham L, Tranos P, Hiscott P, et al. The use of silicone oil-RMN3 (Oxane HD) as heavier-than-water internal tamponade in complicated inferior retinal detachment surgery. Graefes Arch Clin Exp Ophthalmol. 2010;248:1225-31.
167. Wong D, Kumar I, Quah SA, et al. Comparison of postoperative intraocular pressure in patients with Densiron-68 vs conventional silicone oil: a case-control study. Eye. 2009;23:190-4.
168. Ang GS, Murphy AL, Ng WS, et al. Oxane HD and retinal detachment surgery in routine clinical practice. Ophthalmologica. 2010;224:347-53.

8 Intraocular Gases in Vitreoretinal Surgery

Shaheeda Mohamed, Timothy YY Lai

Introduction

Vitreous substitutes as surgical adjuncts have been described as early as 1911 when Ohm injected air into the vitreous cavity to treat retinal detachment.[1] In 1938, Rosengren further built on this concept with the technique of internal gas tamponade.[2] Modern vitrectomy techniques introduced by Machemer in the 1970s accelerated the use of vitreous substitutes for intraoperative and postoperative vitreous replacement.[3] Advances in surgical techniques, instrumentation and vitreous substitutes over the past few decades have greatly improved the anatomical and functional success rates of vitreoretinal surgery. The three most common types of vitreous substitutes in use today are intraocular gas, silicone oil and perfluorocarbon liquid (PFCL). This chapter will review the properties, indications of use and complications associated with commonly used intraocular gases in vitreoretinal surgery.

Intraocular Gases and Kinetics

The high surface tension between gas and fluid enables formation of an effective seal around a retinal break, thus allowing the retinal pigment epithelium (RPE) to absorb any remaining subretinal fluid to facilitate reattachment of the retina.[4] Compared with silicone oil and PFCLs, gases provide the highest surface tension. Since the specific gravity of gases is lower than that of water, the intraocular gas bubble has buoyancy that keeps the retina against the RPE. This buoyancy effect is greatest at the apex of the gas bubble.[5] With careful positioning of the patient's head, the buoyancy forces can be directed to the desired manner so that retinal break can be placed at the apex of the bubble, until chorioretinal adhesions created by laser photocoagulation or cryotherapy can be established to seal off the retinal break. In cases of giant retinal tear (GRT), the buoyancy force of intraocular gases may also be used to unroll the edges of a GRT. However, this role has increasingly been supplanted by the introduction of PFCLs.

Four different intraocular gases are commonly used in vitreoretinal surgery; air, sulfur hexafluoride (SF_6), perfluoroethane (C_2F_6) and perfluoropropane (C_3F_8). These gases are colorless, odorless and inert in the vitreous cavity. When injected into the vitreous cavity, air does not expand, while pure SF_6, C_2F_6 and C_3F_8 gas will expand. When the gas is inside the vitreous cavity, three different phases can be distinguished;(1) expansion; (2) equilibrium and (3) dissolution (Fig. 8.1). The initial gas expansion is a result of the absorption of nitrogen, oxygen and carbon dioxide from the surrounding tissue fluid into the gas bubble. The most rapid rate of expansion occurs within the initial 6–8 hours after gas injection. During the equilibrium phase, the partial pressures between the two compartments equilibrate as the diffusion of nitrogen into the gas is balanced by the diffusion of gas into the surrounding fluid. Finally, during dissolution phase, there is a net exit of gases as they are ultimately absorbed into the bloodstream. Absorption of intraocular gas bubbles is described reasonably accurately by first-order kinetics which predicts that a constant volume percentage of

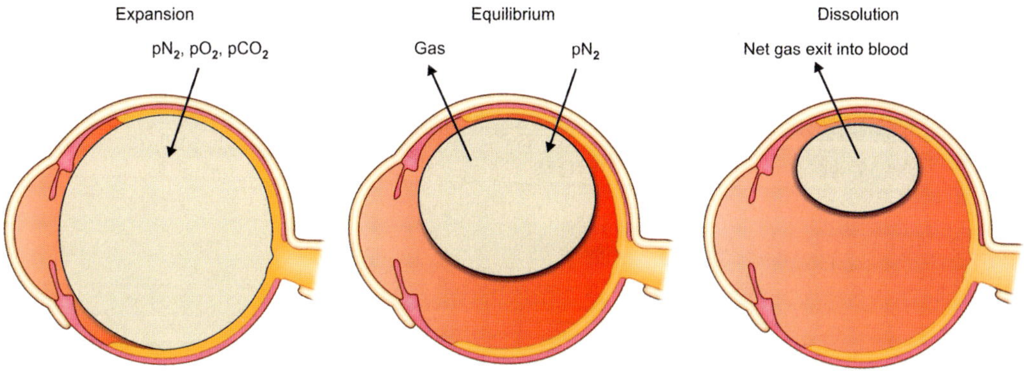

▲ **Figure 8.1**
Phases of intraocular gas kinetics inside the vitreous cavity

the intraocular gas absorbs over a given unit of time.[6-8] The dynamics of intraocular gas bubble depend on a number of factors including initial gas concentration and volume, lens status and history of prior vitrectomy.

The physical properties and gas dynamics are summarized in Table 8.1. A pure SF_6 bubble expands by about two times its injected volume within 24–48 hours with an average effective duration of 1–2 weeks. A pure C_3F_8 bubble expands to about four times its original volume within 72–96 hours and lasts within the vitreous cavity for 6–8 weeks. The maximum effective duration of the tamponade is approximately equal to 3 half-lives.[9]

Intraocular gases can be used in office or operative settings. Following vitrectomy surgery for retinal detachment, most vitreoretinal surgeons use a nonexpansile gas fill that allows placement of a large gas bubble to tamponade a large area of retina. In contrast, pneumatic retinopexy involves the injection of a small, usually pure, expansile intraocular gas bubble in a nonvitrectomized eye in order to provide focal tamponade over a retinal break. Intraocular gas may also be used as an adjunct in scleral buckling procedures known as pneumatic buckle. Superior tears with retinal detachment without proliferative vitreoretinopathy (PVR) can be treated with air or short-acting gases such as SF_6. Longer-acting gas, such as C_3F_8, can be used for retinal detachment with inferior tears, GRTs, or more complex rhegmatogenous and tractional retinal detachment cases with PVR, except when silicone oil is preferred.

Techniques of Fluid-Air Exchange and Intraocular Gas Injection

Following vitrectomy, intraocular gases are usually injected via the pars plana infusion line after fluid (e.g. balanced salt solution) in the vitreous cavity is replaced by air. This fluid-air exchange may be performed by passive or active aspiration under direct visualization. With passive aspiration, a silicone tip or flute needle is used and the pressure of air entering the vitreous cavity through the infusion cannula causes the

TABLE 8.1: Physical properties and dynamics of commonly used gases in vitreoretinal surgery

Gas	*Molecular weight*	*Maximal expansion*	*Duration*	*Nonexpansile concentration*	*Expansivity (times)*
Air	29	Not applicable	5–7 days	Not applicable	0
SF_6	146	24–48 hrs	1–2 weeks	20%	2
C_2F_6	138	36–60 hrs	4–5 weeks	16%	3.3
C_3F_8	188	72–96 hrs	6–8 weeks	12%	4

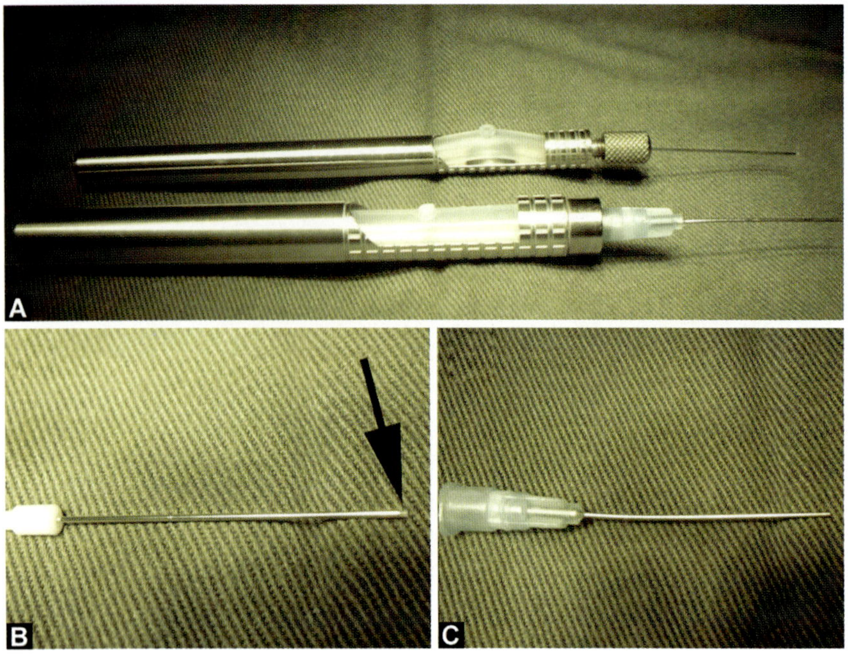

Figures 8.2A to C

(A) Photographs of silicone tip needle (above) and flute needle (below); (B) Close up view of the silicone tip needle. The soft silicone tip (arrow) has a smaller lumen and is less likely to cause trauma to the retina on touching the retina; (C) Close up view of the flute needle tip which has a wider lumen compared with the silicone tip and thus has a faster aspiration rate

intraocular fluid to egress through the lumen of the aspiration needle, which is vented to the atmosphere (Figs 8.2A to C). Fluid-air exchange with active aspiration into the vitrectomy cassette is more rapid, but may result in hypotony if the aspiration of fluid is faster than the inflow of air. Subretinal fluid in eyes with a retinal detachment is usually removed during surgery via the retinal break or a drainage retinotomy created in a more posterior location.

The introduction of PFCLs in vitreoretinal surgery has further enhanced the surgical techniques.[10] PFCLs have a higher specific density than water and thus allowing displacement of subretinal fluid anteriorly via the retinal break to flatten the retina. Their low viscosity permits easy injection and withdrawal through instruments. PFCLs are also optically clear, and tamponade using PFCLs can facilitate application of endolaser, especially with more posterior breaks. PFCLs are intended for long-term vitreous substitutes and they can be exchanged with air and gas or directly with silicone oil.

When preparing the gas for injection, a sterile filter (e.g. 0.22 μm Millipore) is recommended to prevent microbial contamination of the gas. A 50 ml syringe is flushed several times with the pure gas to avoid dilution of the desired concentration with residual air. As diffusion will alter the effective gas concentration, the gas should not be left in the syringe for a prolonged period of time prior to injection. For traditional 20-gauge vitrectomy, one sclerotomy site is closed and the second sclerotomy site is sutured without tying the knot (Figs 8.3A to D). The second sclerotomy site is closed temporarily and the infusion tubing is clamped to maintain the eye at a constant pressure. The gas syringe is then attached to the infusion tubing and the clamp is removed with gentle opening of the sclerotomy. Approximately, 35–40 ml of the gas mixture is gently lavaged through the eye as air in the vitreous cavity is expelled through the open sclerotomy. The suture is then tied to close the second sclerotomy site. Finally, the infusion cannula is removed and a suture is used to close the final infusion line sclerotomy site. For 23- or 25-gauge vitrectomy, gas can be injected via the infusion cannula while the trocars are in place. The trocars can then be removed after injection of 35–40 ml of the gas mixture and the integrity of the wound can be assessed.

Another technique of injecting gas following vitrectomy is to close the second sclerotomy site completely, followed by lavage of gas into the eye via the infusion cannula while the air is expelled using a 25-gauge needle, inserted through the pars plana. If the eye becomes soft during closure of the third sclerotomy site, additional gas can be injected at the pars plana via a 30-gauge needle attached to a smaller 3 ml syringe containing the gas mixture.

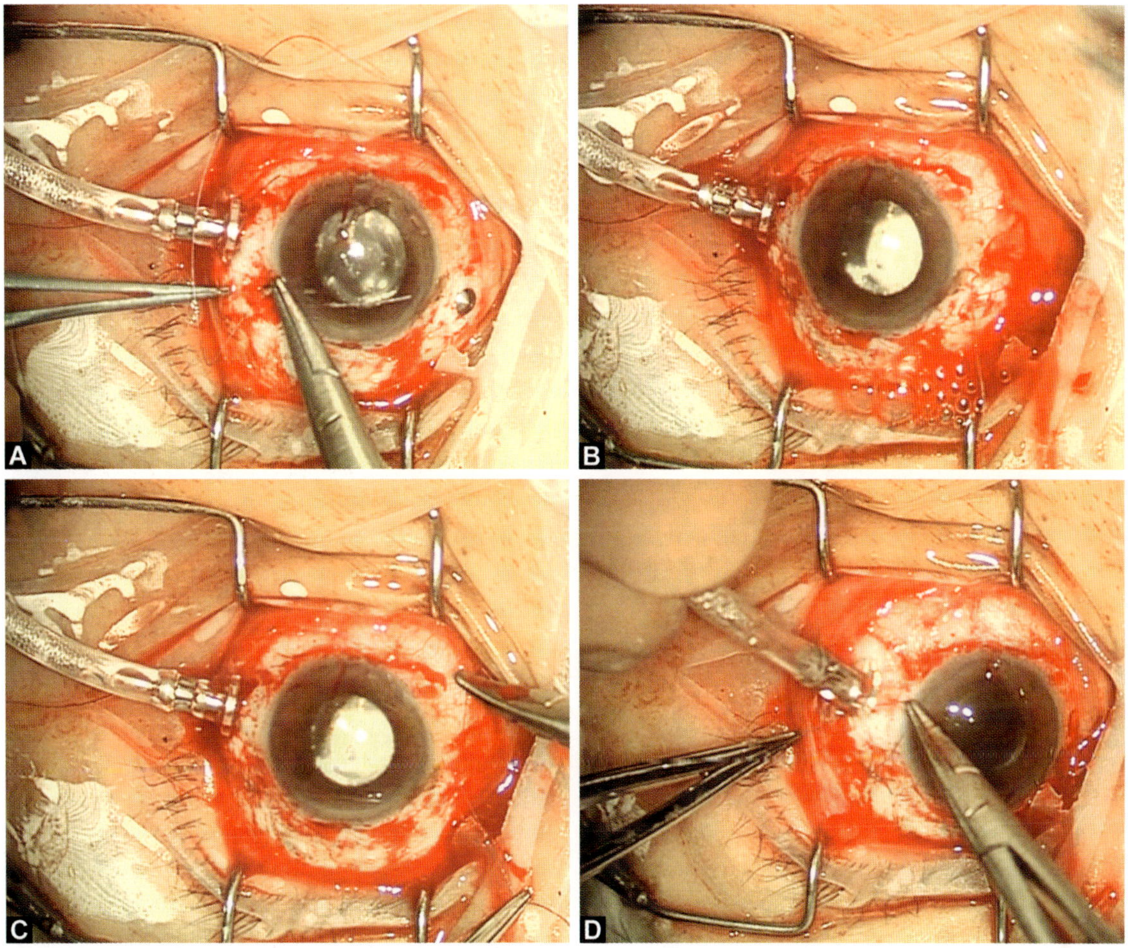

▲ **Figures 8.3A to D**

Steps involved in air or gas exchange during vitreoretinal surgery. (A) Closure of one sclerotomy site with suture; (B) Gentle opening of the temporary knot at the second sclerotomy site to allow air to escape while gas mixture is being injected via the infusion tubing into the eye; (C) Closure of the second sclerotomy site; (D) Removal of the infusion tubing and closure of the infusion sclerotomy site

Uses of Intraocular Gases

▶ Pneumatic Retinopexy

Pneumatic retinopexy is primarily indicated for uncomplicated retinal detachment with retinal breaks involving the superior 8 clock hours of the fundus. The multicenter pneumatic retinopexy trial and other studies have shown that despite lower single operation success rates (about 74%) with pneumatic retinopexy as compared to scleral buckling procedures, the final surgical success (about 96%) is not disadvantaged by the initial pneumatic retinopexy.[11,12] Complications of this technique include subretinal passage of gas, iatrogenic retinal breaks, progression of detachment with macular involvement and PVR.

The technique involves the injection of intraocular gas before or after retinopexy, retinopexy of retinal breaks with cryotherapy or laser and maintenance of specific head posture by the patient after surgery. The desired volume of gas (usually 0.3–0.5 ml) is injected rapidly into the vitreous cavity in order to minimize formation of small "fish-egg" bubbles (Fig. 8.4). The intraocular pressure (IOP) is monitored by digital palpation as the gas is injected into the eye. If the eye is already hypotonous after drainage of subretinal fluid, gas

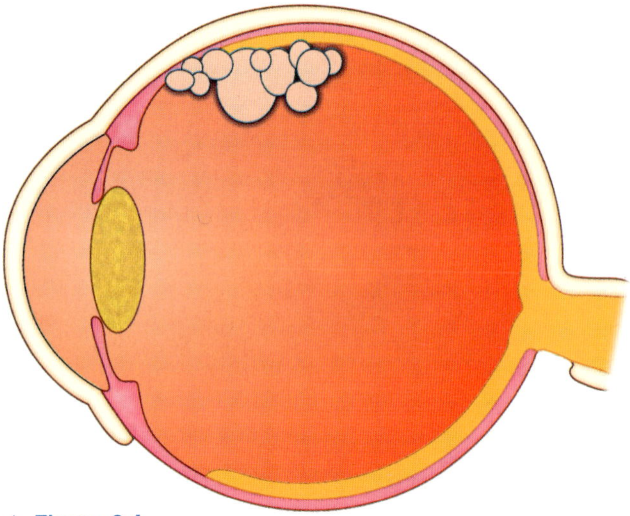

▲ **Figure 8.4**

"Fish egg" bubble formation from gas injection in pneumatic retinopexy

may be injected with a 30-gauge needle attached to a 3 ml syringe via the pars plana. If the eye is normotensive, vitreous or aqueous fluid must be removed to allow injection of more than 0.2 ml of gas, which is the maximum volume of gas that can be injected into a normotensive eye. The first method involves making a limbal anterior chamber paracentesis with a slit-knife or 30-gauge needle for aqueous drainage after gas injection. A repeat paracentesis after 5–10 minutes may normalize the pressure if the IOP remains elevated. The second method involves the aspiration of vitreous fluid before gas injection, using a 22–25-gauge needle attached to a 1 ml or 3 ml syringe placed via the pars plana. This method allows a larger volume of gas to be injected than the first technique of paracentesis. However, the latter method might potentially increase the risk of retinal complications during the vitreous aspiration.[13]

Intraocular gases can also be injected in association with sclera buckling procedures, especially when there is substantial residual subretinal fluid.

Macular Hole Surgery

In the original description of macular hole (MH) repair by Kelly and Wendel, the surgery has been suggested to be a five step procedure; (1) posterior vitrectomy, (2) posterior hyaloid removal, (3) internal limiting membrane removal, (4) intraocular gas tamponade and (5) one week of face down posturing postoperatively (Figs 8.5A to D). The presence of intraocular gas provides isolation or waterproofing of the MH from the vitreous cavity by surface tension of the gas-liquid interface. It may also mechanically tamponade the hole and can provide a template over which nascent bridging membrane forms. The duration of gas tamponade that is required for MH closure has come under debate in recent years. Recent reports have shown that hole closure can occur as early as the first postoperative day, suggesting that prolonged gas tamponade and face-down posturing may be unnecessary. Similar MH closure rates have been reported in studies comparing air versus 20% SF_6 and with 20% SF_6 versus 12–16% C_3F_8.[5,14,15]

Pneumatic Displacement of Submacular Hemorrhage

Submacular hemorrhage can result in sudden dramatic visual loss and has many causes, such as choroidal neovascularization, polypoidal choroidal vasculopathy, trauma and retinal artery macroaneurysm. The visual prognosis might be poor, especially if there is delayed presentation, thick hemorrhage, foveal involvement and an underlying choroidal neovascularization. The technique of pneumatic displacement involves the injection of an expansile pure C_3F_8 gas (about 0.2–0.3 ml) via the pars plana at 3.5 mm from the limbus with a 30-gauge needle, followed by face down and prone positioning for 5–7 days (Figs 8.6A to C). Intravitreal tissue plasminogen activator (tPA) or intravitreal antivascular endothelial growth factor (anti-VEGF) agents may also be injected at the same setting with the expansile gas as adjuvants.[16-21]

Unrolling the Edges of a Giant Retinal Tear

A GRT may be unrolled using an intraocular gas bubble by placing the patient in a prone position and injecting gas via the infusion cannula, while removing fluid from the anterior vitreous cavity at the same time (upside down fluid-gas exchange). The gas bubble will expand in the vitreous cavity and push the retina against the underlying RPE, unrolling the edges of the GRT as the subretinal fluid moves to the anterior vitreous and is removed through an aspiration needle via the sclerotomy, which is in a dependent position. The patient is then returned to a supine position. Postoperatively, the patient should remain in a prone position to avoid slippage

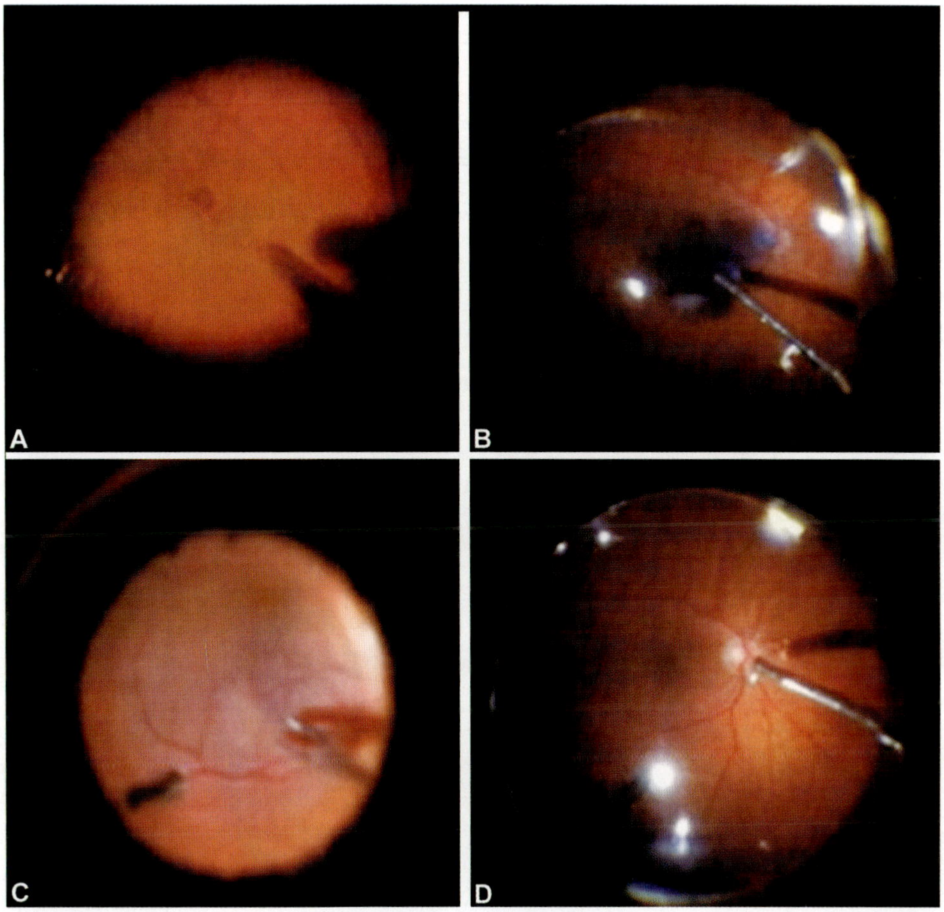

▲ **Figures 8.5A to D**

Steps in a patient undergoing macular hole surgery. (A) Induction of posterior vitreous detachment, if necessary and vitrectomy; (B) Injection of trypan blue dye for staining of internal limiting membrane (ILM) under air; (C) Internal limiting membrane peeling using forceps; (D) Fluid or air exchange using a flute needle

of the GRT edge. The use of PFCLs has allowed a more convenient technique for unrolling the edges of a giant tear.

Postoperative Positioning and Duration of Positioning

Appropriate postoperative positioning is dictated by the size of the intraocular gas bubble, the location of the retinal tear and lens status. Prone positioning in phakic patients can potentially reduce prolonged gas contact with the posterior lens surface. Pseudophakic and aphakic patients with retinal breaks in the superior periphery may avoid prolonged prone positioning because the gas bubble will provide good tamponade in the upright position.

The duration of postoperative positioning is determined by the location of the retinal breaks and the absorption rate of the intraocular gas bubble. An appropriate gas concentration is chosen to provide adequate duration of tamponade. Superior retinal breaks without retinal detachment may be treated with air and shorter-acting gas mixtures (e.g. 5% C_3F_8 or 20% SF_6) may be used to treat superior retinal breaks associated with retinal detachment. Inferior retinal breaks associated with retinal detachment may be treated with longer-acting 12% C_3F_8, so that the gas bubble will remain large enough for at least 10 days in order to provide adequate tamponade for the inferior retinal break to close. Complex retinal detachments with PVR or GRTs usually require prolonged gas tamponade with 10–15% C_3F_8 gas mixture.

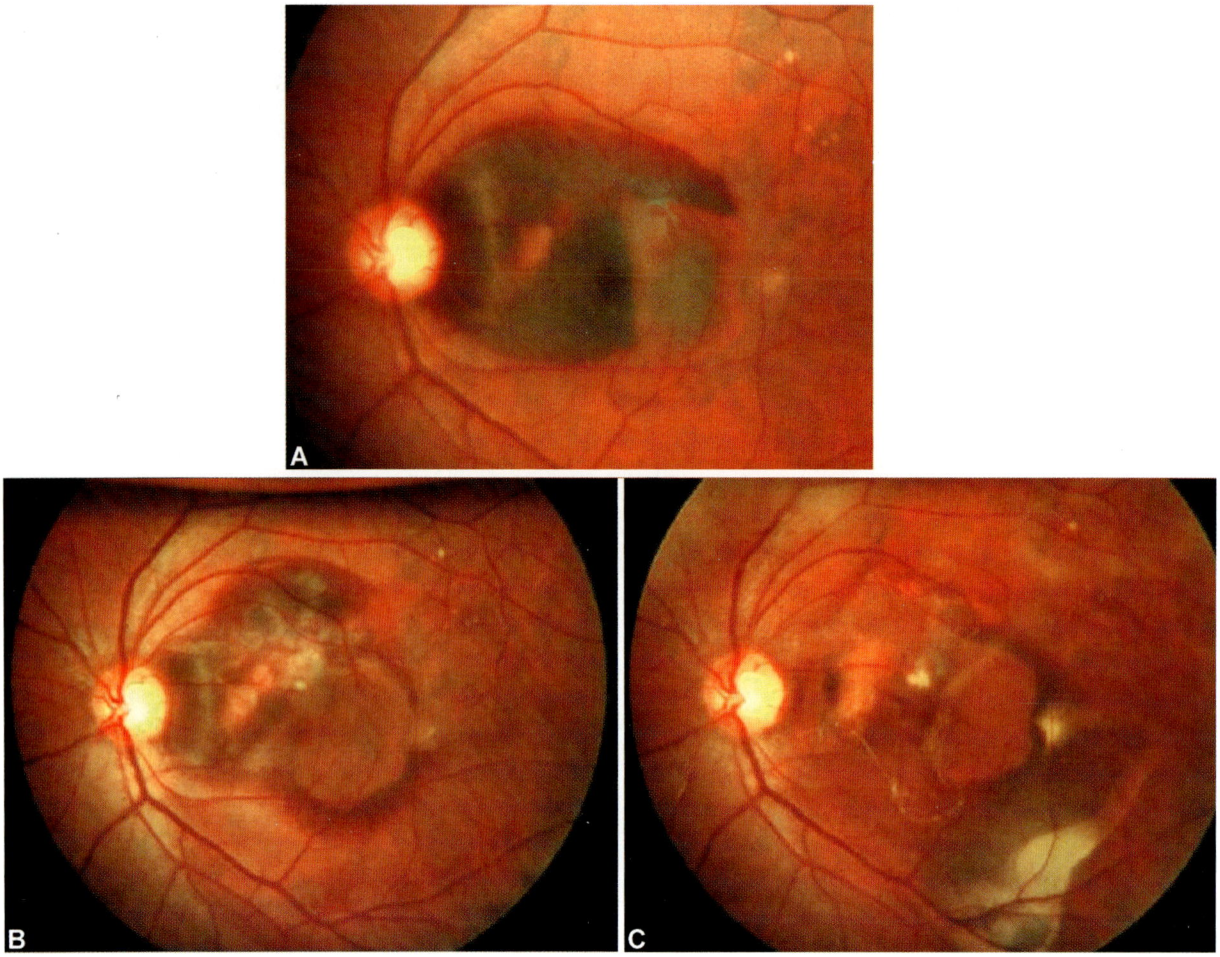

▲ **Figures 8.6A to C**

Gas displacement of submacular hemorrhage. (A) Fundus photograph of a patient with submacular hemorrhage secondary to polypoidal choroidal vasculopathy; (B) Fundus photograph at 3 days after injection of 0.3 ml 100% C_3F_8. The meniscus of the gas bubble can be seen superiorly and the submacular hemorrhage is being displaced away from the macula; (C) Fundus photograph at 14 days after gas injection showing the submacular blood has displaced inferiorly

Contraindications for Intraocular Gas

Postoperatively, patients with intraocular gases *in situ* should be advised against air travel or travelling to high altitudes, since the reduced atmospheric pressure under these conditions will lead to expansion of the intraocular gas bubble and cause considerable increase in intraocular pressure. Early cases may manifest with pain and decreased vision and may be treated by prompt lowering of the altitude of travel. In extreme cases, the rise in IOP can result in retinal vascular occlusions and even globe explosion via the surgical wounds. Experimental studies and clinical observations suggested that less than 0.6–1.0 ml of residual gas might be safe for air travel.[22,23] However, it is still advisable for patients to avoid any air travel when there is residual intravitreal gas bubble.

Patients with intraocular gases *in situ* should also avoid diving. At sea level, the body is exposed to an ambient pressure of one atmosphere absolute (ATA). When diving, the absolute pressure is expressed by the formula ATA = [Depth (in feet of sea water) + 33]/33. Hyperbaric pressures that occur during scuba diving cause the intraocular gas bubble to decrease in size according to Boyle's law, leading to hypotony and partial globe collapse. As the eye goes from hyperbaric conditions to normal sea-level atmospheric pressure during the ascent to the surface, expansion of the intraocular gas bubble occurs and can cause large increase in IOP. Pressure-induced changes in the volume of the gas bubble can also result in choroidal hemorrhage.[24]

Nitrous oxide anesthesia must also be avoided in patients with intraocular gas bubbles. Since nitrous oxide in the blood is highly water-soluble, it enters the intraocular gas bubble and can lead to increase in IOP as the sclerotomies are closed. Later, as the nitrous oxide in the gas bubble returns to the bloodstream, the eye may become hypotonous. If nitrous oxide anesthesia is used during eye surgery, it should be discontinued at least 30 minutes prior to intraocular gas injection to allow clearance of nitrous oxide from the bloodstream and tissues.[25]

Complications of Intraocular Gases

Elevated Intraocular Pressure

Elevation of the IOP is one of the more common complications in eyes with an intraocular gas bubble. Predisposing factors include pre-existing glaucoma, anterior synechiae and impaired aqueous outflow at the drainage angle by hemorrhage, pigment, inflammation, or neovascularization.[26] In the majority of eyes, the elevation in IOP is usually transient and can be managed with topical or systemic antiglaucomatous agents. If the intraocular gas bubble expands to such an extent that the lens-iris diaphragm is shifted forward, leading to iatrogenic angle closure glaucoma, gas aspiration from the vitreous cavity via the pars plana may be indicated. Injection of viscoelastics may help in reformation of the flat anterior chamber. Aphakic eyes may be more prone to angle closure with a very large intraocular gas bubble because the iris can easily be pushed forward, especially when the patient is lying supine. Poor compliance with prone positioning may precipitate this complication. Subsequent evaluation of the anterior chamber angle of the operated eye and the fellow eye by gonioscopy will help to determine whether a laser peripheral iridotomy is indicated.

Cataract

Vitrectomy alone can lead to progressive nuclear sclerosis cataract due to oxidative stress to the crystalline lens or surgical trauma. Prolonged contact of the intraocular gas with the posterior lens surface can lead to gas-induced cataract, presenting typically as "lens feathering" with branching pattern of posterior subcapsular lens changes (Figs 8.7A and B). It usually develops in the first few postoperative days in a patient who is poorly compliant to prone positioning. The posterior subcapsular feathering may be reversible by diligent prone positioning, but if the patient remains noncompliant with prone positioning for more than a week, permanent lens changes, such as lens vacuolation or a diffuse posterior subcapsular cataract, may develop.[27]

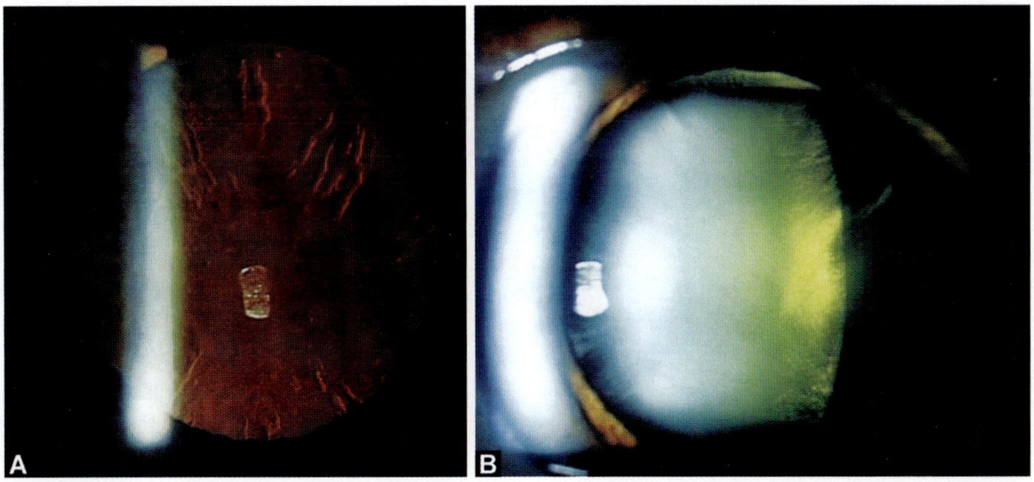

Figures 8.7A and B

Postoperative lens changes with intraocular gas *in situ*. (A) Lens feathering; (B) Posterior subcapsular cataract

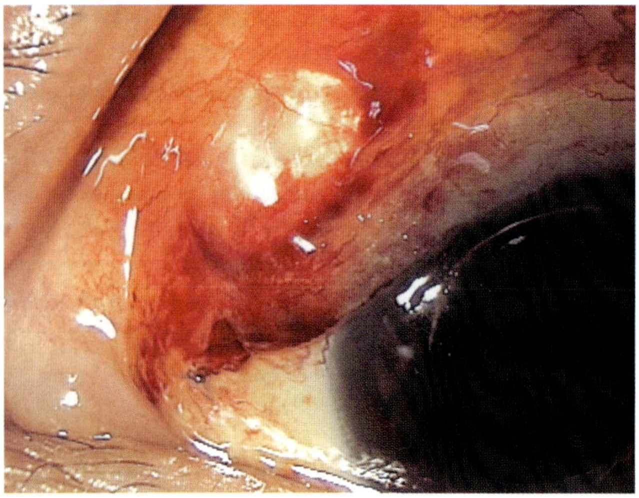

▲ Figure 8.8
Migration of intraocular gas into the subconjunctival space

Migration of the Intraocular Gas Bubble

The intraocular gas bubble can rarely migrate into the subretinal space in pneumatic retinopexy if the tear is larger than the bubble, during fluid-gas exchange when there is unrelieved traction on the retina, or when the gas is injected accidentally into the subretinal space. Although the subretinal intraocular gas bubble will eventually absorb, the retinal break may not be properly sealed by the gas bubble and thus redetachment of the retina can occur. Intraocular gas can also migrate out of the sclerotomy into the subconjunctival space if the sclerotomy wound integrity is not secured at the end of surgery (Fig. 8.8). In phakic or pseudophakic patients, intraocular gas bubble may also migrate into the anterior chamber via weakened zonules or large posterior capsulotomy. Prolonged contact of gas with the corneal endothelium in aphakic eyes may lead to corneal decompensation.[28] These patients should be reminded to avoid sleeping in a supine position.

Inadequate Gas Bubble Size

Inadequate gas fill may develop if the surgery is completed with a smaller than desired intraocular gas bubble. This may occur if inadequate vitreous or subretinal fluid is removed and exchanged with air, or if intraocular gas escapes through the sclerotomy during the perioperative period, leading to loss of intravitreal gas and hypotony. Inadequate gas bubble size may also be caused by premature absorption of the gas due to errors with the reconstitution of gas mixture.

Other Complications

Iatrogenic retinal breaks and PVR are important causes of surgical failure after injection of intraocular gases. Other complications include visual field defects, which have been reported in eyes following MH surgery. Prolonged contact of the intraocular gas bubble with the nerve fiber layer has been postulated to have a role, although other reports have associated these visual field defects with surgical trauma or the use of certain intraoperative stains like indocyanine green.

The intraocular gas bubble is one of the most useful surgical adjuncts in vitreoretinal surgery. A thorough understanding of the properties, indications and potential complications of intraocular gases is essential to optimizing the outcomes of vitreoretinal surgery.

References

1. Olm J. Über die Behandlung der Netzhautablösung durch operative Entleerung der Subretinalen Flüssigkeit und Einspritzung von Luft in den Glaskörper. Albrecht von Graefes Arch Ophthalmol. 1911;79:442-65.
2. Rosengren B. Results of treatment of detachment of the retina with diathermy and injection of air into the vitreous. Acta Ophthalmol. 1938;16:573-9.
3. Machemer R, Buettner H, Norton EW, et al. Vitrectomy: a pars plana approach. Trans Am Acad Ophthalmol Otolaryngol. 1971;75:813-20.
4. de Juan E, McCuen B, Tiedeman J. Intraocular tamponade and surface tension. Surv Ophthalmol. 1985;30:47-51.
5. Gupta D. Face-down posturing after MH surgery. Review. Retina. 2009;29:430-3.
6. Abrams GW, Edelhauser HF, Aaberg TM, et al. Dynamics of intravitreal sulfur hexafluoride gas. Invest Ophthalmol Vis Sci. 1974;13:863-8.
7. Lincoff A, Haft D, Liggett P, et al. Intravitreal expansion of perfluorocarbon bubbles. Arch Ophthalmol. 1980;98:1646.
8. Lincoff H, Mardirossian J, Lincoff A, et al. Intravitreal longevity of three perfluorocarbon gases. Arch Ophthalmol. 1980;98:1610-1.
9. Thompson JT. Kinetics of intraocular gases. Disappearance of air, sulfur hexafluoride, and perfluoropropane after pars plana vitrectomy. Arch Ophthalmol. 1989;107:687-91.
10. Chang S. Low viscosity liquid fluorochemicals in vitreous surgery. Am J Ophthalmol. 1987;103:38-43.
11. Chan CK, Lin SG, Nuthi AS, et al. Pneumatic retinopexy for the repair of retinal detachments: a comprehensive review (1986-2007). Surv Ophthalmol. 2008;53:443-78.
12. Han DP, Mohsin NC, Guse CE, et al. Comparison of pneumatic retinopexy and scleral buckling in the management of primary rhegmatogenous retinal detachment. Southern Wisconsin Pneumatic Retinopexy Study Group. Am J Ophthalmol. 1999;127:741-3.

13. Hilton GF, Das T, Majji AB, et al. Pneumatic retinopexy: principles and practice. Indian J Ophthalmol. 1996;44:131-43.
14. Hasegawa Y, Hata Y, Mochizuki Y, et al. Equivalent tamponade by room air as compared with SF(6) after macular hole surgery. Graefes Arch Clin Exp Ophthalmol; 2009.
15. Kim SS, Smiddy WE, Feuer WJ, et al. Outcomes of sulfur hexafluoride (SF_6) versus perfluoropropane (C_3F_8) gas tamponade for macular hole surgery. Retina. 2008;28:1408-15.
16. Ohji M, Saito Y, Hayashi A, et al. Pneumatic displacement of subretinal hemorrhage without tissue plasminogen activator. Arch Ophthalmol. 1998;116:1362-72.
17. Daneshvar H, Kertes PJ, Leonard BC, et al. Management of submacular hemorrhage with intravitreal sulphur hexafluoride: a pilot study. Can J Ophthalmol. 1999;34:385-8.
18. Mahesh G, Giridhar A, Saikumar SJ, et al. Intravitreal gas for submacular haemorrhage. Indian J Ophthalmol. 2003;51:349-50.
19. Ogawa T, Kitaoka T, Mera A, et al. Treatment of submacular hemorrhage in the macula. Retina. 2000;20:684-5.
20. Gopalakrishan M, Giridhar A, Bhat S, et al. Pneumatic displacement of submacular hemorrhage: Safety, efficacy, and patient selection. Retina. 2007;27:329-34.
21. Chawla S, Misra V, Khemchandani M. Pneumatic displacement and intravitreal bevacizumab: a new approach for management of submacular hemorrhage in choroidal neovascular membrane. Indian J Ophthalmol. 2009;57:155-7.
22. Mills MD, Devenyi RG, Lam WC, et al. An assessment of intraocular pressure rise in patients with gas-filled eyes during simulated air flight. Ophthalmology. 2001;108:40-4.
23. Lincoff H, Weinberger D, Stergiu P. Air travel with intraocular gas. II. Clinical considerations. Arch Ophthalmol. 1989;107:907-10.
24. Butler F. Diving and hyperbaric ophthalmology. Surv Ophthalmol. 1995;39:347-66.
25. Fu AD, McDonald HR, Eliott D, et al. Complications of general anesthesia using nitrous oxide in eyes with pre-existing gas bubbles. Retina. 2002;22:569-74.
26. Gedde SJ. Management of glaucoma after retinal detachment surgery. Curr Opin Ophthalmol. 2002;13:103-9.
27. Chang S, Lincoff HA, Coleman DJ, et al. Perfluorocarbon gases in vitreous surgery. Ophthalmology. 1985;92:651-6.
28. Lee DA, Wilson MR, Yoshizumi MO, et al. The ocular effects of gases when injected into the anterior chamber of rabbit eyes. Arch Ophthalmol. 1991;109:571-5.

9 Perfluorocarbon Liquids and Vitreoretinal Surgery

Anna Gabrielian, Seenu M Hariprasad

Introduction

Perfluorocarbon liquids (PFCLs) were initially introduced into medicine as novel blood substitutes, given their impressive capacity to transport oxygen. This unique property, as well as the biological inertness of PFCLs, prompted further investigations into their potential uses in surgery.

The initial experimental use of PFCLs in ophthalmology as vitreoretinal substitutes occurred in the early 1980's, in an attempt to aid the closure of inferior retinal breaks in tamponade.[1,2] In 1987, these substitutes were first used in humans by Chang[3] as an intraoperative tool in the management of complex retinal detachments. Since then, a number of diverse uses have been reported, establishing PFCLs as essential components in the armamentarium of today's vitreoretinal surgeon.

Chemical and Physical Properties

Chemical Properties

Perfluorocarbon liquids are synthetic analogs of hydrocarbons and are fully fluorinated with carbon-fluorine bonds. When saturated, these bonds are very stable, even at temperatures as high as 400–500°C and are responsible for the biologic inertness of these substances. Though there are perfluorochemicals that contain heteroatoms such as nitrogen, oxygen and hydrogen, the maximum stability of these liquids is rendered by the carbon-fluorine bonds.[4] Partially fluorinated hydrocarbons have also been used in vitreoretinal surgery in the recent years, given their solubility with silicone oil secondary to the hydrocarbon moiety and a lower specific gravity compared with the fully fluorinated hydrocarbons.[5,6] However, these liquids have not yet been approved by the US Food and Drug Administration for intraocular use in vitreoretinal surgery.

Physical Properties

Perfluorocarbon liquids have high density (specific gravity of 1.6–2.1) and low viscosity (2–3 centistokes at 25°C).[4] The high density allows for hydrokinetic manipulation of detached retina in the removal of subretinal fluid through peripheral retinal breaks. The low viscosity allows easy injection and aspiration with small gauge instruments. PFCLs have low surface tension and a high interfacial tension—properties which decrease the likelihood of subretinal migration and keep the liquids cohesive in a large bubble.[7]

Perfluorocarbon liquids are immiscible, colorless, odorless and optically clear.[7] Their refractive indices are only slightly different from saline and thus allow the use of conventional contact lenses, free of optical aberrations. At the same time, the difference in the refractive index from that of water provides a visible interface when it is injected into the vitreous cavity. Immiscibility of these substances with balanced salt solution (BSS) or silicone oil provides the needed visibility when performing PFCL-air exchange and PFCL-silicone exchange.[7] The optical clarity also allows for the application of laser intraoperatively, and the high boiling point of these liquids prevents intraocular vaporization when laser is applied.[8]

Indications for Use

Perfluorocarbon liquids have been used in a wide variety of situations, from giant retinal tear to complex retinal detachment repairs in patients with proliferative vitreoretinopathy and/or trauma, to intraocular foreign body manipulation and retrieval, including dislocated lenses and in the management of suprachoroidal and submacular hemorrhages (Figs 9.1A to D). Though traditionally, PFCLs have been used in large gauge vitrectomy systems, most recently, these liquids have been successfully used in a transconjunctival 23- and 25-gauge systems, even in complicated cases.[9]

Giant Retinal Tears

A number of diverse techniques have been tried in the repair of giant retinal tears (GRT) prior to the use of PFCLs. Perhaps the most dramatic of these techniques was the turning of the patient into a prone position intraoperatively to allow the unfolding of the inverted flap by the intraocular gas bubble, as it was injected into the eye.[10] Additionally, the other heavy liquids such as silicone oil (whose tamponade force is six times less than that of the PFCLs), fluorosilicone oil and sodium hyaluronate 1%, have been manipulated in GRT repairs.[11,12]

The use of PFCLs by far prevails in the GRT repair today, as it allows for gentle manipulation of the tear [with minimal retinal pigment epithelium (RPE) dispersion], so that retinopexy can be performed with the retina oriented in the proper position.[13] After the core vitrectomy and epiretinal membrane dissection, the PFCL is initially infused over the optic nerve to stabilize the macula and mobilize the posterior flap. Perfluorocarbon liquid is then added to reach the edge of the tear to flatten the peripheral retina. Any further membranes that need to be dissected can be done at this time. Peripheral vitrectomy is then performed while the PFCL is

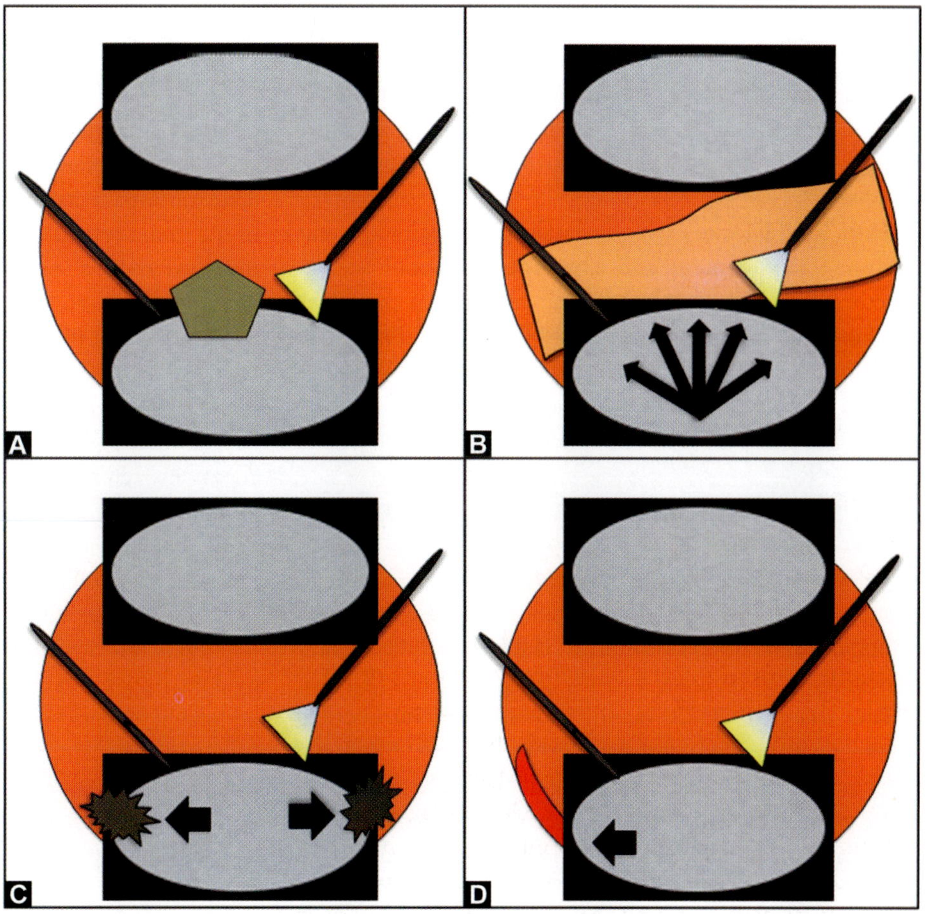

Figures 9.1A to D

Simplified diagrams showing common uses of perfluorocarbon liquids. (A) Protection of retina during retrieval of retained lens fragment; (B) Unfolding of giant retinal tear; (C) Visualization of preretinal membranes to facilitate membrane peeling; (D) Displacement of subretinal blood tamponading. Additional PFCL can then be added above the level of the tear and endophotocoagulation is then applied along the posterior edge of the GRT.[7]

Since long-term intraocular tamponade is needed in all of these cases, with either gas or silicone oil, air-fluid exchange is typically performed where PFCL is exchanged with air. To decrease the chances of retained PFCL, it is directly aspirated in exchange with air, while leaving a layer of BSS above it to maintain PFCL in one bubble until it is fully aspirated. To ensure no slippage has occurred, the area of the break should periodically be aspirated, to ensure that it remains dry. A rinse with BSS is done by some surgeons to ensure complete washout of PFCL from the vitreous cavity. Following this, air can be exchanged with the tamponading agent of choice, be it air or silicone oil. Alternatively, PFCL can be exchanged with silicone oil through an automated infusion system. The incoming oil meniscus will engage the edge of the tear as the PFCL is removed.

Proliferative Vitreoretinopathy

The use of PFCLs has revolutionized the management of PVR by stabilizing the macula and allowing a gentle manipulation of the retina, as well as allowing a more thorough removal of membranes and shortening the duration of the surgery. All this has resulted in improved visual and anatomic outcomes.[14-17]

In PVR, PFCL can exert its tamponade effect by opening the funnel detachment and exposing preretinal and/or subretinal membranes, which appear as areas of persistent elevation and/or traction under the PFCL bubble. PFCL can then allow the displacement of subretinal fluid, obviating the need to create a posterior drainage retinotomy, which in its turn reduces the risk of iatrogenic retinal damage and further PVR.[7]

The PFCL is injected over the cleared optic nerve head after the core vitrectomy once the posterior hyaloid has been separated and membranes have been peeled. As the retina flattens under PFCL, additional liquid is added and further membrane dissection is performed. If a relaxing retinotomy is needed, it can be made anterior to the level of PFCL.[7]

Just like with GRT repair, if long-term intraocular tamponade is needed with perfluorocarbon gas, PFCL-air exchange is performed. Photocoagulation can be performed at any point intraoperatively, whether it is during the PFCL tamponade, or after PFCL-air or PFCL-fluid exchange.[7]

Rhegmatogenous Retinal Detachment without Proliferative Vitreoretinopathy

PFCLs can be used as tamponading agents even in some cases of rhegmatogenous retinal detachments without PVR. These liquids can reveal the location of occult breaks by exerting a flattening force that displaces the subretinal fluid through the occult breaks. This displacement of fluid exhibits a phenomenon called schlieren—seen when two liquids of differing refractive index are mixed. The direction of the flow of schlieren will manifest the occult breaks.[7] Additionally, by flattening a bullous detachment, areas of obscured breaks can be exposed.

When all the breaks have been identified, PFCL can be added until its bubble meniscus reaches the posterior edge of the most anterior retinal break. At this point, laser endophotocoagulation can be applied. Just like before, air-PFCL exchange is performed with drainage of fluid through the most anterior break and removing the PFCL at its most anterior interface with BSS. If necessary, a long-term tamponading agent can be then infused as previously.[7]

Tractional Retinal Detachments in Proliferative Diabetic Retinopathy

Vitreous surgery has become the standard of care in end-stage diabetic retinopathy, when tractional retinal detachments develop in patients.[18-20] PFLCs have been used as adjuncts in tractional retinal detachment repairs, both as part of the modified en bloc technique[21,22] and in as infusion substitute in perfluoron-perfused vitrectomies (PFPV).[23,24]

Historically, the en bloc excision of fibrovascular tissue utilizes the posterior hyaloid to lift and immobilize the membrane as it is excised with horizontally cutting scissors.[25] Fibrovascular proliferation was reported to be more commonly removed via this technique prior to the advent of microincisional surgery.[26] However, a big disadvantage of this techniques has been the increased risk of iatrogenic retinal breaks, both posteriorly, given a strong retinal adherence of the fibrovascular tissue and in the periphery, secondary to traction at the vitreous base exerted by the retained posterior hyaloid, as well as a thinner and relatively more ischemic peripheral retina.[27]

A modification of the en bloc technique has used PFCL to enforce posterior counter-traction for membrane peeling at the midperiphery and at other anterior locations.[27,28] This technique involves PFCL injection into the vitreous cavity until the posterior hyaloid starts to exert traction on the retina, allowing it to be delaminated with the suction cutter.[27] The posterior hyaloid membrane, including the proliferative tissues adherent to it, is then lifted and peeled away from the posterior to the peripheral retina, until the former is completely separated from the retina. This is possible because the tissue planes remain immobilized and mechanically separated by the PFCL.[27]

Yet another modification of the en bloc technique has been described for the separation of the epiretinal tissue from the subjacent retina.[21] In this technique, a hole is made in the midperipheral posterior hyaloid to inject PFCL between the retina and the posterior hyaloid. This has been reported to allow for easier dissection of epiretinal membranes, as well as better visualization of vitreous and intraocular structures, a faster retinal reattachment and less bleeding improved blood confinement.[21]

Though it did not gain wide popularity, PFCL has also been used as a substitute for the continuous balanced salt solution infusion in PFPV, given its high oxygen-carrying capacity (useful during surgery on an ischemic retina), high oxygen affinity and thus theoretically higher intraocular pressure and hence hemorrhage-free surgery.[23,24]

All in all, PFCL certainly represents an advance in the surgical treatment of tractional retinal detachments in severe proliferative diabetic retinopathy.

Ocular Trauma and Foreign Bodies

Perfluorocarbon liquid's utility in ocular trauma is multi-fold. Retinal detachments resulting from penetrating trauma are usually highly mobile and complicated by vitreous, subretinal and/or choroidal hemorrhage. The increased mobility of the retina increases the risk of iatrogenic retinal breaks. PFCL can be useful in stabilizing this highly mobile retina and obviate the need for posterior retinotomy. In cases with vitreous or subretinal hemorrhage, PFCL can be used to displace it anteriorly, where in the case of subretinal hemorrhage; it can then be aspirated through a peripheral retinal break.[7]

Some cases of severe ocular trauma can cause retinal incarceration despite adequate surgical closure. Resulting traction at the incarceration site can lead to retinal detachment. Instead of a relaxing retinotomy, placement of PFCL over the incarceration site can be tried to help relieve traction.[29]

Intraocular foreign bodies, if organic, can be floated anteriorly on the surface of PFCLs. Metallic foreign bodies, on the other hand, though heavier than PFCL, can still be aided by these heavy liquids, since they are easier to grasp once fixated by PFCL.[7]

Finally, dislocated lenses, nuclear fragments and intraocular lenses can be captured and removed with the use of PFCLs.[30-32] After freeing the vitreous adhesions to the dislocated lenses via pars plana vitrectomy, PFCL can be injected into the vitreous cavity beneath the dislocated lens, to float the lens onto the anterior surface of the heavy liquid meniscus. The advantage of PFCL use in this situation is to prevent posterior and/or subretinal migration of the lens and securing the grasping of the lens, while at the same time flattening the posterior retina. Pars plana fragmentation can then be used to remove the subluxed lens, or in the case of dislocated intraocular lens, it can be delivered through a limbal incision.[7,30-33]

Submacular and Suprachoroidal Hemorrhages

Submacular hemorrhage can be seen in the setting of choroidal neovascularization, as well as after trauma, either in association with retinal detachment or without, in high myopia and in retinal vascular disorders. Regardless of etiology, large submacular hemorrhages have poor natural history, given the irreversible foveal damage that occurs. PFCL may facilitate the removal of submacular hemorrhage by displacing it away from the fovea, after performing core vitrectomy and removing of the posterior hyaloid.[34] Posterior retinotomy is performed near the edge of the hemorrhage, preferably as far away from the fovea as possible and a bubble of PFCL is then injected over the macula. The heavy liquid then exerts a tamponade effect on the submacular blood and the latter is then displaced to be aspirated through the retinotomy. PFCL is then removed from the eye as described previously. Tissue plasminogen activator can be used as an adjunct to liquefy the fresh clot and assist with easier removal through the retinotomy.[35]

Suprachoroidal hemorrhage is a dreaded complication of intraocular surgery. Wound closure is an initial management of suprachoroidal hemorrhage. This may then followed by draining of the suprachoroidal blood via posterior sclerotomies. PFCLs can be used as a tamponading agent in suprachoroidal hemorrhage when placed through anterior sclerotomies and may even allow for a more complete removal of the blood than air or gas tamponade.[36,37]

PFCL-Assisted Vitreous Biopsy

Perfluorocarbon liquids have been used experimentally as adjunctive surgical tools in a number of vitreoretinal surgeries and manipulations. For example, PFCLs have been reported useful in obtaining large undiluted vitreous biopsy samples for histology, cytology and research of the vitreous composition.[38] For this, PFCL is placed in a syringe connected to the infusion line and is injected into the vireous cavity as the vitreous is aspirated by the vitrectomy probe. Vitreous is then collected from the aspiration line of the vitrectomy probe by another syringe. Since the specific gravity of the PFCL is different from that of the vitreous, the clear interface between the two substances can be observed and subsequent separation of the vitreous from the PFCL could then be performed at the pathology laboratory.

Drawbacks of PFCL Use

Traditional postoperative endotamponades used in ocular surgery include silicone oil, air and expansive gases—all of which are lighter than water.[39-41] Though heavy liquids could theoretically be better long-term postoperative endotamponading agents than the currently available agents in certain surgical cases, the toxicity of the heavy liquids has precluded the use of these substances in the long term.[42]

The toxicity and the tendency of the PFCLs to disperse are perhaps the greatest drawbacks of the heavy liquids. The toxicity is related to the concentration of polar impurities in the heavy liquids,[43] which alter the PFCL interface and cause fibroblastic reaction with formation of preretinal membranes.[44] Additionally, PFCL can be proinflammatory when left in the eye for longer than one week, based on animal studies as well as clinical case reports.[44-49] In any case, since assessment of any subtle decline in retinal function which can be attributed to extended PFLC tamponade is difficult in the clinical setting,[50] currently extended postoperative tamponade is not recommended with PFCLs.

The most common complication of PFCL use, however, is its tendency to disperse into small bubbles at the PFCL-vitreous fluid interface.[7,50,51] These small droplets can then migrate subretinally[8] and/or into the anterior chamber and cause secondary complications such as corneal endothelial cell damage, trabecular obstruction and macrophage response resulting in cellular deposits on the lens, ciliary body and peripheral retina.[7,42,52-55] The dispersed droplets can also affect the optical clarity of the PFCL intraoperatively. Once dispersed, that portion of the heavy liquid has minimal tamponading effect.[50] The rate of dispersion is related to the specific solubility of the given PFCL, as well as its viscosity and the turbulence which it encounters.[55]

Another consideration in the use of PFCL would be its interaction with silicone oil. Even though the solubility of PFCLs in silicone oil is low, when the latter is removed from the eye, large quantities of PFCLs have still been found present.[56] Residual droplets of PFCL in the vitreous cavity have been reported to occur at rates between 1–11%.[57] This is because when silicone oil is infused into the eye, any remnant droplets of PFCLs are attracted and spread over the surface of the oil. Subsequently, inertial forces from eye movements can cause microsuspension of the small droplets of PFCL within silicone oil.[58]

The incidence of PFCLs retention in the eye, regardless of prior silicone oil injection, can have grave consequences, especially if the PFCL bubble has migrated into the subfoveal space. Most commonly this occurs in cases where large peripheral retinotomies are made, and in the absence of a saline rinse during the fluid-air exchange upon PFCL removal.[59] Clinical reports have shown that functional changes form retained subfoveal PFCLs range from permanent scotomas at the site of the retained bubble,[60] to subsequent underlying RPE atrophy and overall poor central vision.[61,62] Animal studies have shown that injection of subretinal heavy liquids causes local retinal necrosis with loss of photorecepter inner and outer segments.[63]

A final consideration in the use of PFCL is its high cost, which can be a major drawback, limiting its use, especially in the perfluoron-perfused perfluoron-perfused vitrectomies, where an average of 87 ml per procedure is used, instead of the 5–7 ml used in conventional surgery.[9,24] Needless to say that many retinal detachments can be repaired with the incorporation of a posterior drainage retinotomy (for which PFCLs are not required) instead of the anterior approach.

The introduction of PFCLs as an intraoperative tool has represented a major progress in the management of complex vitreoretinal surgical cases. The diversity of the surgical cases which benefit from PFCLs is growing. Though the association of complications with extended postoperative PFCL tamponade currently limits these liquids to intraoperative use, further the safety and efficacy of postoperative PFCL vitreoretinal tamponade.

References

1. Haidt SJ, Clark LC, Ginsbeg J. Liquid perfluorocarbon replacement of the eye. Invest Ophthalmol Vis Sci. 1982;22: 233.
2. Zimmerman NJ, Faris D. The use of N-perfluorocarbon amines in complicated retinal detachments. Invest Ophthalmol Vis Sci. 1984;25:258.
3. Chang S. Low viscosity liquid fluorochemicals in vitreous surgery. Am J Ophthalmol. 1987;103:38-43.
4. Miyamoto K, Refojo MF, Tolentino FL, et al. Fluorinated oils as experimental vitreous substitutes. Arch Ophthalmol. 1986;104:1053-6.
5. Meinert H, Roy T. Semifluorinated alkanes—a new class of compounds with outstanding properties for use in ophthalmology. Eur J Ophthalmol. 2000;10:189-97.
6. Zeana D, Becker J, Kuckelkorn R, et al. Perfluorohexloctane as a long term vitreous tamponade in the experimental animal. Experimental perfluorohexyloctane substitution. Int Ophthalmol. 1999;23:17-24.
7. Chang S, Kwun RC. Perfluorocarbon liquids in vitreoretinal surgery. In: Ryan SJ, Hinton DR, Schachat AP, Wilkinson CP (Eds). Retina. Mosby; 2003. pp. 2179-90.
8. Bourke RD, Simpson RN, Cooling RJ, et al. The stability of perfluoro-N-octane during vitreoretinal procedures. Arch Ophthalmol. 1996;114:537-44.
9. Quiroz-Mercado H, Garcia Aguirre G, Ustáriz-González O, et al. Perfluorocarbon-perfused vitrectomy using a transconjunctival 25-gauge system. Retina. 2007;27:926-31.
10. Michels RG, Rice TA, Blankenship G. Surgical techniques for selected giant retinal tears. Retina. 1983;3:139-53.
11. Leaver PK, Cooling RJ, Feretis EB, et al. Vitrectomy and fluid-silicone oil exchange for giant retinal tears: results at 6 months. Br J Ophthalmol. 1984;68:432-8.
12. Brown GC, Benson WE. Use of sodium hyaluronate for the repair of giant retinal tears. Arch Ophthalmol. 1989;107:1246-9.
13. Kreiger AE, Lewis H. Management of giant retinal tears without scleral buckling: use of radical dissection of the vitreous base and perfluoro-n-octane and intraocular tamponade. Ophthalmology. 1992;99:491-7.
14. Banker AS, Freeman WR, Vander JF, et al. Use of Perflubron as a new temporary vitreous substitute and manipulation agent for vitreoretinal surgery. Retina. 1996;16:285-91.
15. Carroll BF, Peyman GA, Mehta NJ, et al. Repair of retinal detachment associated with proliferative vitreoretinopathy using perfluoroperhydrophenanthrene (Vitreon). Can J Ophthalmol. 1994;29:66-9.
16. Coll GE, Chang S, Sun J, et al. Perfluorocarbon liquid in the management of retinal detachment with proliferative vitreoretinopathy. Ophthalmology. 1995;102:630-8.
17. Han DR, Rychwalski PJ, Mieler WF, et al. Management of complex retinal detachment with combined relaxing retinotomy and intravitreal perfluoro-n-octane injection. Am J Ophthalmol. 1994;118:24-32.
18. Thompson JT, de Bustros S, Michels RG, et al. Results and prognostic factors in vitrectomy for diabetic traction retinal detachment of the macula. Arch Ophthalmol. 1987;105:497-502.
19. Thompson JT, de Bustros S, Michels RG, et al. Results and prognostic factors in vitrectomy for diabetic traction-rhegmatogenous retinal detachment of the macula. Arch Ophthalmol. 1987;105:503-7.
20. Rice TA, Michels RG, Rice EF. Vitrectomy for diabetic rhegmatogenous retinal detachment. Am J Ophthalmol. 1983;95:34-44.
21. Arevalo JF. En bloc perfluorodissection for tractional retinal detachment in proliferative diabetic retinopathy. Ophthalmology. 2008;115:e21-5.
22. Arevalo JF. En bloc perfluorodissection in vitreoretinal surgery: a new surgical technique. Retina. 2008;28:653-6.
23. Quiroz-Mercado H, Suarez-Tata L, Magdalenic R, et al. Perfluorocarbon perfused vitrectomy: animal studies. Am J Ophthalmol. 2004;137:287-93.
24. Quiroz-Mercado H, Guerrero-Naranjo J, Agurto-Rivera R, et al. Perfluorocarbon-perfused vitrectomy: a new method for vitrectomy—a safety and feasibility study. Graefes Arch Clin Exp Ophthalmol. 2005;243:551-62.
25. Abrams GW, Williams GA. "En bloc" excision of diabetic membranes. Am J Ophthalmol. 1987;103:302-8.
26. Han DR, Murphy ML, Mieler WF. A modified en bloc excision technique during vitrectomy for diabetic traction retinal detachment. Results and complications. Ophthalmology. 1994;101:803-8.
27. Yadarola MB, Gramajo AL, Arrambide MP, et al. Perfluorocarbon liquid vitreous delamination and wide-angle viewing system in the management of complicated diabetic retinal detachment. Eur J Ophthalmol. 2009;19:452-9.
28. Maturi RK, Merrill PT, Lomeo MD, et al. Perfluoro-N-octane (PFO) in the repair of complicated retinal detachments due to severe proliferative diabetic retinopathy. Ophthalmic Surg Lasers. 1999:30:715-20.
29. Peyman GA, Schulman JA, Sullivan B. Perfluorocarbon liquids in ophthalmology. Surv Ophthalmol. 1995;39:375-95.
30. Rowson NJ, Bacon AS, Rosen PH. Perfluorocarbon heavy liquids in the management of posterior dislocation of the lens nucleus during phacoemulsification. Br J Ophthalmol. 1992;76:169-70.
31. Lewis H, Blumenkranz MS, Chang S. Treatment of dislocated crystalline lens and retinal detachment with perfluorocarbon liquids. Retina. 1992;12:299-304.
32. Liu KR, Peyman GA, Chen M, et al. Use of high-density vitreous substitutes in the removal of posteriorly dislocated lenses or intraocular lenses. Ophthalmology. 1991;22:503-7.
33. Brod RD, Flyn HW, Clarkson JG, et al. Management options for retinal detachment in the presence of a posteriorly dislocated intraocular lens. Retina. 1990;10:50-6.
34. Lambert HM, Capone A, Aaberg TM, et al. Surgical excision of subfoveal neovascular membranes in age-related macular degeneration. Am J Ophthalmol. 1992;113:257-62.
35. Johnson MW, Olsen KR, Hernandez E. Tissue plasminogen activator thrombolysis during surgical evacuation of

experimental subretinal hemorrhage. Ophthalmology. 1992;99:515-21.

36. Lakhanpal V, Schocket SS, Elman MJ, et al. A new modified vitreoretinal surgical approach in the management of massive suprachoroidal hemorrhage. Ophthalmology. 1989;96:793-800.
37. Desai UR, Peyman GA, Chen CJ. Use of perfluoroperhydrophenanthrene in the management of suprachoroidal hemorrhage. Ophthalmology. 1992;99:1542-7.
38. Quiroz-Mercado H, Rivera-Sempertegui J, Macky TA, et al. Performing vitreous biopsy by perfluorocarbon-perfused vitrectomy. Am J Ophthalmol. 2005;140:1161-3.
39. Giordano GG, Refojo MF. Silicone oils as vitreous substitutes. Prog Polym Sci. 1998;23:509-32.
40. Saxena S, Gopal L. Fluid vitreous substitutes in vitreo-retinal surgery. Indian J Ophthalmol. 1996;44:191-206.
41. Soman N, Banerjee R. Artificial vitreous replacements. Biomet Mater Eng. 2003;13:59-74.
42. Matteucci A, Formisano G, Paradisi S, et al. Biocompatibility assessment of liquid artificial vitreous replacements: relevance in vitro studies. Surv Ophthalmol. 2007;52:289-99.
43. Keese C, Giaver I. Cell growth on liquid interfaces: role of surface active compounds. Proc Natl Acad Sci USA. 1983;80:5622.
44. Sparrow JR, Ortiz R, MacLeish PR, et al. Fibroblast behavior at aqueous interfaces with perfluorocarbon, silicone, and fluorosilicone liquids. Invest Ophthalmol Vis Sci. 1990;31: 638-46.
45. Chang S, Sparrow JR, Iwamoto T, et al. Experimental studies of tolerance to intravitreal perfluoro-n-octane liquid. Retina. 1991;11:367-74.
46. Elsing SH, Fekrat S, Green WR, et al. Clinicopathologic findings in eyes with retained perfluoro-n-octane liquid. Ophthalmology. 2001;108:45-8.
47. Conway MD, Peyman GA, Karacorlu M, et al. Perfluorooctylbromide (PFOB) as a vitreous substitute in non-human primates. Int Ophthalmol. 1993;17:259-64.
48. Devin F, Jourdan T, Saracco JB, et al. Experimental tolerance to perfluorodecalin used in prolonged intraocular tamponade. Ophthalmologica. 1995;209:306-14.
49. Singh J, Ramaesh K, Wharton SB, et al. Perfluorodecalin-induced intravitreal inflammation. Retina. 2001;21:247-51.
50. Kirchhof B, Wong D, Meurs JV, et al. Use of perfluorohexyloctane as long-term internal tamponade agent in complicated retinal detachment surgery. Am J Ophthalmol. 2002;133:95-101.
51. Hiscott P, Magee RM, Colthurst M, et al. Clinicopathological correlation of epiretinal membranes and posterior lens opacification following perfluorohexyloctane tamponade. Br J Ophthalmol. 2001;85:179-83.
52. Mertens S, Bernarz J, Engelmann K. Evidence of toxic side effects of perfluorohexyloctane after vitreoretinal surgery as well as in previously established in vitro models with ocular cell types. Graefes Arch Clin Exp Ophthalmol. 2002;240:989-95.
53. Schatz B, El-Shabrawi Y, Haas A, et al. Adverse side effects with perfluorohexyloctane as a long-term tamponade agent in complicated vitreoretinal surgery. Retina. 2004;21:247-51.
54. Vote B, Wheen L, Cluroe A, et al. Further evidence for proinflammatory nature of perfluorohexyloctane in the eye. Clin Experiment Ophthalmol. 2003;31:408-14.
55. Nakamura K, Refojo MF, Crabtree DV. Factors contributing to the emulsification of intraocular silicone and fluorosilicone oils. Invest Ophthalmol Vis Sci. 1990;31:647-56.
56. Friberg TR, Siska PE, Somayajula K, et al. Interactions of perfluorocarbon liquids and silicone oil as characterized by mass spectrometry. Graefes Arch Clin Exp Ophthalmol. 2003;241:809-15.
57. Scott IU, Murray TG, Flynn, HW, et al. Outcomes and complications associated with perfluoro-n-octane and perfluoroperhydrophenanthrene in complex retinal detachment. Ophthalmology. 2000;107:860-5.
58. Hoerauf H, Fraude F, Menz DH, et al. Determination of the solubility of perfluorocarbon liquids in silicone oil in vitro and in vivo. Retina. 2002;22:163-8.
59. Garcia-Valenzuela E, Ito Y, Abrams GW. Risk factors for retention of subretinal perfluorocarbon liquid in vitreoretinal surgery. Retina. 2004;24:746-52.
60. Lesnoni G, Rossi T, Gelso A. Subfoveal liquid perfluorocarbon. Retina. 2004;24:172-6.
61. Blinder KJ, Peyman GA, Desai UR, et al. Vitreon, a short-term vitreoretinal tamponade. Br J Ophthalmol. 1992;76:525-8.
62. Lee GA, Finnegan SJ, Bourke RD. Subretinal perfluorodecalin toxicity. Aust N Z J Ophthalmol. 1998;26:57-60.
63. Berglin L, Ren J, Algvere PV. Retinal detachment and degeneration in response to subretinal perfluorodecalin in rabbit eyes. Graefes Arch Clin Exp Ophthalmol. 1993;231: 233-7.

Chromovitrectomy

10

Milton Nunes de Moraes-Filho, Eduardo Buchele Rodrigues,
Carsten H Meyer, Mauricio Maia, Eduardo Dib,
Elaine de Paula Fiod Costa, Michel Eid Farah

Introduction

"Chromovitrectomy" is the intraocular application of dyes to assist visualization of preretinal tissues during vitreoretinal surgery. It has been introduced with the goal of avoiding ocular complications related to internal limiting membrane (ILM) peeling, poor removal of the vitreous and incomplete removal of the epiretinal membrane (ERM). Thereby, leading to improvement in the postoperative visual acuity. Since 2000, chromovitrectomy has become a popular approach among vitreoretinal specialists.[1,2] The first vital dye used in chromovitrectomy, indocyanine green (ICG), facilitated the identification of the fine and transparent ILM. Following ICG, trypan blue (TB) has been introduced as an appropriate agent to identify ERM and triamcinolone acetonide (TA) has been found to stain the vitreous well. Recently, additional vital dyes such as infracyanine green (IfCG) and patent blue (PB) have been proposed for intraocular application during vitrectomy.[3] In this chapter, the current knowledge involving the use of dyes in chromovitrectomy will be discussed. In order to minimize the risk of toxic effects of dyes in chromovitrectomy, surgical recommendations are presented.

Use of Vital Dyes for Internal Limiting Membrane

Internal limiting membrane (ILM) peeling to treat idiopathic macular holes (MH) was first described by Eckardt et al. in 1997. A large meta-analysis of published nonrandomized studies involving 1,654 eyes suggested that ILM-maculorhexis increases anatomic and functional success rates of IMH surgery.[4] However, surgical removal of ILM may lead to retinal damage. The two main complications of ILM removal are visual field defects and retinal pigment epithelium (RPE) damage. Visual field defects after ILM removal mainly located temporal to the macula could be related to mechanical trauma to optic disc, to the fluid-air exchange or to direct trauma to the retina. Macular retinal pigmentary epithelial hyperpigmentation or hypofluorescence on angiography could be induced by surgical trauma or phototoxicity.[3] In order to try to minimize complications related to surgical trauma and to better visualization of ILM, most common dyes are presented.

▶ Indocyanine Green

The application of intravitreal ICG was first reported in cadaveric eyes to improve the visualization of the ILM. Since then, many articles have been released regarding the use of ICG as a surgical adjuvant of the identification and removal of the ILM in macular surgery (Fig. 10.1).

ICG adheres well to the extracellular matrix components of the ILM, such as collagen type 4, laminin and fibronectin.[5] In a porcine model, ICG with light exposure produces a significant increase in biomechanical stiffness, thereby facilitating ILM peeling.[6] Many authors have reported easier and less traumatic ICG-guided peeling with good clinical results. MH closure rate may be achieved in 74–100% of patients using ICG-guided ILM peeling.[3,7]

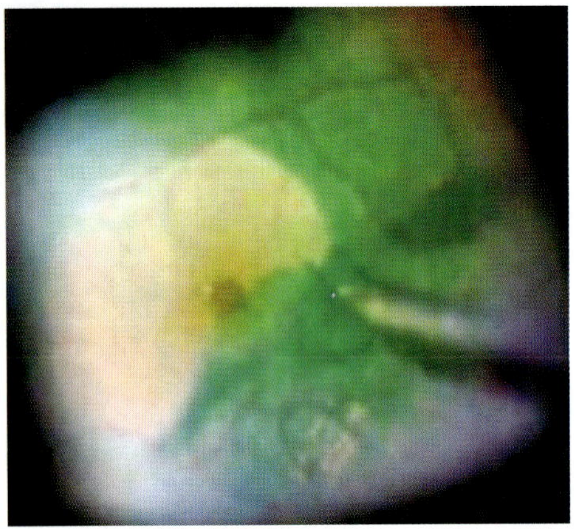

▲ Figure 10.1

ILM peeling guided by ICG staining in MH surgery. Peeling is facilitated because ICG produce an ILM stiffness and a good contrast to the retina

However, the potential for toxic effects of ICG on the retina has been suggested.[8-10] ICG may persist after macular hole surgery for up to 36 months.[3] In addition, ICG could also migrate to subretinal space through the MH, causing retinal damage.[11-13] Complications of ICG-assisted chromovitrectomy include RPE changes, visual field defects and optic nerve atrophy.[3,14]

Few controlled studies have been performed to compare ILM removal with and without ICG staining in MH surgery. Some authors found significantly worse visual outcomes when ICG was used.[15-17] The better outcomes in recent papers may be explained by a more careful ICG-injection technique.[3,18]

In comparing studies of ICG-assisted MH surgery criteria such as dye incubation time, concentration and osmolarity should be noted. Incubation time, the time that the dye remains in the vitreous cavity before aspiration, may vary from immediate removal to 5 minutes. RPE changes have been found mainly in studies reporting incubation time over 30 seconds. RPE toxicity is more common when the ICG solution has an osmolarity below 270 mOsm and concentration above 0.5%.[3]

The first use of ICG in MH surgery was with a dye concentration of 0.5%. A lower concentration was thought to be safer after RPE changes and visual field defects appeared. Low ICG concentration (0.125%) found no signs of retinal toxicity, with good anatomical and visual results.[19] In contrast, Engelbrecht et al.[20] using the same ICG concentration observed RPE changes in 54.5%. The difference could be related to the solution osmolarity, which was 299 mOsm in the former and 250 mOsm in the latter. Maia et al.[8] observed 27.5% of RPE abnormalities after 0.5% of ICG used with osmolarity of 270 mOsm. This high rate of RPE abnormalities may be related to the ICG concentration, technique of application, ICG exposure to light or a combination of factors. Recently studies have utilized ICG in a concentration of 0.05% and osmolarity around 290 mOsm with few or no signs of RPE toxicity.[3]

A meta-analysis of ICG application for ILM peeling in 837 eyes showed similar anatomic, but worse functional, outcomes when ICG has been used in chromovitrectomy.[21] Most of the studies in this meta-analysis used ICG in high concentrations and volumes.

ICG has been also used to facilitate ILM peeling in other diseases. Its use in diabetic macular edema (DME) revealed no sign of retinal toxicity, but visual outcome was similar to vitrectomy without ICG.[22] ICG compared to triamcinolone acetonide (TA) in patients with diffuse DME showed no differences.[23] Radetzky et al.[24] evaluated ILM peeling with ICG for persistent macular edema due to central retinal vein occlusion, DME, Irvine-Gass syndrome and vitreomacular traction syndrome. Significant improvement in visual acuity was observed only in patients with DME. Large-scale randomized trials should evaluate the benefit and safety of ICG-guided ILM peeling in other diseases.[3]

▶ Infracyanine Green

Infracyanine green (IfCG) is the modified version of ICG that does not contain 5% sodium iodide used for the lyophilized form necessary for dye-solubility. It stains ILM homogenously, but not epiretinal membranes, a cellular tissue. Similar to ICG, this iodine-free dye also binds with high affinity to the ILM and facilitates its visualization. The dilution of IfCG in glucose 5% generates an iso-osmotic solution (294–314 mmol/kg), thereby reducing the risks of hypo-osmotic-induced toxicity previously reported with ICG. Indeed, osmolarity changes at the vitreoretinal interface or subretinal space induced by various types of solutions have been shown to be toxic to retinal cells and tissue.[3]

Several clinical investigations have shown little or no retinal toxicity with IfCG application. IfCG-assisted ILM peeling demonstrated closure rates over 90% of MH and an improvement in visual acuity.[25,26] In surgical ILM removal for DME, IfCG appeared to be safe and to promote good clinical results.[27] Nevertheless, controlled clinical studies showed that IfCG-guided peeling did not significantly improve the results of MH surgery.[7,28]

Immunohistochemical analysis of the ILM peeled with IfCG showed the presence of remnants of footplates from Muller, glial cells and neural or ganglion cells.[29] This could explain why in cadaver eyes, IfCG as well as ICG followed by illumination may alter the cleavage plane at inner retinal layers of the ILM.[30] Therefore, although IfCG and ICG may facilitate ILM removal, they may produce undesired retinal alterations in the neurosensory retina and RPE leading to visual field defects.[30,31] In summary, a safer IfCG profile may make it a better alternative than ICG for chromovitrectomy in humans, since IfCG in the concentration of 0.5 mg/ml allows ILM identification with fewer toxic effects.

Brilliant Blue

Brilliant Blue G (BBG), also known as Coomassie or Acid Blue, is a synthetic dye that has been certified as safe food additive in Europe and may be used as protein gel electrophoresis marker in cardiovascular and neurologic diseases.[7] In chromovitrectomy the safety profile of BBG was investigated in preclinical experiments with no significant retinal alterations at low dosage of 0.5 mg/ml at ILM peeling in primates.[32]

In humans, BBG produced appropriate ILM staining in an iso-osmolar solution of 0.25 mg/ml when used for idiopathic ERM and MH treatment. Eighty-five percent of eyes improved at least two Snellen lines with no signs of toxicity.[33] Similar outcomes were reported even using multifocal electroretinogram to evaluate retinal toxicity.[34] Since this dye has good affinity for the ILM, BBG double staining may help simultaneous ERM and ILM peeling with no apparent effect on visual acuity. Moreover this technique appears to reduce subsequent ERM recurrence.[35]

BBG is emerging as a good alternative for ICG and IfCG in chromovitrectomy because of its remarkable affinity for ILM (Fig. 10.2), although the data on its toxicity are limited.

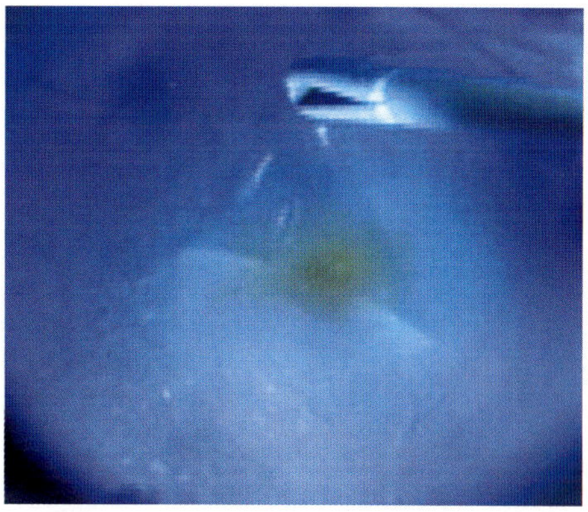

Figure 10.2
ILM peeling guided by BBG staining in an optic disc pit retinal detachment repair (André Maia, MD)

Triamcinolone Acetonide

Kimura et al. first used TA for ILM peeling, observing that the white specks and crystals deposit over the ILM, thereby facilitating its identification and removal. They obtained good clinical results and observed no adverse effects after three months. Subsequent pathology disclosed the presence of ILM in specimens after TA-assisted peeling, thereby showing that is possible to remove ILM and not just vitreous.[2,7] Since then other studies have confirmed that TA-assisted ILM removal gives good results.[36-38] Compared to ICG-guided ILM removal, a noncontrolled study indicates that TA has the same closure rate with significantly better visual results with no side effects.[39]

Crystals of TA have been detected until 40 days post surgery with chromovitrectomy for MH surgery. Some authors suggest that this persistent TA could slow the healing process necessary for MH closure.[3] A recent study compared ILM peeling with and without the use of TA. During a mean follow-up of 7.3 months, no recurrence of the MH was observed.[37] Despite of this concern, preservative-free TA appears to be a preferred agent in chromovitrectomy.[40]

Trypan Blue

Soon after its introduction in cataract surgery, TB was proposed as a stain for chromovitrectomy.[3] However, TB does not enhance ILM visualization as well as ICG; and TB is recommended mainly for ERM-staining.[7] In addition, ILM visualization with TB is much more difficult than with ICG-guided.[2,41] If TB is used for ILM staining, the dye should be kept in contact with the ILM for a longer period of time than ICG.

Two comparative studies showed same rate of closure stage II to IV idiopathic MH using ICG or TB. However, vision was significantly better only in the TB-group.[41,42]

Although many clinical studies reveal that TB exerted little or no toxic effect to the retina, TB-staining may produce retinal damage, especially at higher concentrations. [3,43,44] In the future, clinical investigations should clarify the role of TB in combination with other vital dyes in chromovitrectomy, the so-called double staining and elucidate the safe dose of intravitreal TB for chromovitrectomy.[45]

Vital Dyes for Epiretinal Membranes

▶ Trypan Blue

Trypan blue is commonly used in microscopy for cellular counting for staining of the reticuloendothelial system and the kidney tubules. In the late 1990s, TB was shown to have a great affinity to the anterior capsule of the lens which facilitated capsulorhexis in cataract surgery. Soon thereafter, TB was tried as a stain for preretinal tissues such as the ILM and ERM in chromovitrectomy. The vital stain may traverse cell membranes only in dead cells thereby coloring dead tissues or cells blue; live cells or tissues with intact cell membranes are not colored since their selective control of cellular membrane transport does not allow TB-binding. Thereby, TB exhibits a strong affinity for ERM because of the many dead glial cells within those membranes.[7] Various investigators, including our group, agree that TB is indicated for recognition of ERMs in vitrectomy, as the blue dye enables complete identification of the entire ERM surface.[7] Trypan blue staining of the ERM may minimize mechanical trauma to the retina during ERM removal and allows recognition of the extent of the ERM (Fig. 10.3).

Postoperatively median visual acuity difference after macular pucker surgery with and without the use of 0.15% TB was not statistically significant for a follow-up of 4–6 months in 20 patients. However, four of 10 patients without and seven of 10 patients with TB-staining experienced an improvement of visual acuity of 2 lines or more.[43] One comparative study with TB and ICG for ERM removal also gave results favoring the application of TB.[46]

No RPE defects or signs of retinal toxicity have been reported in most studies. However, in one case report of inadvertent subretinal migration of TB away from the fovea, RPE changes were noted at the migration site, but did not compromise visual acuity.[47] Histopathological analysis of excised ERM showed no retinal cells on the retinal side of the ERM and no signs of apoptosis.[48] Multifocal ERG found no retinal toxicity.[49] Finally, electron microscopy of the TB-stained ERM showed fragments of ILM in all specimens.[46] Interestingly, Smiddy and coworkers showed that without the use of any dye, epiretinal membrane fragments contain ILM fragments in 76% of cases.[3] The clinical relevance of those ultrastructural findings remains to be determined; however, future controlled studies should clarify if TB has any toxicity.

To enhance dye penetration onto retinal surface in an air-fluid-exchange, TB may be mixed with glucose, thereby creating a dye solution denser than water (Table 10.1, Fig. 10.4). Lesnik Oberstein et al.[50] used TB and 10% glucose isovolumetrically in osmolarity of 320 mOsm/L to evaluate ERM staining without fluid-air exchange. Just 25% of eyes needed a reapplication of the solution to achieve ERM staining. In addition all patients exhibited improved visual

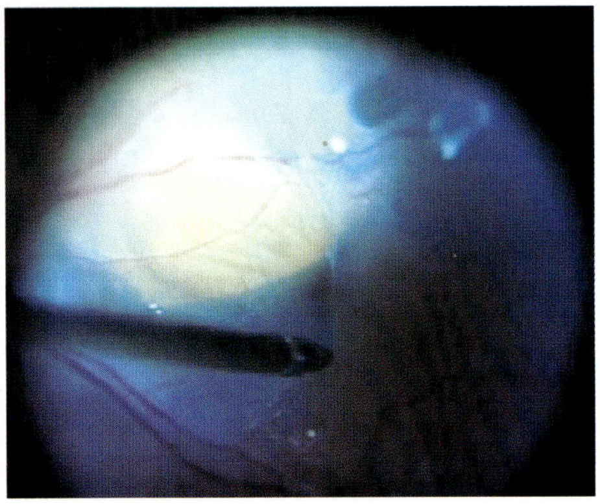

▲ **Figure 10.3**

ERM removal using TB 0.05% (diluted in glucose 5%). TB has a strong affinity of dead glial cells within ERM (André Maia, MD)

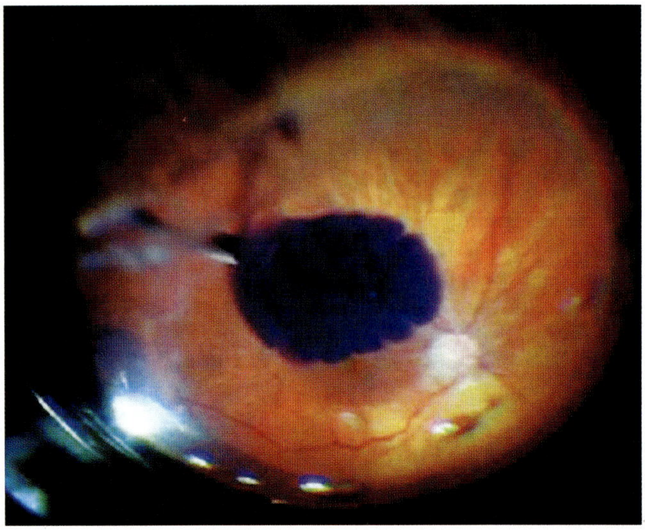

▲ **Figure 10.4**

A TB and glucose-mixed solution injected in a fluid-filled technique. This dye solution is denser than water that might avoid contact at the posterior capsule of the lens and helps to maintain selective staining of posterior pole (André Maia, MD)

TABLE 10.1: Comparison of substances currently used in chromovitrectomy[7, 18]

Substance	*Dilution/ Osmolarity*	*Affinity for intraocular structures*	*Avoiding RPE/ Retina toxicity*	*High cost*	*Chemical properties*
Triamcinolone acetonide 40 mg/ml 4%	No dilution	Vitreous	Use a preservative-free solution	+	Triamcinolone is a synthetic nonsoluble steroid (C24H31FO6; 434 daltons)
Trypan blue 1.2 mg/ml 0.12%	No dilution or mix with glucose 1.2 mg/ml (0.12%)/310 mOsm	ERM	Use with no dilution or mix 0.3 ml with 0.1 ml glucose 5% for better ERM identification	+	Trypan blue is an anionic hydrophilic azo dye (C34H24N6Na4O14S4; 960 daltons)
Patent blue 2.5 mg/ml 0.25%	No dilution or mix with glucose 2.5 mg/ml (0.25%)/290 mOsm	ERM	Use with no dilution or mix 0.3 ml with 0.1 ml glucose 5% for better ERM identification	++	Patent blue is a triarylmethane dye (C27H31N2NaO6S2; 582 daltons)
Brilliant blue 0.25 mg/ml 0.025%	No dilution/ 280 mOsm	ILM	Use with dilution	+++	Brilliant blue is a blue anionic aminotriarylmethane compound (C47H48N3S2O7Na; 854 daltons)
Indocyanine green 5 mg, 0.5%; 25 mg, 2.5%; 50 mg, 5.0%	Less than 0.5 mg/ml (0.05%) Dissolve in small amount of distilled water. Dilution: use large amount of BSS	ILM	Add 1 ml distilled water to 1 vial 5 mg Take 0.1 ml of the solution and mix with 0.9 ml BSS	++++	Indocyanine green is a tricarbocyanine dye (C43H47N2NaO6S2; 775 daltons) and contains 3% to 5% iodine
Infracyanine green 5 mg, 0.5%, 25 mg, 2.5%	Less than 0.5 mg/ml (0.05%) Dissolve in glucose 5%/290 mOsm	ILM	Add 1 or 2 ml glucose 5% to 1 vial of 5 mg	+++++	Infracyanine green has the same chemical formula as ICG but contains no sodium iodine

BSS = Balanced salt solution; ERM = Epiretinal membrane; ICG = Indocyanine green; ILM = Internal limiting membrane; RPE = Retinal pigment epithelium

acuity with no signs of retinal toxicity. However, higher glucose concentrations should be avoided. Injection of 0.05 ml of a 1000 mOsm solution in animals caused rapid whitening of the posterior retina, followed by the development of a large detachment and permanent retinal degeneration. An ERG showed immediate loss of the c-wave and a slower decline of the a- and b-waves.[51,52] Osmolarity should be considered in planning any vitreous injection of dyes and drugs.

Patent Blue

Patent blue is a fluorescent marker that enables lymph nodes removal and *in vitro* fungi specimens identification. The dye has been has been certified for capsule staining during cataract surgery at concentration of 0.24%.[3]

Animal studies and preliminary clinical data demonstrate moderated affinity of PB to ERM and vitreous, but poor affinity to the ILM.[2,7] Nevertheless, our recent clinical data revealed that PB is as appropriate a vital dye for coloring ERM as TB.[53]

There is conflicting data regarding the retinal toxicity of PB. In one study PB induced only mild and reversible retinal toxicity,[54] whereas RPE-cells exposed *in vitro* to PB showed no toxicity.[53] Our rabbit subretinal toxicity model demonstrated that subretinal injection of PB resulted only in mild ultrastructural retinal damage during follow-up; the histological damage induced by TB was more severe than by PB. Most studies to date indicate a safer profile for PB compared to TB, particularly in neuroretinal cells. However, the safe dosage range for intravitreal PB injection remains unclear yet.

Bromophenol Blue

Bromophenol blue (BroB) has been used as acid-base indicator and as marker of gel electrophoresis procedures. In comparison to six biological stains (light green yellowish, E68, Chicago blue, Rhodamine, rhodulinblau-basic) BroB has stained the ERM and ILM better with no RPE-cell *in vitro* toxicity or primary proliferation at concentrations of 0.2% and 0.02%.[55] *In vivo* studies in rodent and porcine eyes demonstrated that BroB at concentrations of 0.5% and 0.02% promoted less retinal toxicity as assessed by histology and ganglion cell counts in comparison to three other vital dyes (Light-green, Chicago blue and E68). Moreover BroB at concentrations of 1% and 2% promoted enhanced ILM coloring and identification.[3]

Its first use in humans using 0.2% concentration showed good staining properties in ERM and vitreous remnants with a good safety profile in a short follow-up.[56] BroB also helped to visualize posterior hyaloid membrane in MH surgery and to remove vitreous base during retinal detachment surgery.[57]

Indocyanine Green

Indocyanine green has been proposed to allow better visualization of ERMs in vitrectomy for proliferative diabetic vitreoretinopathy (PDVR), idiopathic ERMs and proliferative vitreoretinopathy (PVR).[2,58] However, the green dye may stain the acellular ILM best and ERM-staining by other vital stains may be better.[7] Foster et al.[59] described a case of recurrent macular hole surgery where ICG stained ILM except in an inferior area with an ERM. The same phenomena was observed in ERM surgery for PVR, where ICG stains ILM but not the ERM facilitating the identification and removal by negative staining.[60]

Epiretinal membrane peeling with and without ICG showed no difference in visual acuity or retinal toxicity. More recently, the effect of ILM peeling with and without ICG staining for idiopathic ERM removal demonstrated no difference in preoperative or postoperative visual acuity, reduction of macular edema, or incidence of recurrent ERM.[3]

Subretinal Vital Dye for Facilitation of Retinal Breaks Visualization

Exact localization of retinal breaks is a critical step in the surgical treatment of rhegmatogenous retinal detachment (RD).[61] Despite clear visualization of the fundus, in 2.2–4% of phakic RDs, the retinal breaks may not be found. In aphakic and pseudophakic RDs, the incidence of nonvisualized breaks may be even higher ranging from 7–16% and 5–22.5%, respectively.[62]

Early in the 20th century, numerous experiments were performed to investigate staining retinal breaks during retinal surgery. In 1939, Sorsby used intravenous Kiton-Fast-V-Green in patients with RD to detect a greenish retina with an unstained retinal break. In the 1950s, other researchers described the use of intravenous fluorescein for the same procedure and described a colored edge in the tears.[3]

Clinical Application of Vital Dyes for Subretinal Breaks Identification

The first use of subretinal application of dyes to stain retinal breaks was made in 1947 by Black. He used methylene blue through a transcleral needle. This vital dye application was considered unsuccessful by Hruby and Gass because of its absorption in the RPE. Later, Kutschera showed that systemic infusion of PB enabled both understanding of retinal metabolism and absorption in animals, which provided further evidence for the role of staining agents in the recognition of retinal breaks. Recently, Jackson et al.[3,61] applied subretinal 0.15% TB with a 41-gauge cannula to identify retinal breaks in patients with RD and no identifiable tears during surgery. Retinal breaks were identified in 4 of the 5 patients and no retinal toxicity was seen in this study. However, the small number of patients does not allow assessment of the risks and potential toxicity.

Vital Dyes for Vitreous

The vitreous plays a very active and important role in several vitreoretinal diseases, including macular holes, macular edema, diabetic retinopathy and retinal detachment. In vitreoretinal surgery for therapy of those diseases, complete removal of the vitreous gel may enhance surgical outcomes.

Triamcinolone Acetonide

Triamcinolone acetonide (TA) deposition onto the vitreous surface was initially reported by Peyman et al. in 2000. The

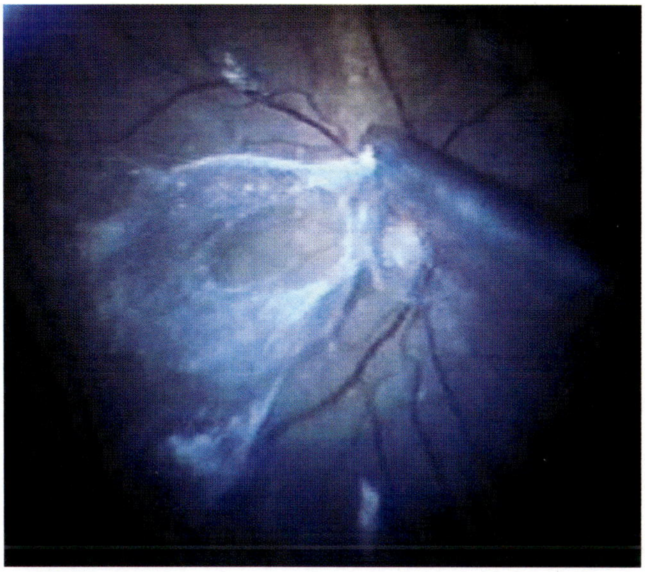

▲ **Figure 10.5**

Triamcinolone acetonide-guided posterior hyaloid dissection. Note that TA crystals deposit to the acellular vitreous gel, providing a clear visualization of the posterior vitreous cortex

crystals of the crystalline steroid adhere to the acellular tissue, thereby enabling a clear contrast between the empty vitreous cavity and the areas where the vitreous fibers are still present (Fig. 10.5). Nowadays, TA is the most used dye for vitreous staining. The current technique application consists of a simple injection of the agent into the vitreous cavity. Following the initial report, a number of studies confirmed the efficacy of TA for staining the transparent vitreous, whereas anatomic or functional signs of complications have rarely been observed.[3,7] In addition to its effect on the vitreous visualization, a TA injection during vitrectomy may prevent fibrin reaction and postoperative PVR. The use of intra-operative TA during vitreoretinal surgery showed decreased risk of postoperative RD, but increased need for postoperative antiglaucoma eye drops, with TA-application.

The safety of TA to the retina has been demonstrated by several *in vitro* and *in vivo* studies.[7] Intravitreal injection of TA in high concentration (up to 30 mg) yielded no relevant retina toxicity, while our investigation disclosed no damage to the retinal tissue after subretinal preservative-free TA-injection in rabbits.[63] It has been recently proposed that the preservative benzyl alcohol present in TA-vehicle induce most retinal damage.[64]

▶ Sodium Fluorescein

Hydrophilic sodium fluorescein (SF) is exceedingly well absorbed by the vitreous. Improved visualization of clear vitreous fibers by intravitreal SF 0.6% showed no complications.[65] Comparison of four different vital vitreous stains found that fluorescein was inferior to the TA.[66] Currently, the main use of SF in chromovitrectomy is vitreous staining. Future clinical investigations should determine its role to improve visualization of membranes during vitreoretinal surgery.

▶ Fluorometholone Acetate

The fluorometholone acetate (FMA) white to creamy powder may be prepared for ophthalmic suspension. The white steroid may be indicated for use in the treatment of steroid-responsive inflammatory conditions of the conjunctiva, cornea and anterior segment of the eye. The safety of intravitreal or subretinal FMA to retina has been recently examined in rat and primate eyes. The researchers found neither remarkable reduction in any ERG waves, nor histological changes and concluded the steroid FMA was a useful alternative to TA during chromovitrectomy.[67] Further clinical experience should elucidate the advantages and disadvantages of FMA in comparison to TA and other newer vital dyes.

▶ Trypan Blue

Intracameral or intravitreal injection of TB has been used to highlight vitreous. The blue dye in various doses may improve detection of both prolapsed vitreous in the anterior chamber and that remaining in the vitreous cavity. 0.15% TB used for staining the vitreous produced no toxicity.[7] TB may allow visualization of the margins of the vitreous strands during vitreoretinal surgery.[68] However, in one comparative analysis TB stained the vitreous less well than TA and FS.[66] For this reason TB application for vitreous visualization has not gained much popularity.

Surgical Techniques for Dye Application during Vitreoretinal Surgery

▶ Double Staining Technique

The double staining technique (Fig. 10.6) is an elegant procedure that may facilitate the identification of the posterior

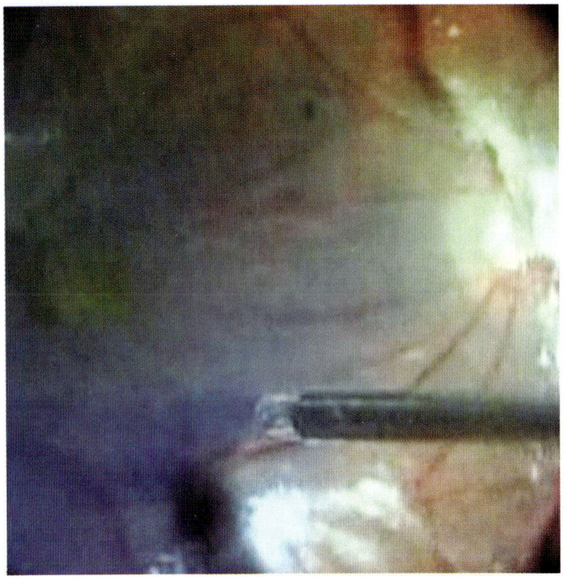

▲ Figure 10.6

Technique of "double staining" using BBG and triamcinolone acetonide (TA) injected over the retinal surface using a soft tip cannula while the BSS infusion remained closed

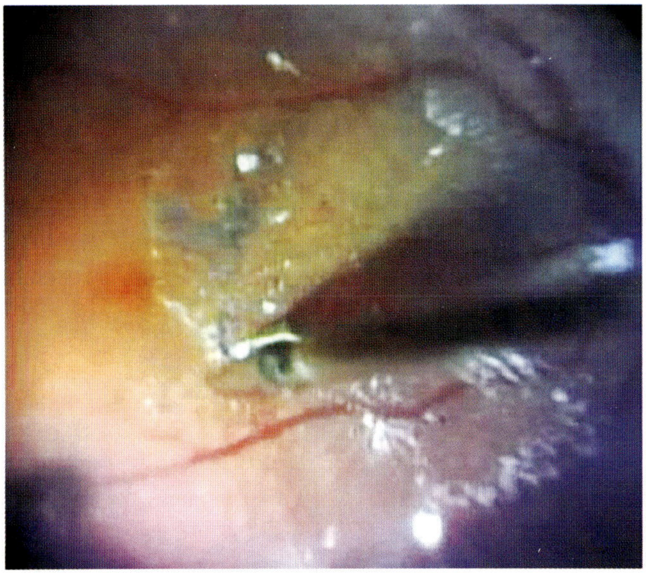

▲ Figure 10.7

ILM peeling guided by the double staining technique after ERM removal. Staining was performed with 0.2 ml of 40 mg/ml TA along with 0.2 ml of 0.25% BBG

hyaloid and ERM as well as the posterior hyaloid and ILM. In this technique, the initial step consists in the injection of a dye with high affinity to the vitreous to enable vitreous removal, followed by a second injection of a dye such as infracyanine green, ICG, TB or BBG to stain and peel pre-retinal membranes.[7,18] As an alternative technique, two dyes may be injected initially before both peeling procedures (Fig. 10.7). Some authors do prefer to name double staining as injection of a dye to peel ERM followed by an additional injection of another dye for ILM peeling.[45] Double staining can be performed with either different dyes or in some instances the same coloring agent can be used to stain two intraocular tissues.[35]

▶ Reconstitution, Dilution and Concentration

Careful selection of the best solvents for vital dyes for chromovitrectomy should be performed, especially regarding those agents provided as a powder for reconstitution by the surgeon in the operating room, such as ICG.

ICG contains iodine to enhance its solubility and must be dissolved in pure water to avoid precipitation and diluted again with BSS to avoid a hypo-osmolar solution. IfCG does not contain iodine, precipitates in water and glucose 5% is rather used as solvent. Thereby, IfCG is an alternative to avoid hypo-osmolar effect on the retina.[18]

Staining with minimum concentrations should be enough to distinguish transparent tissues for removal with the underlying semitransparent retina over an orange-reddish background. A low concentration has also the rationale to cause minimal or no toxic effects to retina, RPE or loss of vision (Table 10.1).

▶ Dye Injection

Several different techniques have been used to inject vital dyes in the vitreous cavity. One has been named the "dry method" or "air-filled technique". Whatever, this consists of removing the fluid in the vitreous cavity by a fluid-gas exchange before dye injection. While this has the advantage of concentrating the dye in the posterior pole and avoiding contact at the posterior capsule of the lens, it may expose the retinal surface to a higher concentration of dye.[2] When the eye is air filled, the full concentration of dye injected into the vitreous cavity reaches the retinal surface.

The second technique is called the "wet method" or "fluid-filled technique". In this approach, the intravitreal fluid (usually balanced salt solution) is left inside the vitreous cavity while the surgeon injects the dye. The concentration of the dye in contact with the retinal surface is lower because it is diluted by the fluid in the vitreous cavity. The disadvantage to this technique is the possible dispersion of the dye leading to unwanted staining of the retina elsewhere. Comparison of the two methods in a porcine model concluded that the air-filled technique induced a higher incidence of RPE atrophy and outer retinal degeneration.[69] A further concern is incubation time of the dye on the retinal surface. Since early dye washout minimizes exposure on retinal tissue, there is a trend to washout the dye a few seconds after its injection.[70]

To avoid an unnecessary and nonselective staining of the entire retina, we developed a new applicator for chromovitrectomy. A prototype was constructed of a metal cannula enclosed in an adjustable silicone tube, giving the instrument a 20-guage outer diameter, with a brush-like proximal end containing multiple, long silk filaments. Subsequently, a commercially available instrument called VINCE (Vitreoretinal Internal limiting membrane Color Enhancer, Dutch Ophthalmic, The Netherlands) has been produced (Figs 10.8A to C). It consists of a modified backflush needle, containing an adjustable silicone tube, which is surrounded by metal cannula. This new device may allow a better visualization of fine, delicate, semitransparent preretinal tissues, while avoiding the uncontrolled staining of the RPE in the MH and peripheral retina.[71]

Macular Hole Protection

There are some ways to avoid dye injection directly through the MH: slow injection of the dye, selective painting instrument (VINCE), or placing substances over the MH such as perfluorocarbons liquids (PFCL), autologous whole blood, or sodium hyaluronate.

In chromovitrectomy, PFCL has been used as a protective agent for the macular hole to avoid the entrance of ICG into

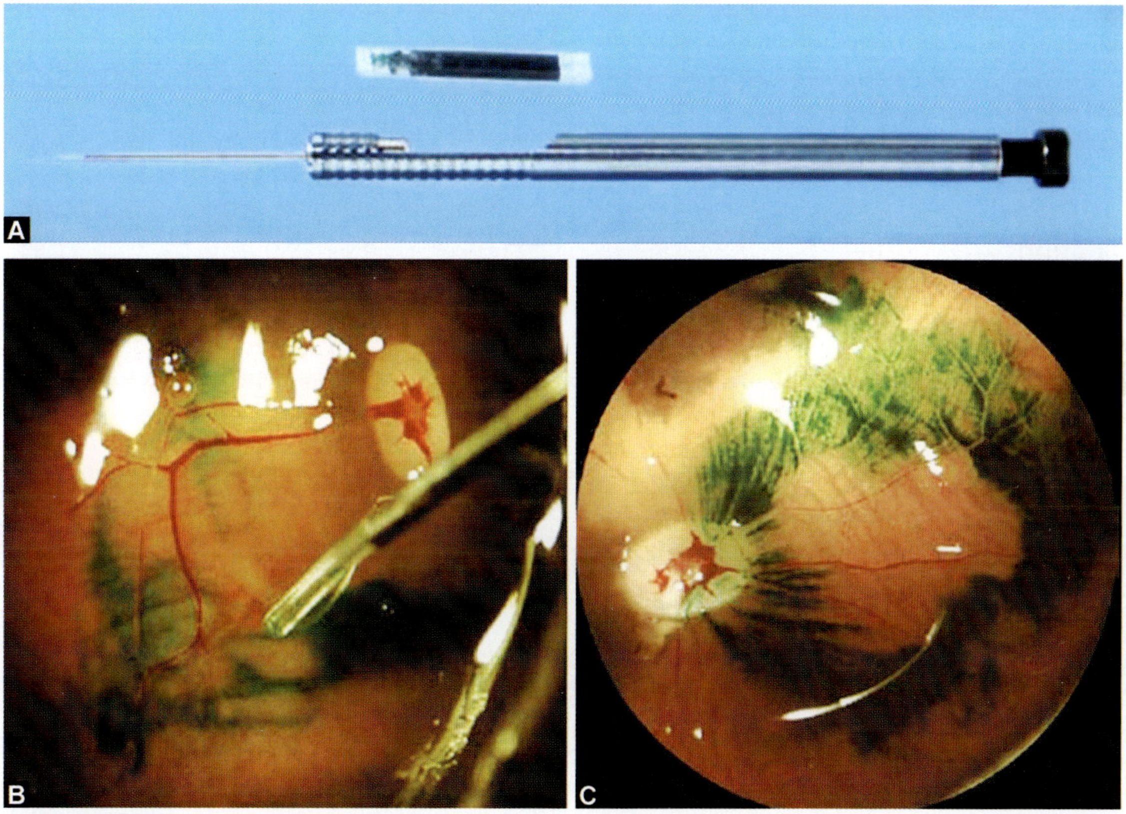

Figures 10.8A to C

The Vitreoretinal Internal limiting membrane Color Enhancer (VINCE) device applicator for chromovitrectomy. (A) A modified 20-gauge backflush needle containing an adjustable silicone tube that is connected to a reservoir in the handpiece, which is filled with the readily prepared and diluted vital dye; (B) The selective circular staining limited to the planned edge of the ILM rhexis may strictly prevent any dye from reaching the center of the macula and peripheral retina; (C) Selective painting the subretinal space. Olson et al.[3] described this surgical approach and proved the immiscibility of PFCL and ICG *in vitro*. Scupola et al.[3] reported the 1 year outcomes of eight patients using chromovitrectomy with PFCL and found no signs of RPE defects and a final median best corrected visual acuity of 20/50. The use of PFCL increases the costs and operative time, while the meticulous use of a small-tip fluted needle is essential to prevent retained PFCL that could lead to retinal toxicity.

Autologous blood has been used as a protective agent during ICG-assisted MH surgery. Lai et al.[3] suggested that, at least *in vitro*, blood could partially protect RPE cells from ICG toxicity. The authors observed that reduced cell viability was greater in the group without blood exposure and no difference was observed when comparing whole blood, plasma, or packed red blood cells. Clinically, a small uncontrolled case series showed that whole blood used in ICG-assisted vitrectomy for MH surgery is apparently safe, with no signs of retinal damage or residual ICG after one month.[72]

Kadonosono et al.[3,73] first described the use of viscoelatics for this purpose. Viscoelastic can be used to control where the dye settles on the retinal surface to avoid staining outside the macular region. Although good visual and anatomic outcomes could be achieved with this technique, it requires more surgical time.

▶ Illumination

Vital dyes are small chemical substances that pass freely through retinal tissue and may play a role in or exacerbate retinal phototoxicity from intraoperative light exposure. Photosensitizing dyes could enhance phototoxicity by increasing levels of free radicals, creating a photoproduct that could be harmful to retinal cells and shifting light absorbance from one site of the retina to another. Clinically, consecutive experiments have shown histologic and functional damage to the retina after light plus ICG exposure in comparison to light without dye application.[74-76]

To analyze the risk for dye-induced light damage, the spectral overlap between light source emission and vital dye absorbance should be known.[74] Haritoglou et al.[76] proposed that a shift in the absorbance band of ICG during vitreoretinal surgery induces photosensitizing effects on the retinal surface. They demonstrated that the absorbance spectrum of ICG overlaps partially with the emission spectrum of one type of halogen light source and that ICG absorbance varies, depending on solvent and osmolarity. Notably, ICG in glucose 5% shifts the absorbance bands to higher wavelengths compared with ICG prepared in balanced salt solution (BSS), thereby decreasing the risk for spectral overlap with the light emission source.[74]

The light pipe should be kept far from the retina and turned off when possible to minimize ICG-related decomposition and thermal damage.[18] Additionally, safer profiles of light sources may be used by the surgeon.[74]

Vital dyes for chromovitrectomy are emerging tools that may enable better visualization of transparent and fine intraocular tissues. The intraoperative staining facilitates surgical removal and thereby better surgical success. The choice of adequate dye for specific surgical cases and membranes should be considered based on fine visibility and lesser chance of ocular toxicity. Dye concentration, pH, osmolarity, type of solvent, injection and illumination techniques are important factors to improving surgical approach in chromovitrectomy.

References

1. Burk SE, Da Mata AP, Snyder ME, et al. Indocyanine green-assisted peeling of the retinal internal limiting membrane. Ophthalmology. 2000;107:2010-4.
2. Rodrigues EB, Meyer CH, Kroll P. Chromovitrectomy: a new field in vitreoretinal surgery. Graefes Arch Clin Exp Ophthalmol. 2005;243:291-3.
3. Rodrigues EB, Costa EF, Penha FM, et al. The use of vital dyes in ocular surgery. Surv Ophthalmol. 2009;54:576-617.
4. Mester V, Kuhn F. Internal limiting membrane removal in the management of full-thickness macular holes. Am J Ophthalmol. 2000;129:769-77.
5. Gandorfer A, Haritoglou C, Kampik A, et al. Ultrastructure of the vitreoretinal interface following removal of the internal limiting membrane using indocyanine green. Curr Eye Res. 2004;29:319-20.
6. Wollensak G, Spoerl E, Wirbelauer C, et al. Influence of indocyanine green staining on the biomechanical strength of porcine internal limiting membrane. Ophthalmologica. 2004;218:278-82.
7. Rodrigues EB, Maia M, Meyer CH, et al. Vital dyes for chromovitrectomy. Curr Opin Ophthalmol. 2007;18:179-87.
8. Maia M, Haller JA, Pieramici DJ, et al. Retinal pigment epithelial abnormalities after internal limiting membrane peeling guided by indocyanine green staining. Retina. 2004;24:157-60.
9. Maia M, Kellner L, de Juan E, et al. Effects of indocyanine green injection on the retinal surface and into the subretinal space in rabbits. Retina. 2004;24:80-91.
10. Maia M, Margalit E, Lakhanpal R, et al. Effects of intravitreal indocyanine green injection in rabbits. Retina. 2004;24:69-79.

11. Arevalo JF, Garcia RA. Macular hole surgery complicated by accidental massive subretinal indocyanine green, and retinal tear. Graefes Arch Clin Exp Ophthalmol. 2007;245: 751-3.
12. Brazitikos PD, Androudi S, Tsinopoulos I, et al. Functional and anatomic results of macular hole surgery complicated by massive indocyanine green subretinal migration. Acta Ophthalmol Scand. 2004;82:613-5.
13. Hirata A, Inomata Y, Kawaji T, et al. Persistent subretinal indocyanine green induces retinal pigment epithelium atrophy. Am J Ophthalmol. 2003;136:353-5.
14. Rodrigues EB, Meyer CH, Farah ME, et al. Intravitreal staining of the internal limiting membrane using indocyanine green in the treatment of macular holes. Ophthalmologica. 2005;219:251-62.
15. Brasil OM, Brasil OF. Comparative analysis of macular hole surgery followed by internal limiting membrane removal with and without indocyanine green staining. Arq Bras Oftalmol. 2006;69:157-60.
16. Horio N, Horiguchi M. Effect on visual outcome after macular hole surgery when staining the internal limiting membrane with indocyanine green dye. Arch Ophthalmol. 2004;122:992-6.
17. Sheidow TG, Blinder KJ, Holekamp N, et al. Outcome results in macular hole surgery: an evaluation of internal limiting membrane peeling with and without indocyanine green. Ophthalmology. 2003;110:1697-701.
18. Farah ME, Maia M, Rodrigues EB. Dyes in ocular surgery: principles for use in chromovitrectomy. Am J Ophthalmol. 2009;148:332-40.
19. Lai MM, Williams GA. Anatomical and visual outcomes of idiopathic macular hole surgery with internal limiting membrane removal using low-concentration indocyanine green. Retina. 2007;27:477-82.
20. Engelbrecht NE, Freeman J, Sternberg P, et al. Retinal pigment epithelial changes after macular hole surgery with indocyanine green-assisted internal limiting membrane peeling. Am J Ophthalmol. 2002;133:89-94.
21. Rodrigues EB, Meyer CH. Meta-analysis of chromovitrectomy with indocyanine green in macular hole surgery. Ophthalmologica. 2008;222:123-9.
22. Kamura Y, Sato Y, Isomae T, et al. Effects of internal limiting membrane peeling in vitrectomy on diabetic cystoid macular edema patients. Jpn J Ophthalmol. 2005;49:297-300.
23. Bardak Y, Cekic O, Tig SU. Comparison of ICG-assisted ILM peeling and triamcinolone-assisted posterior vitreous removal in diffuse diabetic macular oedema. Eye. 2006;20: 1357-9.
24. Radetzky S, Walter P, Fauser S, et al. Visual outcome of patients with macular edema after pars plana vitrectomy and indocyanine green-assisted peeling of the internal limiting membrane. Graefes Arch Clin Exp Ophthalmol. 2004;242: 273-8.
25. Lanzetta P, Polito A, Del Borrello M, et al. Idiopathic macular hole surgery with low-concentration infracyanine green-assisted peeling of the internal limiting membrane. Am J Ophthalmol. 2006;142:771-6.
26. Rivett K, Kruger L, Radloff S. Infracyanine-assisted internal limiting membrane peeling in macular hole repair: does it make a difference? Graefes Arch Clin Exp Ophthalmol. 2004;242:393-6.
27. Kolacny D, Parys-Vanginderdeuren R, Van Lommel A, et al. Vitrectomy with peeling of the inner limiting membrane for treating diabetic macular edema. Bull Soc Belge Ophtalmol. 2005;296:15-23.
28. Husson-Danan A, Glacet-Bernard A, Soubrane G, et al. Clinical evaluation of the use of indocyanine green for peeling the internal limiting membrane in macular hole surgery. Graefes Arch Clin Exp Ophthalmol. 2006;244:291-7.
29. La Heij EC, Dieudonne SC, Mooy CM, et al. Immunohistochemical analysis of the internal limiting membrane peeled with infracyanine green. Am J Ophthalmol. 2005;140:1123-5.
30. Haritoglou C, Gandorfer A, Gass CA, et al. Histology of the vitreoretinal interface after staining of the internal limiting membrane using glucose 5% diluted indocyanine and infracyanine green. Am J Ophthalmol. 2004;137:345-8.
31. Kodjikian L, Richter T, Halberstadt M, et al. Toxic effects of indocyanine green, infracyanine green, and trypan blue on the human retinal pigmented epithelium. Graefes Arch Clin Exp Ophthalmol. 2005;243:917-25.
32. Enaida H, Hisatomi T, Goto Y, et al. Preclinical investigation of internal limiting membrane staining and peeling using intravitreal brilliant blue G. Retina. 2006;26:623-30.
33. Enaida H, Hisatomi T, Hata Y, et al. Brilliant blue G selectively stains the internal limiting membrane/brilliant blue G-assisted membrane peeling. Retina. 2006;26:631-6.
34. Cervera E, Diaz-Llopis M, Salom D, et al. Internal limiting membrane staining using intravitreal brilliant blue G: good help for vitreo-retinal surgeon in training. Arch Soc Esp Oftalmol. 2007;82:71-2.
35. Shimada H, Nakashizuka H, Hattori T, et al. Double staining with brilliant blue G and double peeling for epiretinal membranes. Ophthalmology. 2009;116:1370-6.
36. Horio N, Horiguchi M, Yamamoto N. Triamcinolone-assisted internal limiting membrane peeling during idiopathic macular hole surgery. Arch Ophthalmol. 2005;123:96-9.
37. Kampougeris G, Cheema R, McPherson R, et al. Safety of Triamcinolone acetonide (TA)-assisted pars plana vitrectomy in macular hole surgery. Eye. 2007;21:591-4.
38. Shah GK, Rosenblatt BJ, Blinder KJ, et al. Triamcinolone-assisted internal limiting membrane peeling. Retina. 2005;25: 972-5.
39. Karacorlu M, Ozdemir H, Arf Karacorlu S. Does intravitreal triamcinolone acetonide-assisted peeling of the internal limiting membrane effect the outcome of macular hole surgery? Graefes Arch Clin Exp Ophthalmol. 2005;243:754-7.
40. Maia M, Penha FM, Farah ME, et al. Subretinal injection of preservative-free triamcinolone acetonide and supernatant

vehicle in rabbits: an electron microscopy study. Graefes Arch Clin Exp Ophthalmol. 2008;246:379-88.
41. Lee KL, Dean S, Guest S. A comparison of outcomes after indocyanine green and trypan blue assisted internal limiting membrane peeling during macular hole surgery. Br J Ophthalmol. 2005;89:420-4.
42. Beutel J, Dahmen G, Ziegler A, et al. Internal limiting membrane peeling with indocyanine green or trypan blue in macular hole surgery: a randomized trial. Arch Ophthalmol. 2007;125:326-32.
43. Haritoglou C, Eibl K, Schaumberger M, et al. Functional outcome after trypan blue-assisted vitrectomy for macular pucker: a prospective, randomized, comparative trial. Am J Ophthalmol. 2004;138:1-5.
44. Narayanan R, Kenney MC, Kamjoo S, et al. Trypan blue: effect on retinal pigment epithelial and neurosensory retinal cells. Invest Ophthalmol Vis Sci. 2005;46:304-9.
45. Stalmans P, Feron EJ, Parys-Van Ginderdeuren R, et al. Double vital staining using trypan blue and infracyanine green in macular pucker surgery. Br J Ophthalmol. 2003;87:713-6.
46. Kwok AK, Lai TY, Li WW, et al. Trypan blue- and indocyanine green-assisted epiretinal membrane surgery: clinical and histopathological studies. Eye. 2004;18:882-8.
47. Uno F, Malerbi F, Maia M, et al. Subretinal trypan blue migration during epiretinal membrane peeling. Retina. 2006;26: 237-9.
48. Balayre S, Boissonnot M, Fernandez B, et al. Ultrastructural study of epiretinal membrane stained by trypan blue: 15 case reports. J Fr Ophtalmol. 2005;28:159-67.
49. Balayre S, Boissonnot M, Paquereau J, et al. Evaluation of trypan blue toxicity in idiopathic epiretinal membrane surgery with macular function test using multifocal electroretinography: seven prospective case studies. J Fr Ophtalmol. 2005;28:169-76.
50. Lesnik Oberstein SY, Mura M, Tan SH, et al. Heavy trypan blue staining of epiretinal membranes: an alternative to infracyanine green. Br J Ophthalmol. 2007;91:955-7.
51. Marmor MF. Retinal detachment from hyperosmotic intravitreal injection. Invest Ophthalmol Vis Sci. 1979;18:1237-44.
52. Negi A, Marmor MF. Effects of subretinal and systemic osmolality on the rate of subretinal fluid resorption. Invest Ophthalmol Vis Sci. 1984;25:616-20.
53. Mennel S, Meyer CH, Tietjen A, et al. Patent blue: a novel vital dye in vitreoretinal surgery. Ophthalmologica. 2006;220: 190-3.
54. Luke C, Luke M, Sickel W, et al. Effects of patent blue on human retinal function. Graefes Arch Clin Exp Ophthalmol. 2006;244:1188-90.
55. Haritoglou C, Yu A, Freyer W, et al. An evaluation of novel vital dyes for intraocular surgery. Invest Ophthalmol Vis Sci. 2005;46:3315-22.
56. Haritoglou C, Schumann RG, Strauss R, et al. Vitreoretinal surgery using bromphenol blue as a vital stain: evaluation of staining characteristics in humans. Br J Ophthalmol. 2007;91: 1125-8.
57. Haritoglou C, Strauss R, Priglinger SG, et al. Delineation of the vitreous and posterior hyaloid using bromophenol blue. Retina. 2008;28:333-9.
58. Hillenkamp J, Saikia P, Herrmann WA, et al. Surgical removal of idiopathic epiretinal membrane with or without the assistance of indocyanine green: a randomised controlled clinical trial. Graefes Arch Clin Exp Ophthalmol. 2007;245: 973-9.
59. Foster RE, Petersen MR, Da Mata AP, et al. Negative indocyanine green staining of epiretinal membranes. Retina. 2002;22:106-8.
60. Sakamoto H, Yamanaka I, Kubota T, et al. Indocyanine green-assisted peeling of the epiretinal membrane in proliferative vitreoretinopathy. Graefes Arch Clin Exp Ophthalmol. 2003;241:204-7.
61. Jackson TL, Kwan AS, Laidlaw AH, et al. Identification of retinal breaks using subretinal trypan blue injection. Ophthalmology. 2007;114:587-90.
62. Salicone A, Smiddy WE, Venkatraman A, et al. Management of retinal detachment when no break is found. Ophthalmology. 2006;113:398-403.
63. Ruiz-Moreno JM, Montero JA, Bayon A, et al. Retinal toxicity of intravitreal triamcinolone acetonide at high doses in the rabbit. Exp Eye Res. 2007;84:342-8.
64. Morrison VL, Koh HJ, Cheng L, et al. Intravitreal toxicity of the kenalog vehicle (benzyl alcohol) in rabbits. Retina. 2006;26:339-44.
65. Das T, Vedantham V. Intravitreal sodium fluorescein enhances visualization of clear vitreous during vitreous surgery for macular hole: a safety and efficacy study. Clin Experiment Ophthalmol. 2004;32:55-7.
66. Guo S, Tutela AC, Wagner R, et al. A comparison of the effectiveness of four biostains in enhancing visualization of the vitreous. J Pediatr Ophthalmol Strabismus. 2006;43:281-4.
67. Hata Y, Enaida H, Sassa Y, et al. Preclinical investigation of fluorometholone acetate as a potential new adjuvant during vitreous surgery. Graefes Arch Clin Exp Ophthalmol. 2007;245:1019-25.
68. Verma L, Prakash G, Tewari HK. Trypan blue enhanced vitrectomy in clear gel vitrectomy. Indian J Ophthalmol. 2003;51: 106.
69. Czajka MP, McCuen BW, Cummings TJ, et al. Effects of indocyanine green on the retina and retinal pigment epithelium in a porcine model of retinal hole. Retina. 2004;24:275-82.
70. Schmidt JC, Rodrigues EB, Meyer CH, et al. A modified technique to stain the internal limiting membrane with indocyanine green. Ophthalmologica. 2004;218:176-9.
71. Meyer CH, Rodrigues EB. A novel applicator for the selective painting of pre-retinal structures during vitreoretinal surgery. Graefes Arch Clin Exp Ophthalmol. 2005;243:487-9.
72. Rizzo S, Belting C, Genovesi-Ebert F, et al. Modified technique for safer indocyanine-green-assisted peeling of the internal limiting membrane during vitrectomy for macular hole repair. Graefes Arch Clin Exp Ophthalmol. 2006;244:1615-9.

73. Cacciatori M, Azzolini M, Sborgia M, et al. Sodium hyaluronate 2.3% prevents contact between indocyanine green and retinal pigment epithelium during vitrectomy for highly myopic macular hole retinal detachment. Retina. 2004;24:160-1.
74. Costa Ede P, Rodrigues EB, Farah ME, et al. Vital dyes and light sources for chromovitrectomy: comparative assessment of osmolarity, pH, and spectrophotometry. Invest Ophthalmol Vis Sci. 2009;50:385-91.
75. Rodrigues EB, Meyer CH, Mennel S, et al. Mechanisms of intravitreal toxicity of indocyanine green dye: implications for chromovitrectomy. Retina. 2007;27:958-70.
76. Haritoglou C, Priglinger S, Gandorfer A, et al. Histology of the vitreoretinal interface after indocyanine green staining of the ILM, with illumination using a halogen and xenon light source. Invest Ophthalmol Vis Sci. 2005;46:1468-72.

11 Endophotocoagulation and Safe Intravitreal Injection Technique

Carsten H Meyer, Anne Fung, Neha Sinha, Sandeep Saxena

Introduction

The term laser was coined by Gordon Gould. It was Albert Einstein who gave the concept of LASER in 1917. Charles Towne gave the practical approach in 1950 when he first produced microwaves using stimulated emission. Its use in ophthalmics came in 1961 when first pulsed ruby laser was used coupled with monocular direct ophthalmoscopic delivery system.The introduction of Endolasers to ophthalmology has radically changed the level of care that we can provide to our patients. Through endolaser probe laser energy is delivered to retina via a fiber optic cable introduced through the pars plana route.

Principle

In photocoagulation, temperature rise in tissue is proportional to the amount of light absorbed by the tissue. Melanin, xanthophyll, hemoglobin can absorb laser energy to produce photocoagulation. Sufficiently high temperature, 40 degree or more can be attained that causes denaturation of proteins. Melanin in the retinal pigment epithelium (RPE) and choroid absorbs all wavelengths and is responsible maximally for photocoagulation effect. Gradual decrease in melanin absorption with increasing wavelength leads to increased depth of chorioretinal burns. Thus a lightly pigmented fundus will require laser of higher power. Hb in blood vessels and hemorrhages and absorbs maximally in yellow light. Xanthophyll is present in inner and outer plexiform layers of macula. It absorbs blue light maximally.

A system was developed for transvitreal application of photocoagulation using a fiber optic probe attached to a portable console. The system is activated by a footswitch, and the probe tip is positioned near the retina after performing a pars plana vitrectomy. This technique can be used to treat posterior retinal breaks, apply scatter retinal photocoagulation in certain diabetic eyes, and treat some of the ciliary processes in eyes with neovascular glaucoma.[1]

Parts of Endolaser

- Laser console
- Endoprobe

LASER Console

Laser console comprises of:

- Active medium
- Resonator cavity with mirrors at each end
- Pumping source to introduce energy into active medium to achieve population inversion.

Active Medium

It is the material that contains atoms which will be stimulated to produce laser. Lasers typically are named after the material that makes up the active medium.

The mediums are:

- Nd: YAG laser
- Diode laser.[2]

Endoprobes

The probes produce a reliable, consistent, and focused laser beam at a safe focal distance from the treatment area. An endophotocoagulation probe has a probe tip adapted for insertion into the eye of a subject, and includes an optical fiber for carrying light, and a lens for focusing the light from the end of the fiber onto target tissue at a desired working distance. The lens forms a convergent beam with the waist of the beam providing a spot of maximum power density whose size is independent of the ocular medium.

Cone Angle

Cone angle refers to the degree the laser beam disperses from the aperture of the probe.

Types of Endoprobes

1. *Straight endoprobe:* It provides direct access to the treatment site and facilitates easy insertion and extraction at the sclerotomy (Fig. 11.1).
2. *Angled endoprobe:* It is used for treatment of the peripheral retina. It provides greater flexibility when utilizing a wide field viewing system and allows easier access around the eye and less chance of hitting the lens in phakic eyes. It consists of a tapered needle tip for added visibility of the treatment area and easier insertion into the eye (Fig. 11.2).
3. *Fluted endoprobe (passive aspirating):* It has an added advantage of flute needle for subretinal fluid aspirartion seen in tears and detachments. It provides the utility of passive aspiration and endophotocoagulation into one device. It is an optimal device for surgeons who prefer to control the rate of fluid extrusion with their finger rather than using the mechanical aspiration of a vitrectomy system (Fig. 11.3).
4. *Aspirating endoprobe (active):* This type of probe provides utility of active aspiration and endophoto-coagulation into one device. Eliminates the need for an extrusion needle and frees hand for illumination (Fig. 11.4).
5. *Stepped angled endoprobe:* It has a smooth, gently tapered needle which permits angled tip to be inserted through standard 25-gauge instrumentation and 20-gauge cannulas. Rigid, fixed angle provides sturdy alternative to flex-tip directional probes. 20-24-gauge model offers an alternative to a standard angled probe for surgeons who prefer top work through a cannula or who prefer a smaller diameter tip (Fig. 11.5).
6. *Illuminating endoprobe:* It provide white illumination with laser delivery in one convenient handpiece. It combines seven illumination fibers and 1 laser fiber to allow high transmission and unparalleled brightness. Homogenous illumination is obtained from high quality glass fibers and geometry of fiber bundle. Laser and illumination fibers are flush at probe tip to avoid shadows in the illuminated field. Only one hand is required for illumination and laser delivery, allowing the other hand to operate additional instruments. It requires fewer instrument insertion during surgery.

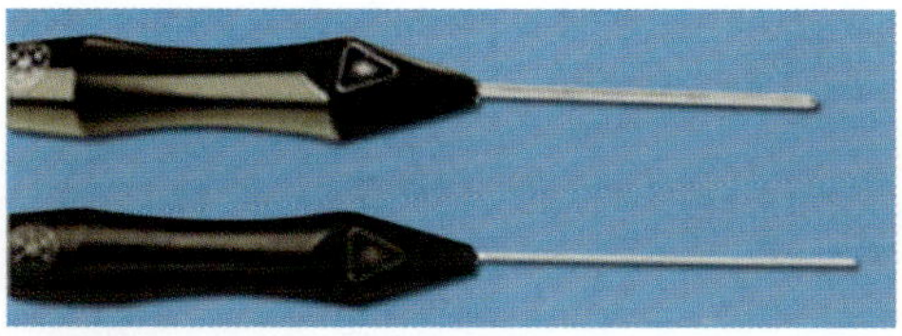

▲ **Figure 11.1**
Straight endoprobe

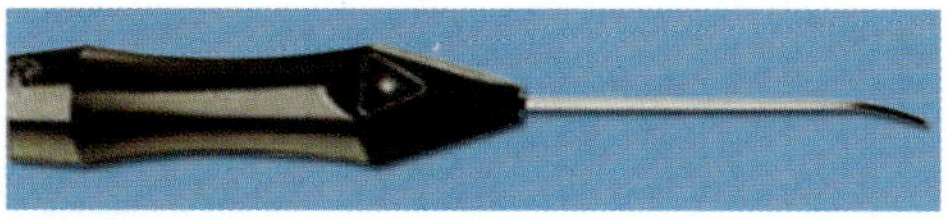

▲ **Figure 11.2**
Angled endoprobe

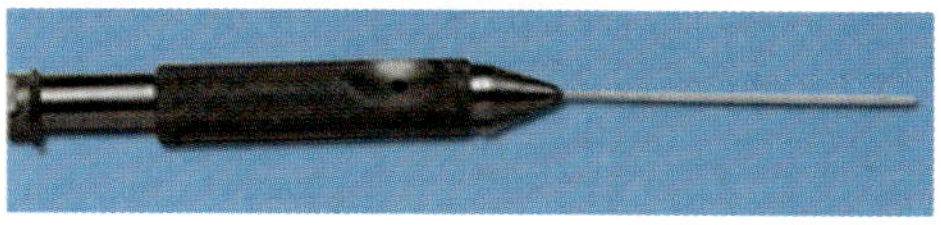

▲ **Figure 11.3**
Fluted endoprobe

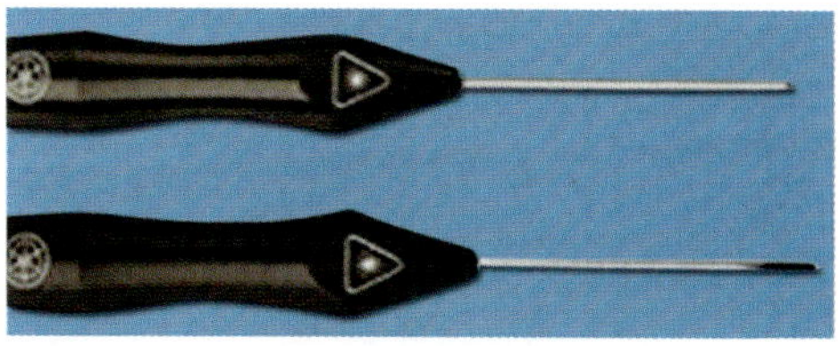

▲ **Figure 11.4**
Aspirating endoprobe

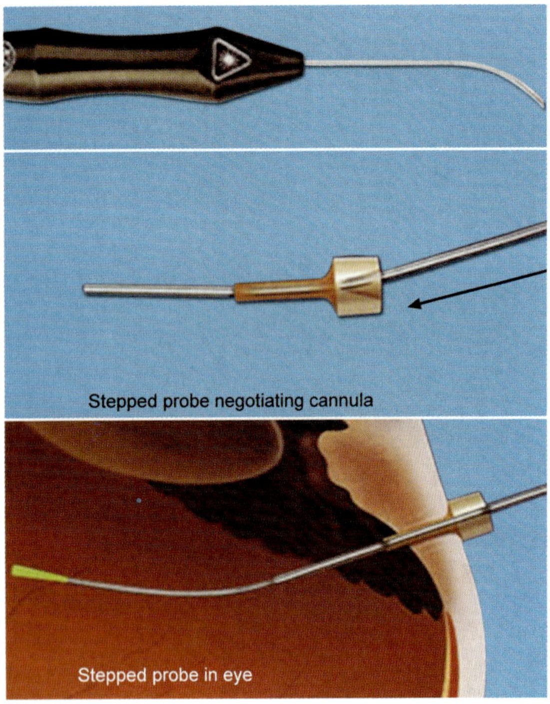

▲ **Figure 11.5**

Stepped angled endoprobe

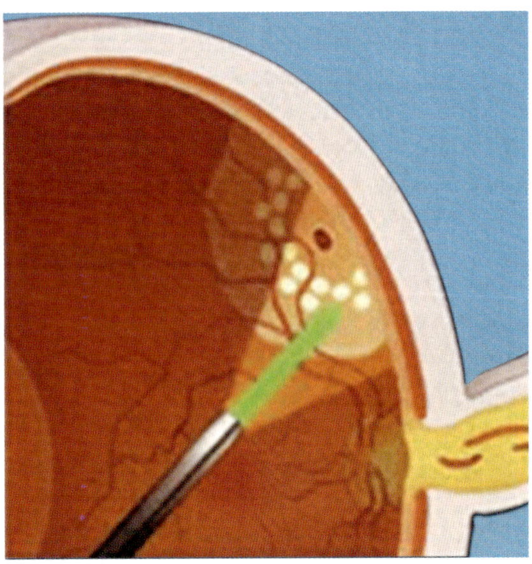

▲ **Figure 11.6**

Illuminating endoprobe

The illuminating endoprobe is indicated for endophotocoagulation for treatment of diabetic retinopathy, retinal breaks and detachments and neovascular glaucoma (Fig. 11.6).

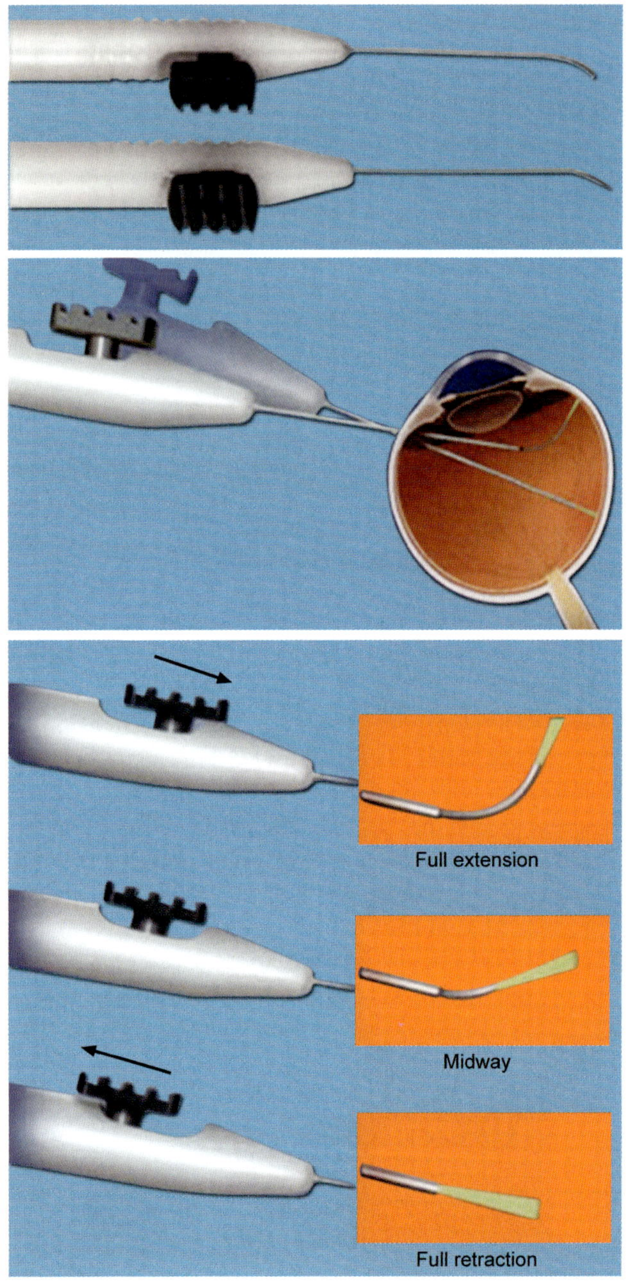

▲ **Figure 11.7**

Endo-ocular probes

7. *Endo-ocular probes:* Fiber optic can be continuously adjusted over a wide range of angles (0-90) for full coverage of peripheral retina without removing the probe from the eye. Fiber optic extends in a logical motion and bends more sharply as slider is pushed forward. The advantage of this probe is consistent mode quality and spot size across all angles (Fig. 11.7).

Indications

1. Barrage laser
2. Pan retinal photocoagulation (PRP) during vitrectomy[3]
3. Neovascular glaucoma[4]
4. Ciliary body destruction[4]
5. Choroidal neovascularization.[5]

Laser photocoagulation is applied around retinal breaks and lattice; in general, two to three rows of treatment are adequate. In more advanced cases of retinal detachment, such as proliferative vitreoretinopathy, laser spots may be placed contiguously in two or three rows on the anterior slope of the scleral buckle. In proliferative diabetic retinopathy and venous occlusion, pan or scatter photocoagulation is applied peripherally to reduce the risk of neovascular glaucoma.

Endophotocoagulation with Indirect Ophthalmoscopy

Endophotocoagulation may not be possible in some eyes due to the poor view afforded by the operating microscope. This limitation is avoided by viewing through filter goggles with the indirect ophthalmoscope while applying treatment with the endophotocoagulation argon laser probe through a pars plana entry site. This method has proved particularly helpful in the gas-filled eye, for treatment over a preexisting scleral buckle, or for a more complete peripheral pan retinal photocoagulation.[6]

Microendoscope Endophotocoagulation

The ophthalmic laser microendoscope has been used to illuminate and view the retina and to deliver diode laser energy in the management of posterior retinal breaks, proliferative retinopathies, and proliferative vitreoretinopathy. The technique of endophotocoagulation was similar to that used routinely in vitreoretinal surgery. The photocoagulation lesions that were created were identical to those delivered by standard endophotocoagulation probes. Intraoperative complications were few, consisting of transient mild retinal or choroidal hemorrhages. Severe postoperative complications related to endophotocoagulation or to use of the ophthalmic laser microendoscope have not been observed.[7]

Safe Intravitreal Injection Technique

Significant advances have been made in optimizing the delivery of drugs to target tissues within the eye and in maintaining effective drug doses within those tissues.

Retinal drug delivery is still a challenging area in the field of ophthalmic drug delivery. A variety of approaches have been described for drug delivery into the vitreous cavity. Intravitreal injection was first reported by Ohm in 1911 as a technique to introduce air for retinal tamponade and repair of retinal detachment.[8] Intravitreal administration of pharmacotherapies dates to the mid-1940s with the use of penicillin to treat endophthalmitis. Since that time, use of the intravitreal injection technique has progressively increased, with its usage being focused primarily on the treatment of retinal detachment, endophthalmitis and cytomegalovirus (CMV) retinitis.

The increasing efficacy and safety of intravitreal injections, in conjunction with the development of pharmacotherapies, has led to a recent rapid increase in the use of this technique for the administration of various pharmacotherapies, including bevacizumab, ranibizumab, pegaptanib sodium and intravitreal triamcinolone acetonide.[9] An intravitreal drug application has been suggested to achieve therapeutic levels locally, with prolonged effective concentrations (Fig. 11.8).[10,11]

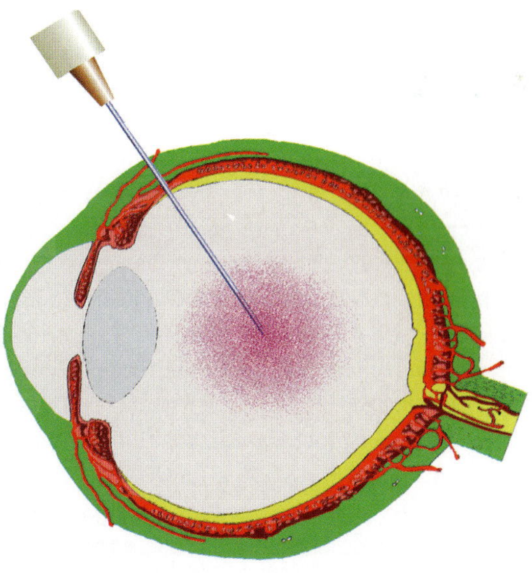

Figure 11.8

Intravitreal injections via the pars plana route into the mid-vitreous

Intravitreal Drug Delivery

The advantage of intravitreal drug administrations is an immediate therapeutic effect at the intended tissue. With the widespread use of intravitreal injections, there has been an increased interest regarding the best application technique. Clinical experience with intravitreal injection has provided physicians with an outline of avoidable risks.

All injections should be performed under sterile conditions. While European countries recommend applying the injection in an operating room, other countries, including the US and India, perform the injection in minor surgery or conventional examining rooms under sterile conditions.[12]

Anticoagulation and Intravitreal Injections

A major concern associated with preoperative discontinuation of anticoagulation therapy is the increased risk of thromboembolic or cerebrovascular events.[13] The ranibizumab study trials observed a low incidence of ocular hemorrhages in patients maintaining warfarin. In the MARINA trial there were a total of 60 warfarin-treated patients, receiving a mean of 22.0 + 3.6 injections.[14] No ocular bleeding was observed in over 1,300 consecutive injections. Intraocular injections in warfarin-treated patients are unlikely to cause ocular hemorrhages.

Surface Preparation with Betadine

The risk of infectious endophthalmitis following intravitreal injection is small. The role of topical antibiotics to prevent postinjection endophthalmitis remains controversial around the world. Topical antibiotics may be applied after the injection for a few days, as the break in the conjunctiva and sclera takes time to completely heal and water-seal. In addition there may be a synergistic effect between topical antibiotics and povidone-iodine. There is no study demonstrating that a reduced conjunctival bacterial load may result in a lower risk for endophthalmitis.[15] Treatment of any active external infection, including significant blepharitis, is mandatory prior to each intravitreal injection.[11,15] The primary goal of any infectious prophylaxis is to minimize the present bacterial flora around the surgical entry site. This can be achieved with the topical application of povidone-iodine, eyelid hygiene, proper isolation of the surgical site and optional postoperative antibiotics.[16-18]

One key step to reducing the risk of endophthalmitis is a sufficient disinfection of the skin, eye lashes and conjunctiva. The eyelids and lashes are usually disinfected with a povidone-iodine (10%) scrub. A sterile speculum is placed between the lids. Various methods of applying povidone-iodine preoperatively have been studied. Most American investigators apply two drops of 0.5% povidone-iodine placed on the ocular surface over the intended site of the injection. Some physicians place three drops of povidone-iodine (5%), three times several minutes apart over the ocular surface preventing dessication and abrasion of the cornea with antibiotic eye drops or sterile saline solution. European investigators have advocated irrigating the conjunctival sac with 1% or 5% povidone-iodine to decrease conjunctival colonization; however it remains unknown whether the application of povidone-iodine drops versus a flush is more effective in preventing endophthalmitis. Preinjection antibiotic drops may be applied according to the label of the applied drug, although there is no evidence supporting its use before intravitreal injections.

Local Topical Anesthesia

Satisfactory pain relief may be achieved with topical lidocaine. Local anesthesia may be induced by applying 3–4 sterile cotton swabs (for 30 seconds each) soaked in sterile 4% lidocaine to the injection area.[19] Alternatively, lidocaine may be applied with 2% eye drops, gel or as a subconjunctival injection. The effective relief of pain with lidocaine for intravitreal injection seems to be independent of its mode of application (gel vs. subconjunctival injection). However, topical applications of lidocaine causes less chemosis compared with subconjunctival anesthesia. Most centers have stopped using gel on a regular basis as topical eye drops seem to induce a sufficient anesthesia.

The Injection Procedure and Recommended Technique

The injection site should be located 3.5–4 mm posterior to the limbus. The injection site may differ in repeated injections by approximately one clock hour.[11,20] This avoids a double penetration through the same site, inducing a persisting scleral hole with consecutive leaking or vitreous incarceration "vitreous wick".

The angle of the incision through the sclera may be directed in an oblique, tunneled fashion (Figs 11.9 and 11.10), as rectangular radial incisions may remain open inducing

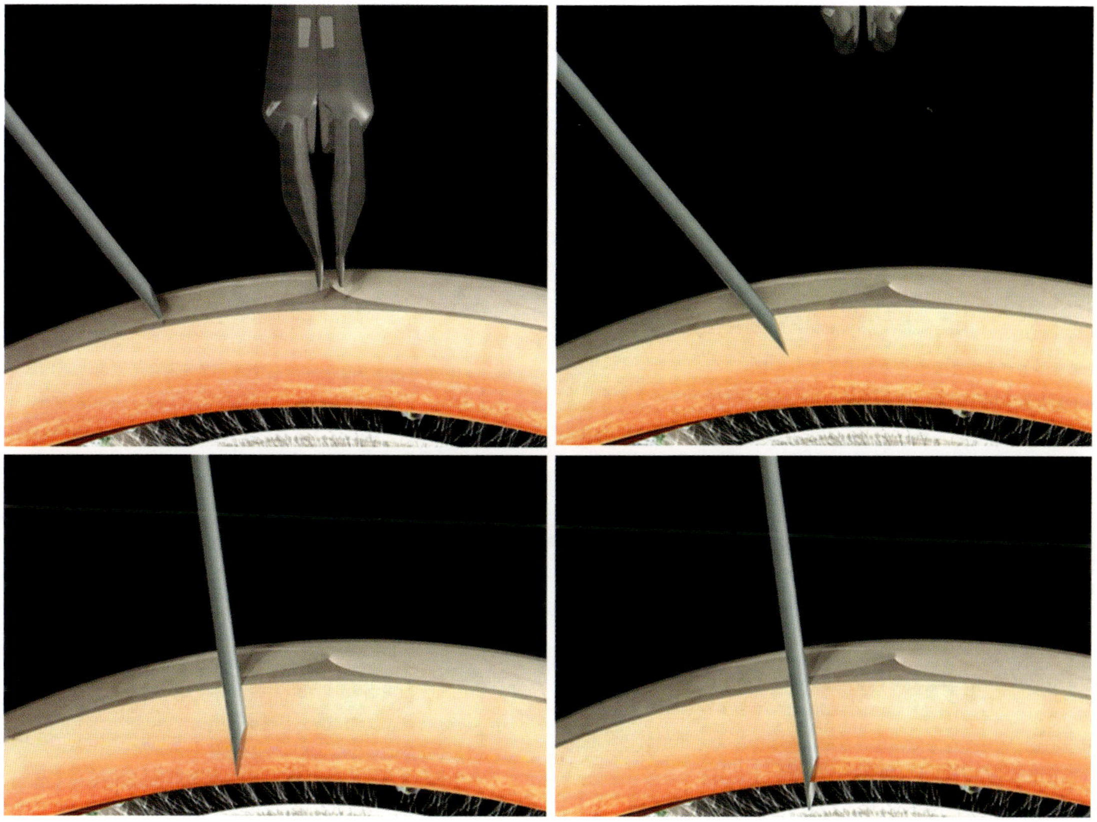

▲ **Figure 11.9**

Schematic drawing of the injection procedure: the conjunctiva is moved upwards, so that the conjunctival hole and the site of the scleral penetration are not on top of each other. After an initial lamellar penetration of the outer sclera, the needle is moved upwards for a full thickness penetration

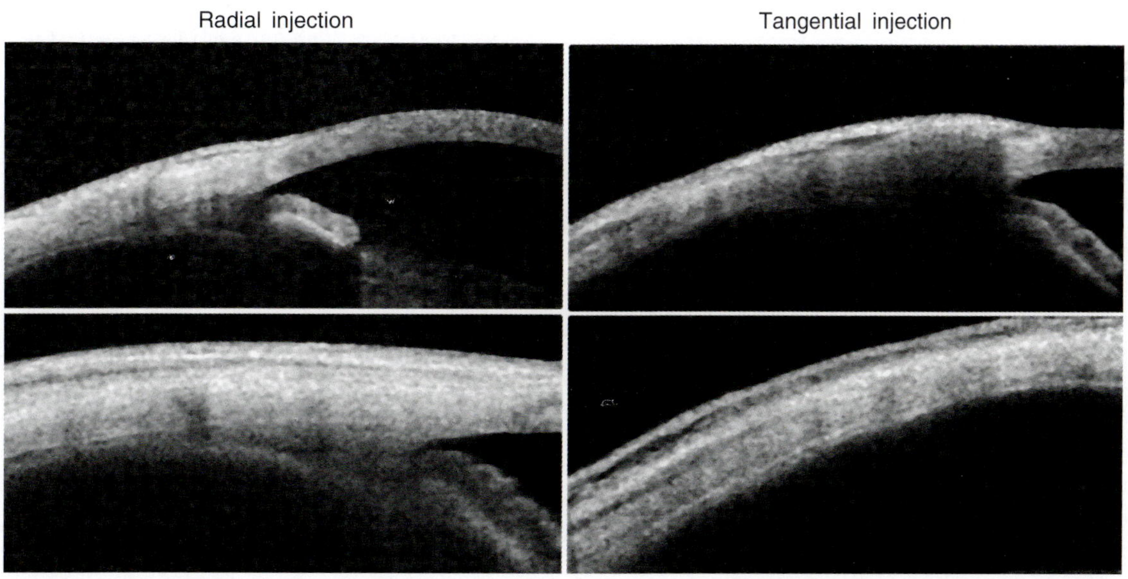

▲ **Figure 11.10**

Examination of the injections site 15 minutes after the injection with the anterior segment OCT scan (Visante): the radial injection remains open and visible, whereas the tangential oblique injection is not detected on OCT vitreous or drug reflux under the conjunctiva as well as severe chemosis and even hypotony in vitrectomized eyes.[21,22] Persistent unsealed sclerotomies following radial injections using a 30-gauge needle, require secondary suturing to seal the penetrating scleral wound. The depth of the insertion may vary between 5–7 mm, so that the tip of the needle is placed in the mid-vitreous. The drug is then gently injected into the vitreous cavity.

The diameter of the needle should be smaller than 27-gauge to reduce the risk of wound leakage or injury. Injections with crystalline TA are frequently applied with 27-gauge needles, while most liquid injections are performed with 30-gauge needles. The required force to penetrate the sclera is almost twice as much using 27-gauge needles compared with 30-gauge or even 31-gauge.[23] Larger needles may not necessarily induce more pain to the patient; however they may induce more reflux or subconjunctival hemorrhage. In addition, blunting of the needle tip, as found in some prefilled syringes, was observed to cause a deeper inpouching and visible indentation of the eye wall during the injection that may have caused the patient more discomfort.[24,25]

The injected volume should be limited up to 0.15 ml without a routine paracentesis releasing an elevated ocular pressure. Administration of rTPA, anti-VEGF and SF_6 gas as triple injection for the management of subretinal hemorrhage requires frequently a paracentesis to release the elevated eye pressure.[26]

Ocular Complications

A survey on ocular complications reported an overall prevalence for retinal detachments of 3.9% per eye or 0.9% per injection and a prevalence of endophthalmitis (including pseudo-endophthalmitis) of 0.3% per injection and 0.9% per eye.[9]

The rational for intravitreal drug application is an immediate and increased therapeutic delivery to the targeted tissue. Some parts of the injection procedure (use of adequate anesthetics, povidone-iodine and a lid speculum; not injecting patients with active eyelid or ocular infections, avoiding extensive massage of eyelid meibomian glands, avoiding prophylactic or postinjection paracentesis) are supported by consensus agreement in all countries while other aspects have less agreement (e.g. most investigators advocate gloves, most prefer povidone-iodine drops over flush, most use no sterile drape). There is no agreement regarding the use of preinjection or postinjection topical antibiotics, as well as a specific intraocular pressure level that should not be exceeded before the injection. Intravitreal drug application is a safe and effective procedure. Side effects, e.g. elevated intraocular pressure, cataract formation and endophthalmitis are limited.

References

1. Charles S. Endophotocoagulation. Retina. 1981;1:117-20.
2. Sasoh M, Smiddy WE. Diode laser endophotocoagulation. Retina. 1995;15:388-93.
3. Zhao P, Wang W, Chen Q. Endolaser photocoagulation in vitrectomy surgery. 1996;32:123-5.
4. Sears JE, Capone A, Aaberg TM, January B. Ciliary body endophotocoagulation during pars plana vitrectomy for pediatric patients with vitreoretinal disorders and glaucoma. Am J Ophthalmol. 1998;126,723-5.
5. Koch FHJ, Mercado HQ, Hattenbach LO, et al. Pigment epithelium endoscopic laser surgery for treatment of choroidal neovascularization. Ophthalmologica ;218:162-75.
6. Hampton GR. Argon Endophotocoagulation With Indirect Ophthalmoscopy. Arch Ophthalmol. 1987;105:132.
7. Uram M. Ophthalmic laser microendoscope endophotocoagulation. Ophthalmology 1992;99:1829-32.
8. Ohm J. Über die Behandlung der Netzhautablösung durch operative Entleerung der subretinalen Flüssigkeit und Einspritzen vom Luft in den Glaskörper. Graefe Arch Klin Ophthalmol. 1911:79:442-50.
9. Fung AE, Rosenfeld PJ, Reichel E. The International Intravitreal Bevacizumab Safety Survey: using the internet to assess drug safety worldwide. Br J Ophthalmol. 2006;90: 1344-9.
10. Kaiser PK, Brown DM, Zhang K, et al. Ranibizumab for predominantly classic neovascular age-related macular degeneration: subgroup analysis of first-year ANCHOR results. Am J Ophthalmol. 2007;144:850-7.
11. Fung AE, Lalwani GA, Rosenfeld PJ, et al. An optical coherence tomography-guided, variable dosing regimen with intravitreal ranibizumab (Lucentis) for neovascular age-related macular degeneration. Am J Ophthalmol. 2007;143:566-83.
12. Schmidt-Erfurth UM, Richard G, Augustin A, et al. European Society for Retina Specialists' Guidelines Committee (EURETINA). Guidance for the treatment of neovascular age-related macular degeneration. Acta Ophthalmol Scand. 2007;85:486-94.
13. Meyer CH, Callizo J, Mennel S, et al. Perioperative management of anticoagulated patients undergoing repeated intravitreal injections. Arch Ophthalmol. 2007;125:994.
14. Charles S, Rosenfeld PJ, Gayer S. Medical consequences of stopping anticoagulant therapy before intraocular surgery or intravitreal injections. Retina. 2007;27:813-5.
15. Scott IU, Flynn HW. Reducing the risk of endophthalmitis following intravitreal injections. Retina. 2007;27:10-12.
16. Safar A, Dellimore MC. The effect of povidone iodine flush versus drops on conjunctival colonization before intravitreal injections. Int Ophthalmol. 2007;27:307-12.

17. Meyer CH, Mennel S, Eter N. Incidence of endophthalmitis after intravitreal Avastin injection with and without postoperative topical antibiotic application. Ophthalmologe. 2007;104:952-7.
18. Ta CN, Egbert PR, Singh K, et al. Prospective randomized comparison of 3-day versus 1-hour preoperative ofloxacin prophylaxis for cataract surgery. Ophthalmology. 2002;109: 2036-41.
19. Kaderli B, Avci R. Comparison of topical and subconjunctival anesthesia in intravitreal injection administrations. Eur J Ophthalmol. 2006;16:718-21.
20. Aiello LP, Brucker AJ, Chan S, et al. Evolving guidelines for intravitreous injections. Retina. 2004;24;S3-19.
21. Rodrigues EB, Meyer CH, Grumann A, et al. Tunneled scleral incision to prevent vitreal reflux after intravitreal injection. Am J Ophthalmol. 2007;143:1035-7.
22. Rodrigues EB, Meyer CH, Schmidt JC, et al. Unsealed sclerotomy after intravitreal injection with a 30-gauge needle. Retina. 2004;24:810-12.
23. Pulido JS, Pulido CM, Bakri SJ, et al. The use of 31-gauge needles and syringes for intraocular injections. Eye. 2007;21: 829-30.
24. Kozak I, Dean A, Clark TM, et al. Prefilled syringe needles versus standard removable needles for intravitreous injection. Retina. 2006;26:679-83.
25. Hochman MN, Friedman MJ. An in vitro study of needle force penetration comparing a standard linear insertion to the new bidirectional rotation insertion technique. Quintessence Int. 2001;32:789-96.
26. Meyer CH, Scholl HP, Eter N, et al. Combined treatment of acute subretinal haemorrhages with intravitreal recombined tissue plasminogen activator, expansile gas and bevacizumab: a retrospective pilot study. Acta Ophthalmol. 2008;86:490-4.

SECTION 2

Retinal Detachment

Scleral Buckling

12

Hermann D Schubert

Introduction

Any discussion of scleral buckling has to recognize that the procedure is not practiced much anymore except by a small group of enthusiasts.[1] On September 29th, 2007, at the 40th annual meeting of the Retina Society in Boston, a symposium in honor of Charles Schepens, entitled "Where It All Began", discussed "Changing Trends in Retinal Detachment Surgery", and "Scleral Buckles and the Dodo Bird". These trends were likened to pasta con tonno, a dish that was popular in rural Sicily in the last century; the Dodo bird referred to a toy that was once popular in the United States, but now is obsolete. During an earlier conference dealing with retinal detachment, author was embarrassed by vocal opponents of scleral buckling who strongly expressed the opinion that this technique should not be mentioned any more to "our young people". These "young people" were sitting quietly in the back of a conference room in Marburg, Germany, perhaps wondering what might happen next. It has become common for the users of this procedure to have a defensive attitude toward scleral buckling, which generally is perceived as the insufficiently advanced approach of another generation, retired or almost gone.[2]

There is no shortage of comprehensive and detailed texts on reasons to perform scleral buckling[3] and how to do it.[4-7] The following presents a brief personal perspective supporting those who, after seeing many vitrectomies promote cataracts,[8] have become curious about the lost art of buckling, a procedure that not only preserves phakia, but expands the surgeon's armamentarium.

Who is a Potential Candidate for Scleral Buckles?

The short answer is that all of those who like their natural lens and do not opt for cataract surgery during or after retinal detachment repair are candidates for scleral buckles. Any vitrectomy, no matter how completely and elegantly performed, promotes cataract and may lead to earlier need for cataract removal.[8] Three groups of patients may benefit from keeping their natural lens: young myopes with clear lenses, accommodation and attached vitreous; moderate to high myopes of any age who, after removal of vitrectomy-induced cataracts, become anisometropes with compromised binocularity that is difficult or impossible to refract; individuals under the age of 59 years who have modest accommodation left, allowing comfortable midrange vision and binocularity.[9] All of these people would benefit from a procedure that preserves the lens, accommodation, midrange vision and natural visual perception. In addition, in some countries and locations, such as, for example, Kyrgyzstan (A E. Eshmanbetov, June 19th, 2010, personal communication) not a single vitrectomy machine is available. In those places, hundreds of patients with retinal detachment could be helped by skillfully performed scleral buckling procedures, done using available technology and financial resources.

A Brief History of Scleral Buckling

Historically, there were two schools of scleral buckling. The Custodis-Lincoff school advocated buckling a break to "cork" it with a localized external indentation, placing one or more breaks on the crest of the buckle to allow subretinal fluid to be spontaneously absorbed.[10] This procedure was preferably done with radial buckles emphasizing precise localization, particularly as to the longitude of the break. Careful study, including scleral depression, was mandatory, as was double patching to reduce the amount of subretinal fluid and allow better localization of the breaks. Drainage or injection of gas was the exception with this approach.

The Arruga-Schepens school, which preferred to use limbus-parallel encircling buckles, required detailed preoperative study, particularly as to the latitude of breaks that had to lie on the crest or the anterior slope of the encircling buckle.[11,12] The longitude of the break was less critical than with radial buckles, even though Schepens[4] took preoperative study of his patients and careful drawing of the retina to an unprecedented level. Apart from buckling and perhaps "corking" the break, the circling element was used to relieve broad-based vitreous traction in a manner similar to tamponade and to wall off the "porous area" between the ora serrata and the equator of the eye from the useful posterior retina. Transscleral drainage of subretinal fluid was necessary to create space for these buckles, which often were large.[12,13] Thus, one main difference between the two methods was how they dealt with the initial separation between the pigment epithelium and the retina. The Custodis-Lincoff procedure advocated preoperative reduction of subretinal fluid by patching and immobilization. In contrast, the Schepens method required accumulation of copious subretinal fluid to allow for reduction of volume by external drainage.

For a variety of reasons, the encircling operation caught on, making scleral buckling almost synonymous with encircling and drainage in a majority of publications. This procedure has survived as the ubiquitous 3.5 mm silicone band used in combination with modern vitrectomy. In a well-known study of scleral buckling versus primary vitrectomy in rhegmatogenous retinal detachment, buckle combined with vitrectomy was shown to be the most effective procedure for pseudophakic eyes.[14] The risky transscleral subretinal fluid drainage of the past was replaced by internal drainage using retinotomy and/or perfluorocarbon liquids.

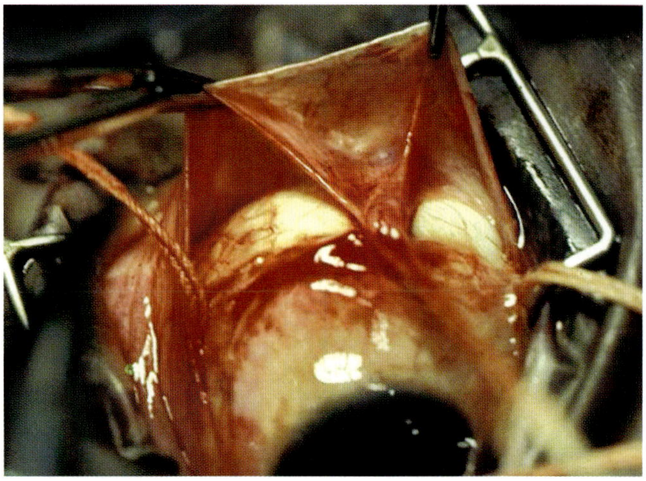

▲ **Figure 12.1**

The conjunctival incision is made parallel to the limbus and 4 mm posterior to it. After placement of the buckle, the intermuscular septae and Tenon's capsule should be reattached in their original position

Orbital Issues

Scleral buckles are intraorbital, episcleral, subtenon and subtendinous foreign bodies applied through a combination of episcleral, anterior orbital and muscle surgery. Of all of these basic surgical techniques, the maneuvers of strabismology may be the most important for proper handling of tissues. Depending on the buckle size, motility problems have been frequently noted.[15] Any episcleral surgery involving Tenon's capsule and intermuscular septae risks destabilizing the orbital pulley system. The cotton tip applicator is often used to push anterior tissues into the posterior orbit. Respect for the septae of Guerin and the intermuscular septae is mandatory, as is careful dual layer closure (Fig. 12.1). In eyes requiring reoperation, author has often found Tenon's capsule recessed to the equator. In addition to motility problems, dry eye can be promoted by scarred episcleral tissues and compromised goblet cells deprived of their natural subepithelial vascular environment. Moreover, preexisting phorias may become tropias related to vision loss associated with the retinal detachment, i.e. even without any iatrogenic orbital scarring, these eyes are at risk for diplopia.

Topographic Considerations

The emmetropic eye has a diameter of 24 mm at its equator, which is located 14 mm posterior to the limbus. The projection of the ora serrata largely coincides with the spiral of Tillaux, which is 5.5–7.9 mm posterior to the limbus. Posterior vitreous insertion and most breaks occur between the ora serrata and the equator. Schepens therefore called

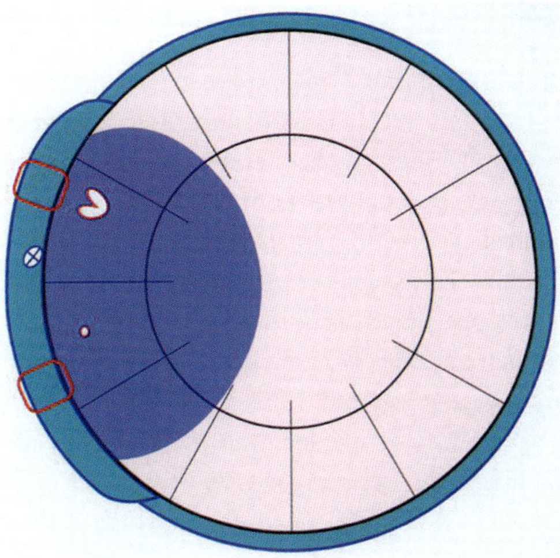

▲ **Figure 12.2**

Schematic of an encircling and drainage operation. The 7.5 mm solid silicone explant covers the ora serrata to the equator for the entire extent of the retinal detachment. Drainage or injection of air is often necessary to reduce the epithelioretinal interspace

this region the "porous zone". The circumference of an emmetropic eye at the latitude of the ora serrata is 60 mm; at the equator, it is 72 mm. Statistically, when measured from the limbus, most breaks are found at 13 mm latitude in phakic eyes and 12 mm in aphakic eyes. Lincoff[16] divided the area anterior to the equator into 12 squares of 6 x 6 mm each. A 7.5 mm explant (#277)[17]will cover this area (Fig. 12.2). In general, cases of uncertain localization of breaks will require larger buckles and/or buckling of the entire extent of the retinal detachment. The ocular circumference of 72 mm allows placement of a theoretical maximum of 9 radial 5 mm buckles. Custodis was known to have placed up to five individual segmental buckles on one eye. Author has done the same, but does not recommend it. Placing so many buckles usually is unnecessary, since 50% of all detachments have one break and only 30% have more than one break.[18]

Preoperative Examination

A 90-diopter lens is used to examine the macula to determine whether or not it is detached and whether the 12 o'clock meridian is attached or detached. The indirect ophthalmoscope shows the extent and contours of the retinal detachment, as well as the obvious breaks. Once the convex contours have been established, the Lincoff rules (Fig. 12.3) can be applied to reexamine and focus on the probable locations of causative breaks.[19,20]

▶ Contact Lens and Scleral Depression at the Slit Lamp

An indirect contact lens and scleral depression at the slit lamp are used for a detailed peripheral retinal examination (Fig. 12.4). The slit lamp has to be defocused (pulled toward the examiner) and then focused (gently pushed forward toward the patient), which the examiner accomplishes by

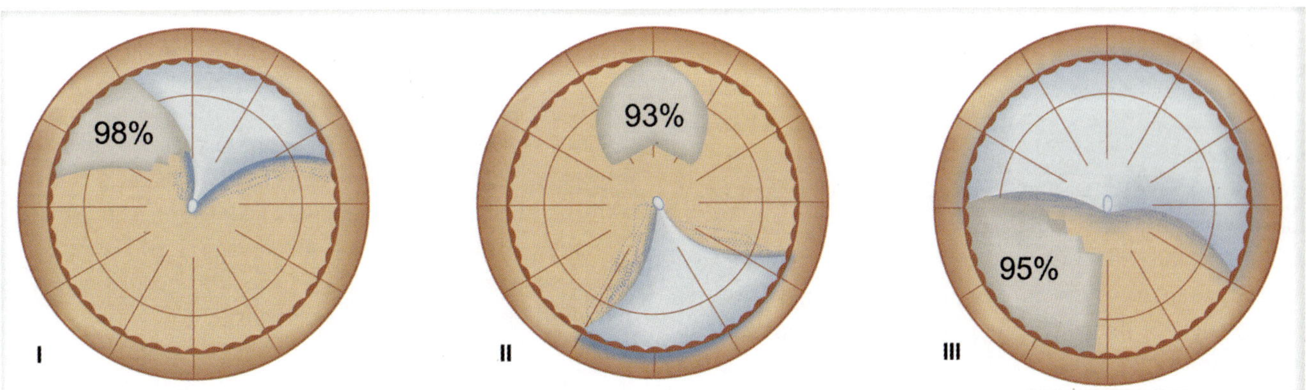

▲ **Figure 12.3**

Schematic representation of the use of Lincoff rules to find the primary break

I. Superior temporal or nasal detachments: In 98% the primary break lies within 1½ clock hours of the highest border.
II. Total or superior detachments that cross the 12 o'clock meridian: In 93% the primary break is at 12 o'clock or in a triangle, the apex of which is at the ora serrata and the sides intersect the equator 1 hour to either side of 12 o'clock.
III. Inferior detachments: In 95% the higher side of the detachment indicates on which side of the 6 o'clock radian an inferior break lies.
When an inferior detachment is bullous the primary break lies above the horizontal meridian

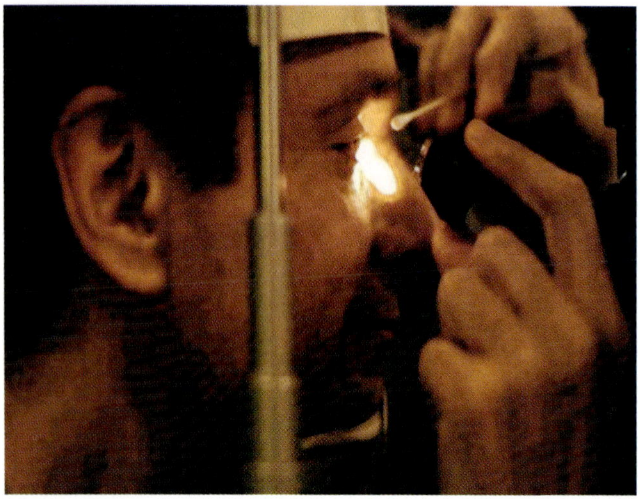

▲ **Figure 12.4**

Scleral depression at the slit lamp. The examiner's hands move the lens and scleral depressor; the examiner's forehead is used to move and focus the slit lamp

pushing the slit lamp with his or her eyebrows and head until the image is focused. This technique, in which the examiner also uses one hand for the contact lens and the other hand for the scleral depressor, is difficult to master. Handedness, size of nose, deeply set eyes and lack of patient cooperation can all be obstacles. Diagnostically, however, it makes all the difference in finding small aphakic breaks.[19]

▶ Drawing

According to Schepens, a drawing should be made to "commit oneself" to the findings and to allow comprehensive and rational preoperative planning.[4] The drawing may, in fact, show that a procedure other than scleral buckling will be of most benefit to the patient. The drawing, placed on the wall of the operating room during surgery, is later supplemented by the addition of intraoperative findings, including reassessment of the latitude and longitude of breaks, scleral localizations, missed breaks, sites of drainage, scleral bites, injection sites and final placement of the buckle. Having a record of the critical sutures allows less traumatic removal of the buckle through minimal conjunctival incisions, should that become necessary. In my practice, the first examination takes up to 40 minutes and, if the findings are still uncertain, the patient's eye is double-patched overnight[21] and reexamined the following morning for 30 minutes.

▶ Double Patching

Double patching immobilizes the eye and reduces the amount of subretinal fluid.[21] This is associated with a decrease in the epithelial retinal interspace, thereby reducing parallax and facilitating precise localization of the break on the sclera, as well as initial apposition of the retina on the crest of the scleral buckle. The reduction of subretinal fluid also makes it possible to regain the contour of a detached retina that corresponds to causative breaks, thus allowing more precise application of the Lincoff rules than would otherwise be possible (Fig.12.3). If the location of retinal breaks is still uncertain, the likely procedure will be a vitrectomy with wide-angle viewing and scleral depression, which permits more detailed examination during retinal repair.

Practical Considerations: Nuts and Bolts

Phakic or aphakic patients with known holes (clear-hole situation) should be considered for a scleral buckle. Statistically, 50% of patients will require one radial buckle; 30% will require two radial buckles or one circumferential segmental buckle if the holes are spaced more closely than 1½ clock hours.[7] The 20% of patients with three holes or more will require combinations of buckles, including limbus parallel segmental buckles. Author does not recommend using more than three segmental buckles. Indeed, even one or two segmental buckles may be considered an eccentric therapeutic approach. An encircling buckle and/or vitrectomy seem to be preferable in this complex situation. Parallel limbus buckles are likely to be centered at 13 mm posterior to the limbus in phakic eyes and at 12 mm in pseudophakic eyes. In general, author uses 5 × 3 mm, 5 × 5 mm and 7 × 3 mm soft silicone sponges and a 3.5 mm and 7.5 mm solid silicone encircling element. The 5 × 5 mm sponge should be reserved for the equatorial radial buckle, since it may cause excessive distortion of the globe and astigmatism.

▶ Radial Buckles

The circumference of the emmetropic eye, depending in its latitude, is 60–72 mm. Breaks should be carefully localized, particularly as to longitude and marked on the sclera. If a break is closer to the ora serrata than it is to the equator, a 5 × 3 mm sponge fixated with a 7 mm mattress suture may be sufficient, particularly since breaks tend to be smaller than

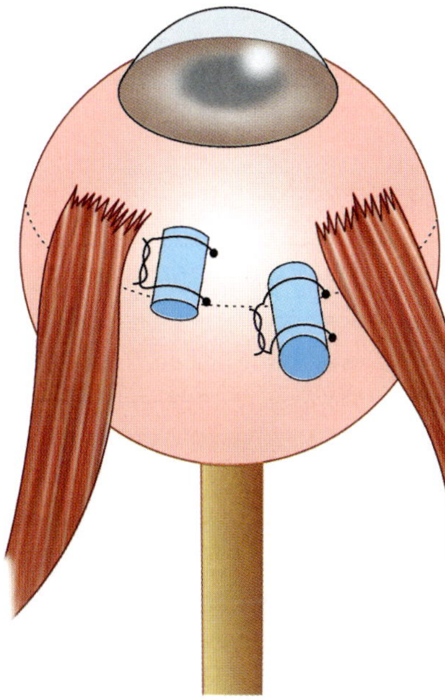

▲ **Figure 12.5**

5 x 3 mm radial sponges are used near the ora serrata; 5 x 5 mm sponges are used near the equator. The width of the mattress sutures is 7 mm and 8 mm, respectively

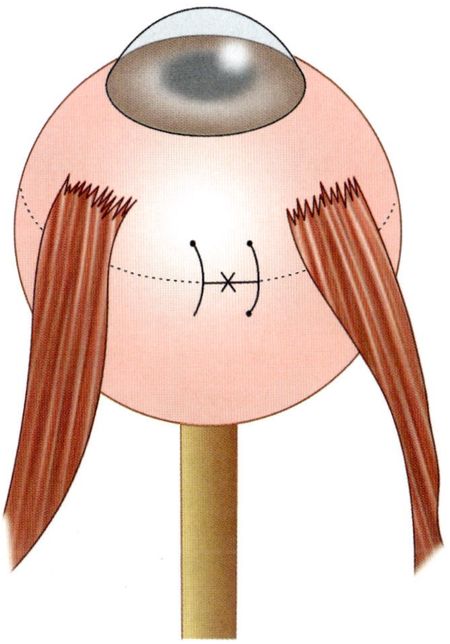

▲ **Figure 12.6**

The scleral mark is straddled by equidistant mattress sutures with intrascleral passes 4 mm in length forming an "H"

2.5 mm in diameter. If the break is closer to the equator, a 5 × 5 mm sponge with an 8 mm mattress suture will provide greater buckle height (Fig. 12.5). Trimmed 7 × 3 mm sponges can also be placed radially. However, the use of such sponges is the exception in my practice. The typical scleral pass of a spatulated needle is 4 mm. Intrascleral passes should be radial and equidistant from the scleral mark; the horizontal portion of the "H" should straddle them (Fig. 12.6).

▶ Circumferential Segmental Buckles

The preferred buckles are a soft silicone 5 × 3 mm sponge or a trimmed 7 × 3 mm sponge (Fig. 12.7).

To avoid "fishmouthing" (redundant retinal folds across the buckle), sponges of both types should not cover more than four clock hours of circumference. In phakic eyes, the buckle crest is likely to be centered at a point 13 mm posterior relative to the limbus; in aphakic eyes, it is likely to be centered at 12 mm relative to the limbus. Despite these averages, the crest of the buckle ideally will be exactly at the latitude of the break. The size and height of the buckle should be moderate; that is, they should not totally deform the globe.

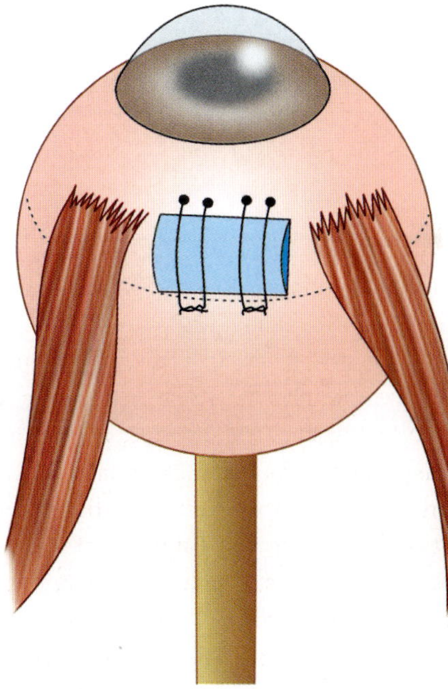

▲ **Figure 12.7**

Circumferential segmental 5 x 3 mm sponges are used for breaks of similar latitude that are separated from each other by less than 1 and 1/2 clock hours, or 9 mm

Encircling Buckles

The 3.5 mm band (#41)[17] and the 7.5 mm solid silicone explant (#277)[17]without a band are used to encircle the eye. The wider 7.5 mm explant is used in myopes with larger eyes; it is also used in eyes with breaks at different latitudes. The encircling bands can be centered at 12 or 13 mm to support the breaks, particularly if they are inferiorly located. Even in "buckle-vits", author marks all breaks and select an encircling buckle that supports the entire break or at least the anterior horns of the breaks. The benefit of meticulously closing breaks with a 3.5 mm encircling band is that it either shortens or eliminates the need for postoperative tamponade. Thus, air can be used instead of SF_6 and saline instead of air. This not only eliminates the need to place the patient in the prone position after surgery, but dramatically reduces postoperative recovery time. Constriction of the buckle has to be modest. Lincoff[22,23] and others have shown that constrictions above 10% interfere with ocular circulation. In general, the encircling buckle is shortened by 5 mm. In the case of a 7.5 mm solid silicone explant, it is passed around the eye and cut flush. At that time, 5 mm are removed from one end of the explant and the ends connected with either a nonabsorbable nylon suture or an absorbable vicryl suture, resulting in a 6–7% constriction. The buckle is sutured in place using the usual 5.0 nylon mattress sutures, one in each quadrant and two in the quadrant where the ends meet (Figs 12.8A and B).

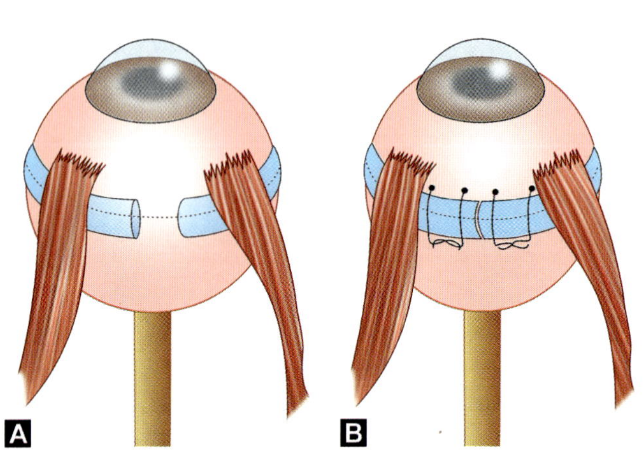

▲ Figures 12.8A and B

(A) A circumferential 7.5 x 3 mm buckle has been cut flush, then shortened by 5 mm, resulting in a 6–7% constriction; (B) If the ends of the buckle are secured with mattress sutures, the closure can be absorbable (7.0 vicryl shown here), allowing for improved ocular circulation

After absorption of the sutures, the ends will separate slightly, decreasing constriction and improving ocular pulse and circulation.

Attention to Detail

The conjunctiva and Tenon's capsule incision are placed in midquadrant, 4 mm posterior to the limbus and parallel to it, in the conjunctival vascular watershed. This incision is away from the anterior ciliary vessels; it respects the corneal stem cells in the palisades of Vogt, as well as the recurrent limbal conjunctival vessels that supply the limbal and perilimbal bulbar conjunctiva. The limbus-parallel incision is enlarged circumferentially to expose the quadrant (or quadrants) of interest. A Gass hook is used to keep incisions as short as possible. Also, caruncular conjunctiva is left intact whenever possible (Figs 12.9A and B).

Relaxing incisions are placed to prevent tearing of the tissues and "popping" of fat by applicators. Breaks are localized on the sclera and marked. However, localization may be impossible in bullous superior retinal detachments that do not respond to double patching, in which case partial drainage, preoperative injection of 0.25 ml of room air on the day before surgery, or localization according to best-estimate "dead reckoning" are options.

In cases of detachments that include the macula, cryopexy should be deferred to prevent the subfoveal migration of pigment, which could impair final visual outcome. After suturing and tying the mattress sutures, the buckle is trimmed to minimal size and carefully covered with Tenon's capsule, which is anchored in its original position. Dual layer closure may take more time than placing the buckle. If possible, patients should be given intravenous steroids during the procedure, as well as the usual periocular steroids, to minimize the risk of proliferative vitreoretinopathy.

Postoperative eye movement exercises will reduce periocular adhesions and the risk of diplopia. After retinal reattachment, a laser beam is applied to retinal breaks. If ocular motility or refractive changes are a persistent problem, the buckles can be removed after a month or two, guided by the postoperative retinal drawing to minimize the size of the conjunctival incision.

Expected Outcomes

One recent retrospective study based on 4,325 cases placed the success rate of retinal buckling surgery at 83–87% and

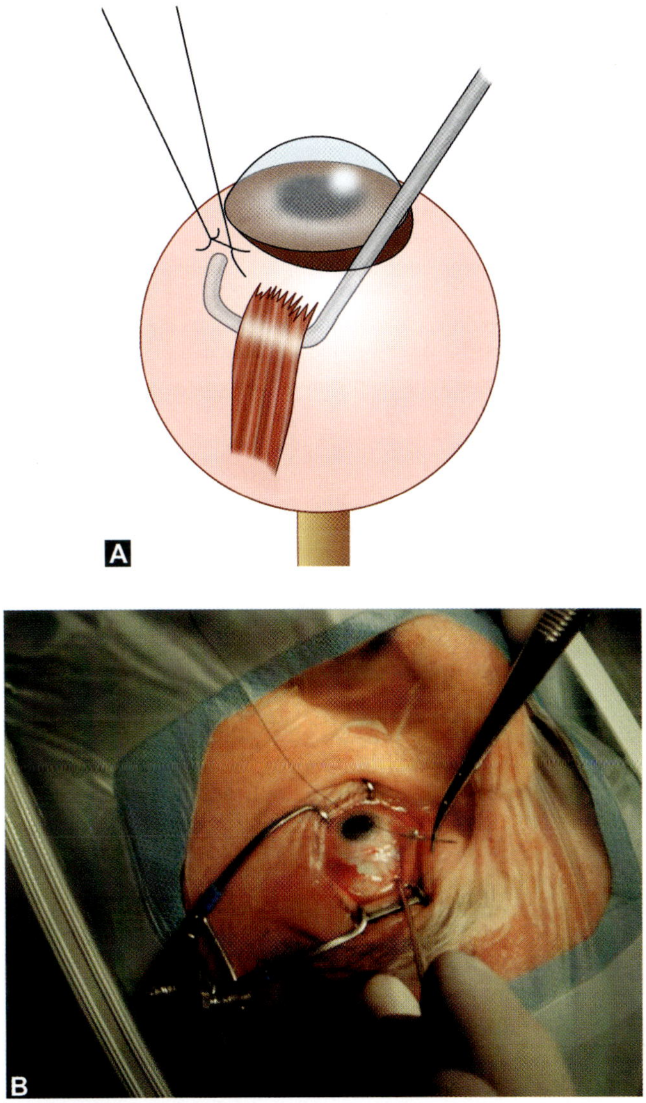

▲ **Figures 12.9A and B**

(A) Schematic drawing of a Gass hook that has been passed underneath a rectus muscle, which is covered by intact conjunctiva; (B) Passing the traction suture through conjunctiva minimizes incision length and postoperative discomfort

found no significant influence of pseudophakia.[24] An 82% success rate of scleral buckling was maintained long-term.[25] In general, however, it seems prudent to allow 10% for pseudophakia and another 10% if the study is prospective and randomized with independent standardized observation.[26] A primary success rate of less than 65% is reason for concern.

Obstacles to Teaching the Lost Art of Scleral Buckling

The tertiary-care university referral center trains most residents and fellows, but does not receive the bulk of primary retinal detachments. Trainees, therefore, are rarely exposed to uncomplicated retinal detachments. Leaders and moderators on the public stages of ophthalmology generally have not been supportive of scleral buckling.[27] Now, in the age of managed care, there is little time to examine, double-patch, and reexamine. Moreover, the 2010 Medicare rates allowed $1,679.28 for a vitrectomy and only $1,285.15 for a scleral buckle, thus providing an official notion of the diminished value of the buckling procedure.

As stated, scleral buckling is not the procedure of choice for every rhegmatogenous retinal detachment. Like this one, many articles have given scleral buckling a place that is amply supported by evidence[13,18] of its merit. Yet all this writing promoting rationality and balance has been ineffective, still moving the buckle toward extinction, making of it a Dodo bird. A few old barking dogs cannot hold up a caravan of young vitrectomists. Despite clear indications of the benefits of scleral buckling, the frequency of use of this procedure has dramatically decreased a trend that is unlikely to be reversed. Some of the reasons for this trend are practical, beginning with the fact that the basics of scleral buckling are no longer taught in training programs.

Beyond that, reasoning that "if it is good for the complicated case, it must be good for the uncomplicated case" leads to "one size fits all" treatments.[28] Jules Gonin had this to say about one size fits all: "*Ce n'est pas avec une seule et meme arme que l'on peut gagner toutes les batailles; il faut pouvoir les varier selon les exigences de la tactique: l' essentiel est que le plan d'etat-major soit le bon.*[29] (It is not with one and the same weapon that can win all the battles. We must be able to vary the requirements of tactics: the point is that the plan of staff is the right).

Author has worked with residents and fellows for many years, during which surgical procedures have generally changed for the better, becoming faster, safer and more efficient. Nevertheless, in author's judgment we should resist the tendency to treat all retinal detachments by just one method. Author is concerned about the disappearance of the careful preoperative study, the drawing and the postoperative assessment that so strongly enhanced individual understanding of what worked and what did not. As so often is the case, the keys to success are patient selection, careful study and meticulous attention to detail in performing the procedure. If one is convinced that comfortable binocularity, accommodation and the presence of a patient's natural lens are important, then promoting cataracts and glaucoma by the lack of diverse surgical skills may not be the best practice.

References

1. Lincoff H, Kreissig I. Changing Patterns in the Surgery for Retinal Detachment: 1929 to 2000. Klin Monatsbl Augenheilkd. 2000;216:352-9.
2. McLeod D. Is it time to call time on the scleral buckle? Br J Ophthalmol.2004;88:1357-9.
3. Kreissig I. Primary retinal detachment. Options for repair. Berlin, Heidelberg: Springer; 2005.
4. Schepens C. Retinal detachment and allied diseases. Philadelphia: WB Saunders Company; 1983.
5. Bonnet M. Microsurgery of retinal detachment. Field and Wood New York: WW Norton and Company, Inc; 1989.
6. Michaels RG, Wilkinson CP, Rice TA. Retinal Detachment. St Louis: CV Mosby Company; 1990.
7. Kreissig I. Minimal Surgery for retinal detachment. Stuttgart, New York: Thieme; 2000.
8. Thomson JT. The role of patient age and intraocular gas use in cataract progression after vitrectomy for macular holes and epiretinal membranes. Am J Ophthalmol. 2004;137(2):250-7.
9. Hayashi K, Hayashi H. Comparison of amplitude of apparent accommodation in pseudophakic eyes with that of normal accommodation in phakic eyes in various age groups. Eye. 2006;20:290-6.
10. Custodis E. Bedeuted die Plombenaufnaehung auf die Sklera einen Fortschritt in der operativen Behandlung der Netzhautabloesung? Ber Dtsch Ophthalmol Ges. 1953;58:102-5.
11. Arruga MH. Le cerclage equatorial pour traiter le decollement retinien. Bull Soc Franc Ophtal. 1958;71:571-80.
12. Schepens CL, Okamura ID, Brockhurst, RJ. The scleral buckling procedures. 1. Surgical techniques and management. Arch Ophthalmol. 1957;58:797-811.
13. Thompson JT, Michels RG. Volume displacement of scleral buckles. Arch Ophthalmol. 1985;103:1822-4.
14. Heimann H, Bartz-Schmidt KU, Bornfeld N, et al. Scleral buckling versus primary vitrectomy in rhegmatogenous retinal detachment: a prospective randomized multicenter clinical study. Ophthalmology. 2007;114:2142-54.
15. Schrader WF, Hamburger G, Lieb B, et al. Motility and binocular function after radial episcleral buckle. Klin Monbl Augenheilkd. 1995;207:224-31.
16. Lincoff H, Rosberger D, Kreissig I. A new chart for planning retinal surgery. Retina. 1998;18:415-9.
17. MIRA Vitreoretinal Implants. Mira Inc., Waltham, MA.
18. Heimann H, Hellmich M, Bornfeld N, et al Scleral buckling versus primary vitrectomy in rhegmatogenous retinal detachment (SPR study): design issues and implications. SPR Study report no.1. Graefes Arch Clin Exp Ophthalmol. 2001;239:567-74.
19. Lincoff H, Kreissig I. Finding the retinal hole in the pseudophakic eye with detachment. Am J Ophthalmol. 1994;117:442-6.
20. Basic and Clinical Science Course 12. American Academy of Ophthalmology. 2009-2010. p. 294.
21. Lincoff H, Stopa M, Kreissig I. Ambulatory binocular occlusion. Retina 2004;24:246-53.
22. Lincoff H, Kreissig I, Parver L. Limits of constriction in the treatment of retinal detachment. Arch Ophthalmol. 1996; 94:1473-7.
23. Lincoff H, Stopa M, Kreissig I, et al. Cutting the encircling band. Retina. 2006;26:650-4.
24. Thelen U, Amler S, Osada N, et al. Success rates of retinal buckling surgery: relationship to refractive error and lens status: results from a large German case series. Ophthalmology. 2010;117:785-90.
25. Schwartz SG, Kuhl DP, McPherson AR, et al. Twenty-year follow-up for scleral buckling. Arch Ophthalmol. 2002; 120:325-9.
26. Amadieh H, Moradian S, Faghihi H, et al. Anatomic and visual outcomes of scleral buckling versus primary vitrectomy in pseudophakic and aphakic retinal detachment. Ophthalmology. 2005;112:1421-9.
27. D'Amico DJ. Primary retinal detachment. NEJM. 2008;359: 2346-54.
28. Johansson K, Malmsjo M, Ghosh F. Tailored vitrectomy and laser photocoagulation without scleral buckling for all primary rhegmatogenous retinal detachments. Br J Ophthalmol. 2006;90:1286-91.
29. Gonin J. Discussion of Arruga H. Le repos apres l'operation du decollement de la retine. Bull Mem Soc Fr Ophtalmol. 1934;47:358.

Pneumatic Retinopexy

13

Paul E Tornambe

Introduction

Pneumatic retinopexy is an operation for reattaching the retina by injecting an expanding gas bubble and using laser and/or cryopexy. Since its introduction in 1985 by Hilton and Grizzard[1] in the United States and by Dominguez[2] in Spain, Pneumatic Retinopexy (PR) has gained acceptance as an alternative to scleral buckling (SB) for selected retinal detachments.[3,4] Over 100 reports have appeared in the world literature, describing several thousand cases.[5]

It is the purpose of this chapter to report the 25 year experience of one surgeon, describing how case selection and the procedure has evolved, with the goal of detecting which cases respond most favorably and which surgical techniques are associated with the highest success rates.

Previous reports have addressed risk factors that affect success rates using the original inclusion criteria and surgical technique described by Hilton and Grizzard.[6-19] This chapter is novel because it reports the largest reported series of eyes treated with PR by a single surgeon with follow-up exceeding one decade. Unlike previous reports, it not only addresses case selection and preoperative risk factors, but also evaluates different pneumatic surgical techniques and cost.

Much of this data has been published previously in the Transactions of the American Ophthalmological Society, Vol XCV, 1997. Furthermore the reader is referred to "YouTube" and asked to search "pneumatic retinopexy, George Hilton". In his honor author has uploaded a digital version of Dr Hilton as he performed and narrated pneumatic retinopexy circa 1991. Author performs the procedure differently today (SF_6 used instead of C_3F_8, a paracentesis prior to gas bubble injection, staged PR with focal and 360° laser) but it is a piece of history worth reviewing.

The Philosophy of Pneumatic Retinopexy

The reason we operate on eyes with retinal detachment is to restore predetachment vision. Of course we must reattach the retina to accomplish this goal but most reports regarding the surgical treatment of retinal detachment emphasize single operation success as the primary criteria for success. This is wrong. The patient does not really care about the number of operations, they care about the return of vision. Incidentally, vision is not the same as visual acuity. Visual acuity is how one perceives a chart in a dark room, vision is how one perceives their environment. The reason author performs PR is because he believes it has the best chance to restore pre-detachment vision. Other very important concerns include the safety of the operation and the morbidity to the eye and patient. Author performs PR in the office with subconjunctival anesthesia. PR does not change the refractive error of the eye and does not ever result in strabismus. The second reason author advocates PR is because it is the safest retinal detachment procedure we can perform. This of course assumes the procedure is performed appropriately and that failures are promptly recognized and treated. If the surgeon uses excessive cryopexy and then waits a week or two to reoperate a failure, inflammation, pucker and proliferative vitreoretinopathy (PVR) are likely. One can usually determine if a case is failing by the second or third day. If excessive cryopexy has not been performed and eyes are reoperated promptly, no harm is done. Finally cost is a huge factor. In the US PR is performed in the office therefore the cost of performing the procedure is a fraction of scleral buckling or vitrectomy, even if reoperations are considered. Let's assume the PR success rate is 70% (which is low if you properly select the case and properly perform the operation). Let us assume the SB or Pars plana vitrectomy (PPV) success rate is 90%. Therefore 7 of 10 patients will be cured with PR alone while 9 of 10 will be cured with a SB or PPV. Is it therefore logical to do SB or PPV purely on a single operation success basis? To attach two more eyes, 7 are subjected to a more extensive, higher morbidity, more costly operation which results in poorer vision. We also must factor another operation in phakic eyes in patients over 50 treated with vitrectomy cataract surgery. PR has the best of both worlds, better vision, lower morbidity and less cost.

Author would like to review with us his experience treating of several hundred eyes. We learn most from our failures, so hopefully we do not repeat our mistakes. Author will share with us how he performs PR today, do it "my way" and your results will improve.

All retinal detachments consecutively treated by author with PR between 1985 and 1995 were reviewed. For each detachment, many parameters were evaluated to answer questions regarding case selection and surgical technique. Salient features, noted in Tables 13.1 and 13.2 include: the type, number and location of retinal breaks, lattice degeneration, macular detachment, the extent of subretinal fluid, the phakic status of the eye, the status of the posterior capsule, preoperative acuity, age, gas type and volume, retinopexy type, sequence, extent of treatment (Tables 13.3 to 13.6), operative and postoperative complications (Tables 13.7 and 13.8), new or missed breaks (Tables 13.9 and 13.10), PVR (Table 13.11), reoperations (Tables 13.12 and 13.13), anatomic retinal attachment (Tables 13.14 to 13.16) and visual acuity recovery (Tables 13.5 and 13.6). Optimal case selection and the most successful surgical techniques are determined. (Tables 13.6 and 13.7). A cost analysis is made (Tables 13.13 and 13.14).

PR evolved with time and experience. At first, a variety of detachments were attempted. Case selection may be divided into two broad groups. The Clinical Trial Group (CTG) consists of eyes with the inclusion criteria described by Hilton and Grizzard[1] and used in the randomized prospective Pneumatic Retinopexy Clinical Trial[9,10] that compared PR with scleral buckling. The CTG eyes have retinal detachments not associated with PVR, clear media and one or more breaks not larger than one clock hour. Tear(s) are located in the upper two-thirds of the fundus. The CTG eyes may include lattice degeneration (not exceeding three clock hours), pseudophakia and a retinal detachment of any size. The amount of subretinal fluid is not a consideration, but the detachment must extend at least three disc diameters from the break(s) (Figs 13.1 and 13.2). The second group is eyes that exceed the CTG criteria and may contain break(s) which extend more than one clock hour, inferior breaks, star folds in up to two retinal quadrants (PVRC2) and other retinal pathology that might limit the view of the entire retina such as vitreous blood or media change.

TABLE 13.1: Salient features: Preoperative

Salient features	*Number of eyes*	*Percent*
Number of eyes	310	100%
Follow-up 6 months	302	98%
Follow-up 12/24/60/ 120 months	233/142/54/12	77%/47%/18%/ 4%
Remain attached	287	95%
Average age	65	
Male/Female	184/118	61%/39%
Right/Left	170/132	56%/44%
Phakic/Pseudophakic-Aphakic	133/167	45%/55%
Macula attached/ Detached	136/166	45%/55%
Macula off <8 days	128/166	77%
Meets clinical trial	194	64%
Exceeds clinical trial	112	36%
One break	183	61%
Lattice	71	24%
RD extent >6 clock hrs	124	41%
Fellow eye pathology	57	19%

Initially, the operation was done in one session. Cryopexy was applied to the retinal break(s), the bubble injected and a paracentesis sometimes performed. The technique evolved into a staged operation; using the laser indirect ophthalmoscope (LIO) delivery system, photocoagulation is applied to attached retina in a scatter fashion between the posterior insertion of the vitreous base and the ora serrata. Cryopexy may be applied to detached retinal break(s) if they are not

TABLE 13.2: Salient features: Operative and postoperative

Salient features	*Number of eyes*	*Percent*
SF_6/ C_2F_6/ C_3F_8	172/ 33/ 93	57%/ 11%/ 31%
Focal laser/Cryopexy	181	60%
360° laser/Cryopexy	121	40%
Paracentesis	197	65%
SOS: male vs female	123/184 vs 79/118	67% vs 67%
SOS: case selection = none Treatment = all techniques	205	68%
Plus laser and/or Cryopexy	30	10%
plus PPV/SB	51	17%
Overall attachment	286	95%
SOS: case selection = CTG Treatment = Focal	69/110	63%
SOS: case selection = CTG Treatment 360° retinopexy	78/86	91%
Group = Mac Off <15 days and VA >20/50 at the last examination	121	100%
VA >20/50 @ 6 months	114	94%
VA >20/50 @ 3 months	96	79%
VA >20/50 @ 6 weeks	94	78%

TABLE 13.3: Characteristic vs single operation success

Characteristic	*Single operation success #eyes (%)*	*p*
Horseshoe tear vs	146/207 (71%)	0.05
Hole	56/95 (59%)	
Phakic vs	100/133 (75%)	0.013
Nonphakic	102/167 (61%)	
Capsule intact vs	22/34 (64%)	0.69
Capsule open	80/133 (61%)	
<0.3 cc gas vs	91/147 (62%)	0.06
>0.3 cc gas	112/155 (72%)	
SF_6	123/172 (72%)	0.06
C_2F_6	22/33 (67%)	1.00
C_3F_8	55/93 (59%)	0.06

highly elevated. Following a paracentesis, 0.5 cc of SF_6 gas is injected through the pars plana away from large breaks. The patient is positioned so that the bubble is opposed to the break for 24–48 hours. As the remainder of the retina attaches,

TABLE 13.4: Single operation success: Preoperative characteristic-focal vs 360° retinopexy

Characteristic	*SOS-focal treatment*	*SOS-360° retinopexy*	*p*
Phakic	46/76 (61%)	53/57 (93%)	0.0001
Nonphakic	53/104 (51%)	49/63 (77%)	0.0006
Number of preoperative retinal breaks			
1	130/183 (71%)	68/76 (89%)	0.0012
2	46/73 (63%)	23/28 (82%)	0.09
3	16/26 (62%)	8/10 (80%)	0.44
>4	9/18 (50%)	4/7 (57%)	1.0
% Detached #eyes			
<25% 60	22/33 (67%)	25/27 (93%)	0.025
26–50% 178	58/99 (59%)	63/79 (80%)	0.0035
51–75% 36	11/24 (46%)	11/12 (92%)	0.01
76–100% 28	13/31 (42%)	9/9 (100%)	0.002
Lattice # eyes			
Lattice 70	24/36 (67%)	29/34 (85%)	0.09
No lattice 232	75/144 (52%)	73/88 (83%)	0.0001

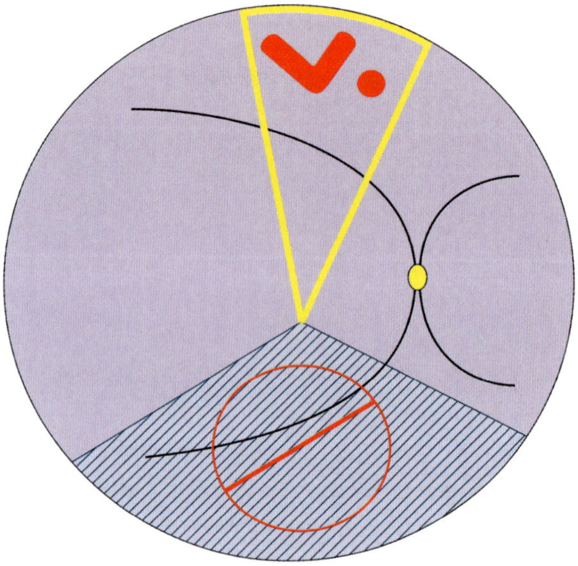

▲ **Figure 13.1**

Clinical Trial Group (CTG) inclusion criteria. CTG eyes have retinal detachments not associated with PVR, clear media and one or more breaks not larger than one clock hour. Tear(s) are located in the upper two-thirds of the fundus. CTG eyes may include lattice degeneration (not exceeding three clock hours), pseudophakia and a retinal detachment of any size. The amount of subretinal fluid is not a consideration, but the detachment must extend at least three disc diameters from the break(s)

TABLE 13.5: Preoperative characteristics vs visual acuity return to ≥20/40

Detachment characteristic	*# Eyes VA return >20/40*	*p*
Macula on	116/136 (85%)	0.0002
Macula off	110/166 (66%)	
Duration of macular detachment (days)		
<1	25/37 (68%)	
<2	44/60 (73%)	
<3	58/82 (71%)	
<7	93/128 (73%)	0.03
8–14	12/21 (57%)	0.0003
15–21	2/4 (50%)	0.0001
>21	4/17 (24%)	0.001
Preoperative VA 20/50–20/200	34/44 (77%)	0.07
Preoperative VA worse than 20/200	75/122 (61%)	
Single operation success	175/204 (86%)	<0.0001
Failed first operation	51/98 (52%)	
No new breaks	176/246 (72%)	0.007
New breaks	29/56 (62%)	
Phakic	103/133 (77%)	0.50
Nonphakic	123/167 (74%)	

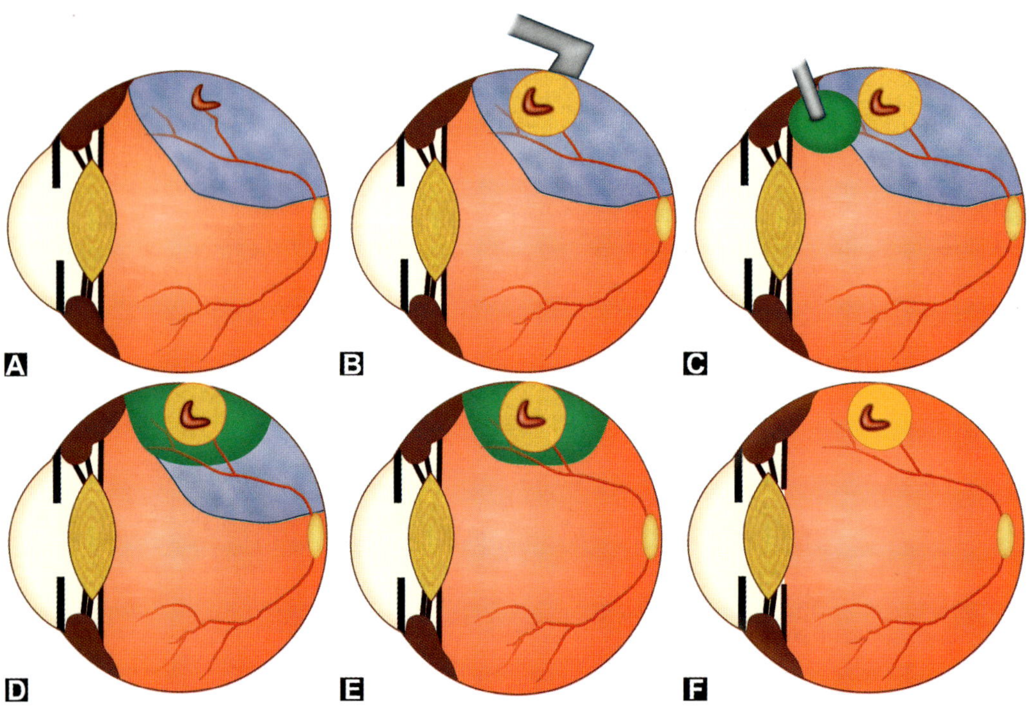

▲ **Figures 13.2A to F**

Pneumatic retinopexy-focal treatment. (A) A superior retinal detachment with a horseshoe tear is present; (B) Cryopexy is applied to the retinal break; (C) The bubble is injected and the patient positioned so the bubble covers the tear; (D) The bubble expands, closes the break; (E) The subretinal fluid resorbs; (F) The bubble resorbs

TABLE 13.6: Age vs visual acuity recovery to ≥20/40

Characteristic	*# Eyes VA return >20/40*	*p*
Patient age (macula off <8 days)		
<65 y/o	46/56 (82%)	0.04
>65 y/o	47/71 (66%)	
Patient age		
<40	8/13 (62%)	0.33
41–50	28/31 (90%)	
51–60	54/62 (87%)	
61–70	63/84 (75%)	
71–80	57/88 (65%)	
81–90	14/24 (58%)	

TABLE 13.7: Operative complications

Operative complication	*Number of eyes (%)*
Anterior hyaloid gas	4 (1.3%)
Hyphema	2 (0.6%)
Subretinal gas	1 (0.3%)

TABLE 13.8: Postoperative complications

Postoperative complication	*Number of eyes (%)*
New breaks	56 (19%)
Missed breaks	43 (14%)
PVR grade C,D	9,20 (10%)
Delayed resorption of subretinal fluid	15 (5%)
Epimacular membrane	8 (3%)
Choroidal detachment	5 (2%)
Cystoid macular edema	4 (1%)
Macular hole	2 (1%)
Cataract	2 (1%)
Ischemic optic neuropathy	1 (1%)

peripheral laser photocoagulation is completed for 360° (Figs 13.3A to C).

Positioning is continued for 3–5 days for 16 hours per day. Activity, including reading, is restricted until the bubble has resorbed.

Preoperatively, great efforts are made to ensure that the patient and family understand the importance of proper

TABLE 13.9: Gas type: Failure, new breaks, missed breaks

Gas type	*Failed cases*	*p*	*New breaks vs missed*	*p*
SF_6	49/172	0.062	28 (57%) 21 (43%)	1.00
C_2F_6	12/33	1.00	6 (50%) 6 (50%)	0.75
C_3F_8	38/93	0.062	21 (55%) 17 (45%)	1.00

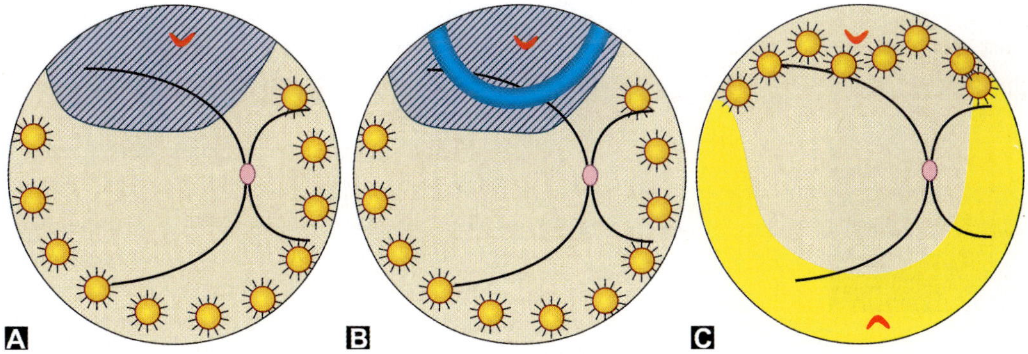

▲ Figures 13.3A to C

Pneumatic retinopexy with twelve hours of retinopexy. (A) Scatter peripheral photocoagulation is applied to attached retina between the insertion of the vitreous base and ora serrata; (B) The bubble is injected and the patient positioned; (C) Once the superior retina attaches photocoagulation is completed. If a new break develops within the laser treatment area (tear at 6 o'clock), a retinal detachment will not occur

TABLE 13.10: Postoperative result, focal vs 360° retinopexy

Postoperative characteristic	*Focal retinopexy*	*360° retinopexy*	*p*
Failed 1st PR	81/180 (45%)	18/122 (15%)	<0.0001
Phakic eyes new and missed breaks	30/76 (39%)	4/57 (7%)	<0.0001
Phakic eyes new vs missed breaks	16/30 vs 14/30 (53%) (57%)	4/4 vs 0/4 (100%) (0%)	0.03
Nonphakic eyes new and missed breaks	51/104 (49%)	14/63 (22%)	<0.0001
Nonphakic new vs missed breaks	25/51 vs 26/51 (49%) (51%)	11/14 vs 3/14 (79%) (21%)	0.0001
Eyes failed to attach, fluid persisted following 1st PR	6 (5%)	5 (4%)	

TABLE 13.11: Proliferative vitreoretinopathy: Gas type. Gas vs pexy sequence, laser vs cryopexy

	# eyes with PVR	*p*
SF_6	12/29 (41%)	0.33
C_2F_6	6/29 (21%)	0.09
C_3F_8	11/29 (38%)	0.63
Gas first	8/68 (12%)	0.48
Pexy first	21/234 (9%)	
Cryopexy	26/261 (10%)	0.78
Laser only	3/41 (7%)	

positioning. They are educated with a videotape presentation, followed by a detailed question and answer period with the surgeon. Following gas bubble injection, a circular level with

TABLE 13.12: First reoperation vs time following pneumatic retinopexy

Days post PR to 1st reoperation	*#eyes (% cumulative)*
0–7	25 (27%)
8–14	19 (49%)
15–21	10 (60%)
22–30	8 (70%)
31–60	12 (82%)
60–90	5 (87%)
90–120	5 (93%)
120–180	4 (97%)
180–360	4 (99%)
>360	2 (100%)

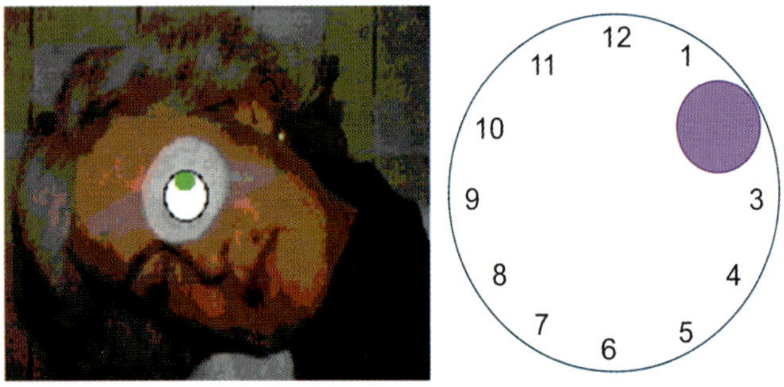

▲ **Figure 13.4**

A "pneumo-level" (Escalon Trek Medical) is attached to the eye patch. The patient is instructed to maintain their head in a position that places the bubble against a certain clock hour on the level. In this example, at 2 o'clock

clock hours is attached to the eye patch. The patient and family are shown how to assume and maintain the proper position and the importance of positioning is stressed (Fig. 13.4).

Three hundred ten patients were treated with PR, five were lost to follow-up and three died before the 6 month follow-up visit. Salient features are summarized in Tables 13.1 and 13.2. Of the 302 eyes followed for at least 6 months, 194 (64%) met the CTG inclusion criteria. The average age was 65, 184 were male, 170 were right eyes and 133 (45%) were phakic. The macula was detached in 166 (55%) and more than half the retina was detached in 41%. Seventy-seven percent were followed for 1 year, 47% for 2 years, 18% for 5 years and 4% for more than 10 years.

TABLE 13.13: The cost of reoperations. Pneumatic retinopexy vs scleral buckling (using PRCT Data[9])

	Number (%)	*MCare payment/ operation*	*OR, supplies, Lab, Meds, H and P anesthesia/ procedure*	*Total Cost— All reoperations*
PR study all eyes	302			
PR failures	99			
PC/cryopexy	32 (21%)	$ 500		$16,000
PR	33 (22%)	$1100	$50	$37,950
SB	22 (15%)	$1400	$3000	$96,800
PPV/SB	64 (42%)	$2000	$3500	$352,000
Total procedures	151 (100%)			$502,750
Average # reop/failed case	1.5			
PRCT-SB, all eyes (extrapolated)	302			
SB failures	54			
PC/cryopexy	6 (11%)	$ 500		$3,000
PR	25 (45%)	$1100	$ 50	$28,750
SB	3 (5%)	$1400	$3000	$13,200
PPV/SB	22 (39%)	$2000	$3500	$121,000
Total procedures	56 (100%)			$165,900
Average # reops/failed case	1.03			

TABLE 13.14: Cost of pneumatic retinopexy vs scleral buckling including reoperations for 302 retinal detachments

Primary procedure	*SOS rate # eyes*	*SOS cost*	*Cost of reoperations*	*Total cost for 302 eyes*	*% SB cost*
SBP	82% (248)	$1,091,200	$165,900	$1,257,100	100%
PR all cases, all techniques	68% (203)	$ 233,450	$502,750	$ 736,200	59%
PR-CTG case selection, with 360° pexy	91% (275)	$ 316,250	$ 29,700	$ 345,950	28%

TABLE 13.15: Anatomic success: subgroup-CTG with 360° pexy, phakic vs nonphakic

Procedure	*All eyes (n=84)*	*Phakic (n=39)*	*Nonphakic (n=45)*
PR CTG and 360° pexy	76 (91%)	38 (97%)	38 (84%)
Laser/Cryo/PR	1 (1%)	1 (laser) (3%)	0
SBP/PPV	6 (7%)	0	6 (13%)
Final attachment	83 (99%)	39 (100%)	44 (98%)

TABLE 13.16: Single operation success: The influence of experience, case selection and surgical technique

	SOS all eyes overall	*SOS meets clin trial and focal pexy*	*SOS meets clin trial and 360° pexy*	*SOS exceeds clin trial and 360° pexy*
First 100 eyes	54/100 (54%)	34/60 (57%)	1/1 (100%)	0
Second 100 eyes	72/100 (72%)	24/34 (71%)	25/27 (93%)	9/13 (69%)
Last 102 eyes	78/100 (78%)	11/16 (69%)	52/58 (90%)	15/22 (68%)

TABLE 13.17: Retinal detachment characteristics vs probability of single operation success

Retinal detachment characteristics	*Probability of single operation success*
Condition 1: A RD involving: <25% of the retina, with 1 break less than one clock hour in size in the superior 2/3 of the fundus, in a phakic eye, with clear media with PVR < B. Treatment includes 360° retinopexy	97%
Condition 2: Condition 1, but in an eye with >50% of the retina detached	subtract 10%
Condition 3: Condition 1, but with >2 retinal breaks	subtract 10%
Condition 4: Condition 1, but in a pseudophakic/aphakic eye	subtract 10%
Condition 5: Condition 1, but Treatment includes only focal retinopexy	subtract 20%

Results: Data Analysis

Anatomic Success

Factors that favor one operation success include: 360° peripheral retinopexy, phakic eyes, a less extensive retinal detachment, fewer retinal breaks and eyes that meet the CTG criteria for admission (Tables 13.3, 13.4, 13.10, 13.15 and 13.6).

Without regard to case selection or surgical technique, the single operation success (SOS) for all 302 eyes was 68%. Additional non-incisional intervention including laser and/or cryotherapy, or reinjection of gas (two eyes), increased the attachment rate to 78%. The addition of buckling surgery and/or vitrectomy resulted in an overall success rate of 95% (Table 13.2)

The attachment rate for eyes treated with 360° PR between the insertion of the vitreous base and ora serrata was compared to those eyes treated with focal retinopexy applied only to visible retinal pathology such as tears, holes, or lattice degeneration. In every category of increased risk for failure, including pseudophakia, a more extensive detachment, or more retinal breaks, 360° retinopexy improved SOS. Complete PR also improved the outcome for eyes associated with more favorable SOS rates such as phakic eyes, eyes with a single break, or a localized one quadrant detachment. In the subgroup of eyes that met the CTG inclusion criteria, SOS was attained in 63% (69/110) of eyes treated with focal retinopexy and in 91% (78/86) of eyes treated with 360° PR (Table 13.16).

Factors not influencing SOS included: the type of tear, the presence of lattice degeneration (not exceeding three clock hours), the type, volume or duration of gas, or the type of retinopexy used (i.e. laser or cryopexy). The order between gas injection and retinopexy (before or following retinopexy) did not affect outcome (Tables 13.3, 13.4, 13.9 and 13.11). Gender did not influence SOS (Table 13.2).

Visual Recovery

Factors favoring better visual return included single operation success, better preoperative acuity, macular attachment, detachment of the macula less than one week and younger age (Tables 13.5 and 13.6). At the 6 month postoperative visit, 86% of eyes cured with one operation versus 52% of eyes cured with more than one operation recovered more than equal to 20/40 acuity. ($p < 0.0001$) Seventy-seven percent of eyes with preoperative acuity 20/50–20/200 versus 61% of eyes with preoperative acuity 20/200 or worse attained 20/40 or better acuity postoperatively. ($p = 0.007$) Eighty-five percent of eyes with preoperative macular attachment and 66% of eyes with preoperative macular detachment recovered more than equal to 20/40 acuity. The likelihood of visual recovery to more than equal to 20/40 decreased if the macula was detached for more than 1 week [($p = 0.0003$) Table 13.4]. Eighty-two percent of patients less than 65 years old versus 64% of patients more than equal to 65 attained more than equal to 20/40 acuity. [($p = 0.04$) Table 13.6] Visual acuity recovery was rapid. In the macula detached group, at 6 months, 69% (114/166) of eyes attained 20/50 or better acuity. Of these eyes, 87% (94/114) attained this acuity by the 6 week postoperative visit. (Table 13.2) Pseudophakic eyes recovered vision as well as phakic eyes.

Complications

▶ Operative Complications

The most common complication was injection of gas anterior to the anterior hyaloid space into the space of Petit. This gives the appearance at the injection site of an anterior loculated, oval bubble (sausage sign) that usually does not move with head position. As the loculated gas bubble expands over 24–48 hours, it breaks through the anterior hyaloid face and enters the vitreous cavity without creating new tears. This complication is avoided by injecting deeper into the center of the vitreous cavity, which ensures penetration of the anterior hyaloid face. Subretinal gas occurred in one eye. After placing the patient supine, the bubble was repositioned back through the hole into the vitreous cavity with scleral depression without an unfavorable outcome (Table 13.7).

▶ Postoperative Complications

New Breaks

The most common postoperative complication was new break formation. An attempt was made to distinguish "new" retinal breaks from "missed" breaks. If a new break was noted, the break was considered a "new break". If the retina never reattached and a previously unnoticed break was detected within the area of detachment at the time of the reoperation, the break was considered a missed break. Using this definition, 19% (56/302) of breaks were new and 14% (43/302) were missed (Table 13.8).

No association was established between new break formation and gas bubble size, duration or the type of gas used (Table 13.3). New break formation and reoperations were analyzed to learn when new tears or redetachment developed. Seventy percent of reoperations were done within the first month and 87% within 3 months (Table 13.12).

Proliferative Vitreoretinopathy

Ten percent (29 eyes) developed PVR, one-third (9 eyes) of these were Grade C. The frequency of PVR was analyzed to find out if the gas bubble (either size or duration), or the type of retinopexy used (cryopexy or laser), or the retinopexy order in relation to gas insertion and retinal flattening influenced the incidence of PVR. No association was established (Table 13.11).

Epimacular Membrane Formation

Visually significant macular pucker developed in 3% (eight eyes). Peripheral 360° retinopexy was not associated with an increased incidence of visually significant macular pucker (Table 13.7).

Choroidal Detachment, CME, Macular Hole, Cataract

Choroidal detachment (2%), cystoid macular edema (1%), macular hole (1%) and cataract (1%) developed infrequently which helps explain why eyes treated with PR rapidly recover vision (Table 13.7).

▶ Reoperations

Ninety-nine eyes failed the first operation and 151 additional procedures were done, which successfully attached all but 15 eyes. The additional operations included laser or cryotherapy (43%), repeat PR (22%), a scleral buckle (15%) and vitrectomy with a scleral buckle [(42%) Table 13.13].

Discussion

Twelve hundred retinal surgeons from around the world attended the 1996 Retina Symposium preceding the annual meeting of the American Academy Ophthalmology (AAO). Sixty percent said they currently use PR for a superior, single quadrant, phakic retinal detachment associated with a single horseshoe tear. The response the preceding year was 28%.

PR is gaining recognition as an alternative to scleral buckling.[3,4] However, there is a significant trend towards vitrectomy without a scleral buckle. At the 2010 Vail Vitrectomy Meeting one European retina specialists stated his opinion that "in 5 years neither scleral buckling nor vitrectomy would be performed". He was saying that only pars plana vitrectomy will be done in the future. Unfortunately scleral buckling may become a lost art. Many training programs provide little exposure to scleral buckling. Although PR is also less frequently performed in training programs, in author's experience, these graduates pursue PR in their private practices. A clever mind will always overcome a poor education. It is very important to realize that there are many ways to "skin a cat". The operation must be customized to the eye and the patient. The operation selected should give the best chance of recovery of vision, provide the least risk to the eye and patient, provide the most rapid recovery so patients can return quickly to their predetachment lifestyle and be cost conscious.

The literature suggests a wide range of successful one operation success rates with pneumatic retinopexy[5,7-9,11-17,19-25] with some reports suggesting a lower success rate than scleral buckling. How can this variability be explained? The definition of single operation success may differ. Some authors include supplemental photocoagulation or laser treatment as part of the primary operation. The ability to identify all retinal pathology preoperatively may vary between surgeons; an unrecognized retinal break usually results in failure. The surgeon cannot be separated from the surgery. The most notable explanation for variability is including cases with different preoperative conditions. Many studies enrolled eyes using the CTG inclusion criteria as a guide and assume that similar cases are being compared. However, this report clearly shows that eyes meeting the CTG criteria may also exhibit other conditions such as pseudophakia, more retinal breaks, or a more extensive detachment, which may significantly influence one operation success. As author mentioned earlier, the purpose of this chapter is to analyze 302 retinal detachments treated with PR by one surgeon to detect preoperative conditions and define PR techniques that give the best results. Factors that decrease the chances for a successful outcome are also described. Using this information, probabilities for success, for a particular detachment, can be estimated (Table 13.17).

Anatomic Success

In this report, anatomic single operation success (SOS) is defined as one procedure success. Initially, the pneumatic operation was done in one sitting, with focal cryopexy followed by gas insertion.[1] Additional treatment, such as supplemental laser treatment, regardless how minor, to previously treated or new pathology was considered a reoperation.[9,10] When PR evolved to a staged operation, treatment to pathology not planned during the initial evaluation was judged a reoperation. Thus, peripheral scatter treatment to recently attached retina a few days following gas insertion is not considered a reoperation, while supplementary treatment at any time to a new break is considered additional surgery and not part of the staged operation. If meaningful comparisons are desired between studies, reoperation and one operation success must be clearly defined.

Analysis of this report's subgroups also suggests a broad range of success, showing many different outcomes are possible (even with a single surgeon) if case selection and surgical techniques vary. For example, the average SOS rate for the entire study group of 302 eyes is 68%, but with additional laser or cryotherapy, the success rate increases to 78%. This approaches the world literature's reported average SOS rate of approximately 80% for sclera buckles.[5] Selected CTG phakic eyes treated with 360° PR have a 97% one operation success rate. But CTG, pseudophakic eyes treated with the same extent of PR have a lower, but very acceptable 84% SOS rate (Table 13.15). As the number of retinal breaks increases, or the extent of the detachment enlarges, or eyes exceeding the CTG criteria are included, the likelihood for one operation success decreases. Table 13.17 suggests a formula to estimate SOS preoperatively. Selecting eyes with the best chance for SOS is important for they recover the greatest amount of acuity (Table 13.5).

Visual Recovery

Visual recovery is highest in eyes cured with one pneumatic procedure. Eighty-six percent of eyes attached with one pneumatic operation attained more than equal to 20/40 acuity, compared to 52% of eyes requiring additional treatment. The eye is not disadvantaged by a failed PR attempt. Several reports[7,8,9,10] have reviewed cases that failed a pneumatic procedure and were then subsequently reattached with a scleral buckle. These failed pneumatic eyes recovered similar levels of visual acuity as eyes treated successfully with a single scleral buckle (SB).

This report and others 6 suggest a good predictor of postoperative acuity is preoperative acuity (Table 13.5). Seventy-seven percent of eyes with 20/50–20/200 preoperative acuity versus 61% of eyes with less than equal to 20/200 preoperative acuity attained more than equal to 20/40 acuity by the 6 month postoperative visit. If the macula is detached for less than 1 week, about 75% will recover more than equal to 20/40 acuity. Visual acuity return is rapid following PR with most sight returning within the first 6 weeks (Table 13.2). Patients less than 65 years old have a better chance of recovering vision than those older than 65 (Table 13.6).

Prognostic Indicators

▶ Pseudophakia

Pseudophakic retinal detachments are associated with lower single operation success than phakic detachments whether treated with PR or SB.[9]

Pseudophakic detachments are associated with small breaks that are difficult to detect, especially if the peripheral capsule is not clear. Unlike previous reports,[8] an open posterior capsule did not negatively influence one operation success (Table 13.3).

▶ Retinal Detachment Size

The extent of the retinal detachment influences SOS, more extensive detachments are associated with lower SOS. A small undetected, untreated defect in attached retina may remain closed following PR, while a small undetected, untreated defect in detached retina will usually result in failure. Grizzard[6] notes that poor preoperative acuity correlates with increased failure. This is understandable because more extensive detachments frequently involve the macula.

▶ The Type and Number of Retinal Defects

The type of retinal defect does not influence success, horseshoe tears respond as favorably as round breaks (Table 13.3). The number of retinal defects does influence success. More retinal breaks are associated with lower SOS probably because more breaks suggest more vitreoretinal interface pathology.

Lattice degeneration (up to three clock hours), either as part of the retinal detachment or in attached retina does not negatively influence the outcome. Lattice degeneration was present in 24% of cases. Eyes with lattice degeneration did as well as eyes without lattice (Table 13.4). Grizzard using scleral buckling, reported that eyes with lattice degeneration were associated with a higher success rate than eyes that did not have visible lattice degeneration.[6]

▶ Gas

The gas bubble type, volume injected and duration did not affect the development of new breaks. C_3F_8 is now used only in more complex cases, such as large eyes or to address multiple breaks in multiple, oblique, or inferior (4 and 8 o'clock) quadrants. PVR was not influenced by either cryopexy or laser, nor by the sequence of retinopexy versus gas bubble injection (Table 13.11). Experimental investigations by Singh implied that cryopexy to elevated retina may enhance liberation and transformation of RPE cells into PVR producing fibroblasts.[26] This suggests cryopexy or laser treatment done after the tear attaches may decrease the incidence of PVR and new break formation. This series did not confirm a relationship between gas sequence and type of retinopexy used and the development of PVR. Grizzard reported less success among men.[6] This series showed no difference in SOS regarding the patient's gender and emphasizes the importance of preoperative education to maximize positioning compliance.

Optimal Case Selection Combined with the Most Effective Surgical Technique

Table 13.17 lists retinal detachment characteristics and surgical techniques determined by this study to influence single operation success. Pseudophakia, more than one retinal break and retinal detachments involving more than 50% of the retina, each reduce SOS by approximately 10%. Compared with focal retinopexy, peripheral 360° retinopexy improves SOS 20%.

Eyes most likely to succeed with a single pneumatic attempt include phakic eyes with clear media with one retinal break, not larger than one clock hour, located in the upper two-thirds of the fundus, not exceeding PVR Grade B. Less extensive retinal detachments are associated with higher success rates probably because fewer breaks are overlooked. Detachments associated with many retinal breaks have a lower SOS rate; more breaks may be a signpost of extensive vitreoretinal interface pathology.

New breaks occur in areas where the vitreous is firmly adherent to the retina. Tears develop as the vitreous continues to physiologically separate. Focal retinopexy to visible retinal pathology does not deal with areas of vitreoretinal interface adherence. Peripheral 360° prophylactic photocoagulation treatment between the insertion of the vitreous base and ora serrata is an effective means of addressing this problem.

Peripheral encircling retinopexy may improve the success rate in two ways. First, it prophylactically treats missed breaks. Second, it prevents the accumulation of subretinal fluid if a new break occurs within the treated area (Fig. 13.3.) Just as an encircling buckle relieves traction on overlooked pathology, scatter peripheral photocoagulation may prophylactically manage overlooked retinal defects. Most retinal detachment repair studies assume all breaks are identified, naively suggesting that all surgeons will find all the retinal breaks. Variability between previous pneumatic studies may be explained by variability among surgeons to consistently identify all pathology. Just as an encircling buckle may act as an "equalizer" to treat an overlooked break, scatter peripheral photocoagulation may provide the same benefit. The incidence of new or missed breaks is three times higher in eyes treated with focal retinopexy than eyes treated with 360° retinopexy (Table 13.10). Laser photocoagulation provides an immediate chorioretinal adhesion.[27] Following prophylactic photocoagulation between the insertion of the vitreous base and the ora serrata, an early new break may not accumulate fluid and progress to retinal detachment.

The application of peripheral 360° retinopexy favorably influenced the outcome in this study. In every subcategory, such as phakic versus pseudophakic or aphakic, extent of detachment, or number of breaks, 12 hours of retinopexy significantly improved SOS (Tables 13.4, 13.10 and 13.15). PR requires two or more sittings suggesting that PR should be considered a staged procedure. Laser photocoagulation should not be delivered to slightly elevated retina because intense burns may cause secondary iatrogenic retinal necrotic holes. Preoperatively, all pathology must be accurately documented for once the bubble is introduced and the retina flattens retinal defects become difficult to locate.

Follow-up Recommendations

We confirm other reports that note most unsuccessful PR attempts fail within the first few postoperative months.[6,7] Fifty percent of reoperations were done within the first 2 weeks, 70% within the first month, 82% in the first 2 months and 87% by the end of the 3 month. This suggests that eyes treated with PR should be followed very closely (every week or two) during the first month, and every 3–4 weeks for the next 2 months. Patients may be released after the 3 month but should be given the warning symptoms of retinal redetachment and told there is approximately a 10% chance they may require more treatment within the first year. Redetachment after the first year is unusual (2 eyes) and was reported in the PR Clinical Trial as 1%[10] (Table 13.12).

Quality and Cost-effective Measurements

Single Operation Success (SOS) can be used as a measure of quality and cost effectiveness. Although it is less costly to treat a population with PR than with a primary scleral buckle (SB), it is yet less costly if pneumatic reoperations are reduced. This may be accomplished with better patient selection and improved surgical technique. Tables 13.13 and 13.14 compare the cost of treating 302 eyes with either PR or SB as the first operation. The PRCT data is used to decide the cost of SB and SB reoperations.[9] In the PRCT there were 95 eyes randomized to SB. The SOS rate was 82%. In Table 13.17 of the PRCT report,[9,18] reoperations are noted. Unfortunately, only the most invasive reoperation for each SB failure is stated, so the following calculations will underestimate the actual total cost of all SB reoperations.

The calculations assume laser photocoagulation, cryopexy and PR are done in an office environment, and all incisional operations are done in an outpatient ambulatory care facility.

Using this information the total cost, including reoperations, of treating a group of eyes first with PR approaches half the cost of treating a similar group first with scleral buckling. Using ideal case selection and proper surgical technique, PR is approximately one quarter the cost of scleral buckling (Tables 13.13 and 13.14).

The Learning Curve

PR has a learning curve and results improve with experience, case selection, and improved surgical techniques. Some cases approached with PR in the past would not be treated with PR today. The SOS rate was 54% for the first one hundred cases, 72% for the second 200 eyes and 78% for the last 102 eyes. Selecting only CTG eyes and adding 360° retinopexy to the PR procedure increased the SOS rate from approximately 63–91% (Table 13.16). PR can repair more complex detachments, but the one operation success rate is lower.[11,12,25] The SOS rate for all eyes that exceed the CTG criteria treated with circumferential retinopexy is 68% (Tables 13.15 and 13.16). Although this may be lower than the scleral buckling success rate for these more complex groups of eyes, it still implies that seven out of ten more difficult detachments can be cured without an incisional procedure.

The literature suggests that a failed pneumatic attempt does not disadvantage the eye's anatomic or visual outcome, had that same eye been treated first with a scleral buckle.[7,8,9,10] This report suggests that PR, including reoperations, is still less expensive than treating all eyes primarily with a scleral buckle. A first attempt with PR appears reasonable even for less favorable cases because no harm is done. SOS for vitrectomy should be higher that PR or SB for the vitreous traction is removed. Even so the vitrectomy single operation success rate is not 100%, visual acuity outcomes have not been shown to be superior to PR, cataract surgery is almost always required within a few years of the vitrectomy, and there is significantly more operative morbidity and cost.

Comparison with Other Surgical Techniques

PR has been compared with conventional scleral buckling[28-32] and with the temporary balloon buckle.[33-38] There have been no studies prospectively comparing PPV with PR. Correlating results between studies is difficult and usually not valid for preoperative characteristics and terms, such as the definition of single operation success, may differ. Some studies regard postoperative laser or cryopexy "enhancements" and not reoperations, others include "partial reattachment" as a successful operation. This chapter underscores the significant influence of preoperative conditions and illustrates how reports may be biased by selecting eyes with different preoperative characteristics. Variable preoperative circumstances also help explain why the literature records a spectrum of one operation success rates with pneumatic retinopexy: 63%,[17] 69%,[6] 71%,[36,22] 73%,[7,9,10] 75%,[11] 77%,[8] 80%,[5] 82%,[16] 84%,[32] 87%,[21] 90%.[1] Many of these reports include eyes meeting "CTG criteria"; however, even CTG groups of eyes can differ by the number of breaks, extent of detachment and phakic status of individual eyes that form the group. These factors significantly influence outcome and invalidate comparisons.

Preoperative conditions, especially the incidence of aphakia or pseudophakia also influence SOS using conventional scleral buckling or temporary balloon buckling procedures. In two balloon studies by the same authors, Lincoff and Kreissig report 69% aphakic SOS[33] and approximately 91% phakic SOS.[34] This emphasizes the importance of considering preoperative conditions, such as pseudophakia, before drawing conclusions between studies.

There are many ways to reattach the retina; however, the goal of retinal detachment surgery is not one operation success but restoration of predetachment vision. The best operation is one that restores the most sight. Vision includes visual acuity and other qualitative measures such as anisometropia, diplopia, comfort, ptosis, metamorphopsia, color vision and contrast sensitivity. PR restores vision more often and more quickly with lower morbidity than other retinal operations.[9,10] Although single operation pneumatic success is desirable because it is associated with the highest level of visual acuity return, a failed pneumatic attempt does not disadvantage visual outcome when compared to scleral buckling.[7,8] This review shows that with careful case selection and proper surgical technique, eyes treated with PR enjoy high anatomic and visual success. In addition, PR may be the most cost-effective means to repair a retinal detachment (Tables 13.13 and 13.14). With critical patient selection and 360° retinopexy, PR may cost 25–50% as much as SB.

Better vision may result with PR because SRF is removed promptly with PR. There has been a laxidazical trend in the literature to wait up to 7–10 days with a macula off detachment. Today surgeons may wait several days before operating on macula off detachment which has been detached for several days. Vision may be better with PR because the macula is usually attached sooner with PR for eyes are operated upon more promptly. Author usually performs PR at the first patient encounter. This may result in less cell damage and death.

Three hundred two retinal detachments repaired with PR were evaluated. The following observations were made:

- Success with PR depends upon case selection and surgical technique. Most favorable cases include phakic eyes with less extensive detachment, secondary to a superior retinal break less than one clock hour in size and no PVR. The most successful pneumatic approach includes peripheral retinopexy placed between the insertion of the vitreous base and ora serrata for 360°. Under these conditions, the expected SOS rate approaches 97%.

- More complex detachments can be cured with PR but the SOS rate decreases. Factors negatively influencing single operation anatomic success includes pseudophakia, an increased number of retinal breaks and a greater area of detached retina. Factors not influencing outcome include the presence of lattice degeneration (less than three clock hours), the type of retinal break, the type or volume of gas used, the type of retinopexy (laser or cryotherapy), the sequence of gas insertion versus retinopexy application, the status of the posterior capsule and gender.
- SOS with PR is desirable for these eyes attain the best postoperative acuity. Other factors positively affecting final visual acuity include preoperative acuity, macular attachment, duration of the detachment less than 8 days and a younger age. Visual acuity return is rapid with 87% of eyes attaining their 6 month acuity level by the 6 week postoperative PR.
- Seventy percent of reoperations are done within the first month and 87% within the first 3 months. Redetachment after 1 year is unusual. Therefore, close follow-up is advised for the first 3 months, with examinations every week or two during the 1 month.
- PR is more cost effective, including reoperations, than scleral buckling. If case selection and surgical techniques are appropriately exercised, PR is 75% less costly than scleral buckling.

References

1. Hilton GF, Grizzard WS. Pneumatic retinopexy. A two-step outpatient operation without conjunctival incision. Ophthalmology. 1986;93:626-41.
2. Dominquez DA. Cirugia precoz y ambulatoria del desprendimento de retina. Arch Soc Esp Ottalmol. 1985;48:47-54.
3. Ai E, Gardner TW. Current patterns of intraocular gas use in North America. Arch Ophthalmol. 1993;111:331-2.
4. Snyder WB, Bloome MA, Birch DG. Pneumatic retinopexy versus scleral buckle. Preferences of Vitreous Society members; 1990. Retina. 1992;12:43-5.
5. Hilton GF, Tornambe PE. The Retinal Detachment Study Group. Pneumatic retinopexy. An analysis of intraoperative and postoperative complications. Retina. 1991;11:285-94.
6. Grizzard WS, Hilton GF, Hammer ME, et al. Pneumatic retinopexy failures. Cause, prevention, timing, and management. Ophthalmology. 1995;102:929-36.
7. Boker T, Schmitt C, Mougharbel M. Results and prognostic factors in pneumatic retinopexy. Ger J Ophthalmol. 1994;3:73-8.
8. Ambler JS, Meyers SM, Zegarra H, et al. Reoperations and visual results after failed pneumatic retinopexy. Ophthalmology. 1990;97:786-90.
9. Tornambe PE, Hilton GF. The Retinal Detachment Study Group. Pneumatic retinopexy. A multicenter randomized controlled clinical trial comparing pneumatic retinopexy with scleral buckling. Ophthalmology. 1989;96:772-83.
10. Tornambe PE, Hilton GF. The Pneumatic Retinopexy Study Group. Pneumatic retinopexy. A two-year follow-up study of the multicenter clinical trial comparing pneumatic retinopexy with scleral buckling. Ophthalmology. 1991;98:1115-23.
11. Tornambe PE, Hilton GF, Kelly NF, et al. Expanded indications for pneumatic retinopexy. Ophthalmol. 1988;5:597-600.
12. McAllister IL, Zegarra H, Meyers SM, et al. Treatment of retinal detachments with multiple breaks by pneumatic retinopexy. Arch Ophthalmol. 1987;105:913-6.
13. Poliner LS, Grand GG, Schoch LH, et al. New retinal detachment after pneumatic retinopexy. Ophthalmology. 1987;94:315-8.
14. Rashed O, Sheta S. Evaluation of the functional results after different techniques for treatment of retinal detachment due to macular holes. Graefes Arch Clin Exp Ophthalmol. 1989;227:508-12.
15. Skoog KO, Textorius O, Wrigstad A. Pneumatic retinopexy in 50 patients. Acta Ophthalmol. 1989;67:103-5.
16. Lowe MA, McDonald HR, Campo RV, et al. Pneumatic retinopexy. Surgical results. Arch Ophthalmol. 1988;106:1672-6.
17. Algvere P, Hallnas K, Palmqvist BM. Success and complications of pneumatic retinopexy. Am J Ophthalmol. 1988;106:400-4.
18. Freeman WR, Lipson BK, Morgan CM, et al. New posteriorly located retinal breaks after pneumatic retinopexy. Ophthalmology. 1988;95:14-8.
19. Hilton GF, Kelly NE, Salzano TC, et al. Pneumatic retinopexy. A collaborative report of the first 100 cases. Ophthalmology. 1987;94:307-14.
20. Algvere PV, Gjotterberg M, Olivestedt G, et al. Results of pneumatic retinopexy with air. Acta Ophthalmol. 1992;70:632-66.
21. Sebag J, Tang M. Pneumatic retinopexy using only air. Retina. 1993;13:8-12.
22. Bochow TW, Olk RJ, Hershey JM. Pneumatic retinopexy perfluoroethane (C_2F_6) in the treatment of rhegmatogenous retinal detachment. Arch Ophthalmol. 1992;110:1723-4.
23. Termote H. Pneumatic retinopexy. Analysis of the first 20 cases Retinopexie pneumatique. Analyse des 20 premiers cas. Bull Soc Belge Ophthalmol. 1989;231:107-16.
24. Melgen SE, Michels M. Pneumatic retinopexy for the treatment of giant retinal dialyses. Am J Ophthalmol. 1994;118:762-5.

25. Irvine AR, Lahey JM. Pneumatic retinopexy for giant retinal tears. Ophthalmology. 1994;101:524-8.
26. Folk JC, Sneed SR, Folberg R, et al. Early retinal adhesion from laser photocoagulation. Ophthalmology. 1989;96: 1523-5.
27. Singh AK, Michels RG, Glaser BM. Scleral indentation following cryotherapy and repeat cryotherapy enhance release of viable retinal pigment epithelial cells. Retina. 1986;6: 176-8.
28. O'Malley P, Swearingen K. Scleral buckle with diathermy for simple retinal detachments. 100 pneumatic retinopexy eligible eyes. Ophthalmology. 1992;99:269-77.
29. Poliner LS, Grand MG, Schoch LH, et al. New retinal detachment after pneumatic retinopexy. Ophthalmology. 1987;94:315-8.
30. McDonald HR, Abrams GW, Irvine AR, et al. The management of subretinal gas following attempted pneumatic retinal reattachment. Ophthalmology. 1987;94:319-26
31. McAllister IL, Zegarra H, Meyers SM, et al. Treatment of retinal detachments with multiple breaks by pneumatic retinopexy. Arch Ophthalmol. 1987;105:913-6.
32. Chan CK, Wessels IF. Delayed subretinal fluid absorption after pneumatic retinopexy. Ophthalmol. 1989;96:1691-700.
33. Lincoff H, Kreissig I, Farber M. Results of 100 aphakic detachments treated with a temporary balloon buckle: a case against routine encircling operations. Br J Ophthalmol. 1985;69:798-804.
34. Kreissig I, Failer J, Lincoff H, et al. Results of a temporary balloon buckle in the treatment of 500 retinal detachments and a comparison with pneumatic retinopexy. Am J Ophthalmol. 1989;107:381-9.
35. McAllister IL, Meyers SM, Zegarra H, et al. Comparison of pneumatic retinopexy with alternative surgical techniques. Ophthalmology. 1988;95:877-83.
36. Binder S. Repair of retinal detachments with temporary balloon buckling. Retina. 1986;6:210-4.
37. Lincoff H, Kreissig I. Results with a temporary balloon buckle for the repair of retinal detachment. Am J Ophthalmol. 1981;92:245-51.
38. Green SN, Yarian DL, Masciulli L, et al. Office repair of retinal detachment using a Lincoff temporary balloon buckle. Ophthalmology. 1996;103:1804-10.

14

Primary Vitrectomy for Retinal Detachment

Heinrich Heimann

Introduction

Over the past years, primary vitrectomy has become the most popular surgical method to treat rhegmatogenous retinal detachments. Worldwide, there has been an extraordinary shift away from scleral buckling surgery and pneumatic retinopexy towards primary vitrectomy.[1,2] In the USA, about 70% of cases are now treated with primary vitrectomy.[3] In this chapter, the evolution of primary vitrectomy, the techniques and the clinical studies on the subject are reviewed.

Evolution of Primary Vitrectomy

About 100 years ago, Leber, Gonin and others first identified vitreoretinal traction and retinal break formation as the key steps preceding the development of retinal detachment.[4] The results of the first surgical attempts to treat this disease were disappointing. One early interesting approach published by Deutschmann in the first decades of the 20th century touched on the pathophysiological descriptions previously described by Leber with an "ab interno" approach to counteract traction through dissection of vitreoretinal adhesions.[5] Success rates were quoted to be 26% for complete retinal reattachment.[6] However, these techniques never gained any noteworthy popularity and were overtaken by the more successful "ab externo" approach of scleral buckling (SB) surgery that was developed by Jess and Custodis.[4]

It was not until the 1970s that the logical approach of "ab interno" dissection of vitreoretinal adhesions to treat retinal detachment was reintroduced with the development of pars plana vitrectomy (PPV) by Machemer.[7] Some of the very first patients operated on with PPV were patients with retinal detachment and the first case series of primary vitrectomy for retinal detachment was soon published.[8] During the early years of vitrectomy, this technique was reserved for the treatment of complicated redetachments. Klöti was the first to devote a paper specifically on vitrectomy without SB as the initial surgical treatment of retinal detachment and termed it "primary vitrectomy"[9] this was followed by a series in the English medical literature from Escoffery et al.[10]

In the early 1990s, SB surgery was still the standard treatment method for primary retinal detachments. This changed following the introduction of two additional technical advances of vitrectomy: The use of heavy liquids to unfold the detached retina,[11] allowing internal drainage of subretinal fluid, and wide-angle viewing systems.[12] These advances facilitated the handling of challenging situations (e.g. giant retinal tears, multiple and central breaks) and led to enormous boost in popularity of primary vitrectomy. Finally, the innovations of endolaser-photocoagulation to treat breaks and as a 360° laser prophylaxis to avoid an additional encircling band[13] as well as the introduction of small gauge vitrectomy techniques[14] further contributed to the refinements of this technique, whereas no significant advances of SB surgery have been introduced over the same period of time.

The past 20 years have seen a tremendous increase in the number of units equipped with vitrectomy machines and the number of surgeons trained in this technique. The indications for vitrectomy are constantly increasing and the vast majority of vitreoretinal procedures nowadays are pars plana vitrectomies. Surgeons of the latest generation are therefore much more familiar with this technique compared to SB surgery, in particular in challenging cases. These reasons also contribute to the enormous increase in popularity of primary vitrectomy as the most popular choice in the treatment of retinal detachment.

Techniques and Variations of Primary Vitrectomy

The basic steps of primary vitrectomy consist of:

- Core vitrectomy
- Completion or induction of posterior vitreous detachment (PVD)
- Identification of retinal breaks with internal search
- Dissection of all vitreoretinal traction, in particular around retinal breaks
- Trimming of the vitreous base
- Retinal reattachment using heavy liquids or internal drainage with active suction or fluid-air exchange
- Retinopexy with laser or cryotherapy
- Short- or long-acting internal tamponade
- Postoperative posturing according to break localization

Within this basic framework, numerous variations are practiced according to the surgeon´s preferences. The term "primary vitrectomy" therefore encompasses a variety of different techniques with the only common denominator of an "ab interno" approach via the pars plana, removal of vitreous, retinopexy and installation of tamponades. Because of these manifold varieties of the surgical technique, it is problematical to compare different series on primary vitrectomy as even minor variations in technique may have a significant influence on treatment outcome.

The major differences in surgical technique of primary vitrectomy are listed in Table 14.1. Overall, the key differences affect five areas:

- Vitrectomy set-up (20-, 23- or 25-gauge)
- Extent of vitrectomy: "Limited" to the area of the break, "moderate" with core vitrectomy and 360° trimming of vitreous base or "aggressive" with removing as much

TABLE 14.1: Variation in technical details of primary vitrectomy

Surgical Step	*Variations*
Setup-viewing system	• Varying wide angle contact or non-contact viewing systems
Setup-sclerotomies	• 20-gauge • 23-gauge • 25-gauge
Illumination	• Internal handheld endoillumination • Chandelier or illuminated infusion systems for bimanual surgery
Combined cataract surgery	• Only in patients $\geq$60 years or with significant cataract • Always in all phakic patients
Extent of vitrectomy	• Core vitrectomy with limited peripheral vitrectomy in the quadrants with retinal breaks • Trimming of vitreous base over 360° • "Radical" vitrectomy, trying to remove as much vitreous as possible
Endodrainage	• Through the break using heavy liquids • Without heavy liquids using active suction through break • Without heavy liquids through central or peripheral retinotomies
Retinopexy	• Exocryotherapy • Endocryotherapy • Endolaser to breaks only • 360° endolaser
Peeling of the inner limiting membrane	• Never • Always with the aim to prevent macular pucker and PVR • Only in cases with significant epiretinal gliosis
Additional scleral buckling (encircling band)	• Never • Always • In selected patients (pseudophakic, inferior breaks, PVR)
Endotamponade	• No long-term tamponade • Air • Air/gas mixtures (SF_6, C_2F_6, C_3F_8) • Silicone oil 1000-, 2000 or 5000 cts • Heavy silicone oil
Postoperative posturing	• Posture according to break localization • No posture

vitreous as possible, often using triamcinolone to detect vitreous remnants
- Choice of tamponade (air, gas/air mixtures or different silicone oils)
- Prophylactic 360° endolaser
- Additional scleral buckling (usually encircling band).

None of these major variations in techniques have been compared in prospective randomized trials. The choice of technique, therefore, currently depends on training, experience, personal preferences of the individual surgeon and the equipment available. In the extremes, identical retinal detachments could be treated with a 25-gauge set-up, very limited vitrectomy and air tamponade or with an extensive 20-gauge vitrectomy combined with an encircling band and silicone oil; both cases would be classified as "primary vitrectomy" despite the obvious differences in technique and the extent of the surgical trauma.

Most surgeons would currently employ a stepwise approach with small gauge vitrectomy with air or short-acting gas tamponades for localized detachments, longer-acting gas tamponades for retinal detachment with medium difficulty (multiple breaks, significant traction on the break, bullous detachment) and 20-gauge systems with the options of silicone oil tamponades and additional SB for complicated retinal detachment (PVR, total retinal detachment, giant tears, retinal detachment with macular hole). As more and more vitreoretinal surgeons are also trained in anterior segment surgery, combining primary vitrectomy with phacoemulsification and intraocular lens implantation as a standard procedure in phakic patients is also gaining more widespread acceptance.[15] This facilitates trimming of the vitreous base, avoids postoperative visual loss caused by cataract formation and the need for an additional secondary cataract surgery. An additional significant advancement is staining of the vitreous with triamcinolone.[16,17] This facilitates the detection of vitreous remnants and may identify a vitreoschisis with an attached posterior hyaloid face even in cases of rhegmatogenous retinal detachments, in particular in highly myopic patients.

The need for additional SB surgery is a point of ongoing controversy. Despite the rapidly decreasing use of additional encircling bands, even very recent series of primary vitrectomy are still divided with some groups applying encircling bands in all cases of primary vitrectomy.[17,18] In the majority of recent publications, however, additional SB surgery is replaced by prophylactic 360° endolaser.[15,19-21] The use of additional SB surgery has also been investigated in a large randomized trial.[22] Analysis showed that better results could be achieved with additional SB surgery in pseudophakic patients, whereas no advantage could be seen in phakic patients. In this study, the use of additional buckling was based on the surgeons´ individual preferences and was not randomized.

The increasing popularity of 25- and 23-gauge vitrectomies has also contributed to the trend away from SB surgery.[23] More and more retinal detachments at the "easier" end of the spectrum are now treated with small gauge vitrectomy and some units do not use SB anymore.[24,25] The advantages of these techniques are the reduction of the number of entry site tears, shorter operating times and less discomfort for the patient. However, there are also several potential disadvantages of these techniques, in particular in the treatment of retinal detachment: Trimming of the vitreous base is challenging with the more flexible instruments and a trocar guided system[23] and the lower intraocular pressure (IOP) that is associated with these techniques[26] has several disadvantages in the treatment of retinal detachment. First, the IOP plays an important role in retinal (re-) attachment. Second, a temporarily raised IOP following the surgery may lead to leakage of tamponade through the sclerotomies, resulting in a decrease in intraocular tamponade effect and possibly unsupported breaks. And third, a significant postoperative hypotony[20,25,26] may occur, which may result in choroidal hemorrhage.[27] Additional measures (combined SB surgery or silicone oil tamponade) can only be used with difficulties and the threshold for using these additional tools is raised. And finally, one of the key advantages of small gauge vitrectomy, enhanced visual recovery, is negligible because of the visual disturbance caused by the intraocular tamponade and the need for external cryotherapy in phakic patients.[23] In fact, a much faster visual recovery can be observed following SB surgery. Partially caused by these disadvantages of small gauge surgery, the first published results have been disappointing,[23] in particular if compared to the high success rates of SB surgery in this group of patients.[28] However, with increasing experience and refinements of the technique (improved trocars and stiffer instruments), results nowadays seem to match those of 20-gauge vitrectomies (Table 14.1).

Probably the most exciting recent development in the field of primary vitrectomy is the "no tamponade" technique that was introduced by Martinez-Castillo in 2007.[29] During the surgery, a meticulous vitrectomy is performed and an intraoperative complete reattachment is achieved by using temporary heavy liquid tamponade and endolaser around the break. Outstanding anatomical results have been achieved with this technique[29] however, there is no widespread adaption of this technique as yet and publications are confined to one center only.

Clinical Studies and Results of Primary Vitrectomy

Since the publication of the first primary vitrectomy within the very early publications of Norten and Machemer,[7,8] more than 50 studies on primary vitrectomy have been published to date. The majority of publications are retrospective single center series, either describing consecutive case series or focusing on particular subtypes of retinal detachments (for example, pseudophakic patients, inferior breaks, etc.) or technical variations of the procedure (for example, additional SB or small gauge vitrectomies). The latest series of primary vitrectomy including small gauge vitrectomies are outlined in Table 14.2.[17,18,20-22,25,27,30-34,24,29,35-43] Summaries of earlier series of primary vitrectomy have been published elsewhere.[22,31,44,45]

The key outcomes of retinal detachment surgery are the primary success rate (percentage of eyes with successful retinal reattachment with one vitreoretinal procedure), the final success rate (retinal reattachment with one or more vitreoretinal procedures) and the postoperative visual acuity. Additional results that are provided in several clinical studies are the rate of postoperative proliferative vitreoretinopathy (PVR), macular pucker and the number and reasons for secondary surgical interventions.

The outcomes of published series of primary vitrectomy vary significantly (Table 14.2). The major reasons for this is that most studies differ regarding the key variables associated with the anatomical and functional outcome, for example, inclusion and exclusion criteria, technical details of the procedure, follow-up, definition and quantification of outcome variables, etc. Overall, the primary success rates of recent series seem to have improved significantly over the past years and are now around 90% compared to approximately 80% in earlier publications.[22,31,44,45] One has to take into account that these success rates may be flawed by the well known disadvantages of retrospective single center series and the tendency of negative results not being forwarded or accepted for publication. This is underlined by the fact that primary success rates of prospective trials are significantly lower at around 70–80%. Final success rates are close to or at 100% in almost all series. The most common complication of primary vitrectomy is cataract development, which could be documented in 77% of phakic patients within the first postoperative year in a prospective randomized trial.[22] Reported rates of macular pucker are at around 2–5 % and postoperative PVR can be seen in 7–17%.[22,37] The functional outcome varies immensely according to the complexity of the preoperative situation, the macular status, lens status, anatomical success and follow-up. On average, a mean logMAR visual acuity of around 0.3 has been reported. Translated into daily practice, this means that even with primary vitrectomy, about 40% of patients will not achieve reading ability without low vision aids postoperatively. The initial publications of small gauge primary vitrectomies included several disappointing results, in particular for phakic patients.[27,43] With increasing experience and better instruments, the results in recent series now seem to match those of 20-gauge vitrectomy in several comparative series.[20,39,40]

Comparison to Other Methods

Several single-center prospective trials[34,35,46-48] and two large multicenter prospective randomized clinical trials[22,49] have been conducted to compare SB surgery and primary vitrectomy in the treatment of rhegmatogenous retinal detachments. Overall, the majority of these trials demonstrate that primary vitrectomy achieves functional and anatomical results comparable to SB surgery. This is confirmed by a recent analysis of secondary surgeries for failures after primary retinal detachment surgery with various methods in medicare beneficiaries. In this large study, failure rates of around 20% were extracted for both, SB surgery and primary vitrectomy.[50] There also seem to be an association of the lens status and outcome. In phakic patients, anatomical and functional outcomes of primary vitrectomy seem to just reach or are slightly inferior to the results of SB surgery.[22,51] In this group of patients, that compromise about two-thirds of all patients with retinal detachment, primary vitrectomy is associated with worse functional results[22,51] and, as demonstrated in several studies, a higher rate of secondary surgical interventions.[43,52] In contrast, primary vitrectomy seems to achieve better results in pseudophakic patients.[22,53] In this group, primary vitrectomy has an advantage of easier identification of small anterior breaks via internal search, which are more common and harder to find compared to

TABLE 14.2: Results of recent series of primary vitrectomy

First Author, Year	*Focus*	*n, follow-up*	*Primary success*	*Final success*	*Functional success logMAR*
20-gauge primary vitrectomy					
Heimann, 2006	Consecutive series of PPPV	516, min 3 m	71%	98%	median 0.4
Salicone, 2006	PPPV and SBS for RRD with unclear break situation	18, min 1 m, mean 8.3 m	72%	83%	mean 1.1
Weichel, 2006	PPV without buckle for pseudophakic RRD	68, min 3 m, mean 11 m	93%	100%	mean 0.38
Weichel, 2006	PPV with buckle for pseudophakic RRD	84, min 3 m, mean 8.6 m	94%	100%	mean 0.55
Alexander, 2007	PPPV with encircling band and silicone for high-risk cases	33, min 12 m	91%	97%	
Azad, 2007	Phakic patients with RRD	30, 6 m	80%	100%	median 0.6
Johansson, 2007	Consecutive series	131, min 3 m, mean 7 m	87%	95%	median 0.3
Koriyama, 2007	Phakic patients	23, 12 m	91%	100%	mean 0.3
Martinez-Castillo, 2007	20 g without long-term tamponade for pseudophakic RRD	60, min 12 m, mean 16 m	98%	100%	mean 0.48
Smith, 2007	Consecutive series combined with cataract surgery	93, min 4 m, mean 25 m	88%	98%	mean 0.3
SPR study, 2007	PPV for phakic patients	174, 12 m	75%	96%	mean 0.48
SPR study, 2007	PPV for pseudophakic patients	132, 12 m	80%	96%	mean 0.38
Wickham, 2007	Prospective multicenter trial, adjuvant pharmacotherapy for prevention of PVR	615, 6 m	84%	98%	median 0.4
Romano, 2008	PPPV with heavy silicone oil	33, min 3 m	91%	94%	mean 0.5
von Fricken, 2009	20 g vs 25 g for RRD	61, min 3 m, mean 15 m	92%	100%	mean 0.18
Acar, 2010	PPPV ± triamcinolone for staining of vitreous, PVR C	72, min 6 m, mean 14.6 m	83%	96%	mean 1.57
Colyer, 2010	20 g vs 25 g, inferior pseudophakic RRD	48, min 3 m, mean 11.4 m	89%	96%	mean 0.32
Kobayashi, 2010	20 g vs 25 g for primary RRD	47, min 3 m, mean 8 m	92%	98%	mean 0.19
Schatz, 2010	Visual recovery	13, min 6 m	77%	100%	
25- and 23-gauge primary vitrectomy					
Acar, 2008	25 g for pseudophakic RRD	22, min 6 m, mean 10 m	95%	100%	mean 0.4
Lai, 2008	25 g for RRD	53, min 1 m, mean 8 m	74%	100%	mean 0.5
Miller, 2008	25 g for RRD	42, min 3 m	93%	100%	mean 0.23
Tsang, 2008	23 g for RRD	24, min 6 m, mean 10 m	92%	100%	mean 0.1 macula on) mean 0.45 (macula off)

Contd...

contd...

First Author, Year	Focus	n, follow-up	Primary success	Final success	Functional success logMAR
Dayani, 2009	20 g with SBS vs SBS alone, macula-off RRD	63, min 3 m, mean 36 m	82%	98%	median 0.3
von Fricken, 2009	20 g vs 25 g for RRD	64, min 3 m, mean 10 m	91%	100%	mean 0.21
Kapran, 2009	25 g for pseudophakic RRD	23, min 6 m, mean 10 m	91%	95%	mean 0.61
Kapran, 2009	25 g for phakic RRD	13, min 6 m, mean 12 m	61%	84%	mean 1.09
Bourla, 2010	25 g for RRD	42, min 3 m, mean 9 m	98%	100%	mean 0.2 (macula on) mean 0.6 (macula off)
Colyer, 2010	20 g vs 25 g, inferior pseudophakic RRD	30, min 3 m, mean 11.4 m	83%	100%	mean 0.28
Kobayashi, 2010	20 g vs 25 g for primary RRD	119, min 3 m, mean 7.6	93%	98%	mean 0.17
Kunikata, 2010	25 g for RRD	84, min 3 m, mean 6.6 m	95%	100%	mean 0.17

entire group

RRD. Rhegmatogenous retinal detachment; PPV: Pars plana vitrectomy; PVR: Proliferative vitreoretinopathy.

phakic retinal detachments. Additionally, a more aggressive trimming of the vitreous base is possible and the major complication of primary vitrectomy, postoperative cataract development, is irrelevant.

Advantages of Primary Vitrectomy

The major advantages of primary vitrectomy over other methods are that it is easier than SB surgery, in particular in more challenging cases. SB surgery is a very successful method in experienced hands, but, in contrast to primary vitrectomy, is associated with a longer learning curve and remains extremely difficult in more complicated cases of retinal detachment. All challenges of advanced SB surgery (correct identification of all breaks with indirect ophthalmoscopy, correct placement of buckles, suturing buckles onto thin sclera, subretinal drainage or paracentesis in phakic eyes with high pressures, intraocular air- or gas injections) as well as potential complications (subretinal hemorrhage, residual subfoveal fluid, buckle erosion and infection, diplopia) are avoided.[2,54] With primary vitrectomy, surgeons in training very quickly are able to control and master challenging situations of retinal detachment.[45] They are then more likely to stick with this method, even at the cost of a higher rate of secondary surgery, rather than going through the complications that are associated with advanced SB surgery. This is particularly true for pseudophakic retinal detachments, in which also better results are achieved with primary vitrectomy compared to SB surgery. From a teaching perspective, it is also a lot easier to teach primary vitrectomy compared to SB surgery, in particular in more challenging cases. Therefore, a fellow currently training in vitreoretinal surgery will simply not be able to treat complicated cases of rhegmatogenous retinal detachments with SB surgery anymore. In addition, the rate of combined primary vitrectomy with encircling band is constantly falling and will now probably be at around 15% or less in most departments.[37] Therefore, at least for more complicated cases of retinal detachments, SB surgery has already become a "forgotten art".[55]

An additional reason for the increasing popularity of primary vitrectomy is the enormous rise in the number of surgeons trained in vitreoretinal surgery and the units equipped with vitrectomy machines. The introduction of significantly improved wide-angle viewing systems, the rapidly increasing experience with vitrectomy techniques across a variety of different vitreoretinal diseases and the ease and comfort of using small gauge vitrectomy systems are all factors that contribute to the massive trend towards primary vitrectomy.

Disadvantages of Primary Vitrectomy

The major drawback of primary vitrectomy is that it is still associated with significant rates of anatomical and functional failures. Many surgeons may still underestimate the failure rates, because primary vitrectomy achieves almost a 100% of "instant success" (retinal reattachment at the end of the surgical procedure), followed by a "honeymoon period" of weeks to months with the intraocular tamponade in place. Anatomical failures may become apparent only at a later stage compared to SB surgery, where this is usually obvious within the first days after the surgery.

Anatomical failure following primary vitrectomy can be caused by a single or a combination of various factors, including development of new breaks, missed breaks, insufficient tamponade of existing breaks and proliferative vitreoretinopathy (PVR). Disappointing functional outcomes are mainly caused by permanent structural damage to the foveal photoreceptor layer, cystoid macular edema, macular pucker, or failure to reattach the retina.[56] All of these problems are not exclusive to primary vitrectomy; however, neither could a major breakthrough to solve these pertinent problems of retinal detachment surgery be achieved with primary vitrectomy, perhaps with the exception of difficult cases of pseudophakic retinal detachment. The only advantage of primary vitrectomy over SB surgery regarding secondary macular changes is the faster reabsorption of persistent subfoveal fluid compared to SB surgery.[57] However, it is not proven whether this is also associated with a long-term functional advantage.

An additional definite disadvantage of primary vitrectomy is cataract development in phakic patients. This leads to a lot higher rate of reoperations compared to SB surgery [50,52] with the associated problems of decreased vision, changes in refraction, increased costs and multiple follow-up examinations for the patient. Young patients will lose their accommodation and postoperative anisometropia is of particular concern in myopic patients.

The practical disadvantages of primary vitrectomy are the need for specialized equipment including vitrectomy machines and microscopes with wide-angle viewing systems and the associated higher costs compared to SB surgery or pneumatic retinopexy. Due to the enormous increase in units equipped with such facilities, this nowadays seems to be less of a problem. However, it is noteworthy that access to relatively expensive vitrectomy techniques including the use of small gauge systems, heavy liquids, silicone oils, etc. still is problematic in many countries.

Indications and Contraindications

Retinal detachment can present with varying degrees of complexity, ranging from clearly identifiable retinal breaks with little surrounding fluid to total retinal detachments complicated by vitreous hemorrhage, macular hole and PVR grade C.[58] In theory, every retinal detachment can be treated successfully with primary vitrectomy and several authors have proposed to use primary vitrectomy for all primary retinal detachment.[1,2,24] Most surgeons would agree that primary vitrectomy is the best option for retinal detachment complicated by PVR, central breaks or macular holes and giant tears. The same holds true for retinal detachment in pseudophakic patients.[53]

Retinal detachments of medium complexity (multiple breaks, bullous configuration and large breaks) can be treated successfully with SB surgery as well as primary vitrectomy. The SPR study has demonstrated slightly better functional results with SB surgery; however, this technique is extremely challenging in such cases. As most comparative studies demonstrate results of primary vitrectomy that are not inferior to those of SB surgery and primary vitrectomy is technically less challenging in these situation, most surgeons would nowadays opt for primary vitrectomy in this subgroup.

Localized detachments (horseshoe tear, one to two quadrants detached) still compromise the majority of primary retinal detachment.[58] Primary vitrectomy has also gained popularity in this subgroup, in particular, through the widespread use of 25- and 23-gauge vitrectomy techniques. Whether this is a "natural" evolution of surgical techniques or an erroneous trend remains to be seen in the future.[2,23,54,55]

There is no defined group of absolute contraindications for primary vitrectomy; this is partially due to general tendency of not publishing negative results but also to the problems of subgroup analysis under the big umbrella of retinal detachment. There simply are not sufficient numbers of particular subtypes of retinal detachment in published trials to allow a clear correlation of preoperative morphology, surgical method and postoperative success. However, based on clinical experience and results of comparative trials and results achieved with other surgical methods, there are several subgroups of patients in which the disadvantages of primary vitrectomy seem to outweigh its benefits: In patients with retinal detachment and (partially) attached vitreous, SB surgery is able to achieve nearly 100% success with the additional advantage of a much slower cataract progression compared to primary vitrectomy.[59] These are often relatively young, myopic patients with round holes. The persistent vitreous attachment might not be obvious to the inexperienced examiner. Intraoperatively, the surgeon may face several problems, for example, dissecting a sometimes very adherent posterior vitreous face from an already detached retina and the formation of multiple iatrogenic breaks in areas of lattice degeneration just by completion of a posterior vitreous detachment. The same holds true for patients with retinal dialysis[60] and those with localized retinal detachment confined to one quadrant and with a clear single break horseshoe tear situation. SB surgery is a simple and highly successful surgical method in such cases[28] and the surgical steps that potentially create most complications associated with SB surgery, trans-sceral drainage of subretinal fluid and intraocular injections for volume replacement, can usually be avoided. Finally, if SB surgery achieves better functional results in more complicated situations of retinal detachment in phakic patients in a randomized controlled clinical trial,[22] one could speculate that it is highly unlikely that primary vitrectomy would show advantages in less complicated morphology with only localized detachments.

References

1. Chong DY, Fuller DG. The declining use of scleral buckling with vitrectomy for primary retinal detachments. Arch 'Ophthalmol. 2010;128:1206-7.
2. D'Amico DJ. Clinical practice. Primary retinal detachment. N Engl J Med. 2008;359:2346-54.
3. Ramulu PY, Do DV, Corcoran KJ, et al. Use of retinal procedures in medicare beneficiaries from 1997 to 2007. Arch Ophthalmol. 2010;128:1335-40.
4. Dellaporta AN. Retinal detachment surgery: historical notes. Doc Ophthalmol. 1999;99:259-72.
5. Deutschmann R. Zur Kenntnis der Netzhauablösung und ihrer Behandlung. Graefes Arch Clin Exp Ophthalmol. 1910;74: 206-23.
6. Deutschmann R. Über Netzhautrisse, insbesondere über ihre Bedeutung für die Netzhautablösung. Graefes Arch Clin Exp Ophthalmol. 1929;122:359-82.
7. Machemer R, Buettner H, Norton EW, et al. Vitrectomy: a pars plana approach. Trans Am Acad Ophthalmol Otolaryngol. 1971;75:813-20.
8. Norton EW, Machemer R. New approach to the treatment of selected retinal detachments secondary to vitreous loss at cataract surgery. Am J Ophthalmol. 1971;72:705-7.
9. Kloeti R. Retinal detachment surgery without scleral buckling. Primary vitrectomy. Klin Mbl Augenheilk. 1983;182:474-8.
10. Escoffery RF, Olk RJ, Grand MG, et al. Vitrectomy without scleral buckling for primary rhegmatogenous retinal detachment. Am J Ophthalmol. 1985;99:275-81.
11. Chang S. Low viscosity liquid fluorochemicals in vitreous surgery. Am J Ophthalmol. 1987;103:38-43.
12. Ho PC, Mainster MA, Dieckert JP, et al. Fundus contact lenses for closed pars plana vitrectomy. Ophthalmology. 1983;Suppl:106-14.
13. Koh HJ, Cheng L, Kosobucki B, et al. Prophylactic intraoperative 360 degrees laser retinopexy for prevention of retinal detachment. Retina. 2007;27:744-9.
14. Fujii GY, De Juan E, Humayun MS, et al. A new 25-gauge instrument system for transconjunctival sutureless vitrectomy surgery. Ophthalmology. 2002;109:1807-12.
15. Bourla DH, Bor E, Axer-Siegel R, et al. Outcomes and complications of rhegmatogenous retinal detachment repair with selective sutureless 25-gauge pars plana vitrectomy. Am J Ophthalmol. 2010;149:630-4 e1.
16. Schmidt JC, Chofflet J, Horle S, et al. Three simple approaches to visualize the transparent vitreous cortex during vitreoretinal surgery. Dev Ophthalmol. 2008;42:35-42.
17. Acar N, Kapran Z, Altan T, et al. Pars plana vitrectomy with and without triamcinolone acetonide assistance in pseudophakic retinal detachment complicated with proliferative vitreoretinopathy. Jpn J Ophthalmol. 2010;54:331-7.
18. Dayani PN, Blinder KJ, Shah GK, et al. Surgical outcome of scleral buckling compared with scleral buckling with vitrectomy for treatment of macula-off retinal detachment. Ophthalmic Surg Lasers Imaging. 2009;40:539-4
19. Acar N, Kapran Z, Altan T, et al. Primary 25-gauge sutureless vitrectomy with oblique sclerotomies in pseudophakic retinal detachment. Retina. 2008;28:1068-74.
20. Colyer MH, Barazi MK, Von Fricken MA. Retrospective comparison of 25-gauge transconjunctival sutureless vitrectomy to 20-gauge vitrectomy for the repair of pseudophakic primary inferior rhegmatogenous retinal detachment. Retina. 2010;30:1678-84.
21. Schatz P, Andreasson S. Recovery of retinal function after recent-onset rhegmatogenous retinal detachment in relation to type of surgery. Retina. 2010;30:152-9.
22. Heimann H, Bartz-Schmidt KU, Bornfeld N, et al. Scleral buckling versus primary vitrectomy in rhegmatogenous retinal detachment: a prospective randomized multicenter clinical study. Ophthalmology. 2007;114:2142-54.

23. Heimann H. Primary 25- and 23-gauge vitrectomy in the treatment of rhegmatogenous retinal detachment—advancement of surgical technique or erroneous trend? Klin Monatsbl Augenheilkd. 2008;225:947-56.
24. Johansson K, Malmsjo M, Ghosh F. Tailored vitrectomy and laser photocoagulation without scleral buckling for all primary rhegmatogenous retinal detachments. Br J Ophthalmol. 2006;90:1286-91.
25. Kunikata H, Nishida K. Visual outcome and complications of 25-gauge vitrectomy for rhegmatogenous retinal detachment; 84 consecutive cases. Eye. 2010;24:1071-7.
26. Bamonte G, Mura M, Tan HS. Hypotony after 25-gauge vitrectomy. Am J Ophthalmol. 2011;151:156-60.
27. Lai MM, Ruby AJ, Sarrafizadeh R, et al. Repair of primary rhegmatogenous retinal detachment using 25-gauge transconjunctival sutureless vitrectomy. Retina. 2008;28:729-34.
28. O'Malley P, Swearingen K. Scleral buckle with diathermy for simple retinal detachments. 100 pneumatic retinopexy eligible eyes. Ophthalmology. 1992;99:269-77.
29. Martinez-Castillo V, Zapata MA, Boixadera A, et al. Pars plana vitrectomy, laser retinopexy, and aqueous tamponade for pseudophakic rhegmatogenous retinal detachment. Ophthalmology. 2007;114:297-302.
30. Salicone A, Smiddy WE, Venkatraman A, et al. Visual recovery after scleral buckling procedure for retinal detachment. Ophthalmology. 2006;113:1734-42.
31. Heimann H, Zou X, Jandeck C, et al. Primary vitrectomy for rhegmatogenous retinal detachment: an analysis of 512 cases. Graefes Arch Clin Exp Ophthalmol. 2006;244:69-78.
32. Weichel ED, Martidis A, Fineman MS, et al. Pars plana vitrectomy versus combined pars plana vitrectomy-scleral buckle for primary repair of pseudophakic retinal detachment. Ophthalmology. 2006;113:2033-40.
33. Alexander P, Ang A, Poulson A, et al. Scleral buckling combined with vitrectomy for the management of rhegmatogenous retinal detachment associated with inferior retinal breaks. Eye. 2008;22:200-3.
34. Azad RV, Chanana B, Sharma YR, et al. Primary vitrectomy versus conventional retinal detachment surgery in phakic rhegmatogenous retinal detachment. Acta Ophthalmol Scand. 2007;85:540-5.
35. Koriyama M, Nishimura T, Matsubara T, et al. Prospective study comparing the effectiveness of scleral buckling to vitreous surgery for rhegmatogenous retinal detachment. Jpn J Ophthalmol. 2007;51:360-7.
36. Smith M, Raman SV, Pappas G, et al. Phacovitrectomy for primary retinal detachment repair in presbyopes. Retina. 2007;27:462-7.
37. Wickham L, Bunce C, Wong D, et al. Randomized controlled trial of combined 5-Fluorouracil and low-molecular-weight heparin in the management of unselected rhegmatogenous retinal detachments undergoing primary vitrectomy. Ophthalmology. 2007;114:698-704.
38. Romano MR, Stappler T, Marticorena J, et al. Primary vitrectomy with Densiron-68 for rhegmatogenous retinal detachment. Graefes Arch Clin Exp Ophthalmol. 2008;246:1541-6.
39. Von Fricken MA, Kunjukunju N, Weber C, et al. 25-Gauge sutureless vitrectomy versus 20-gauge vitrectomy for the repair of primary rhegmatogenous retinal detachment. Retina. 2009;29:444-50.
40. Kobayashi S, Sato S, Inoue M, et al. Comparison of 20- and 25-gauge vitrectomy for primary repair of rhegmatogenous retinal detachment. Ophthalmic Surg Lasers Imaging. 2010;41:550-4.
41. Miller DM, Riemann CD, Foster RE, et al. Primary repair of retinal detachment with 25-gauge pars plana vitrectomy. Retina. 2008;28:931-6.
42. Tsang CW, Cheung BT, Lam RF, et al. Primary 23-gauge transconjunctival sutureless vitrectomy for rhegmatogenous retinal detachment. Retina. 2008;28:1075-81.
43. Kapran Z, Acar N, Altan T, et al. 25-Gauge sutureless vitrectomy with oblique sclerotomies for the management of retinal detachment in pseudophakic and phakic eyes. Eur J Ophthalmol. 2009;19:853-60.
44. Barrie T, Kreissig I, Heimann H, et al. Repair of a primary rhegmatogenous retinal detachment. Br J Ophthalmol. 2003;87:782.
45. Heimann H, Bartz-Schmidt KU, Bornfeld N, et al. Primary pars plana vitrectomy. Techniques, indications, and results. Ophthalmologe. 2008;105:19-26.
46. Brazitikos P. Scleral buckling versus primary vitrectomy. Ophthalmology. 2006;113:1245.
47. Sharma A, Grigoropoulos V, Williamson TH. Management of primary rhegmatogenous retinal detachment with inferior breaks. Br J Ophthalmol. 2004;88:1372-5.
48. Tewari HK, Kedar S, Kumar A, et al. Comparison of scleral buckling with combined scleral buckling and pars plana vitrectomy in the management of rhegmatogenous retinal detachment with unseen retinal breaks. Clin Experiment Ophthalmol. 2003;31:403-7.
49. Ahmadieh H, Moradian S, Faghihi H, et al. Anatomic and visual outcomes of scleral buckling versus primary vitrectomy in pseudophakic and aphakic retinal detachment: six-month follow-up results of a single operation—report no. 1. Ophthalmology. 2005;112:1421-9.
50. Day S, Grossman DS, Mruthyunjaya P, et al. One-year outcomes after retinal detachment surgery among medicare beneficiaries. Am J Ophthalmol. 2010;150:338-45.
51. Pastor JC, Fernandez I, Rodriguez de la Rua E, et al. Surgical outcomes for primary rhegmatogenous retinal detachments in phakic and pseudophakic patients: the Retina 1 Project—report no. 2. Br J Ophthalmol. 2008;92:378-82.
52. Heussen N, Hilgers RD, Heimann H, et al. Scleral buckling versus primary vitrectomy in rhegmatogenous retinal detachment study (SPR Study): Multiple-event analysis of risk factors for reoperations. SPR Study report no. 4. Acta Ophthalmol; 2009.p.11.

53. Arya AV, Emerson JW, Engelbert M, et al. Surgical management of pseudophakic retinal detachments: a meta-analysis. Ophthalmology. 2006;113:1724-33.
54. McLeod D. Is it time to call time on the scleral buckle? Br J Ophthalmol. 2004;88:1357-9.
55. Lincoff H, Kreissig I. Changing patterns in the surgery for retinal detachment: 1929 to 2000. Klin Monatsbl Augenheilkd. 2000;216:352-9.
56. Wakabayashi T, Oshima Y, Fujimoto H, et al. Foveal microstructure and visual acuity after retinal detachment repair: imaging analysis by Fourier-domain optical coherence tomography. Ophthalmology. 2009;116:519-28.
57. Wolfensberger TJ. Foveal reattachment after macula-off retinal detachment occurs faster after vitrectomy than after buckle surgery. Ophthalmology. 2004;111:1340-3.
58. Feltgen N, Wolf S, Weiss C, et al. Scleral buckling versus primary vitrectomy in rhegmatogenous retinal detachment study (SPR Study). Evaluation of the recruitment list (SPR Study report number 2). Graefes Archive. 2005;submitted.
59. Ung T, Comer MB, Ang AJ, et al. Clinical features and surgical management of retinal detachment secondary to round retinal holes. Eye. 2005;19:665-9.
60. Stoffelns BM, Richard G. Is buckle surgery still the state of the art for retinal detachments due to retinal dialysis? J Pediatr Ophthalmol Strabismus. 2010;47:281-7.

15 Proliferative Vitreoretinopathy

Ryan M Tarantola

Introduction

Despite significant advancements in vitreoretinal surgical techniques, proliferative vitreoretinopathy (PVR) remains the most common cause of failed rhegmatogenous retinal detachment (RD) repair and its incidence has been estimated to be 5–11%.[1-5] PVR can also be encountered following penetrating trauma and has been estimated to occur in approximately 10–44% of eyes following posterior segment penetrating injury with varying incidence depending on the type and extent of injury.[6-9] PVR is characterized by progressive preretinal and subretinal membrane growth with subsequent contraction resulting in traction, retinal breaks and redetachment.[5] There is wide variability in the severity and extent of membrane formation ranging from a mild macular pucker to massive, diffuse proliferation. PVR typically develops within 3 months of primary retinal detachment repair with the greatest risk in the first 2 months following initial surgery.[10] Surgical repair of retinal detachments with associated PVR involves the removal of membranes and placement of a scleral buckle to relieve retinal traction, creating chorioretinal adhesions surrounding all retinal breaks and providing a tamponade to aid in retinal reattachment. Reattachment rates following repair have increased with the development of improved surgical techniques. However, the prevention of primary PVR and reproliferation of PVR membranes following surgery remains a challenge.

Clinical Aspects and Classification

The earliest manifestations of PVR include the presence of pigmented cells and protein flare in the vitreous cavity and pigmented cells or clumps on the retinal surface, most often inferiorly (Figs 15.1 and 15.2). The predisposition and increased severity of PVR located on the inferior retina is felt to be secondary to gravitational settling of cellular elements in the inferior vitreous cavity. These initial stages of PVR development are followed by the formation of early membranes that manifest as stiff retina with associated vascular tortuosity, surface wrinkling and rolled edges of retinal breaks (Fig. 15.3). These membranes are relatively transparent in the early stages of formation. With progression of membrane formation and maturation, membranes become more visible and continue to contract. Full thickness retinal folds can form with multiple potential configurations, locations and extents. Variations in presentation are the result of differences in the location and severity of the proliferative process. Focal contraction of membranes located on the inner retinal surface results in distortion of the retinal architecture known as starfolds (Fig. 15.4). Alternately, there can be diffuse posterior membranes (Fig. 15.5). Contraction of confluent posterior membranes causes extensive retinal folding that can emanate from the optic disc (Figs 15.6 and 15.7). The disc may or may not remain visible. Cellular proliferation can also occur in the subretinal space, resulting

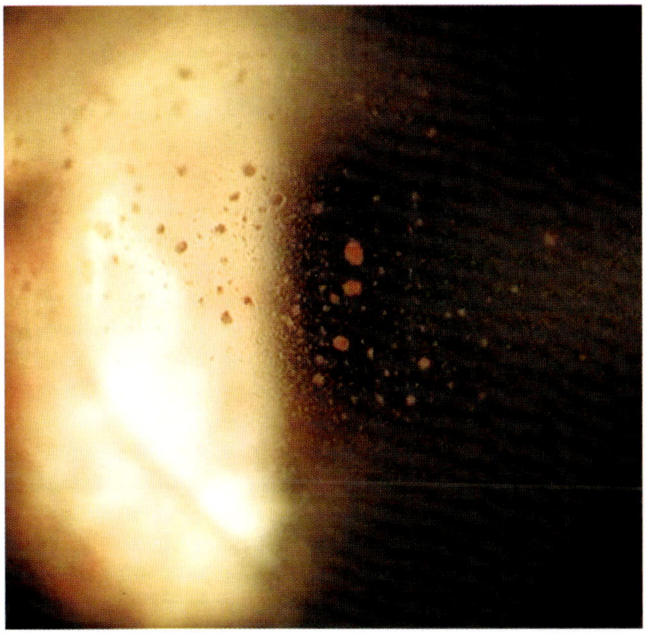

▲ **Figure 15.1**

Grade A PVR with pigment clumps in the vitreous cavity (University of Iowa and EyeRounds.com)

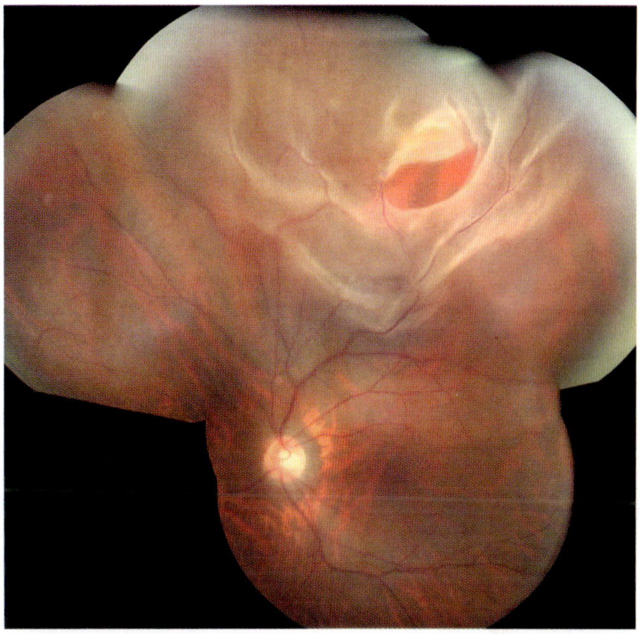

▲ **Figure 15.3**

Grade B PVR with stiff, detached superior retina and a horseshoe retinal tear with a rolled edge (H Culver Boldt, MD)

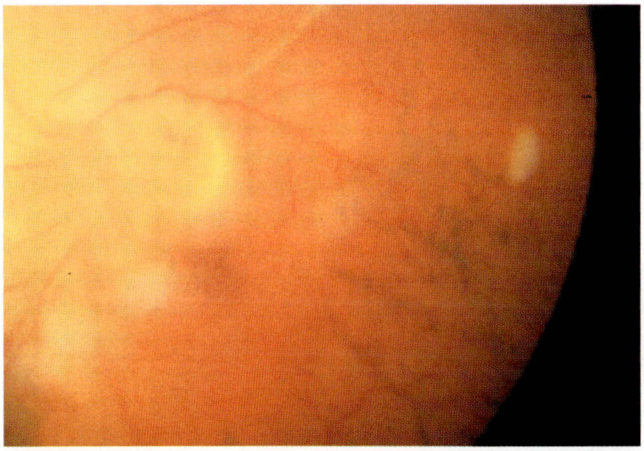

▲ **Figure 15.2**

Grade A PVR with pigment clumps on the retinal surface in the temporal macula (Vinit B Mahajan MD, PhD and James C Folk, MD)

in annular strands near the disc in a "napkin ring" configuration or linear strands resulting in a "clothesline" elevation of the retina (Figs 15.8 and 15.9). PVR membranes located anterior to the equator of the globe are classified as

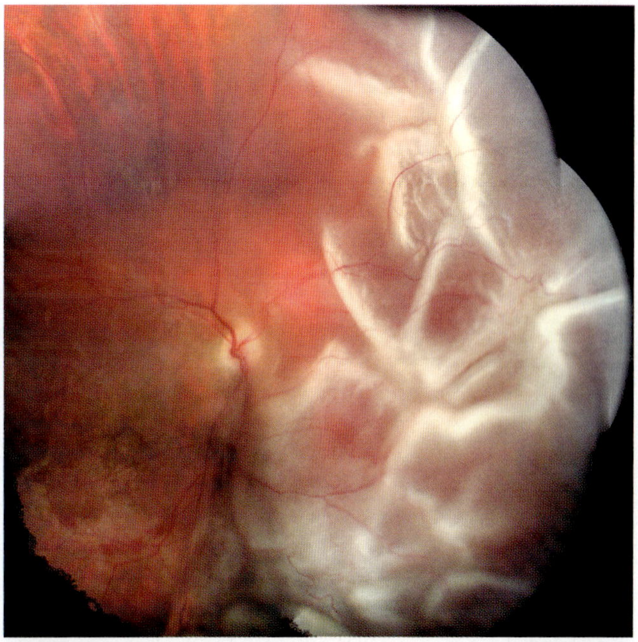

▲ **Figure 15.4**

Grade C type 1 PVR with focal contraction causing several nasal starfolds posterior to the equator (H Culver Boldt, MD)

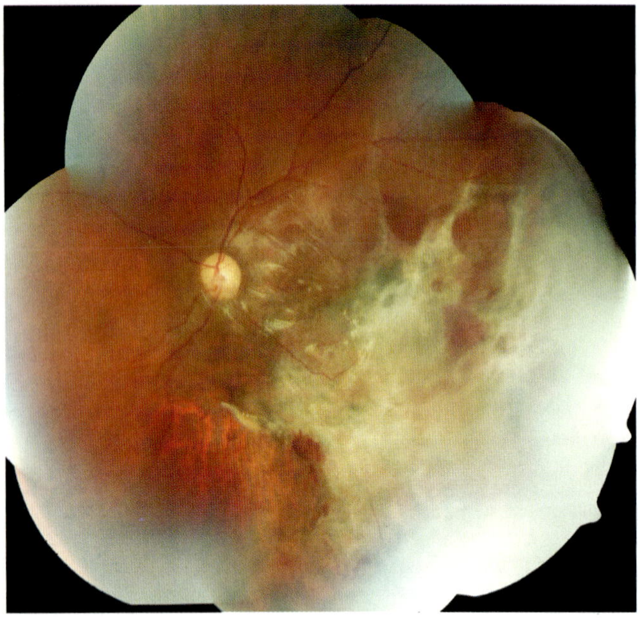

▲ **Figure 15.5**

Grade C type 2 PVR with diffuse posterior membranes in the temporal macula extending into the temporal mid-peripheral retina (Anita Agarwal, MD)

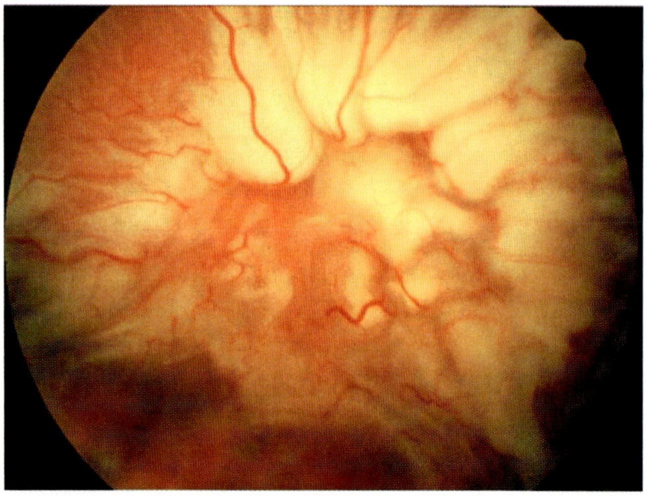

▲ **Figure 15.7**

Severe grade C type 2 PVR emanating from the optic disc with the disc no longer visible (H Culver Boldt, MD)

anterior PVR. These membranes can be located on the retinal surface or over the pars plana, ciliary body, zonules, or the posterior surface of the lens or iris. Formation of anterior PVR on the retinal surface can result in circumferential contraction resulting in irregular radial retinal folds and perpendicular contraction with central displacement of the retina. Contraction of the vitreous base can result in anterior-posterior traction on the peripheral retina, displacing the peripheral retina anteriorly towards the pars plana, stretching

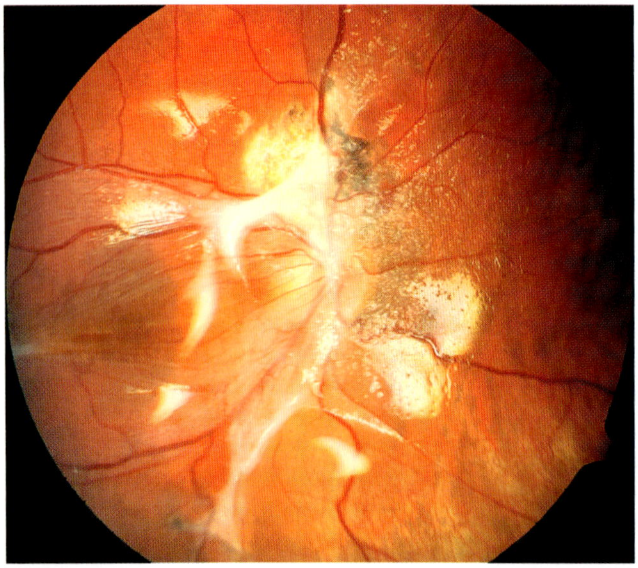

Figure 15.6

Reproliferation of grade C type 1 PVR in an eye filled with silicone oil with membranes emanating from the optic disc and causing traction on the macula (Anita Agarwal, MD)

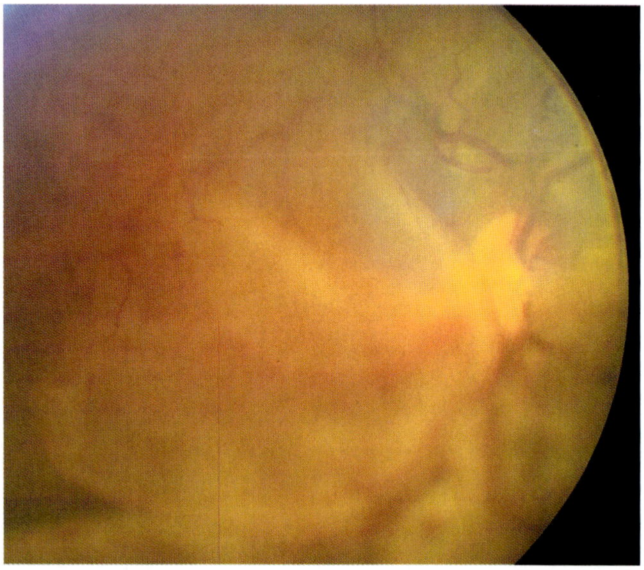

▲ **Figure 15.8**

Severe grade C type 3 subretinal PVR membranes beneath the macula diffusely with "napkin ring" subretinal membrane temporal to the optic disc (H Culver Boldt, MD)

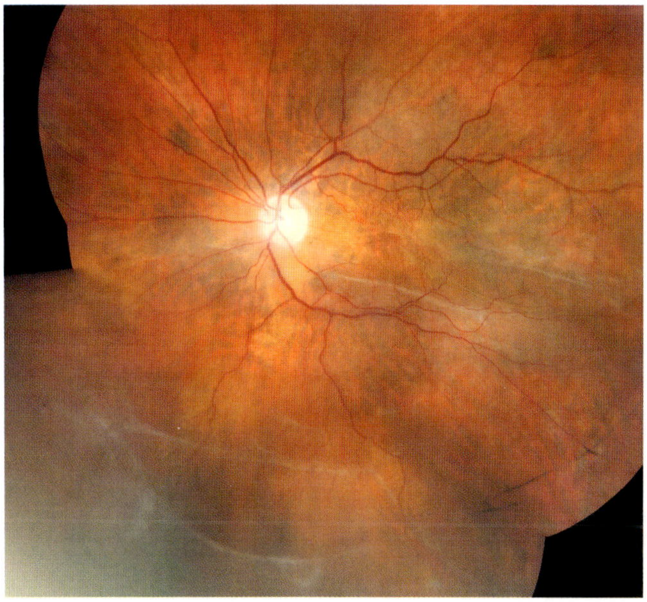

▲ **Figure 15.9**

Mild grade C type 3 linear "clothesline" subretinal PVR membranes in the inferior macula and inferior mid-periphery of an eye with a chronic inferior retinal detachment (Elliott H Sohn, MD)

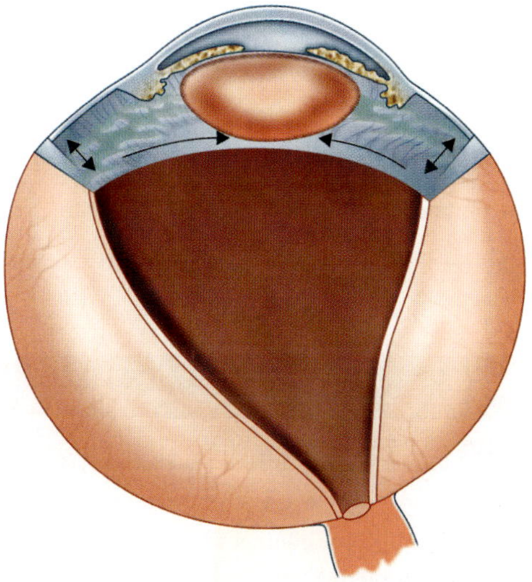

▲ **Figure 15.10**

Showing grade C anterior PVR with circumferential (type 4), perpendicular (type 5), and anterior (type 6) contraction

the ciliary processes and retracting the iris posteriorly with possible resultant hypotony (Fig. 15.10).

The classification of PVR has undergone numerous iterations over time. In 1983, the Retina Society published an initial classification system that has been used widely and

TABLE 15.1: Retina Society classification of PVR

Grade	*Name*	*Clinical signs*
A	Minimal	Vitreous haze, vitreous pigment clumps
B	Moderate	Wrinkling of the inner retinal surface, rolled edge of retinal break, retinal stiffness, vessel tortuosity
C 1-3	Marked	Full thickness fixed retinal folds in 1-3 quadrants
D	Massive	Fixed retinal folds in four quadrants
D-1		Wide funnel shape
D-2		Narrow funnel shape
D-3		Closed funnel (optic nerve head not visible)

Source: The Retina Society Terminology Committee. The classification of retinal detachment with proliferative vitreoretinopathy. Ophthalmology. 1983;90:121-5.

modified the previously published classification proposed by Machemer in 1978 (Table 15.1).[5,11] The initial Retina Society classification system separates PVR into 4 major categories (grade A-D) and subdivides grade C and D based upon extent in quadrants (grade C) and configuration of retinal detachment (grade D). Limitations of this scheme include the failure to address the anterior-posterior location of PVR membranes and the type of contraction present. An alternate classification system was developed for use in the silicone study, a randomized clinical trial comparing the efficacy of silicone oil with gas tamponade as management of RD complicated by PVR. This system was published in 1989 (Tables 15.2 and 15.3).[12] In response, the Retina Society appointed a committee that suggested additional modifications that were published 1991 (Tables 15.4 and 15.5).[13]

TABLE 15.2: Grading of proliferative vitreoretinopathy used in the Silicone Study

Grade	*Clinical signs*
A	Vitreous haze, vitreous pigment clumps
B	Inner retinal wrinkling, rolled edge of retinal breaks
P1-4	Starfold and/or diffuse contraction in posterior retina and/or subretinal membrane in posterior retina involving 1-4 quadrants
A1-4	Circumferential and/or perpendicular and/or anterior traction in anterior retina involving 1-4 quadrants

Source: Lean JS, Stern WH, Irvine AR, et al. Classification of proliferative vitreoretinopathy used in the Silicone Study. The Silicone Study Group. Ophthalmology. 1989;96:765-71.

TABLE 15.3: Classification of proliferative vitreoretinopathy contraction type in the Silicone Study

Type no.	*Type of contraction*	*Location of PVR*	*Summary of clinical signs*
1	Focal	Posterior	Starfold
2	Diffuse	Posterior	Confluent irregular retinal folds in posterior retina; remainder of retina drawn posteriorly; optic disc may not be visible
3	Subretinal	Posterior	"Napkin ring" around disc, or "clothesline" elevation of retina
4	Circumferential	Anterior	Irregular retinal folds in the anterior retina; series of radial folds more posteriorly; peripheral retina within vitreous base stretched inward
5	Perpendicular	Anterior	Smooth circumferential fold of retina at insertion of posterior hyaloid
6	Anterior	Anterior	Circumferential fold of retina at insertion of posterior hyaloid pulled forward; trough of peripheral retina anteriorly; ciliary processes stretched with possible hypotony; iris retracted

Source: Lean JS, Stern WH, Irvine AR, et al. Classification of proliferative vitreoretinopathy used in the Silicone Study. The Silicone Study Group. Ophthalmology. 1989;96:765-71.

TABLE 15.4: Updated Retina Society PVR classification

Grade	*Clinical signs*
A	Vitreous haze; vitreous pigment clumps; pigment clusters on inferior retina
B	Wrinkling of inner retinal surface; retinal stiffness; vessel tortuosity; rolled and irregular edge of retinal break; decreased mobility of vitreous
CP 1-12	Posterior to equator: focal, diffuse, or circumferential full-thickness folds or subretinal strands. Expressed in total number of clock hours
CA 1-12	Anterior to equator, focal, diffuse, or circumferential full-thickness folds, subretinal strands, anterior displacement, or condensed vitreous with strands. Expressed in total number of clock hours

Source: Machemer R, Aaberg TM, Freeman HM, et al. An updated classification of retinal detachment with proliferative vitreoretinopathy. Am J Ophthalmol. 1991;112:159-65.

TABLE 15.5: Updated Retina Society PVR classification of grade C contraction type

Type of contraction	*Location*	*Summary of clinical signs*
1. Focal	Posterior	Starfold posterior to vitreous base
2. Diffuse	Posterior	Confluent starfolds posterior to vitreous base. Optic disc may not be visible
3. Subretinal	Posterior/anterior	Proliferations under the retina: Annular strand near disc; linear strands; motheaten-appearing sheets
4. Circumferential	Anterior	Contraction along posterior edge of vitreous base with central displacement of the retina; peripheral retina stretched; posterior retina in radial folds
5. Anterior displacement	Anterior	Vitreous base pulled anteriorly by proliferative tissue; peripheral retinal trough; ciliary processes may be stretched, may be covered by membrane; iris may be retracted

Source: Machemer R, Aaberg TM, Freeman HM, et al. An updated classification of retinal detachment with proliferative vitreoretinopathy. Am J Ophthalmol. 1991;112:159-65.

The more recent classification systems allow more specific description of anterior-posterior location, describe circumferential extent by clock hours rather than quadrants involved and elaborate on the contraction types present in greater detail. These modifications have allowed for more accurate description of severity and extent of PVR in an individual eye. Despite increased specificity in the ability to describe the characteristics of PVR with newer classification schemes, each eye with PVR presents unique challenges that may not be fully characterized by current grading systems.

Risk Factors

The occurrence of PVR is typically seen in the setting of recent RD repair. However, PVR formation can occur in eyes with chronic retinal detachment, trauma, inflammation, or infection.[9,14] In eyes with a RD, several risk factors have been identified that increase the incidence of PVR development. Preoperative factors that appear to increase the risk of subsequent PVR include giant, large, or multiple retinal tears, signs of uveitis, aphakia, vitreous hemorrhage, choroidal detachment or hemorrhage and anterior chamber flare.[3,10,15-19] Postoperative PVR is associated with the preoperative presence of PVR, uveitis, intra- or postoperative vitreous hemorrhage, excessive cryotherapy, diathermy or photocoagulation, repeated surgical procedures, loss of vitreous during drainage of subretinal fluid, undetected breaks, use of air or sulfur hexafluoride as a tamponade agent in the presence of PVR at the time of RD repair and postoperative choroidal detachment.[3,19-24]

Pathogenesis

The formation of PVR appears to be a modification of the wound healing process involving inflammation, proliferation and scar tissue formation and remodeling.[25]

PVR membranes are characterized by proliferation of glial cells, retinal pigment epithelium (RPE) and inflammatory cells and collagen formation in the vitreous cavity and on the preretinal and subretinal retinal surfaces.[26-30] In response to inflammatory mediators released at the time of rhegmatogenous RD and breakdown of the blood-retinal barrier, RPE and glial cells migrate onto both surfaces of the retina and subsequently proliferate. Remodeling of these membranes leads to contraction. Numerous cytokines including platelet derived growth factor, insulin-like growth factor, transforming growth factor-β, vascular endothelial growth factor and several interleukins have been shown to be present in altered concentration in the vitreous of eyes with PVR and are felt to be part of an elaborate signaling process that ultimately results in membrane formation and contraction.[31-35]

Surgical Management

Primary management of PVR involves surgery. Significant improvements have been made in the surgical care of RDs complicated by PVR over the past 3 decades. Improved techniques, as well as instrumentation have allowed for successful reattachment to be accomplished in up to 90% of cases of severe PVR.[36-43] Surgical goals include placement of a scleral buckle and removal of PVR membranes to relieve retinal traction, prevent reproliferation and support the peripheral retina in the setting of residual traction or membrane reproliferation, creation of a chorioretinal adhesion surrounding all retinal breaks and the use of a tamponade agent to facilitate postoperative attachment of the retina. A sclera buckle is often placed and relaxing retinotomies and retinectomies can be considered if membrane peeling alone does not sufficiently remove traction from the retina. The timing of surgery for RDs with PVR has been controversial. Early PVR often has very transparent membranes that are more difficult to identify and remove. Over several weeks, the membranes appear more white and fibrotic and exert more traction on the retina. Prior recommendations had suggested waiting several weeks so that the membranes mature allowing easier removal.[44] While a delay in surgery may allow for more complete membrane identification and removal, the longer duration of macular detachment will limit postoperative visual potential.[45-47] Therefore we use similar guidelines to repair RDs with and without PVR. Cases where the central macula is attached are typically performed within 24 hours and cases where the macula is detached within 7–10 days.

The initial step in the repair of a RD complicated by PVR is typically placement of a scleral buckle. The goal of buckle placement is to relieve anterior or posterior and circumferential traction from the peripheral retina (Fig. 15.11). The buckle will also support the peripheral retina and help prevent recurrent detachment if PVR membranes reproliferate after surgery. Historically, scleral buckle placement alone has not been sufficient to achieve high rates of successful RD repair in cases of severe PVR.[48,49] Scleral buckle alone is an option

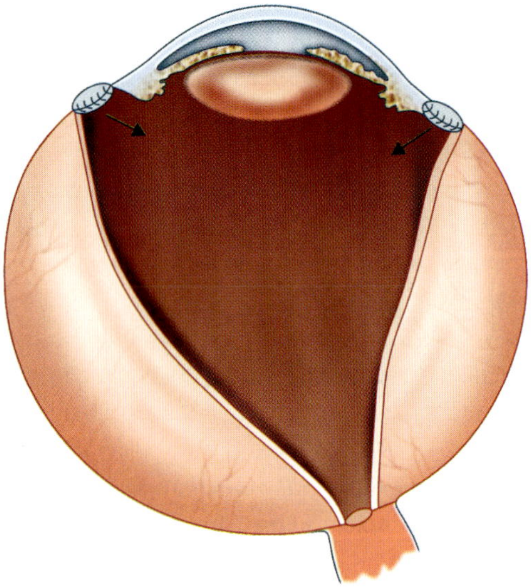

▲ **Figure 15.11**

Showing effect of an encircling scleral buckle providing adequate imbrication to decrease traction created by anterior PVR membranes

for eyes with mild (grade A or B) PVR, but often a vitrectomy or scleral buckle and vitrectomy is chosen in these cases.

A 360° conjunctival peritomy is created, each quadrant is freed from Tenon's attachments by spreading Steven's scissors adjacent to the globe. The 4 rectus muscles are looped with a muscle hook and isolated on 3-0 silk suture. Adequate exposure of each quadrant can then be obtained with a retractor and with counter traction on the silk sutures. Quadrants should be examined for the presence of scleral thinning and the location of vortex veins should be noted. Partial thickness horizontal mattress sutures are then placed through the sclera in each quadrant. Placement of sutures prior to vitrectomy, when the globe is firm and the intraocular pressure is not variable, is technically easier. Suture placement should be approximately 2–3 mm wider than the width of the encircling element chosen to allow adequate scleral imbrication. The anterior mattress suture bite is placed approximately 1 mm posterior to the rectus muscle insertions. We typically use 5-0 nylon suture and either a 42 band or a 506 sponge (grooved or non-grooved) with a suture width of 6 mm and 7 mm respectively. Some surgeons prefer a broader buckle such as a 276 or 287 tire with a 240 band. The encircling element can be placed beneath the muscles, passed through the mattress sutures and a sleeve can be placed prior to vitrectomy, but the buckle sutures are typically not tied until after a vitrectomy has been completed. Alternately, the buckle sutures can be kept out of the surgical field by taping them to the surgical drape with steri-strips and the buckle can be placed around the eye after a vitrectomy has been performed.

Either 20-gauge or small-gauge instrumentation is a reasonable choice in repairing a RD complicated by PVR.[50,51] If removal of the crystalline lens is required, it is often preferable to choose 20-gauge instrumentation to allow phacofragmentation. However, a small-gauge system can be used with enlargement of the superotemporal sclerotomy to accommodate the fragmatome. Presence of the crystalline lens will typically make adequate anterior dissection and vitreous removal difficult, however, if there is minimal anterior PVR the lens can be retained. At the time of lens removal, it is preferable to remove the entire capsule, which may serve as a scaffold for recurrent anterior PVR. Implantation of an intraocular lens is typically deferred until the retina has remained attached following surgery for 4–6 months. Often, an anterior chamber or scleral fixated lens can be placed at the time of silicone oil removal. In cases where inadequate pupillary dilation is present, flexible iris retractors can be useful to achieve improved visualization.[52]

Following sclerotomy creation, a core vitrectomy is performed. After removal of the core vitreous, scleral depression is performed for 360° to assist in the removal of peripheral vitreous. Peripheral vitreous should be removed aggressively since it can serve as a scaffold for reproliferation. Either direct visualization with the operating microscope or a wide field viewing system with scleral depression can allow adequate visualization to extensively remove anterior vitreous.[53] Once a complete vitrectomy has been performed, attention is directed to the PVR membranes. Intravitreal triamcinolone can assist in highlighting these membranes, especially when they are immature, as well as any remaining vitreous.[41,54-56] We prefer to remove posterior membranes initially, stripping membranes anteriorly to avoid undue traction on the peripheral retina. When membranes are immature, using a diamond dusted membrane scraper to brush the retinal surface, elevating a membrane edge and allowing for removal with forceps, can be a useful technique. When membranes are more mature, fixed folds are often present and membranes can be directly engaged with a pick, forceps or both (Figs 15.12 and 15.13). A variety of techniques can be used to successfully remove posterior membranes. Bimanual dissection with either a chandelier light source or an illuminated forceps or pick is helpful allowing counter traction to be placed on the retina with the second instrument

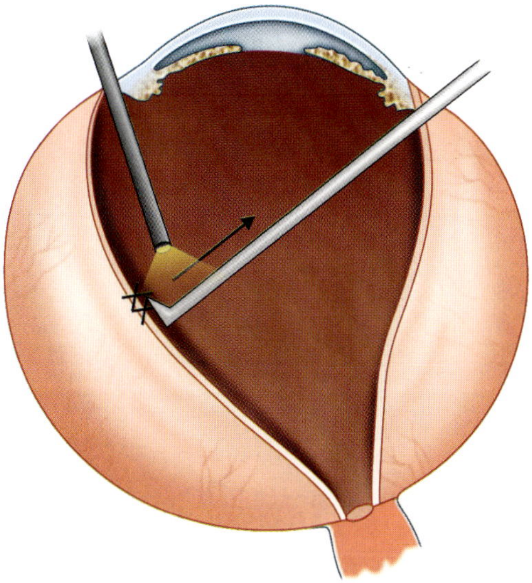

▲ **Figure 15.12**
Showing membrane elevation with a vitreoretinal pick

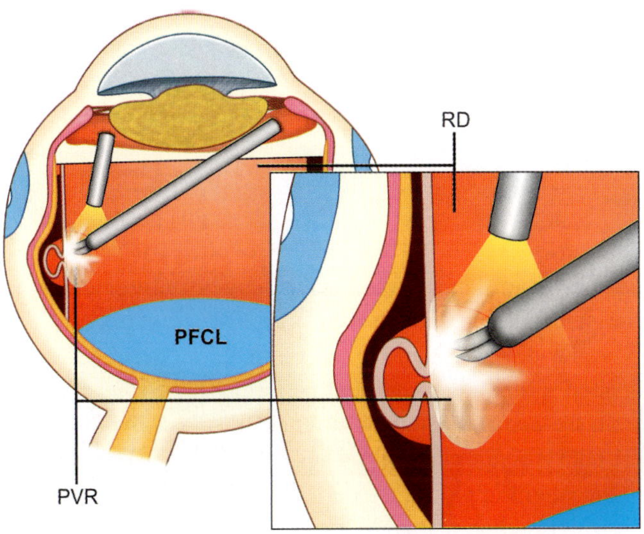

▲ **Figure 15.13**
Showing membrane removal with a forceps

in the non-dominant hand. Additionally, Indocyanine green can be used to stain the ILM and facilitate peeling, ensuring that all posterior membranes have been removed. This technique may prevent the recurrence of membranes postoperatively.[57] It is often difficult to extend the ILM peel more than a few millimeters anterior to the arcades. Once all posterior membranes have been removed, attention can then be directed to removal of anterior membranes.

Perfluorocarbon liquid (PFCL) is often injected over the posterior pole to provide counter traction when addressing the anterior membranes. Additional PFCL can be added as the membrane dissection is carried further anterior to continue to stabilize the retina. Similar membrane peeling techniques are typically used for anterior membranes and bimanual peeling techniques can be very helpful. Use of a wide-field viewing system and an assistant performing sclera depression allows excellent visualization and stereopsis for removal of anterior membranes. Another option is to use direct visualization or place a contact lens with the assistant holding the light pipe obliquely at the external limbus 180° away from the area being addressed to aid in illumination. An alternate technique is to use an endoscope.[58,59] These techniques are particularly useful for very anterior membranes over the ciliary body that can be difficult to view with a wide-field viewing system.

The initial steps to relieve circumferential and anterior-posterior traction are placement of a scleral buckle and extensive membrane removal. In instances where membranes are particularly adherent and sufficient removal is not possible to adequately relieve peripheral traction, or if there is significant retinal foreshortening that persists after membrane removal, a relaxing retinotomy or retinectomy can be performed (Figs 15.14 and 15.15). Instances where there is residual traction causing retinal detachment after air-fluid exchange or if air passes into the subretinal space during air-

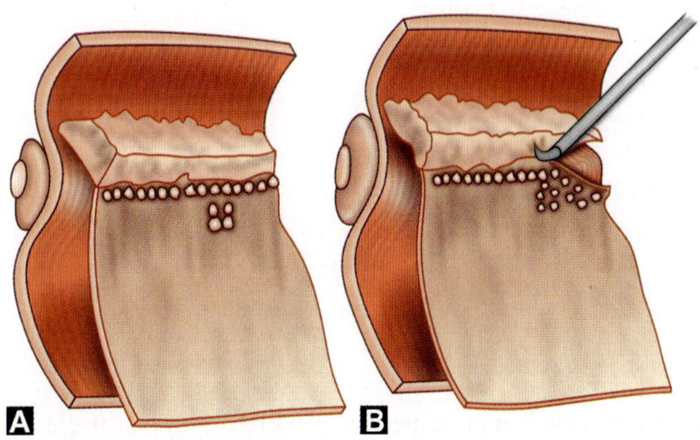

▲ **Figures 15.14A and B**
Showing creation of retinectomy with a vertical scissors following application of diathermy

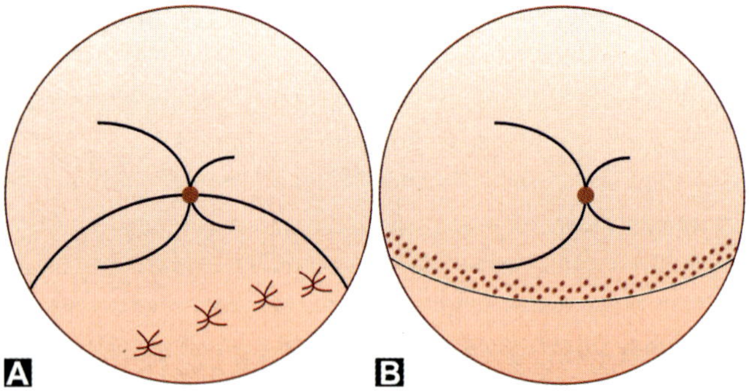

▲ **Figures 15.15A and B**

Showing appearance prior to and following inferior retinectomy (A) Detached retinal with extensive membranes and shortening; (B) Appearance after relaxing retinotomy and removal of remaining anterior retina

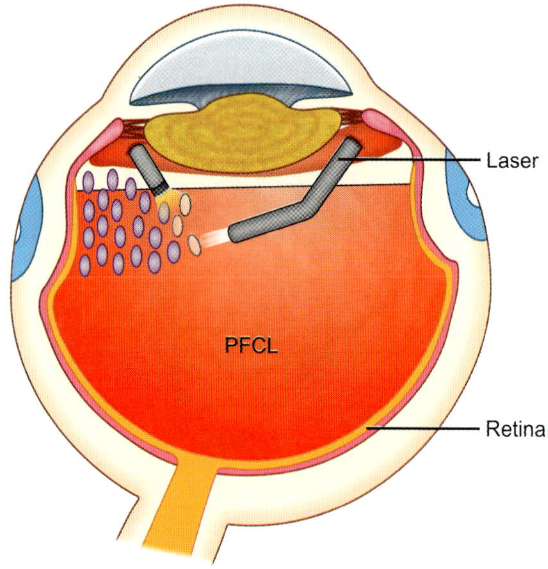

▲ **Figure 15.16**

Showing placement of endolaser under PFCL

fluid exchange suggests that a retinotomy or retinectomy should be performed. This step allows for isolation of the posterior retina from persistent traction in the vitreous base and surgical success can be achieved at high rates using this technique.[43,60-64] Retinotomy or retinectomy should be performed after all membrane removal has been performed. Typically, a relaxing retinotomy is performed when the retina remains foreshortened after membrane removal and a retinectomy is performed when membranes cannot be completely removed from the retinal surface and are excised. Retinotomies can also be used to gain access to subretinal membranes that may prevent appropriate retinal reattachment. Prior to cutting the retina, diathermy should be applied to the area to be cut with particular attention being paid to treating blood vessels in the retina. The posterior retina should be stabilized with PFCL. The retina can then be cut with either the vitreous cutter or vertical scissors along the diathermized retina. Care must be taken to not damage the choroid during cutting. The extent of a retinotomy should extend into normal retina, which is free of PVR membranes. If normal retina at the edges of the retinotomy is attached, it can be aspirated with the cutter using suction prior to excision to separate it from the underlying RPE and decrease the risk of causing choroidal bleeding. The anterior flap of a retinotomy should be excised to avoid any anterior reproliferation in this area causing traction on the ciliary body. Once completed, PFCL can then be injected and extended beyond the edge of the intact retina to allow retinal-RPE apposition and treatment with endolaser. Two or 3 confluent rows of laser should be placed along the edge of the intact retina.

Laser photocoagulation is applied to surround all retinal breaks using either an endolaser probe or the indirect laser ophthalmoscope. We prefer to use an endolaser probe and treat when the retina is coapted to the RPE with PFCL (Fig. 15.16). Alternately, laser can be applied following fluid-air exchange in an air filled eye. Some surgeons elect to place 360° peripheral scatter laser to potentially prevent retinal detachment if new breaks form. It is often easier to apply laser prior to tying of the buckle sutures and tightening of the scleral buckle to prevent any difficulty treating the posterior downslope of the buckle. After all desired laser is applied, a fluid-air exchange is performed removing all PFCL from the eye and resulting in an air-filled eye. At this time, the buckle sutures can be tied and the buckle can be tightened at the band to produce the desired imbrication. Any areas of peripheral retina that were not treated with endolaser under PFCL due to anterior subretinal fluid can be treated at this time.

The choices for intraocular tamponade include a long-acting gas, perfluoropropane (C_3F_8) and silicone oil. In the Silicone Study, there was no major advantage to silicone oil compared with C_3F_8, however, short-acting sulfur hexafluoride (SF_6) was demonstrated to have a lower success rate for retinal reattachment and a higher complication rate.[39,65] Advantages of C_3F_8 include the spontaneous absorption that does not require a second surgery for removal and stronger tamponade strength. Disadvantages include shorter duration of tamponade, possible elevated intraocular pressure, cataract formation and prohibition of air travel. Advantages of silicone oil include extended tamponade, better tamponade in hypotonous eyes and no restrictions on air travel. Disadvantages include refractive changes and limited visual acuity while oil is in place, potential corneal toxicity, oil emulsification, elevated intraocular pressure and the need for a second surgery to remove the oil to achieve best possibly visual acuity. In certain situations either C_3F_8 or silicone oil may be preferable. In patients who cannot reliably maintain a prone position or in eyes that are at high-risk for hypotony (preoperative hypotony, severe anterior PVR, large retinectomies) silicone oil is the preferred tamponade agent. C_3F_8 may be preferable in patients with an irregularly dilated iris or aniridia where silicone oil is more likely to enter the anterior chamber and cause corneal decompensation. Additionally, in eyes with choroidal hemorrhage which precludes an adequate silicone oil fill, or if there is a break at the base of a high scleral buckle where oil may not adequately tamponade the break due to its tendency to retain a spherical configuration, C_3F_8 may be preferable. In eyes where silicone oil is used, an inferior peripheral iridectomy is created in aphakic eyes and in pseudophakic eyes without an intact lens capsule. This step helps to prevent passage of silicone oil into the anterior chamber and allows aqueous to enter the anterior chamber and relieve any pupillary block that may result from the oil.

We typically inject silicone oil into an air-filled eye following removal of PFCL. Alternately, a direct PFCL-silicone oil exchange can be performed. We first close one of the superior sclerotomies and leave the air infusion in place inferotemporally. Alternately, the air infusion can be removed and a 27-gauge needle can be placed on the infusion and it can be inserted through the pars plana superiorly and positioned in the plane of the pupil. We inject the oil through a viscous fluid injection system. Once reflux is noted in the infusion line, an adequate fill has been obtained. In addition, a ½ inch 27-gauge needle on a syringe with the plunger pulled can be placed through the pars plana during injection to help judge the extent of fill as the oil level approaches the pupillary plane and to allow for venting of air in systems that do not reflux through the infusion line. The target intraocular pressure following oil fill is low-normal and the globe should be palpated to determine the pressure, to determine if the eye has been overfilled or underfilled. Prior to the conclusion of surgery, oil may be added or removed to obtain a target intraocular pressure. After closure of all 3 sclerotomies, we thoroughly rinse the surface of the globe with BSS to remove any oil that may subsequently be trapped in the subconjunctival space. Oil should be left in place for at least 3 months postoperatively and may be removed subsequently depending on the appearance of the retina.

Following gas or oil fill and closure of any remaining open sclerotomies, the conjunctiva is then reapproximated and closed. Some surgeons prefer to close Tenon's fascia to the muscle insertions to ensure coverage of the buckling material and possibly reduce the risk of future extrusion or infection. Subconjunctival antibiotic and steroid are then injected. Any desired topical drops including an antibiotic, steroid, or cycloplegic can be placed prior to placing an eye patch and shield. Patients should be placed in the prone position soon after surgery.

Postoperative Care or Complications

Appropriate postoperative care can determine success or failure following surgery for RD complicated by PVR. Directly after surgery, appropriate positioning is critical to obtain adequate tamponade of breaks, allow for the RPE to absorb any residual subretinal fluid and to form an early adhesion in areas where laser photocoagulation was applied. The first evening following surgery, we typically keep all patients in the prone position. In addition to providing tamponade, this will help prevent any pupillary block that may result in increased intraocular pressure. On the first postoperative day, the intraocular pressure and the level of the gas or oil fill are the primary concerns. Elevated pressure in gas or oil-filled eyes is typically treated with topical β-blockers, carbonic anhydrase inhibitors, α-agonists and prostaglandin analogs. Systemic carbonic anhydrase inhibitors can be used in cases of recalcitrant elevated intraocular pressure. In instances where the pressure is extremely high, a gas dilution error must be considered. Gas can be removed from the vitreous cavity and patients should be monitored closely. In patients with a shallow anterior chamber and a pupillary block from either gas or oil, prone positioning may relieve the block. The anterior chamber can be reformed by injecting viscoelastic. In patients with an oil-filled eye and pupillary block due to occlusion of the peripheral iridectomy, recombinant tissue plasminogen activator (3 mg in 0.1 ml) can be injected through the limbus. This is typically done approximately 3 days after surgery to reduce the risk of hemorrhage in the early postoperative period. This can also be done in eyes with excessive postoperative fibrin formation. Eyes that have a silicone oil overfill often require surgical removal to lower the intraocular pressure.

While an overfill of gas or oil can result in elevated intraocular pressure, an inadequate fill can be problematic as well. Ensuring an adequate gas or oil fill is critical for the success of surgery, especially in eyes with inferior retinal breaks. The optimal gas fill will provide tamponade to breaks for a sufficient duration to allow formation of a chorioretinal adhesion at sites where laser was placed. In eyes without sufficient gas, several techniques can be used to perform a fluid-gas exchange and augment the gas fill postoperatively. In aphakic eyes, gas can be injected through the limbus through an inferior paracentesis while fluid escapes the eye around the needle with the patient positioned at the slit lamp. Alternately, this can be done with the patient in a prone position to achieve a greater gas fill. In phakic or pseudophakic eyes, a "push-pull" technique can be used. A syringe with the desired concentration of gas is used to sequentially inject gas via the pars plana and then aspirate a small amount of dependent, inferior fluid. This process is repeated multiple times with the needle withdrawn towards the dependent portion of the vitreous cavity until no additional fluid is able to be removed.

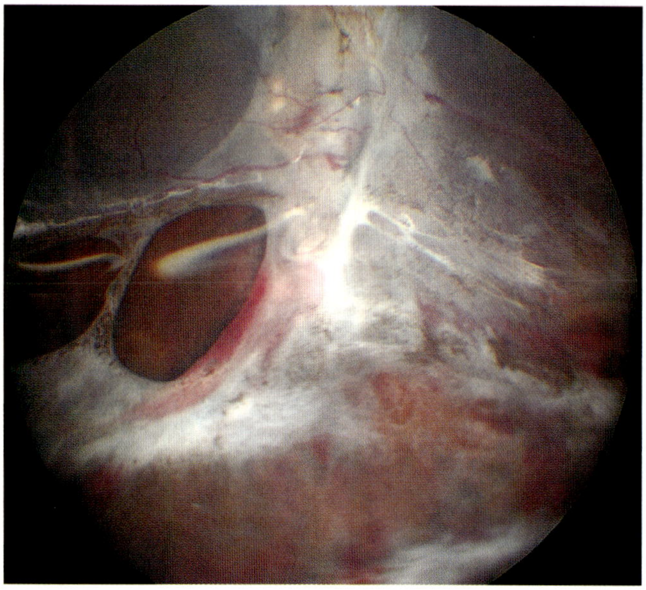

▲ **Figure 15.17**

Preretinal membrane reproliferation and stretch hole formation under silicone oil (Anita Agarwal, MD)

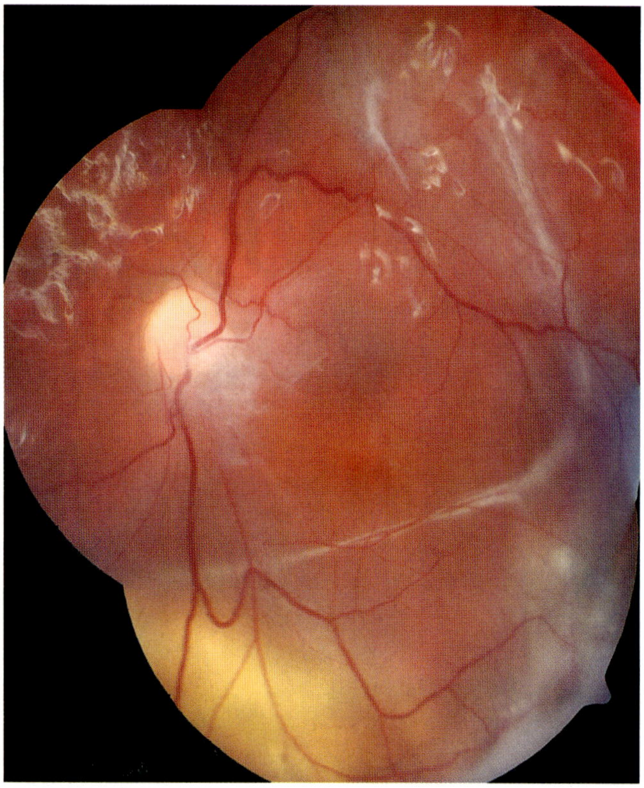

▲ **Figure 15.18**

Preretinal and subretinal membrane reproliferation and recurrent retinal detachment under silicone oil (Anita Agarwal, MD)

Following the initial postoperative period, the primary concern is monitoring for membrane reproliferation and recurrent RD (Figs 15.17 and 15.18). Less severe reproliferation can result in epiretinal membrane formation without recurrent RD (Fig. 15.19). For mild peripheral recurrent detachments without significant traction, additional indirect laser can be placed to demarcate the subretinal fluid. However, if there is significant reproliferation causing traction and retinal detachment, repeat surgery is typically required. Silicone oil should be left in place for a minimum of 3 months. In eyes that are hypotonous, regardless of whether the retina is attached, silicone oil should be left in place to avoid phthisis. Other complications that can occur in the late postoperative period include cataract formation, cystoid macular edema, scleral buckle exposure, rubeosis, hypotony, band keratopathy and phthisis.

Surgical Outcomes

The most useful data regarding surgical outcomes in eyes with RD secondary to PVR comes from the Silicone Study. The Silicone Study was a prospective, randomized clinical trial comparing surgical repair with vitrectomy and either

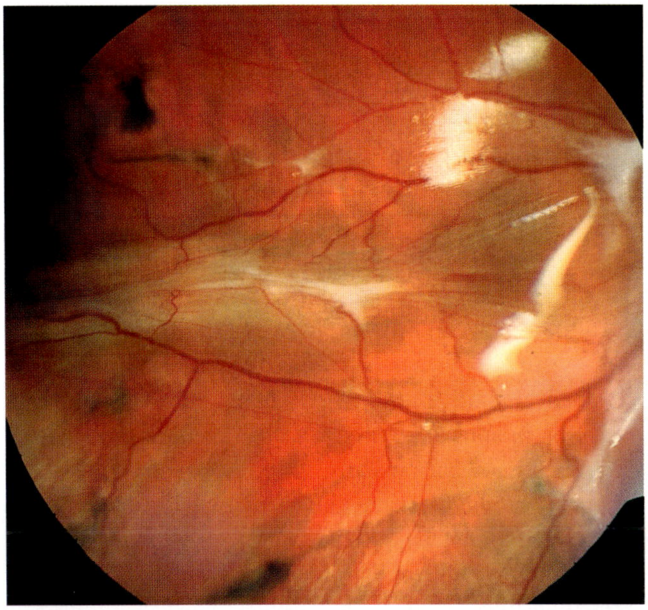

▲ **Figure 15.19**

Preretinal membrane reproliferation without recurrent detachment, but causing traction on the macula (Anita Agarwal, MD)

silicone oil or gas as tamponade in eyes with RD and Grade C3 or greater PVR. Eyes that not had a prior vitrectomy (group 1) and those that had undergone previous vitrectomy outside the study (group 2) were both included. Standardized vitrectomy techniques, postoperative follow-up, fundus photographs and repeat surgery if required were utilized. End points of the study included visual acuity of 5/200 or greater and macular reattachment for 6 months following the final surgical procedure. Outcomes and complications of the two tamponade modalities were compared.

In the Silicone Study Report 1, between 50% and 60% of eyes that received silicone oil had visual acuity better than or equal to 5/200 compared with 30–40% of the eyes that received SF_6.[65] Macula attachment was more frequent in eyes that received silicone oil (80%) than in those that received sulfur hexafluoride gas (60%).[65] The authors concluded that silicone oil was a superior tamponade in cases of RD with severe PVR when compared with SF_6.

The Silicone Study Report 2 showed that the differences between silicone oil and SF_6 tamponade were not found when comparing silicone oil to C_3F_8 tamponade and both silicone oil and C_3F_8 produced superior results compared with SF_6. There was no significant difference between C_3F_8 and silicone oil in achieving visual acuity greater than or equal to 5/200 (43% vs 45% for group 1, 38% vs 33% for group 2) and complete posterior retinal reattachment (73% vs 64% for group 1, 73% vs 61% for group 2).[39] For group 1 eyes followed for at least 18 months, there was an advantage favoring C_3F_8 in achieving complete posterior retinal reattachment (83% vs 60% at 36 months).[39] The rates of reoperation and keratopathy were similar, while hypotony was more prevalent in eyes randomized to C_3F_8 (group 2).[39] Regardless of tamponade, groups 1 and 2 had similar anatomic and visual success. Hypotony was twice as prevalent in group 2 (C_3F_8) and the prevalence of keratopathy increased with follow-up in group 2 (either tamponade).[39]

The Silicone Study Report 3 demonstrated that in eyes which had undergone no prior vitrectomy (group 1) and eyes that had undergone prior vitrectomy with intraocular gas tamponade (group 2), there was no differences in achieving visual acuity of 5/200 or better (44% vs 39%), macular reattachment (78% vs 77%), or complete retinal reattachment (67% for both groups), but keratopathy was more frequent in eyes in group 2.[66] These results suggested that differences in outcomes between group 1 and group 2 eyes were not as great as previously believed.

In Report 4, chronically elevated intraocular pressure was more prevalent in eyes randomized to silicone oil than in those randomized to C_3F_8 gas (8% vs 2%) and chronic hypotony was more prevalent in eyes randomized to C_3F_8 gas than in those randomized to silicone oil (31% vs. 18%).[67]

Report 5 demonstrated that group 1 eyes not undergoing retinotomy or retinectomy had better anatomic and visual outcomes as well as less hypotony and for eyes undergoing retinotomy or retinectomy, silicone oil decreased the likelihood of hypotony.[68]

Report 6 examined eyes that underwent silicone oil removal and concluded that removal of silicone oil in anatomically successful eyes significantly increases the likelihood of improved visual acuity with a slight increase in the likelihood of recurrent retinal redetachment.[69]

Report 7 showed that the incidence of corneal abnormalities at 24 months was 27%, did not differ significantly between treatment groups and the incidence of corneal abnormalities in gas-filled eyes was higher than expected and remained high in oil-filled eyes, despite the use of an inferior iridectomy.[70]

In Report 8, the prevalence of postoperative macular pucker was 15% at 6 months, was 3 times more likely to develop in aphakic or pseudophakic eyes and was not influenced by the choice of intraocular tamponade.[71]

Report 10 demonstrated that eyes with anterior PVR had a worse visual prognosis, higher rates of hypotony and were less likely to have complete reattachment of the retina when compared with eyes with posterior PVR.[72] Eyes with anterior PVR and clinically significant posterior PVR changes had a better visual prognosis if silicone oil was used.[72] In the final report from the Silicone Study Report 11, long-term outcomes (3 year) were examined.[40] The authors concluded that success in the first surgery for PVR is important to optimize visual results and if anatomically and visually successful at 3 years, there is an excellent chance that the results will be maintained over the long-term.[40]

Future Directions

Numerous studies have examined the utility of adjuvant treatments to inhibit formation of PVR membranes. Typical strategies have targeted inflammation, cellular proliferation and membrane formation or maturation through a variety of mechanisms. Corticosteroids have been one of the most studied agents in attempts to reduce PVR formation. In animal models, there have been several studies reporting a reduction in PVR formation using intravitreal Triamcinolone.[73-76] In humans, Jonas et al. performed a pilot study suggesting that intravitreal injection of crystalline cortisone was not toxic to intraocular structures, reduced postoperative intraocular inflammation and may be a potentially useful additional tool in the treatment of PVR.[77] In a noncontrolled study, Cheema et al. suggested that intravitreal Triamcinolone acetonide (TA) at the time of RD repair may have potential as an adjuvant in the treatment of retinal detachment with PVR.[78] However, a more recent prospective, controlled clinical trial did not demonstrate an increase in surgical reattachment rate when comparing eyes with and without adjunctive intravitreal TA at the time of RD repair and concluded the outcomes of surgery for established PVR are not improved significantly by adjunctive TA injection in silicone-filled eyes.[79]

Adjunctive Daunorubicin infused at the time of vitrectomy was investigated in a randomized study that found a significant decrease in reoperations after 1 year of treatment. However, retinal reattachment rates were minimally improved and there was no statistically significant difference in visual acuity between the two groups.[80]

Initial studies examining the use of 5-fluorouracil and low-molecular weight heparin added to the infusion fluid at the time of vitrectomy in high-risk patients showed promising results.[81] However, no benefit was seen in subsequent studies using a similar treatment in eyes with established PVR and in the primary prevention of PVR and a worse visual outcome was observed in patients who presented with macula-sparing retinal detachments following repair in the treatment group.[82,83] Data regarding the use of 5-fluorouracil and low-molecular weight heparin remains inconsistent.[84]

Despite numerous advancements in the understanding of PVR, the primary treatment remains surgical in nature. While there have been promising results in some animal models and early trials in humans, no adjuvant treatment has been consistently show to decrease PVR membrane formation in controlled human trials and thus no proposed treatments have been widely adopted. Several targets for potential therapy remain under investigation and show promise for future adjunctive treatments. Future research and continued progress in understanding this complicated disease process will hopefully lead to preventative treatments that result in improved visual outcomes.

References

1. Speicher MA, Fu AD, Martin JP, et al. Primary vitrectomy alone for repair of retinal detachments following cataract surgery. Retina. 2000;20:459-64.
2. Greven CM, Sanders RJ, Brown GC, et al. Pseudophakic retinal detachments. Anatomic and visual results. Ophthalmology. 1992;99:257-62.
3. Girard P, Mimoun G, Karpouzas I, et al. Clinical risk factors for proliferative vitreoretinopathy after retinal detachment surgery. Retina. 1994;14:417-24.
4. Gartry DS, Chignell AH, Franks WA, et al. Pars plana vitrectomy for the treatment of rhegmatogenous retinal detachment uncomplicated by advanced proliferative vitreoretinopathy. Br J Ophthalmol. 1993;77:199-203.
5. The classification of retinal detachment with proliferative vitreoretinopathy. Ophthalmology. 1983;90:121-5.
6. Nashed A, Saikia P, Herrmann WA, et al. The outcome of early surgical repair with vitrectomy and silicone oil in open-globe injuries with retinal detachment. Am J Ophthalmol. 2011;151:522-8.
7. Cardillo JA, Stout JT, LaBree L, et al. Post-traumatic proliferative vitreoretinopathy. The epidemiologic profile, onset, risk factors, and visual outcome. Ophthalmology. 1997;104:1166-73.
8. Spiegel D, Nasemann J, Nawrocki J, et al. Severe ocular trauma managed with primary pars plana vitrectomy and silicone oil. Retina. 1997;17:275-85.
9. Kruger EF, Nguyen QD, Ramos-Lopez M, et al. Proliferative vitreoretinopathy after trauma. Int Ophthalmol Clin. 2002;42:129-43.

10. Mietz H, Heimann K. Onset and recurrence of proliferative vitreoretinopathy in various vitreoretinal disease. Br J Ophthalmol. 1995;79:874-7.
11. Machemer R. Pathogenesis and classification of massive periretinal proliferation. Br J Ophthalmol. 1978;62:737-47.
12. Lean JS, Stern WH, Irvine AR, et al. Classification of proliferative vitreoretinopathy used in the silicone study. The Silicone Study Group. Ophthalmology. 1989;96:765-71.
13. Machemer R, Aaberg TM, Freeman HM, et al. An updated classification of retinal detachment with proliferative vitreoretinopathy. Am J Ophthalmol. 1991;112:159-65.
14. Yao Y, Jiang L, Wang ZJ, et al. Scleral buckling procedures for longstanding or chronic rhegmatogenous retinal detachment with subretinal proliferation. Ophthalmology. 2006;113:821-5.
15. Yanyali A, Bonnet M. Risk factors of postoperative proliferative vitreoretinopathy in giant tears. J Fr Ophtalmol. 1996;19:175-80.
16. Duquesne N, Bonnet M, Adeleine P. Preoperative vitreous hemorrhage associated with rhegmatogenous retinal detachment: a risk factor for postoperative proliferative vitreoretinopathy? Graefes Arch Clin Exp Ophthalmol. 1996;234:677-82.
17. Bonnet M, Fleury J, Guenoun S, et al. Cryopexy in primary rhegmatogenous retinal detachment: a risk factor for postoperative proliferative vitreoretinopathy? Graefes Arch Clin Exp Ophthalmol. 1996;234:739-43.
18. Dumas C, Bonnet M. Choroidal detachment associated with rhegmatogenous retinal detachment: a risk factor for postoperative PVR? J Fr Ophtalmol. 1996;19:455-63.
19. Cowley M, Conway BP, Campochiaro PA, et al. Clinical risk factors for proliferative vitreoretinopathy. Arch Ophthalmol. 1989;107:1147-51.
20. Bonnet M. The development of severe proliferative vitreoretinopathy after retinal detachment surgery. Grade B: a determining risk factor. Graefes Arch Clin Exp Ophthalmol. 1988;226:201-5.
21. Bonnet M. Clinical factors predisposing to massive proliferative vitreoretinopathy in rhegmatogenous retinal detachment. Ophthalmologica. 1984;188:148-52.
22. Bonnet M, Guenoun S. Surgical risk factors for severe postoperative proliferative vitreoretinopathy (PVR) in retinal detachment with grade B PVR. Graefes Arch Clin Exp Ophthalmol. 1995;233:789-91.
23. Campochiaro PA, Kaden IH, Vidaurri-Leal J, et al. Cryotherapy enhances intravitreal dispersion of viable retinal pigment epithelial cells. Arch Ophthalmol. 1985;103:434-6.
24. Singh AK, Michels RG, Glaser BM. Scleral indentation following cryotherapy and repeat cryotherapy enhance release of viable retinal pigment epithelial cells. Retina. 1986;6:176-8.
25. Weller M, Wiedemann P, Heimann K. Proliferative vitreoretinopathy—is it anything more than wound healing at the wrong place? Int Ophthalmol. 1990;14:105-17.
26. Ryan SJ. The pathophysiology of proliferative vitreoretinopathy in its management. Am J Ophthalmol. 1985;100:188-93.
27. Campochiaro PA. Pathogenic mechanisms in proliferative vitreoretinopathy. Arch Ophthalmol. 1997;115:237-41.
28. Glaser BM, Cardin A, Biscoe B. Proliferative vitreoretinopathy. The mechanism of development of vitreoretinal traction. Ophthalmology. 1987;94:327-32.
29. Laqua H, Machemer R. Glial cell proliferation in retinal detachment (massive periretinal proliferation). Am J Ophthalmol. 1975;80:602-18.
30. Machemer R, Laqua H. Pigment epithelium proliferation in retinal detachment (massive periretinal proliferation). Am J Ophthalmol. 1975;80:1-23.
31. Kon CH, Occleston NL, Aylward GW, et al. Expression of vitreous cytokines in proliferative vitreoretinopathy: a prospective study. Invest Ophthalmol Vis Sci. 1999;40:705-12.
32. Kauffmann DJ, van Meurs JC, Mertens DA, et al. Cytokines in vitreous humor: interleukin-6 is elevated in proliferative vitreoretinopathy. Invest Ophthalmol Vis Sci. 1994;35:900-6.
33. Grant MB, Guay C, Marsh R. Insulin-like growth factor I stimulates proliferation, migration, and plasminogen activator release by human retinal pigment epithelial cells. Curr Eye Res. 1990;9:323-35.
34. Ricker LJ, Kijlstra A, Kessels AG, et al. Interleukin and growth factor levels in subretinal fluid in rhegmatogenous retinal detachment: a case-control study. PLoS One. 2011;6:e19141.
35. Ogata N, Nishikawa M, Nishimura T, et al. Inverse levels of pigment epithelium-derived factor and vascular endothelial growth factor in the vitreous of eyes with rhegmatogenous retinal detachment and proliferative vitreoretinopathy. Am J Ophthalmol. 2002;133:851-2.
36. Smiddy WE, Michels RG, Stark WJ, et al. Cataract extraction after retinal detachment surgery. Ophthalmology. 1988;95:3-7.
37. Lewis H, Aaberg TM. Anterior proliferative vitreoretinopathy. Am J Ophthalmol. 1988;105:277-84.
38. Lewis H, Aaberg TM. Causes of failure after repeat vitreoretinal surgery for recurrent proliferative vitreoretinopathy. Am J Ophthalmol. 1991;111:15-9.
39. Vitrectomy with silicone oil or perfluoropropane gas in eyes with severe proliferative vitreoretinopathy: results of a randomized clinical trial. Silicone Study Report 2. Arch Ophthalmol. 1992;110:780-92.
40. Abrams GW, Azen SP, McCuen BW, et al. Vitrectomy with silicone oil or long-acting gas in eyes with severe proliferative vitreoretinopathy: results of additional and long-term follow-up. Silicone Study Report 11. Arch Ophthalmol. 1997;115:335-44.
41. Acar N, Kapran Z, Altan T, et al. Pars plana vitrectomy with and without triamcinolone acetonide assistance in pseudophakic retinal detachment complicated with proliferative vitreoretinopathy. Jpn J Ophthalmol. 2010;54:331-7.

42. Tan HS, Mura M, Oberstein SY, de Smet MD. Primary retinectomy in proliferative vitreoretinopathy. Am J Ophthalmol. 2010;149:447-52.
43. Quiram PA, Gonzales CR, Hu W, et al. Outcomes of vitrectomy with inferior retinectomy in patients with recurrent rhegmatogenous retinal detachments and proliferative vitreoretinopathy. Ophthalmology. 2006;113:2041-7.
44. Michels RG. Surgery of retinal detachment with proliferative vitreoretinopathy. Retina. 1984;4:63-83.
45. Diederen RM, La Heij EC, Kessels AG, et al. Scleral buckling surgery after macula-off retinal detachment: worse visual outcome after more than 6 days. Ophthalmology. 2007;114: 705-9.
46. Hassan TS, Sarrafizadeh R, Ruby AJ, et al. The effect of duration of macular detachment on results after the scleral buckle repair of primary, macula-off retinal detachments. Ophthalmology. 2002;109:146-52.
47. Ross WH, Stockl FA. Visual recovery after retinal detachment. Curr Opin Ophthalmol. 2000;11:191-4.
48. Grizzard WS, Hilton GF. Scleral buckling for retinal detachments complicated by periretinal proliferation. Arch Ophthalmol. 1982;100:419-22.
49. Yoshida A, Ho PC, Schepens CL, et al. Severe proliferative vitreoretinopathy and retinal detachment. II. Surgical results with scleral buckling. Ophthalmology. 1984;91:1538-43.
50. Oliveira LB, Reis PA. Silicone oil tamponade in 23-gauge transconjunctival sutureless vitrectomy. Retina. 2007;27:1054-8.
51. Shah CP, Ho AC, Regillo CD, et al. Short-term outcomes of 25-gauge vitrectomy with silicone oil for repair of complicated retinal detachment. Retina. 2008;28:723-8.
52. de Juan E, Hickingbotham D. Flexible iris retractor. Am J Ophthalmol. 1991;111:776-7.
53. Murray TG, Boldt HC, Lewis H, et al. A technique for facilitated visualization and dissection of the vitreous base, pars plana, and pars plicata. Arch Ophthalmol. 1991;109:1458-9.
54. Peyman GA, Cheema R, Conway MD, et al. Triamcinolone acetonide as an aid to visualization of the vitreous and the posterior hyaloid during pars plana vitrectomy. Retina. 2000;20:554-5.
55. Ueno A, Enaida H, Hata Y, et al. Long-term clinical outcomes and therapeutic benefits of triamcinolone-assisted pars plana vitrectomy for proliferative vitreoretinopathy: a case study. Eur J Ophthalmol. 2007;17:392-8.
56. Furino C, Micelli Ferrari T, Boscia F, et al. Triamcinolone-assisted pars plana vitrectomy for proliferative vitreoretinopathy. Retina. 2003;23:771-6.
57. Aras C, Arici C, Akar S, et al. Peeling of internal limiting membrane during vitrectomy for complicated retinal detachment prevents epimacular membrane formation. Graefes Arch Clin Exp Ophthalmol. 2009;247:619-23.
58. Uram M. Laser endoscope in the management of proliferative vitreoretinopathy. Ophthalmology. 1994;101:1404-8.
59. de Smet MD, Mura M. Minimally invasive surgery-endoscopic retinal detachment repair in patients with media opacities. Eye. 2008;22:662-5.
60. Machemer R, McCuen BW, de Juan E. Relaxing retinotomies and retinectomies. Am J Ophthalmol. 1986;102:7-12.
61. Han DP, Lewis MT, Kuhn EM, et al. Relaxing retinotomies and retinectomies. Surgical results and predictors of visual outcome. Arch Ophthalmol. 1990;108:694-7.
62. Iverson DA, Ward TG, Blumenkranz MS. Indications and results of relaxing retinotomy. Ophthalmology. 1990;97:1298-304.
63. Han DP, Rychwalski PJ, Mieler WF, et al. Management of complex retinal detachment with combined relaxing retinotomy and intravitreal perfluoro-n-octane injection. Am J Ophthalmol. 1994;118:24-32.
64. Shalaby KA. Relaxing retinotomies and retinectomies in the management of retinal detachment with severe proliferative vitreoretinopathy (PVR). Clin Ophthalmol 2010;4:1107-14.
65. Vitrectomy with silicone oil or sulfur hexafluoride gas in eyes with severe proliferative vitreoretinopathy: results of a randomized clinical trial. Silicone Study Report 1. Arch Ophthalmol 1992;110:770-9.
66. McCuen BW, Azen SP, Stern W, et al. Vitrectomy with silicone oil or perfluoropropane gas in eyes with severe proliferative vitreoretinopathy. Silicone Study Report 3. Retina. 1993;13: 279-84.
67. Barr CC, Lai MY, Lean JS, et al. Postoperative intraocular pressure abnormalities in the Silicone Study. Silicone Study Report 4. Ophthalmology. 1993;100:1629-35.
68. Blumenkranz MS, Azen SP, Aaberg T, et al. Relaxing retinotomy with silicone oil or long-acting gas in eyes with severe proliferative vitreoretinopathy. Silicone Study Report 5. The Silicone Study Group. Am J Ophthalmol. 1993;116: 557-64.
69. Hutton WL, Azen SP, Blumenkranz MS, et al. The effects of silicone oil removal. Silicone Study Report 6. Arch Ophthalmol. 1994;112:778-85.
70. Abrams GW, Azen SP, Barr CC, et al. The incidence of corneal abnormalities in the Silicone Study. Silicone Study Report 7. Arch Ophthalmol. 1995;113:764-9.
71. Cox MS, Azen SP, Barr CC, et al. Macular pucker after successful surgery for proliferative vitreoretinopathy. Silicone Study Report 8. Ophthalmology 1995;102:1884-91.
72. Diddie KR, Azen SP, Freeman HM, et al. Anterior proliferative vitreoretinopathy in the silicone study. Silicone Study Report Number 10. Ophthalmology. 1996;103:1092-9.
73. Tano Y, Chandler D, Machemer R. Treatment of intraocular proliferation with intravitreal injection of triamcinolone acetonide. Am J Ophthalmol. 1980;90:810-6.
74. Chandler DB, Rozakis G, de Juan E, et al. The effect of triamcinolone acetonide on a refined experimental model of proliferative vitreoretinopathy. Am J Ophthalmol. 1985;99: 686-90.
75. Chandler DB, Hida T, Sheta S, et al. Improvement in efficacy of corticosteroid therapy in an animal model of proliferative vitreoretinopathy by pretreatment. Graefes Arch Clin Exp Ophthalmol. 1987;225:259-65.
76. Rubsamen PE, Cousins SW. Therapeutic effect of periocular corticosteroids in experimental proliferative vitreoretinopathy. Retina. 1997;17:44-50.

77. Jonas JB, Hayler JK, Panda-Jonas S. Intravitreal injection of crystalline cortisone as adjunctive treatment of proliferative vitreoretinopathy. Brit J Ophthalmol. 2000;84:1064-7.
78. Cheema RA, Peyman GA, Fang T, et al. Triamcinolone acetonide as an adjuvant in the surgical treatment of retinal detachment with proliferative vitreoretinopathy. Ophthal Surg Las Im. 2007;38:365-70.
79. Ahmadieh H, Feghhi M, Tabatabaei H, et al. Triamcinolone acetonide in silicone-filled eyes as adjunctive treatment for proliferative vitreoretinopathy: a randomized clinical trial. Ophthalmology. 2008;115:1938-43.
80. Wiedemann P, Hilgers RD, Bauer P, et al. Adjunctive daunorubicin in the treatment of proliferative vitreoretinopathy: results of a multicenter clinical trial. Daunomycin Study Group. Am J Ophthalmol. 1998;126:550-9.
81. Asaria RHY, Kon CH, Bunce C, et al. Adjuvant 5-fluorouracil and heparin prevents proliferative vitreoretinopathy - Results from a randomized, double-blind, controlled clinical trial. Ophthalmology. 2001;108:1179-83.
82. Charteris DG, Aylward GW, Wong D, et al. A randomized controlled trial of combined 5-fluorouracil and low-molecular-weight heparin in management of established proliferative vitreoretinopathy. Ophthalmology. 2004;111:2240-5.
83. Wickham L, Bunce C, Wong D, et al. Randomized controlled trial of combined 5-fluorouracil and low-molecular-weight heparin in the management of unselected rhegmatogenous retinal detachments undergoing primary vitrectomy. Ophthalmology. 2007;114:698-704.
84. Sundaram V, Barsam A, Virgili G. Intravitreal low molecular weight heparin and 5-fluorouracil for the prevention of proliferative vitreoretinopathy following retinal reattachment surgery. Cochrane Database Syst Rev. 2010: CD006421.

16 Giant Retinal Tears

Kamalesh J Ramaiya, Kevin J Blinder

Introduction

▶ Background

Giant retinal tears (GRT) are defined as a full-thickness retinal break which extend circumferentially for greater than 90° or 3 clock hours of the peripheral retina (Figs 16.1A and B).[1,2] The incidence of GRT's has been estimated to be 0.05 per 100,000 persons per year.[3] GRT's are always associated with posterior vitreous detachment (PVD) and the peripheral vitreous is strongly adherent to the anterior margin of the tear (Fig. 16.2A). The posterior edge lacks vitreous support

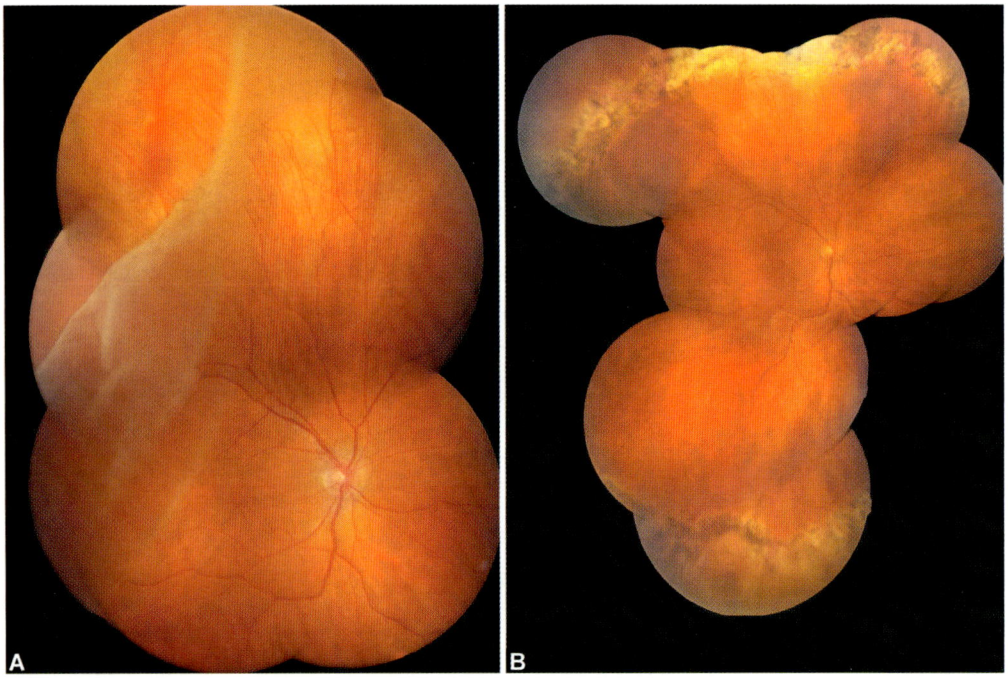

▲ **Figures 16.1A and B**

(A) Preoperative clinical color montage photograph of a giant retinal tear; (B) 6 months postoperatively following pars plana vitrectomy, PFCL insertion, endolaser, PFCL removal, air-fluid exchange and silicone oil injection

Note that the retina is attached and there are circumferential photocoagulation scars present around the periphery

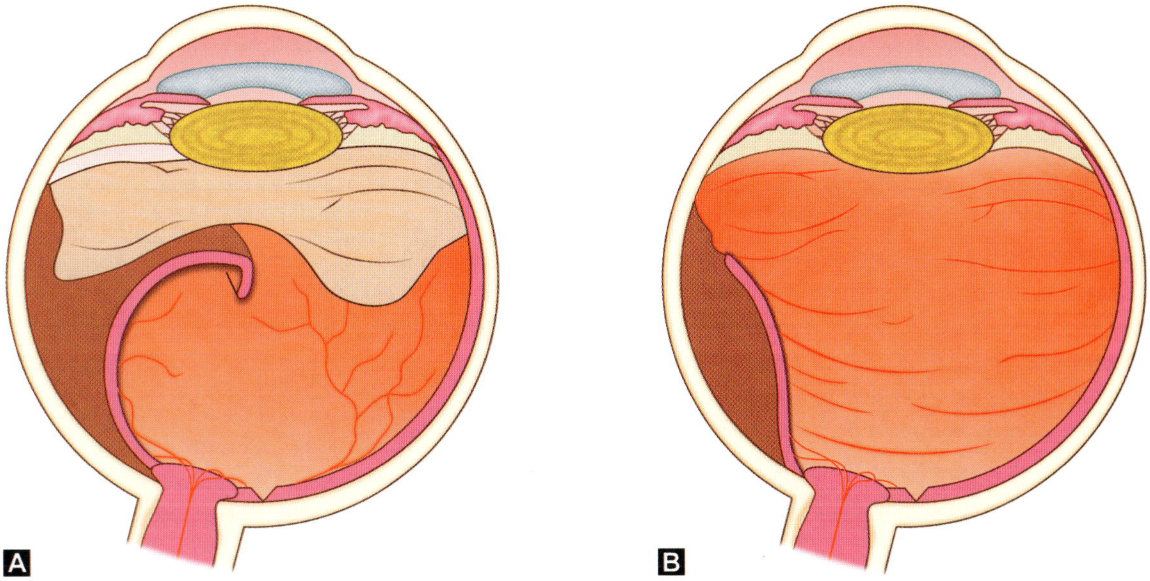

▲ **Figures 16.2A and B**

(A) Schematic diagram showing preoperative appearance of a giant retinal tear; (B) Giant retinal dialysis
Note the differences in vitreous attachments to the tear edges

and susceptible to the effects of gravity and therefore can rotate posteriorly onto itself, resulting in an inverted flap. In some cases, one or both ends of the tear may radialize, increasing the risk of flap formation and inversion. This is in contrast to a giant retinal dialysis (Fig. 16.2B) in which the break is at the ora serrata and vitreous is adherent to both edges of the pathology. This condition is usually amenable to less complex surgical techniques.[4]

Classification, Risk Factors and Etiology

Three classes of GRT's were described by Schepens et al.[5] in 1962 based on etiology. The majority of GRT's were found to be idiopathic (70%) or traumatic (20%) and a small subset was associated with chorioretinal degeneration (10%). Similar distributions of GRT etiologies have been described more recently.[6] Since then other etiologies have been described for GRT's including an association with systemic syndromes such as Sticklers,[7-10] Ehlers-Danlos[11] and Marfans.[12,13] Case reports of iatrogenic GRT's have also described their association with pars plana vitrectomy,[14-16] pneumatic retinopexy,[17] various types of laser and intraocular refractive surgery[18-24] and after retained lens fragment removal with anterior vitrectomy.[25] Additionally, intrinsic ocular conditions that leave the peripheral retina weakened to vitreous forces have also been described as a risk factor for GRT development. These include aniridia,[26] microspherophakia,[27] retinitis pigmentosa,[28,29] retinopathy of prematurity[13] and peripheral vitreo-chorio-retinal pathology such as lattice degeneration. Associations with severe inflammatory ocular conditions has also been described including: endophthalmitis,[30] syphilitic panuveitis[31] and the acute retinal necrosis syndrome.[32] Myopia is seen in 63% of cases with a mean of approximately –7.50 diopters.[11] A significant gender predilection is present with over 75% of GRT's found in males.[33]

Pathogenesis

The pathogenesis of idiopathic GRT is thought to be similar to that of smaller peripheral retinal tears. Core vitreous liquefaction with secondary condensation and contraction of the peripheral vitreous base leads to traction on the peripheral retina. Traumatic GRT's occur almost exclusively secondary to blunt force injury causing an anterior-posterior compression and secondary transverse distention of the globe.[34] These forces act at sites of vitreoretinal adhesion and are sometimes associated with avulsion of the vitreous base.[6] Various etiologies of traumatic tears have been described including nonaccidental trauma[35] and sports related trauma.[36] Since traumatic GRTs tend to occur in younger individuals with formed vitreous, the posterior edge of the break has more support and is less likely to have slipped posteriorly at presentation.

Idiopathic GRT's develop due to manipulation of the vitreous either directly or indirectly, often in the setting of pre-existing retinal pathology (e.g. myopia and peripheral retinal degenerations).[37] Unlike traumatic GRT's, those of the idiopathic variety frequently present with posterior slippage due to a pre-existing liquefied core vitreous. A case report of idiopathic unilateral GRT's occurring within 2 weeks of each other in identical twins suggests a that a genetic predisposition may also contribute to some GRT's.[38]

Preoperative Evaluation

As with other types of retinal tears, a thorough preoperative evaluation should be undertaken prior to repair of GRT's. Slit-lamp examination should be performed with particular attention to pupillary dilation and lens status. Careful indirect ophthalmoscopy should be performed on both eyes to document the extent, location and mobility of the tear and/or detachment, as well as other retinal comorbidities in the affected and fellow eyes. These include proliferative vitreoretinopathy (PVR), as well as lattice degeneration, white without pressure and other peripheral retinal degenerations. If there is a limited view of the fundus due to media opacities, B-scan ultrasonography should be performed to determine the extent of the pathology. The characteristic findings are a discontinuity in the normally linear hyperechoic retina as well as vitreous and vitreoretinal interface changes.[4] This technique has been shown to have high specificity for GRT's. [39]

Surgical Techniques for Repair

The management of retinal detachment secondary to GRT's has remained a significant challenge for vitreoretinal surgeons, even with the development of newer surgical techniques including wide field visualization systems, advanced vitrectomy techniques and modern instrumentation. However, the most notable advance in the surgical repair of GRT's has been the advent of heavy perfluorocarbon liquids (PFCLs) that have proven to be invaluable in the intraoperative manipulation and unfolding of retinal tissue.[40] Because of these improved surgical techniques, the success rate of surgical repair has significantly increased over the last four decades.[11]

Historical Techniques

The earliest techniques utilized in repair of GRT's involved positioning the patient in such a manner as to unfold the flap of the tear. This was first described by Schepens et al.[41] in 1965 with the advent of a "power driven multipositional operating table", but the procedure evolved over the following two decades. Machemer described a technique in 1976 involving vitrectomy followed by gas fluid exchange while the patient is in a prone position with the surgeon operating from underneath.[42] In the 1980's Peyman[43] in the US and Bacin[44] in France modified the technique with the introduction of new rotating tables that somewhat simplified the procedure. Freeman described a variation of this technique utilizing rapid head movements to unfold the tear.[45]

Parallel to the refinement of positioning techniques, intraocular methods of unfolding and fixation of the retina evolved. Intravitreal air-fluid exchange for GRT's was described by Norton as early as 1969. Subsequently techniques attempting to suture the retina in place were proposed by Usui,[46] Federman,[47] and Nishi.[48] Other innovative methods of holding the retina in position were also developed, including cyanoacrylate adhesives,[49] retinal micro incarceration via a penetrating diathermy needle,[50] retinal tacks[51-60] and screws.[33] The intraocular stability of some of these implants after remaining in the eye for over 20 years have been reported recently.[61] With the advent of viscoelastic agents, techniques using sodium hyaluronate to unfold the flap of the tear were also attempted.[62-64]

Perfluorocarbon Liquids

Perfluorocarbon Liquids (PFCLs) (Table 16.1) are biologically and chemically inert synthetic compounds which were initially developed for medical use as blood substitutes due to their oxygen solubility and molecular weight.[65] The PFCLs that are available for ophthalmic use in the United States are Perfluoron (perfluoro-n-octane) and Vitreon (perfluoroperhydrophenanthrene). They continue to be utilized in medical fields outside ophthalmology; for example, in

TABLE 16.1: Perfluorocarbon liquids

• Perfluorooctane (Perfluoron)	C_8F_{18}
• Perfluoroperhydrophenanthrene (Vitreon)	$C_{14}F_{24}$
• Perfluorotributylamine	$C_{12}F_{27}N$
• Perfluorooctylbromide	$C_8F_{17}Br$
• Perfluorodecalin	$C_{10}F_{18}$
• Perfluoroethylcyclohexane	C_2F_6

TABLE 16.2: Physical properties of perfluorocarbon liquids

- Chemically inert
- Low viscosity
- High specific gravity (heavier than water)
- Refractive index similar to water
- Water immiscible
- Good surface tension in aqueous environment
- Nearly 100% transmission of visible light (optically clear)
- Higher boiling point than saline

contrast enhanced ultrasonography,[66] for tissue oxygenation in organ transplantation[67] and as liquid ventilation agents.[68] Their physical properties (Table 16.2) in addition to their biological inertness facilitated their development for intraocular use by Haidt,[69] Zimmerman[70] and Chang[71] in the 1980's. Their low-viscosity allows them to be easily infused into and removed from the vitreous cavity; their high specific gravity (1.76–2.03 times that of water[72]) allows for the anterior displacement of subretinal fluid and drainage through retinal breaks; and their nearly 100% transmission of visible light allows for endolaser photocoagulation while they are present in the vitreous cavity. The refractive indices of most PFCL's are approximately equivalent to water, allowing a good view to the retina through them. These agents have quickly become invaluable tools for indirect retinal manipulation during vitreoretinal surgery. Unfortunately, the eye's poor long-term tolerance of these agents has limited their use as long-acting vitreous substitutes,[73] yet some recent literature suggests that they can be left in the vitreous cavity for up to 5–14 days without significant toxicity.[40,74,75] However, postoperative tamponade with PFCL's is not common practice.

PFCLs have revolutionized the management of GRT's with retinal detachments by providing a technique of easily unfolding the flap of the tear and generating temporary internal tamponade while the tear is treated with cryotherapy or laser photocoagulation. GRT with retinal detachment was one of the first ophthalmic indications for use of these heavy liquids[71] and it remains one of the best clinical indications for their use. Other situations in which PFCLs can be useful include retinal counter pressure while peeling membranes from high stage PVR,[76] subretinal fluid drainage in bullous retinal detachments,[77] tamponade for choroidal hemorrhages[78] and levitating dislocated crystalline lenses or intraocular lens implants.[79]

Surgical Technique

The goals of surgical repair of GRT's are four-fold:

1. Unfold any inverted areas of the retina flap,
2. Flatten the retina either with internal tamponade and/or external support to the vitreous base,
3. Create strong chorioretinal adhesions in areas of pathology to seal any breaks, and
4. Treat high-risk areas of pathology in the fellow eye.

The technique begins with automated core vitrectomy followed by more peripheral vitrectomy. This may be undertaken on either the traditional 20-gauge or newer 23- and 25-gauge platforms.[80] During the peripheral vitrectomy careful shaving of the vitreous base using scleral-depression techniques is essential to eliminate vitreous traction, especially along the anterior tear margin where there is tightly adherent (Fig. 16.3). Wide-angle viewing systems have allowed for much better intraoperative visualization of the retinal periphery so that a complete trimming of the vitreous base is possible. To achieve a thorough peripheral vitrectomy in phakic patients, a lensectomy may be performed at this point; however, the necessity of this has been debated.[81] Care should be taken to preserve the anterior capsule in these cases in order to minimize complications of using vitreous substitutes in a one chambered eye.[82] In addition, good anterior capsular support will allow for future secondary posterior chamber intraocular lens implantation.

Once all vitreoretinal traction has been relieved, the PFCL is injected into the eye in a posterior to anterior direction (Fig. 16.4). The PFCL bubble should first be placed at the posterior pole over the fovea. As the PFCL bubble enlarges it should be directed beneath the inverted retinal flap to unfold it. An effort should be made to keep the tip of the infusion cannula within the original PFCL bubble while enlarging it in order to minimize risk of additional bubbles forming. The weight of the heavy PFCL simultaneously forces the

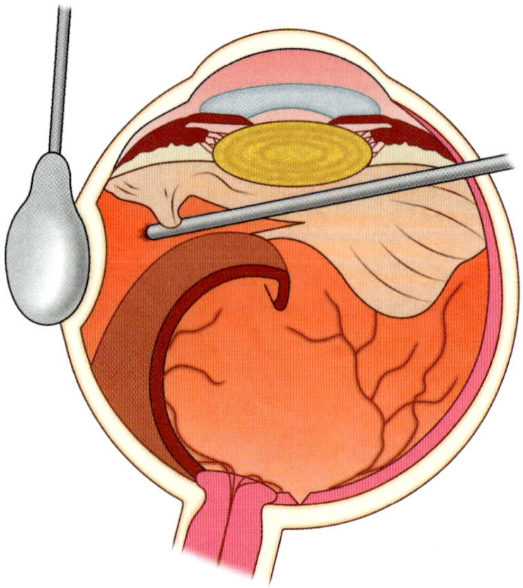

▲ **Figure 16.3**

Thorough shaving of the vitreous base with intraoperative scleral indentation. Completion of this step may require lensectomy (see text)

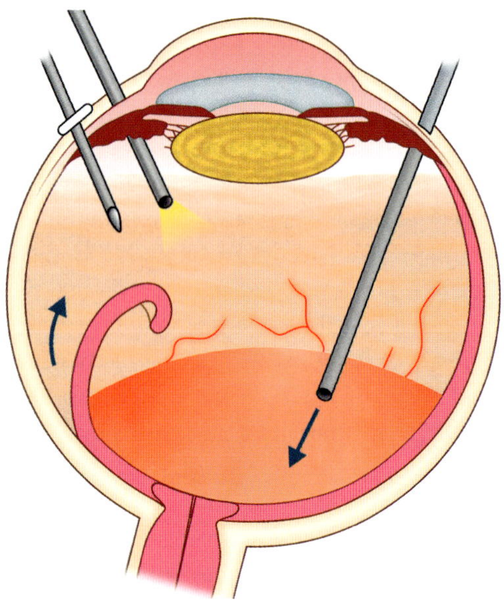

▲ **Figure 16.4**

Injection of PFCL in a posterior to anterior steamroller technique, allowing egress of subretinal fluid through the original break and flattening of the retina

Note the position of the infusion cannula tip within the enlarging PFCL bubble to minimize risk of multiple bubbles and subretinal PFCL

subretinal fluid anteriorly in a steamroller fashion and into the vitreous cavity through the original retinal break, obviating the need for a posterior retinotomy (and its potential complications). The risk of surgical trauma to the retina is also nearly eliminated, as direct manipulation of this tissue is not required with this technique. Once the PFCL bubble reaches the edge of the GRT, the injection should be discontinued (Fig. 16.5A). At this point, the retinal break should be definitively treated with cryotherapy and or endolaser photocoagulation (Fig. 16.5B) prior to the air fluid exchange while the retinal view is good. Laser uptake is also facilitated by the PFCL because of tight apposition between the retina and underlying retinal pigment epithelium (RPE).

An encircling element[83] may now be placed, however buckle-less techniques have been advocated by some.[84-87] In a small study of 34 patients, Verstraeten[81] reported a higher rate of failure (45%) when no encircling element is placed as compared to performing a combination buckle-vitrectomy procedure (15%). If a scleral buckle is utilized, it should be (1) low, and (2) wide enough to cover the vitreous base. Too high a scleral buckle must be avoided as it encourages radial folds and fish-mouthing of the tear which may increase the chances of reaccumulating subretinal fluid and consequently increase the risk of surgical failure.

Removal of the PFCL is then undertaken in a slow, cautious fashion (Fig. 16.6). The eye is rotated toward the tear and aspiration is performed to dry the tear edge completely in order to prevent fluid from re-entering the subretinal space and minimize slippage. Following the air-PFCL exchange, a partial fluid-PFCL exchange followed by air-fluid exchange can be performed to assist in removing any residual PFCL. The air is then exchanged for either long acting 10–15% perfluoropropane (C_3F_8) gas or silicone oil. Some advocate using silicone oil for long-term tamponade in these cases,[88, 89] but others have shown no definite benefit of silicone oil over long acting gas for GRT.[90] Certain indications may require silicone oil such as pediatric patients, monocular patients and those who cannot avoid air travel.[91]

Some surgeons perform direct PFCL-silicone oil exchange, asserting a lower rate of retinal slippage during the exchange.[92, 93] However, direct exchange could result in retained PFCL, as the meniscus between silicone oil and PFCL may be difficult to discern. To reduce this risk, a special instrument described by Peyman and Mehta for PFCL-silicone oil exchange can be utilized.[94] If silicone oil is used, it should be removed after an average of 6 months of successful attachment.[95]

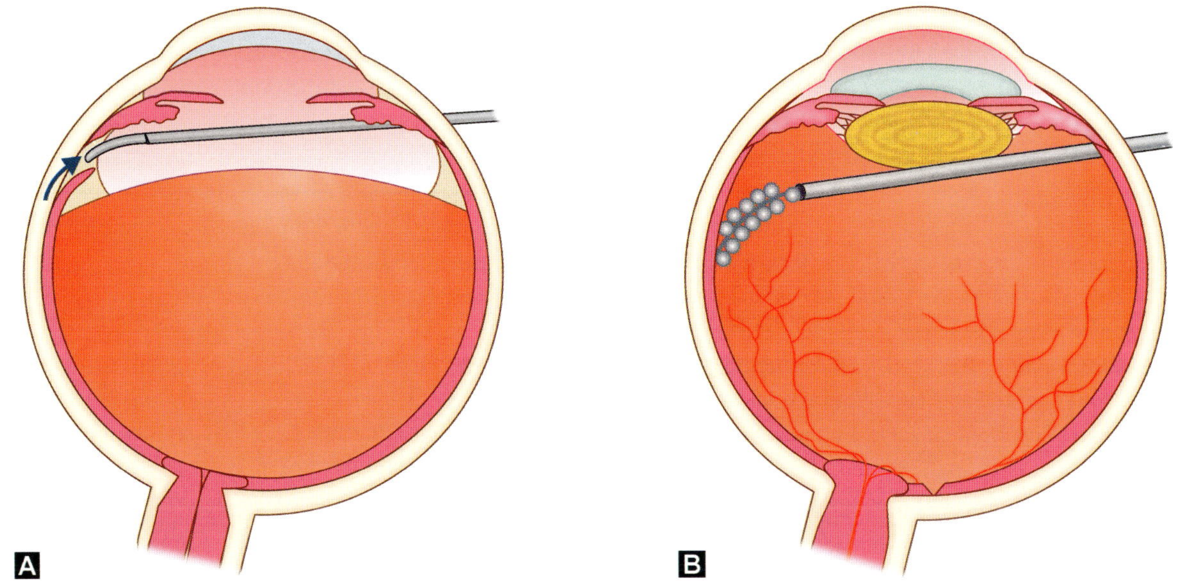

▲ **Figures 16.5A and B**

(A) Air-fluid exchange performed over the intact PFCL bubble, drying the tear edge thoroughly to remove any residual subretinal fluid in order to prevent slippage and allow for definitive treatment of the break with (B) Endolaser

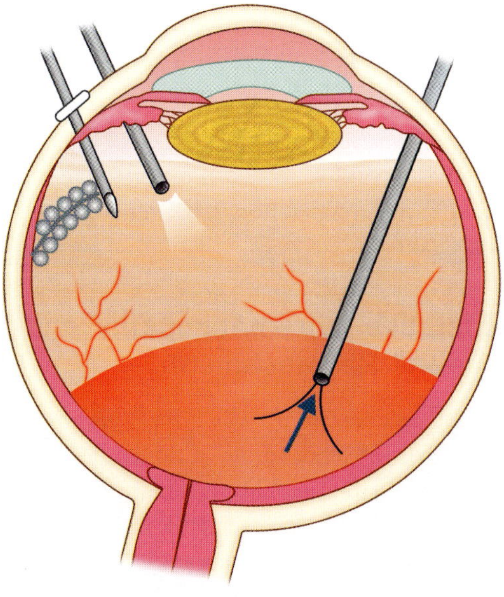

▲ **Figure 16.6**

Air-PFCL exchange. The eye may be rotated toward the tear at this step. The tear edges must be dried completely to prevent slippage. Partial fluid-PFCL exchanges may be performed in order to facilitate removal of any residual PFCL

▶ Giant Retinal Tears with Proliferative Vitreoretinopathy

Giant retinal tears presenting with PVR add yet another level of complexity to the surgical repair and additional factors must be considered when approaching these patients. These include the need for lensectomy, peeling of preretinal membranes, need for retinectomy and placement of encircling elements.

Although the lens may be preserved in cases of GRT without PVR (in the absence of other indications for lensectomy), a lower threshold for this step in the procedure should be observed when PVR is present. Posterior PVR alone may not necessitate lensectomy, but it is essential when anterior PVR is present.

PFCL can be used to the surgeon's advantage, providing countertraction while peeling PVR membranes.[96] This step should be performed with as little PFCL as possible, however, in order to minimize the chance of perfluoron escaping subretinally through the large retinal defect. A complete removal of the membranes is required in order to reduce retinal traction to a minimum.

In very severe cases, it may not be possible to relieve all PVR related traction by membrane peeling and dissection alone. In these situations a circumferential peripheral relaxing retinectomy may be required to flatten the retina.[97] This can be done prior to[98] or under[99] PFCL. Thorough endolaser retinopexy and/or cryopexy must be then applied to the retinectomy margin. Recently, one group has reported a small series of patients with recurrent detachment and very severe PVR in which 360° circumferential retinectomy helped achieve successful reattachment.[100] Peripheral retinectomy may also be indicated if the PFCL is unable to unravel a severely folded edge of the GRT.

In contrast to GRTs without PVR, an encircling element is almost always placed to minimize tractional forces when PVR is present. The element should be positioned such that the entire vitreous base is supported. The buckle does not necessarily need to be posterior enough to cover the posterior margin of the break as this is free from vitreous adhesion.

Prophylaxis of the Fellow Eye

There is no doubt that fellow eyes of patients with GRT's are at higher risk of developing retinal tears, GRT's and retinal detachments. The bilateral sequential GRT rate in the fellow eye has been reported to be 12.8% with an average interval of 3.5 years,[3] up to as high as 74% with 5 year follow-up for equatorial giant tears.[101] Specifically, high-risk eyes with extensive lattice degeneration, white without pressure and Sticklers syndrome have rates of GRT in the fellow eye as high as 90.9%.[102]

The utility of prophylactic intervention in the fellow eye has been somewhat controversial with a spectrum of recommendations ranging from aggressive circumferential 360° treatment with laser,[37,103-105] cryotherapy,[106,107] or prophylactic buckle,[102,108,109] to local treatment in areas of high-risk pathology.[110,111] It should be noted that these recommendations were all based on retrospective studies and none of these interventions were proven to be superior to another. No randomized controlled trials or case control series supporting such interventions have been published to date.[112] Nevertheless, the existing literature definitely suggests that prophylactic therapy, especially in high-risk circumstances, may be effective. When considering prophylactic therapy, the surgeon must keep in mind that no intervention is without risk and treatments do not guarantee complete retinal stability. Detachments have been reported to occur in areas of previously prophylaxed retina.[111]

Given the high-risk of retinal detachment in the fellow eye, we recommend treatment at the time of initial surgery to any areas of high-risk pathology including lattice degeneration, holes, tears and white without pressure. The decision to place a prophylactic encircling element should be dealt with on a case by case basis and it should certainly be considered if extensive enough or progressing pathology is present in the fellow eye. At a minimum, even if there is no visible pathology in the fellow eye, we recommend very close monitoring with thorough scleral depressed examination of the peripheral retina.

Complications

Complications after repair of GRTs are more severe than those resulting from simpler forms of retinal detachment repair. In addition to the known risks associated with vitrectomy (including cataract formation, endophthalmitis, vitreous hemorrhage and postoperative hypotony, etc.), scleral buckling (diplopia, anterior segment ischemia, buckle extrusion, etc.), cryotherapy (epiretinal membrane formation, etc.), silicone oil injection (elevated intraocular pressure, corneal decompensation, emulsification of silicone oil, retained silicone oil droplets,[113] sudden vision loss,[114] etc.) and endodrainage retinotomies,[115] GRT repair is associated with additional risks specific to this pathology.

Slippage of GRT

Slippage of the posterior edge of the GRT flap is not an uncommon complication. This most commonly occurs intraoperatively and repositioning of the flap is required using the techniques described above. Postoperative slippage of the tear may require reoperation, especially if subretinal fluid starts to accumulate.

Proliferative Vitreoretinopathy and Recurrent Redetachment

The proposed mechanism by which PVR occurs in GRTs is the same as that for other forms of retinal detachment with dispersion of subretinal retinal pigment epithelial cells into the vitreous cavity.[116,117] However, PVR rates are much higher in the setting of GRT repair surgery as compared with conventional RD repair. This may be because (1) there is a larger area of exposed RPE and (2) a greater amount of cryotherapy or laser is required to treat a larger defect, increasing the risk of RPE cell dispersion and breakdown of the blood-retinal barrier.[91] In fact, incidence rates of PVR following GRT repair range from 40–78%.[1,37,45,118-120] The presence of vitreous hemorrhage, either visible or subclinical, may also contribute to PVR development.[121,122] Cytokine production, either by the released RPE cells or from blood cells has also been linked with PVR.[123] Management of GRT's with PVR is described above.

Complications of PFCL

Given their relative biological inertness there are relatively few complications associated with the use of PFCLs.[124] The most common complications are secondary to incomplete evacuation of PFCL during the operative procedure. PFCLs can either be retained within the anterior chamber, vitreous cavity, or more dangerously, the subretinal space. A larger sized retinal break is more likely to result in subretinal PFCL retention.[125] Rates of intraocular retention have been reported to be similar for perfluorodecalin and perfluoro-n-octane.[125] However, a study comparing perfluoro-n-octane (Perfluoron) to perfluoroperhydrophenanthrene (Vitreon) in 264 eyes suggests that although overall retention rates are low, the latter has a higher rate of retention, likely due to its greater specific gravity and lower vapor pressure.[126]

Retained PFCL has been shown in numerous studies to be associated with both retinal and corneal toxicity. Histopathologic evidence suggests that retained intraocular PFCL elicits an intraocular inflammatory response characterized by macrophages with intracellular vacuoles containing the PFCL.[127] Subretinal PFCL has been shown in animal studies to result in local damage to the inner and outer segments of photoreceptors.[128] The functional effect of this on vision has been demonstrated by microperimetry, showing dense scotomas in the area of retained PFCL with partial recovery after its evacuation.[129] In addition, recovery of visual function has been described following removal of even chronically retained subretinal PFCL.[130] Retinal hole has also been described as a complication of long-term subretinal PFCL.[131]

Removal of PFCL from the anterior chamber or vitreous cavity is relatively straightforward by utilizing active aspiration. PFCL retained in the subretinal space poses a greater surgical challenge. If the retained material is located in the periphery and is remaining stable and not threatening the fovea, it may be prudent to simply observe. If threatening the macula or more specifically, the fovea, prompt extraction is necessary. Various techniques have been described for removing subretinal PFCL, including the use of 32-gauge[132] or 39-gauge[133] flexible cannulas and 50-gauge glass pipettes.[134] These studies all report both anatomic and visual success following the procedures. Others have reported improvements in visual acuity after displacing subfoveal PFCL into the inferior periphery via creation of a localized retinal detachment with subretinal balanced salt solution followed by air-fluid exchange and face down positioning.[135]

Prognosis

The surgical success rates for GRT repair have thankfully improved significantly over the last 40 years.[11] Today, most surgeons are reporting visual success in the range of 75–95% of patients.[11,37,75,136,137] In a large review of 212 cases from the Bascom Palmer Eye Institute, risk factors for recurrent retinal detachment were found to include female gender, younger age, preoperative PVR, prior vitrectomy, larger size of the giant retinal tear, lack of scleral buckle placement and relaxing retinotomy.[119] Risk factors for good visual outcome (>20/200) were no prior vitrectomy, good preoperative visual acuity and no need for relaxing retinotomy.

References

1. Schepens CL, Freeman HM. Current management of giant retinal breaks. Trans Am Acad Ophthalmol Otolaryngol. 1967;71:474-87.
2. Scott JD. Giant tear of the retina. Trans Ophthalmol Soc UK. 1975;95:142-4.
3. Freeman HM. Fellow eyes of giant retinal breaks. Trans Am Ophthalmol Soc. 1978;76:343-82.
4. Genovesi-Ebert F, Rizzo S, Chiellini S, et al. Echographic study of the vitreoretinal interface in giant retinal tears. Ophthalmologica. 1998;212:89-90.
5. Schepens CL, Dobble JG, Mc MJ. Retinal detachments with giant breaks: preliminary report. Trans Am Acad Ophthalmol Otolaryngol. 1962;66:471-9.
6. Aylward GW, Cooling RJ, Leaver PK. Trauma-induced retinal detachment associated with giant retinal tears. Retina. 1993;13:136-41.
7. Ang A, Poulson AV, Goodburn SF, et al. Retinal detachment and prophylaxis in type 1 Stickler syndrome. Ophthalmology. 2008;115:164-8.
8. Karel I, Dolezalova J, Oudova P. [Stickler's syndrome (dystrophia vitreoretinalis hereditaria). Results of surgery for retinal detachment]. Cesk Slov Oftalmol. 2001;57:147-54.
9. Langmann A, Langmann G, Kainer U, et al. [Vitreoretinal changes in siblings of two patients with Stickler syndrome. Study of two families]. Ophthalmologe. 1993;90:506-9.
10. Spallone A. Empty cavity and giant tears. Surv Ophthalmol. 1989;33:495-501.

11. Lee SY, Ong SG, Wong DW, et al. Giant retinal tear management: an Asian experience. Eye. 2009;23:601-5.
12. Dotrelova D, Karel I, Clupkova E. Retinal detachment in Marfan's syndrome. Characteristics and surgical results. Retina. 1997;17:390-6.
13. Witmer R. Giant retinal tears in retrolental fibroplasia and Marfan's syndrome. Mod Probl Ophthalmol. 1979;20:279-81.
14. Batman C, Cekic O. Giant retinal tears after pars plana vitrectomy. Eye. 1998;12:163-4.
15. Abu el-Asrar AM. Giant retinal tears after pars plana vitrectomy. Eye. 1997;11:325-7.
16. McLeod D. Giant retinal tears after central vitrectomy. Br J Ophthalmol. 1985;69:96-8.
17. Yam JC, Liu DT, Lee VY, et al. Giant retinal tear after pneumatic retinopexy. Acta Ophthalmol. 2008;86:232-3.
18. Georgalas I, Petrou P, Papaconstantinou D. Bilateral giant tear-associated retinal detachment following Artisan phakic intraocular lens implantation for correction of moderate myopia. Acta Ophthalmol. 2010;88:143-4.
19. Aras C, Ozdamar A, Karacorlu M, et al. Retinal detachment following laser in situ keratomileusis. Ophthalmic Surg Lasers. 2000;31:121-5.
20. Farah ME, Hofling-Lima AL, Nascimento E. Early rhegmatogenous retinal detachment following laser in situ keratomileusis for high myopia. J Refract Surg. 2000;16:739-43.
21. Hernaez-Ortega MC, Soto-Pedre E. Giant retinal tear after iris claw phakic intraocular lens. J Refract Surg. 2004;20:839-40.
22. Navarro R, Gris O, Broc L, et al. Bilateral giant retinal tear following posterior chamber phakic intraocular lens implantation. J Refract Surg. 2005;21:298-300.
23. Schipper I, Senn P. Giant retinal tears after photorefractive keratectomy. Retina. 2000;20:225-6.
24. Vilaplana D, Guinot A, Escoto R. Giant retinal tears after photorefractive keratectomy. Retina. 1999;19:342-3.
25. Aaberg TM, Rubsamen PE, Flynn HW, et al. Giant retinal tear as a complication of attempted removal of intravitreal lens fragments during cataract surgery. Am J Ophthalmol. 1997;124:222-6.
26. Dowler JG, Lyons CJ, Cooling RJ. Retinal detachment and giant retinal tears in aniridia. Eye. 1995;9:268-70.
27. Pal N, Sharma YR, Azad R, et al. Isolated bilateral microspherophakia with giant retinal tear and rhegmatogenous retinal detachment. J Pediatr Ophthalmol Strabismus. 2005;42:238-40.
28. Johnston ME, Gonder JR. Giant retinal tears, retinal detachment and retinitis pigmentosa. Can J Ophthalmol. 1985;20:16-8.
29. Kim RY, Schwartz SD, Heckenlively JR, et al. Giant retinal tear and retinal detachment with underlying retinitis pigmentosa and hearing loss. Eye. 1996;10:697-700.
30. Jain K, Lam W. Giant retinal tear and meningococcus endogenous endophthalmitis. J Aapos. 2002;6:259-60.
31. Pournaras JA, Laffitte E, Guex-Crosier Y. Bilateral giant retinal tear and retinal detachment in a young emmetropic man after Jarish-Herxheimer reaction in ocular syphilis. Klin Monatsbl Augenheilkd. 2006;223:447-9.
32. Topilow HW, Nussbaum JJ, Freeman HM, et al. Bilateral acute retinal necrosis. Clinical and ultrastructural study. Arch Ophthalmol. 1982;100:1901-8.
33. Freeman HM. Current management of giant retinal breaks and fellow eyes. In: Schachat A (Ed). Retina, 2nd edition. St. Louis: Mosby; 1994.
34. Weidenthal DT, Schepens CL. Peripheral fundus changes associated with ocular contusion. Am J Ophthalmol. 1966;62:465-77.
35. Lash SC, Williams CPR, Luff AJ, et al. 360 degree giant retinal tear as a result of presumed non-accidental injury. Br J Ophthalmol. 2004;88:155.
36. Duguid IG, Leaver PK. Giant retinal tears resulting from eye gouging in rugby football. Br J Sports Med. 2000;34:65-6.
37. Ghosh YK, Banerjee S, Savant V, et al. Surgical treatment and outcome of patients with giant retinal tears. Eye. 2004;18:996-1000.
38. Chaudhry NA, Flynn HW, Tabandeh H. Idiopathic giant retinal tears in identical twins. Am J Ophthalmol. 1999;127:96-9.
39. Jalkh AE, Jabbour N, Avila MP, et al. Ultrasonographic findings in eyes with giant retinal tears and opaque media. Retina. 1983;3:154-8.
40. Blinder KJ, Peyman GA, Desai UR, et al. Vitreon, a short-term vitreoretinal tamponade. Br J Ophthalmol. 1992;76:525-8.
41. Schepens CL, Freeman HM, Thompson RF. A Power-Driven Multipositional Operating Table. Arch Ophthalmol. 1965;73:671-3.
42. Machemer R, Allen AW. Retinal tears 180 degrees and greater. Management with vitrectomy and intravitreal gas. Arch Ophthalmol. 1976;94:1340-6.
43. Peyman GA. A new operating table for the management of giant retinal breaks. Arch Ophthalmol. 1981;99:498-9.
44. Bacin F, Buffet JM, Raynaud S, et al. [Treatment of detachments caused by giant tears and retinal inversion using a multiple decubitus table]. Bull Soc Ophtalmol Fr. 1983;83:699-702.
45. Freeman HM. Current management of giant retinal breaks. In: Kanski JJ, Morse PH (Eds). Disorders of the Vitreous, Retina, and Choroid. London: Butterworths; 1983.
46. Usui M, Hamazaki S, Takano S. A new surgical technique for the treatment of giant tear: Transvitreoretinal fixation. Jpn J Ophthalmol. 1979;23:206-15.
47. Federman JL, Shakin JL, Lanning RC. The microsurgical management of giant retinal tears with trans-scleral retinal sutures. Ophthalmology. 1982;89:832-9.
48. Nishi O, Ideta H. A new suturing method for the treatment of giant retinal tear. Ophthalmic Surg. 1987;18:359-62.
49. Faulborn J. Treatment of giant retinal tears after perforating injuries with vitrectomy and a cyanoacrylate tissue adhesive. Adv Ophthalmol. 1976;33:204-7.
50. Peyman GA, Rednam KR, Seetner AA. Retinal microincarceration with penetrating diathermy in the manage-

ment of giant retinal tears. Arch Ophthalmol. 1984;102:562-5.
51. Abrams GW, Williams GA, Neuwirth J, et al. Clinical results of titanium retinal tacks with pneumatic insertion. Am J Ophthalmol. 1986;102:13-9.
52. Algvere P, Stenkula S, Crafoord S, et al. Sealing of retinal breaks with metal tacks. Evaluation of a new procedure in retinal reattachment surgery. Acta Ophthalmol. 1986;64: 421-4.
53. Ando F, Kondo J. A plastic tack for the treatment of retinal detachment with giant tear. Am J Ophthalmol. 1983;95:260-1.
54. Ando F, Kondo J. Surgical techniques for giant retinal tears with retinal tacks. Ophthalmic Surg. 1986;17:408-11.
55. Brown GC. The use of tacks for the repair of complicated retinal detachment. Trans Pa Acad Ophthalmol Otolaryngol. 1987;39:578-82.
56. De Juan E, Hickingbotham D, Machemer R. Retinal tacks. Am J Ophthalmol. 1985;99:272-4.
57. De Juan E, McCuen BW, Machemer R. The use of retinal tacks in the repair of complicated retinal detachments. Am J Ophthalmol. 1986;102:20-4.
58. De Juan E, McCuen BW, Machemer R. Mechanical retinal fixation using tacks. Ophthalmology. 1987;94:337-40.
59. O'Grady GE, Parel JM, Lee W, et al. Hypodermic stainless steel tacks and companion inserter designed for peripheral fixation of retina. Arch Ophthalmol. 1988;106:271-5.
60. Whitton S. Managing detachment with retinal tacks. J Ophthalmic Nurs Technol. 1986;5:91-3.
61. Javey G, Schwartz SG, Flynn HW. Lack of toxicity of stainless steel retinal tacks during 21 years of follow-up. Ophthalmic Surg Lasers Imaging. 2009;40:75-6.
62. Brown GC, Benson WE. Use of sodium hyaluronate for the repair of giant retinal tears. Arch Ophthalmol. 1989;107:1246-9.
63. Stenkula S, Ivert L, Gislason I, et al. The use of sodium-hyaluronate (Healon) in the treatment of retinal detachment. Ophthalmic Surg. 1981;12:435-7.
64. Lavin MJ, Leaver PK. Sodium hyaluronate and giant retinal tears. Arch Ophthalmol. 1990;108:480.
65. Clark LC. Perfluorodecalin as a red cell substitute. Prog Clin Biol Res. 1978;19:69-80.
66. Mattrey RF. The potential role of perfluorochemicals (PFCs) in diagnostic imaging. Artif Cells Blood Substit Immobil Biotechnol. 1994;22:295-313.
67. Matsumoto S. Clinical application of perfluorocarbons for organ preservation. Artif Cells Blood Substit Immobil Biotechnol. 2005;33:75-82.
68. Wolfson MR, Shaffer TH. Pulmonary applications of perfluorochemical liquids: ventilation and beyond. Paediatr Respir Rev. 2005;6:117-27.
69. Haidt SJ, Clark LC, Grinsberg J. Liquid perfluorocarbon replacement of the eye. Invest Ophthalmol Vis Sci. 1982;22:233.
70. Zimmerman NJ, Faris D. The use of N-perfluorocarbon amines in complicated retinal detachments. Invest Ophthalmol Vis Sci. 1984;25:258.
71. Chang S. Low viscosity liquid fluorochemicals in vitreous surgery. Am J Ophthalmol. 1987;103:38-43.
72. Peyman GA, Schulman JA, Sullivan B. Perfluorocarbon liquids in ophthalmology. Surv Ophthalmol. 1995;39:375-95.
73. Chang S, Sparrow JR, Iwamoto T. Experimental studies of tolerance to intravitreal perfluoro-n-octane liquid. Retina. 1991;11:367-74.
74. Sirimaharaj M, Balachandran C, Chan WC, et al. Vitrectomy with short term postoperative tamponade using perfluorocarbon liquid for giant retinal tears. Br J Ophthalmol. 2005;89:1176-9.
75. Ventura MC, Melo C, Escariao P. [Perfluoroctane liquid as a short-term vitreous-retinal tamponade in the postoperative period in patients with retinal detachment due to giant tears]. Arq Bras Oftalmol. 2007;70:495-500.
76. LoRusso FJ, Diaz-Rohena R, Lambert HM. Management of giant retinal tears. Semin Ophthalmol. 1995;10:42-8.
77. Abu El-Asrar AM, Al-Kwikbi HF, Kangave D. Prognostic factors after primary vitrectomy and perfluorocarbon liquids for bullous rhegmatogenous retinal detachment. Eur J Ophthalmol. 2009;19:107-17.
78. Feretis E, Mourtzoukos S, Mangouritsas G. Secondary management and outcome of massive suprachoroidal hemorrhage. Eur J Ophthalmol. 2006;16:835-40.
79. Chan CK, Agarwal A, Agarwal S, et al. Management of dislocated intraocular implants. Ophthalmol Clin North Am. 2001;14:681-93.
80. Riemann CD, Miller DM, Foster RE, et al. Outcomes of transconjunctival sutureless 25-gauge vitrectomy with silicone oil infusion. Retina. 2007;27:296-303.
81. Verstraeten T, Williams GA, Chang S, et al. Lens-sparing vitrectomy with perfluorocarbon liquid for the primary treatment of giant retinal tears. Ophthalmology. 1995;102:17-20.
82. MacCumber MW, Packo KH, Civantos JM, et al. Preservation of anterior capsule during vitrectomy and lensectomy for retinal detachment with proliferative vitreoretinopathy. Ophthalmology. 2002;109:329-33.
83. Goezinne F, EC LAH, Berendschot TT, et al. Low redetachment rate due to encircling scleral buckle in giant retinal tears treated with vitrectomy and silicone oil. Retina. 2008;28:485-92.
84. Ambresin A, Wolfensberger TJ, Bovey EH. Management of giant retinal tears with vitrectomy, internal tamponade, and peripheral 360 degrees retinal photocoagulation. Retina. 2003;23:622-8.
85. May DR. Buckle-less repair of giant retinal tears. Ophthalmology. 1992;99:1181-2.
86. Hoffman ME, Sorr EM. Management of giant retinal tears without scleral buckling. Retina. 1986;6:197-204.
87. Kreiger AE, Lewis H. Management of giant retinal tears without scleral buckling. Use of radical dissection of the vitreous base and perfluoro-octane and intraocular tamponade. Ophthalmology. 1992;99:491-7.
88. Unlu N, Kocaoglan H, Acar MA, et al. The management of giant retinal tears with silicone oil. Eur J Ophthalmol. 2003;13:192-5.

89. Azen SP, Scott IU, Flynn HW. Silicone oil in the repair of complex retinal detachments. A prospective observational multicenter study. Ophthalmology. 1998;105:1587-97.
90. Batman C, Cekic O. Vitrectomy with silicone oil or long-acting gas in eyes with giant retinal tears: long-term follow-up of a randomized clinical trial. Retina. 1999;19:188-92.
91. Chang S, Lopez J. Giant retinal tears with proliferative vitreoretinopathy. In: Ryan S, Hinton D, Schachat A, Wilkinson P (Eds). Retina, 4th edition. St. Louis: Mosby; 2005.
92. Mathis A, Pagot V, Gazagne C, et al. Giant retinal tears. Surgical techniques and results using perfluorodecalin and silicone oil tamponade. Retina. 1992;12:7-10.
93. Wong D, Williams RL, German MJ. Exchange of perfluorodecalin for gas or oil: a model for avoiding slippage. Graefes Arch Clin Exp Ophthalmol. 1998;236:234-7.
94. Peyman GA, Mehta NJ. Intravitreal infusion-aspiration instrument for silicone oil-perfluorocarbon liquid exchange. Retina. 1993;13:177-8.
95. Camacho H, Bajaire B, Mejia LF. Silicone oil in the management of giant retinal tears. Ann Ophthalmol. 1992;24:45-9.
96. Carroll BF, Peyman GA, Mehta NJ, et al. Repair of retinal detachment associated with proliferative vitreoretinopathy using perfluoroperhydrophenanthrene (Vitreon). Vitreon Study Group. Can J Ophthalmol. 1994;29:66-9.
97. Morse LS, McCuen BW, Machemer R. Relaxing retinotomies. Analysis of anatomic and visual results. Ophthalmology. 1990;97:642-7.
98. Han DP, Rychwalski PJ, Mieler WF, et al. Management of complex retinal detachment with combined relaxing retinotomy and intravitreal perfluoro-n-octane injection. Am J Ophthalmol. 1994;118:24-32.
99. Greve MD, Peyman GA, Millsap CM. Relaxing retinotomy under perfluorocarbon liquid. Ophthalmic Surg Lasers. 1996;27:154-5.
100. Banaee T, Hosseini SM, Eslampoor A, et al. Peripheral 360 degrees retinectomy in complex retinal detachment. Retina. 2009;29:811-8.
101. Scott JD. Equatorial giant tears affected by massive vitreous retraction. Trans Ophthalmol Soc UK. 1976;96:309-12.
102. Freeman HM. Fellow eye of nontraumatic giant retinal breaks. In: Lewis H, Ryan S, (Eds). Medical and Surgical Retina: Advances, Controversies, and Management. St. Louis: Mosby: 1994.
103. Brasseur G, Charlin JF, Langlois J. [The fellow eye in cases of giant tears of the retina. Preventive attitude]. Bull Soc Ophtalmol Fr. 1985;85:215-8.
104. Girard P, Boscher C, Merad I, et al. [Retinal detachment in the 2d eye. Risk factors]. J Fr Ophtalmol. 1983;6:975-9.
105. Meyer-Schwickerath G. [Prevention and giant tears]. Bibl Ophthalmol. 1967;72:345-6.
106. Wolfensberger TJ, Aylward GW, Leaver PK. Prophylactic 360 degrees cryotherapy in fellow eyes of patients with spontaneous giant retinal tears. Ophthalmology. 2003;110:1175-7.
107. Govan JA. Prophylactic circumferential cryopexy: a retrospective study of 106 eyes. Br J Ophthalmol. 1981;65: 364-70.
108. Freeman HM, Castillejos ME. Current management of giant retinal breaks: results with vitrectomy and total air fluid exchange in 95 cases. Trans Am Ophthalmol Soc. 1981;79:89-102.
109. Glasspool MG, Kanski JJ. Prophylaxis in giant tears. Trans Ophthalmol Soc UK. 1973;93:363-71.
110. Kreissig I, Robert Y. [Prevention, in the contralateral eye, of a giant tear ablation]. Klin Monatsbl Augenheilkd. 1983;182: 121-4.
111. Mastropasqua L, Carpineto P, Ciancaglini M, et al. Treatment of retinal tears and lattice degenerations in fellow eyes in high-risk patients suffering retinal detachment: a prospective study. Br J Ophthalmol. 1999;83:1046-9.
112. Ang GS, Townend J, Lois N. Interventions for prevention of giant retinal tear in the fellow eye. Cochrane Database Syst Rev. 2009:CD006909.
113. Wang LC, Wang TJ, Yang CM. Entrapped preretinal oil bubble: report of two cases. Jpn J Ophthalmol. 2006;50: 277-9.
114. Michel G, Meyer L, Naoun O. [Sudden visual loss following silicone oil removal: Three patients treated for giant retinal tear.] J Fr Ophtalmol. 2009;32:104-11.
115. McDonald HR, Lewis H, Aaberg TM, et al. Complications of endodrainage retinotomies created during vitreous surgery for complicated retinal detachment. Ophthalmology. 1989;96:358-63.
116. Campochiaro PA, Kaden IH, Vidaurri-Leal J, et al. Cryotherapy enhances intravitreal dispersion of viable retinal pigment epithelial cells. Arch Ophthalmol. 1985;103:434-6.
117. Glaser BM, Vidaurri-Leal J, Michels RG, et al. Cryotherapy during surgery for giant retinal tears and intravitreal dispersion of viable retinal pigment epithelial cells. Ophthalmology. 1993;100:466-70.
118. Kertes PJ, Wafapoor H, Peyman GA, et al. The management of giant retinal tears using perfluoroperhydrophenanthrene. A multicenter case series. Vitreon Collaborative Study Group. Ophthalmology. 1997;104:1159-65.
119. Scott IU, Murray TG, Flynn HW, et al. Outcomes and complications associated with giant retinal tear management using perfluoro-n-octane. Ophthalmology. 2002;109:1828-33.
120. Rofail M, Lee LR. Perfluoro-n-octane as a postoperative vitreoretinal tamponade in the management of giant retinal tears. Retina. 2005;25:897-901.
121. Duquesne N, Bonnet M, Adeleine P. Preoperative vitreous hemorrhage associated with rhegmatogenous retinal detachment: a risk factor for postoperative proliferative vitreoretinopathy? Graefes Arch Clin Exp Ophthalmol. 1996;234:677-82.
122. Girard P, Mimoun G, Karpouzas I, et al. Clinical risk factors for proliferative vitreoretinopathy after retinal detachment surgery. Retina. 1994;14:417-24.

123. Kon CH, Occleston NL, Aylward GW, et al. Expression of vitreous cytokines in proliferative vitreoretinopathy: a prospective study. Invest Ophthalmol Vis Sci. 1999;40:705-12.
124. Meffert S, Peyman GA. Intraoperative complications of perfluoroperhydrophenanthrene: subretinal perfluorocarbon, retinal slippage and residual perfluorocarbon. Vitreon Study Group. Can J Ophthalmol. 1999;34:272-80.
125. Garcia-Valenzuela E, Ito Y, Abrams GW. Risk factors for retention of subretinal perfluorocarbon liquid in vitreoretinal surgery. Retina. 2004;24:746-52.
126. Loewenstein A, Humayun MS, de Juan E, et al. Perfluoroperhydrophenanthrene versus perfluoro-n-octane in vitreoretinal surgery. Ophthalmology. 2000;107:1078-82.
127. Elsing SH, Fekrat S, Green WR. Clinicopathologic findings in eyes with retained perfluoro-n-octane liquid. Ophthalmology. 2001;108:45-8.
128. Berglin L, Ren J, Algvere PV. Retinal detachment and degeneration in response to subretinal perfluorodecalin in rabbit eyes. Graefes Arch Clin Exp Ophthalmol. 1993;231:233-7.
129. Tewari A, Eliott D, Singh CN, et al. Changes in retinal sensitivity from retained subretinal perfluorocarbon liquid. Retina. 2009;29:248-50.
130. Lai JC, Postel EA, McCuen BW. Recovery of visual function after removal of chronic subfoveal perfluorocarbon liquid. Retina. 2003;23:868-70.
131. Cohen SY, Dubois L, Elmaleh C. Retinal hole as a complication of long-standing subretinal perfluorocarbon liquid. Retina. 2006;26:843-4.
132. Sakurai E, Ogura Y. Removal of residual subfoveal perfluoro-n-octane liquid. Graefes Arch Clin Exp Ophthalmol. 2007;245:1063-4.
133. Roth DB, Sears JE, Lewis H. Removal of retained subfoveal perfluoro-n-octane liquid. Am J Ophthalmol. 2004;138:287-9.
134. Garcia-Arumi J, Castillo P, Lopez M. Removal of retained subretinal perfluorocarbon liquid. Br J Ophthalmol. 2008;92:1693-4.
135. Le Tien V, Pierre-Kahn V, Azan F, et al. Displacement of retained subfoveal perfluorocarbon liquid after vitreoretinal surgery. Arch Ophthalmol. 2008;126:98-101.
136. Al-Khairi AM, Al-Kahtani E, Kangave D, et al. Prognostic factors associated with outcomes after giant retinal tear management using perfluorocarbon liquids. Eur J Ophthalmol. 2008;18:270-7.
137. Karel I, Michalickova M, Soucek P. Long-term results of pars plana vitrectomy and silicone oil for giant tears. Eur J Ophthalmol. 1996;6:315-21.

SECTION 3

Diabetic Retinopathy

Proliferative Diabetic Retinopathy: Surgical Considerations

17

Nakhleh E Abu-Yaghi, Sophie J Bakri

Introduction

The underlying abnormality in all proliferative vascular retinopathies is retinal ischemia. Proliferative diabetic retinopathy (PDR), retinal venous occlusive disease, sickle-cell retinopathy and retinopathy of prematurity can all share proliferative fibrovascular membranes, vitreous hemorrhage and/or retinal detachment.[1]

Since the first vitrectomy for vitreous hemorrhage from PDR was performed in 1971,[2] indications and techniques of vitreoretinal surgery have changed considerably. High speed vitrectomy instruments, wide-field viewing systems and transconjunctival approaches have facilitated the objectives of diabetic vitrectomy.[3] The introduction of endolaser and better understanding of the vitreoretinal interface pathology have led to a paradigm shift in the surgical treatment of PDR and its complications.

Pathophysiology

Ischemia driven retinal vascular changes are punctuated by the production of angiogenic factors.[4] Vascular endothelial growth factor (VEGF) is the most important factor implicated, with VEGF mRNA localized in retina and neovascular tissue. VEGF expression is enhanced by hypoxia.[5] Sites of VEGF expression include: glial cells (Müller cells), anterior optic nerve cells, retinal astrocytes, retinal pigment epithelial cells, retinal vascular endothelial cells and retinal ganglion cells.[6] Other growth factors include insulin-like growth factor-1 (IGF-1) and basic fibroblast growth factor (bFGF).

Angiogenesis is a cascade of events that may cause:

- Development of neovascular buds (vascular epicenters)
- Proliferation of new vessels in the potential space between the retina and vitreous
- Invasion of the posterior lamellae of the cortical vitreous producing a very firm adhesion
- Fibrous element contraction exerting traction on the friable vascular tissue and the retina, resulting in hemorrhage and tractional retinal detachment
- Formation of retinal breaks (usually near fibrovascular proliferative epicenters) which may result in a combined rhegmatogenous/tractional detachment.

In approaching those cases, a careful assessment of the vitreoretinal interface is paramount.[7] In particular, it is important to assess the degree of posterior vitreous separation and the type of vitreoretinal adhesions.

Degree of Posterior Vitreous Separation

There are four categories:

- No or minimal posterior vitreous separation (manifesting as preretinal hemorrhage, dragged macula, or tractional diabetic macular edema)
- Partial vitreous separation (attached at posterior pole and at mid-peripheral retina)
- Fully detached vitreous at mid-periphery but attached at posterior pole
- Complete posterior vitreous detachment.

Type of Vitreoretinal Adhesions

- *Focal adhesions:* Multiple focal adhesions are the most common. Epiretinal membranes may surround the focal adhesion producing a broader attachment. The vitreous may or may not be separated around the adhesions and a tractional and/or rhegmatogenous retinal detachment may occur around the adhesions.
- *Broad adhesions:* Either associated (more commonly) or not associated with folding of the underlying retina. Vitreoretinal adhesions with underlying retinal folds may have a smooth plaque like appearance but the underlying retina is corrugated and almost always detached. The vitreous around the broad detachment is usually separated, at least in part.

Vitreoretinal attachments may predict visual and surgical outcomes after surgery.[7] Extensive vitreoretinal attachments correlated with higher rates of membrane reproliferation and worse visual outcome.

Other factors affecting the surgical approach include the presence of vitreous hemorrhage and the presence, location and chronicity of retinal detachment, the degree of active neovascularization and previous panretinal photocoagulation.[8]

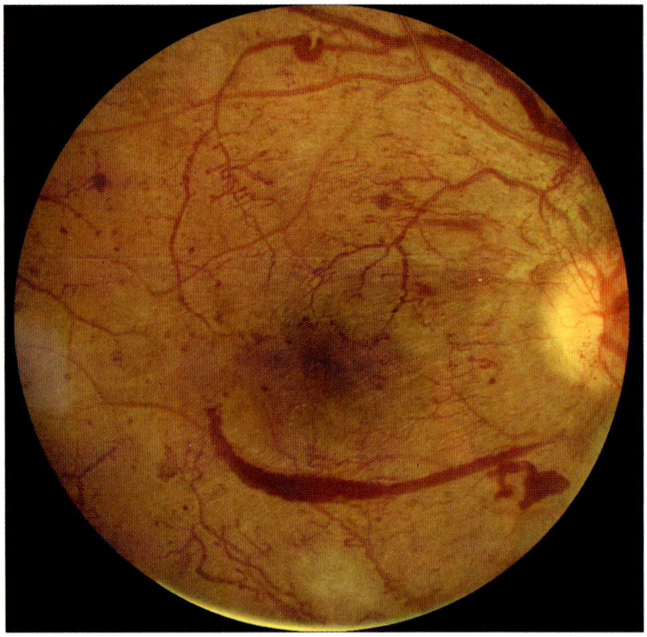

▲ **Figure 17.1**

Color photograph showing severe PDR, as indicated by NVD, NVE, intraretinal microvascular abnormalities and subhyaloid hemorrhage

Surgical Indications

For decades the major indications have remained the same (Figs 17.1 to 17.7):

- Severe non-clearing vitreous hemorrhage
- Tractional retinal detachment involving the macula
- Combined tractional or rhegmatogenous detachment

Early additional indications included progressive fibrovascular proliferation, severe vitreous hemorrhage in the presence of rubeosis and ghost-cell glaucoma.[9]

The first results of the Diabetic Retinopathy Vitrectomy Study (DRVS) were reported in 1985 and provided considerable additional experience and further refined the role of vitrectomy.[10] This study was designed to evaluate the risks and benefits of performing early pars plana vitrectomy in eyes with advanced PDR. It was a multicenter, prospective, randomized clinical trial that comprised three studies. One was a natural history study that included eyes with severe proliferative diabetic retinopathy but without severe vitreous hemorrhage and these eyes were followed with conventional management. The other two studies were randomized clinical

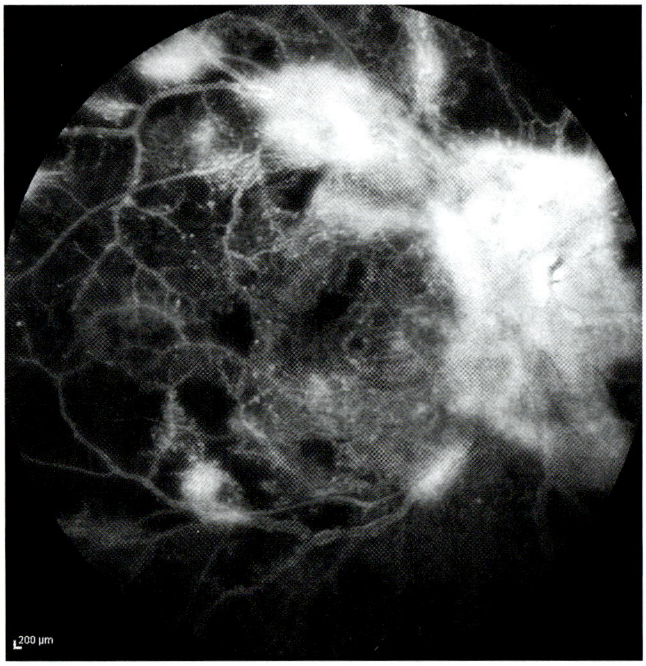

▲ **Figure 17.2**

Fluorescein angiogram of right eye showing leakage from severe NVD and leakage from fibrovascular proliferation on the arcades. There is also capillary nonperfusion in the temporal macula

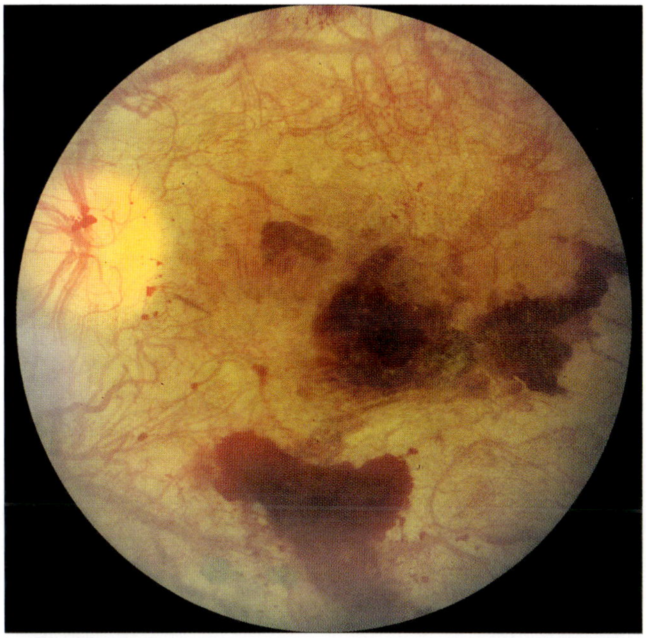

▲ **Figure 17.3**

Color photograph showing severe PDR, as indicated by NVD, NVE, intraretinal microvascular abnormalities and subhyaloid hemorrhage. Note the large hemorrhages are preretinal or subhyaloid and there is a taut thickened posterior hyaloids overlying them

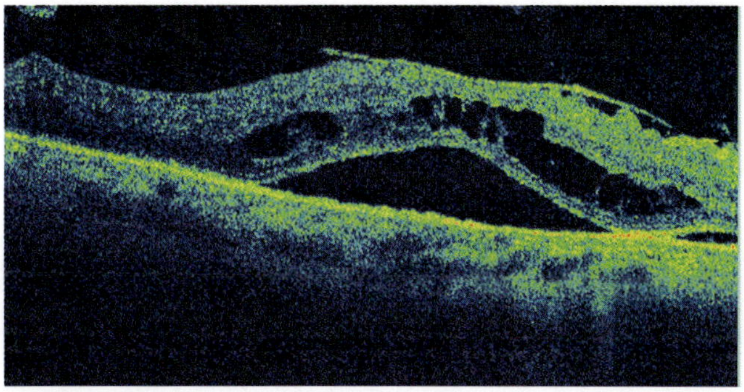

▲ **Figure 17.4**

Optical coherence tomography showing taut posterior hyaloid, with CME and subretinal fluid

trials involving vitrectomy. The first compared early vitrectomy versus deferral of surgery in eyes with severe vitreous hemorrhage and the second compared early vitrectomy versus conventional management in eyes with severe PDR. More recent literature has supported the impression that visual outcomes following diabetic vitrectomy are continually improving with newer techniques.[11]

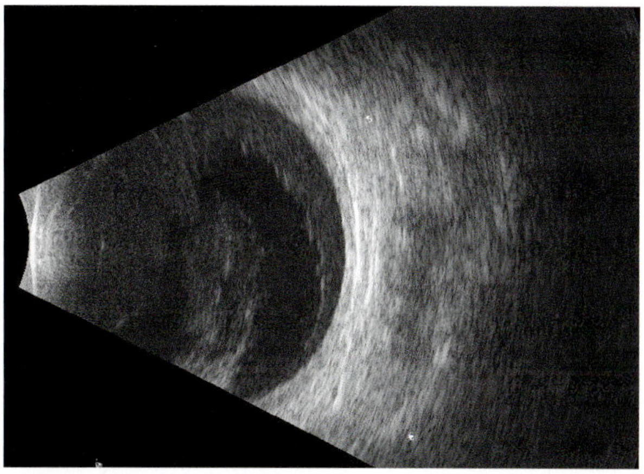

▲ **Figure 17.5**

B scan ultrasound showing traction retinal detachment

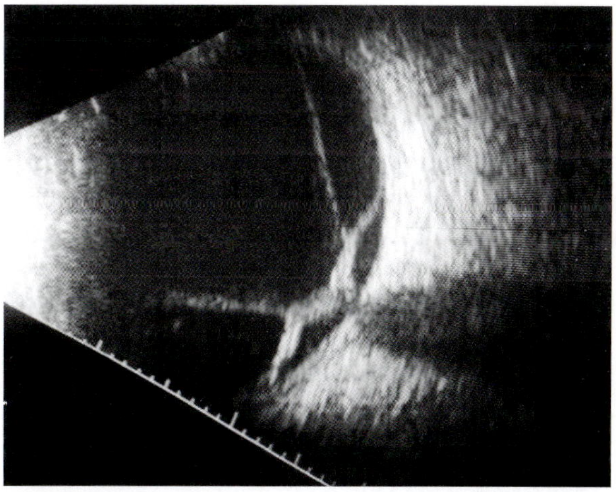

▲ **Figure 17.6**

B scan ultrasound showing subhyaloid hemorrhage and vitreous hemorrhage

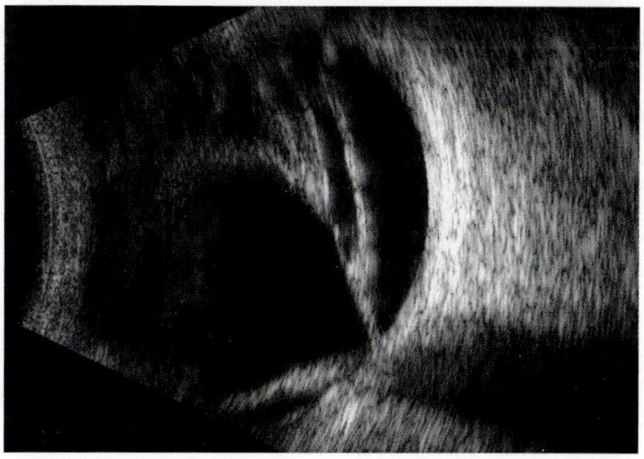

▲ **Figure 17.7**

B scan ultrasound showing funnel retinal detachment

Severe Non-clearing Vitreous Hemorrhage

This remains a major indication for vitrectomy despite the reduction in prevalence after the advent of panretinal photocoagulation.[12-14] Restricting patient activity and elevating the head of the patient's bed are additional conservative measures that are usually initially recommended. B scan ultrasonography is essential if no view of the fundus is available. Vitrectomy is indicated if spontaneous clearing of a dense vitreous hemorrhage does not occur.

Enzymatic vitreolysis has been investigated in patients with vitreous hemorrhage and may emerge as an adjunct in the future.[15-16]

The Diabetic Retinopathy Vitrectomy Study (DRVS) extensively evaluated the timing of vitrectomy for eyes with vitreous hemorrhage. Specifically, it examined the outcome of early (before 6 months) versus deferred (1 year) vitrectomy for severe vitreous hemorrhage, defined as central vitreous hemorrhage reducing visual acuity to 5/200 or less for at least 1 month. Patients were classified as having type 1 diabetes if diabetes was diagnosed at or before age 20 years and if they were receiving insulin at the time of entry into the study. Type 2 diabetes included patients aged 40 years or older at diagnosis (regardless of insulin use) and patients with diabetes diagnosed at a younger age if they were not receiving insulin. An intermediate group comprised patients diagnosed between 21 and 39 years of age, inclusive, who were receiving insulin.

The study demonstrated that in type 1 diabetes patients with vitreous hemorrhage, vitrectomy performed within 6 months gave more favorable visual and anatomic results than did deferral of surgery for 1 year or longer. In the type 2 and intermediate groups, however, the results of vitrectomy performed at these two different intervals were the same. It must be noted that the DRVS was performed before the development of endolaser photocoagulation. Since then vitrectomy instrumentation has continued to improve and it is believed that this has translated to better visual outcomes. Generally, the recommended timing of vitrectomy for severe diabetic vitreous hemorrhage is before 3 months for type 1 diabetics and 6 months for type 2 patients.[16] Surgical goals include removal of vitreous hemorrhage to provide a clear medium, excision of the posterior hyaloid and epiretinal fibrovascular membranes to relieve vitreoretinal traction and application of endolaser photocoagulation to achieve regression of proliferative tissue.

Traction Retinal Detachment Involving or Threatening the Macula

Traction retinal detachment results from progressive fibrovascular proliferation and contraction. This type of detachment typically has a concave appearance, is relatively immobile and is stable or exhibits slow progression. The aim of vitrectomy is to relieve vitreoretinal traction, both anteroposterior and tangential, by removing the posterior hyaloid and epiretinal fibrovascular membranes.[17] The duration and the extent of the detachment, the presence of prior laser treatment and the degree of neovascularization can all affect the surgical outcome.

Extramacular detachments usually do not progress to involve the macula and therefore do not cause severe visual loss. Vitrectomy therefore is not often performed in these cases.[18] Studies have demonstrated that in some patients with progressive traction detachment that threatens the macula, early vitrectomy is beneficial.[19] These patients present with partial vitreous detachment, vitreoretinal traction along the arcades and/or disc, retinal traction lines (striae) extending through the fovea and progressive visual loss. Because of improved surgical techniques and instrumentation, as well as a better understanding of the disease process, many surgeons have taken the indication one step further to include traction detachment threatening the macula or causing macular distortion.

Macular detachment greater than 6 months to 1 year is usually atrophic, tightly adherent and is associated with irreversible photoreceptor loss. Surgery in these cases is of very limited value to visual acuity.

Combined Traction or Rhegmatogenous Retinal Detachment

A combined traction or rhegmatogenous detachments occurs when a retinal break is created by contraction of fibrotic tissue.[20] Sudden visual loss may occur, as a detachment with a rhegmatogenous component often progresses rapidly. In this type of detachment the retina appears convex and it may be bullous and mobile. Careful inspection usually reveals hydration lines and retinal break(s). The retinal break is usually located posterior to the equator and adjacent to or underneath areas of fibrovascular proliferation. The break is often small and may be obscured by vitreous hemorrhage; breaks within previous laser photocoagulation can also occur.

A prompt vitrectomy is needed in these cases. Posterior breaks and persistent traction usually limit the use of scleral buckling. Relief of all traction and closure of all breaks are the goals of surgery. If the rhegmatogenous component extends to involve the macula then the visual prognosis is much worse.

Dense Premacular Hemorrhage

This pertains to intraocular hemorrhage trapped between the macula and the posterior hyaloid face in an incomplete vitreous detachment. This has a round or oval appearance and is usually dense with pronounced drop of vision. If the vitreous completely detaches, the bleeding may break through and disperse. Nd:YAG posterior hyaloidotomy can be attempted to drain the blood in the vitreous cavity and allow subsequent focal laser treatment of the macula.[21]

Progressive fibrovascular proliferation along the posterior surface of the vitreous can ensue, leading to macular detachment. The optimal timing of intervention in these cases is controversial: some studies recommend surgery within 1 month of the onset of a dense premacular hemorrhage.[22] More extensive membrane peeling is required if surgery is delayed and macular distortion often remains. A surgical plane is already established by the hemorrhage, facilitating removal of the posterior hyaloid. Panretinal laser photocoagulation is then added.

Severe Fibrovascular Proliferation

In poorly controlled diabetics with an attached posterior hyaloid, active neovascular and fibrovascular proliferation may progress despite extensive laser treatment. The fibrovascular tissue usually undergoes contraction resulting in vitreous hemorrhage, macular distortion, and/or retinal detachment. Vitrectomy surgery is indicated in some of these cases to excise the posterior cortical vitreous and to reattach the retina.[23]

The DRVS extensively evaluated the timing of vitrectomy for eyes with advanced, active proliferative diabetic retinopathy and useful vision. It compared the outcome of early vitrectomy versus conventional management in eyes with visual acuity of 10/200 or better and extensive, active, neovascular or fibrovascular proliferations. This was defined as severe new vessels (four or more disc areas) and severe fibrous proliferation (two or more disc areas at the disc, or four or more disc areas total); severe new vessels and red vitreous hemorrhage (any preretinal or vitreous hemorrhage); or moderate new vessels (two or more disc areas), severe fibrous proliferation and red vitreous hemorrhage. Conventional management included observation, photocoagulation and vitrectomy only after traction macular detachment or 6 months of non-clearing vitreous hemorrhage. The study demonstrated that early vitrectomy gave more favorable visual and anatomic results than did conventional management.

Diabetic Macular Edema Associated with Posterior Hyaloidal Traction

The lack of posterior vitreous detachment is thought to be one factor in the pathogenesis of macular edema in a subset of diabetic eyes with a diffusely thickened posterior hyaloid. Macular edema in these patients is usually refractory to macular grid laser albeit a good capillary perfusion. One study suggested that spontaneous vitreomacular separation may promote the resolution of diabetic macular edema and improve visual acuity.[24] Vitrectomy with elevation of the posterior hyaloid can resolve the macular edema is select cases.[25]

Hemolytic or Ghost Cell Glaucoma

Old and less pliable blood cells can clog the outflow in the trabecular meshwork and cause elevated intraocular pressure (IOP). Blood-induced open-angle glaucoma may also result from erythrocytic debris and/or macrophages containing erythrocytic debris (hemolytic cells). Ghost cell or hemolytic glaucoma typically occurs in aphakic eyes with a disrupted anterior hyaloid face. It may also occur after surgery for non-clearing vitreous hemorrhage, as the peripheral residual vitreous skirt acts as a reservoir for degenerated erythrocytes and blood products. If IOP cannot be controlled medically, vitrectomy is indicated to manage this problem.[26]

Anterior Segment Neovascularization with Media Opacity

Anterior segment neovascularization arises secondary to retinal ischemia and panretinal photocoagulation is performed to prevent neovascular glaucoma. Dense vitreous hemorrhage in an eye with progressive rubeosis is an indication for vitrectomy. In eyes with established neovascular glaucoma, vitrectomy surgery (usually with lensectomy and endolaser) in conjunction with anterior chamber or pars plana tube implantation is a reasonable approach.[27]

Surgical Objectives and Techniques

Surgery for PDR involves[3]:

- Removal of media opacities
- Relieving anteroposterior and tangential traction
- Delamination of preretinal membranes
- Stopping bleeding and effecting hemostasis
- Closing all retinal breaks
- Delivering adequate laser treatment
- Keeping the retina attached.

Removal of Media Opacities

Standard visualization is achieved by an operating microscope, endoillumination and a wide-angle optical viewing system. The vitreous cutter, extrusion needle and the fragmatome can be used to remove axial opacities. Increasingly complex surgeries are being performed using small gauge systems (23-or 25-gauge vitrectomy). The vitreous cutter combines suction and cutting and the light probe can be combined to a pick, forceps or laser delivery. A multi-port illumination system allows a bimanual approach. Wide-field viewing systems facilitate a global view of the posterior segment and iris retractors can be used to allow a maximum view in patients with small pupils.

Relieving Vitreoretinal Traction

The following techniques mesh to achieve this goal. Although conceptually distinct, surgery is usually a combination of all three approaches[28] (Figs 17.8 to 17.14):

1. *Segmentation:* Involves sequential dissection and removal of traction from anterior to posterior, with dissection of bridging epiretinal traction. This is followed by removing any residual epiretinal membranes.
2. *Delamination:* Entails removal of anteroposterior traction using horizontal instruments to remove preretinal tissue.
3. *"En bloc":* This technique uses the anteroposterior traction of the vitreous as countertraction ("third hand") to remove surface membranes. This "third hand" is removed last with the bulk of the vitreous.

Control of Bleeding

Blood and fibrin will act as media opacities but will also serve as promoters of cellular proliferation. Strategies to affect hemostasis include[29-32]:

- Use of intraocular diathermy
- Increasing the infusion pressure
- Using intraocular thrombin
- Preoperative treatment with an anti-VEGF agent (e.g. intravitreal bevacizumab).

Intraoperative panretinal photocoagulation reduces the rate of postoperative hemorrhage.[32] Silicone oil may block diffusion of vasoproliferative mediators, although this is widely debated. Lensectomy is associated with an increased risk of postoperative rubeosis, although adequate application of laser can prevent this.

Intraoperative Issues

Corneal Edema

Corneal epithelial edema can result from inadequate lubrication of the corneal surface, especially in prolonged procedures. Endothelial damage and elevated IOP can also contribute to this. This may impair visualization and scraping the epithelium gently with a blade may become necessary. Changes in pressure during air-fluid exchange can also produce Descemet folds and hinder visualization. Protecting the endothelium with viscoelastic can help prevent or delay this problem.

Pupillary Constriction

Dilating drops can be applied topically or added to the infusion fluid to prevent or counteract pupillary constriction. This is common in lengthy procedures, after lensectomy or air-fluid exchange. Iris hooks can also be used.[33]

Lens Opacities

Cataracts and lens opacities can occur due to iatrogenic instrument contact with the posterior capsule. Eddie currents from the infusion can also lead to lens opacities especially in long cases. Adding glucose to the infusion fluid can minimize lens feathering in diabetics. Injecting gas or oil in a phakic eye will eventually lead to cataract formation. In patients who have a cataract and require complex diabetic vitrectomy surgery, the lens may be removed prior to vitrectomy[34] by a phacoemulsification approach and implantation of a posterior chamber intraocular lens. Doing this several weeks prior to surgery allows the eye to heal and facilitates dissection and removal of the vitreous especially if work on the peripheral retina is to be performed.

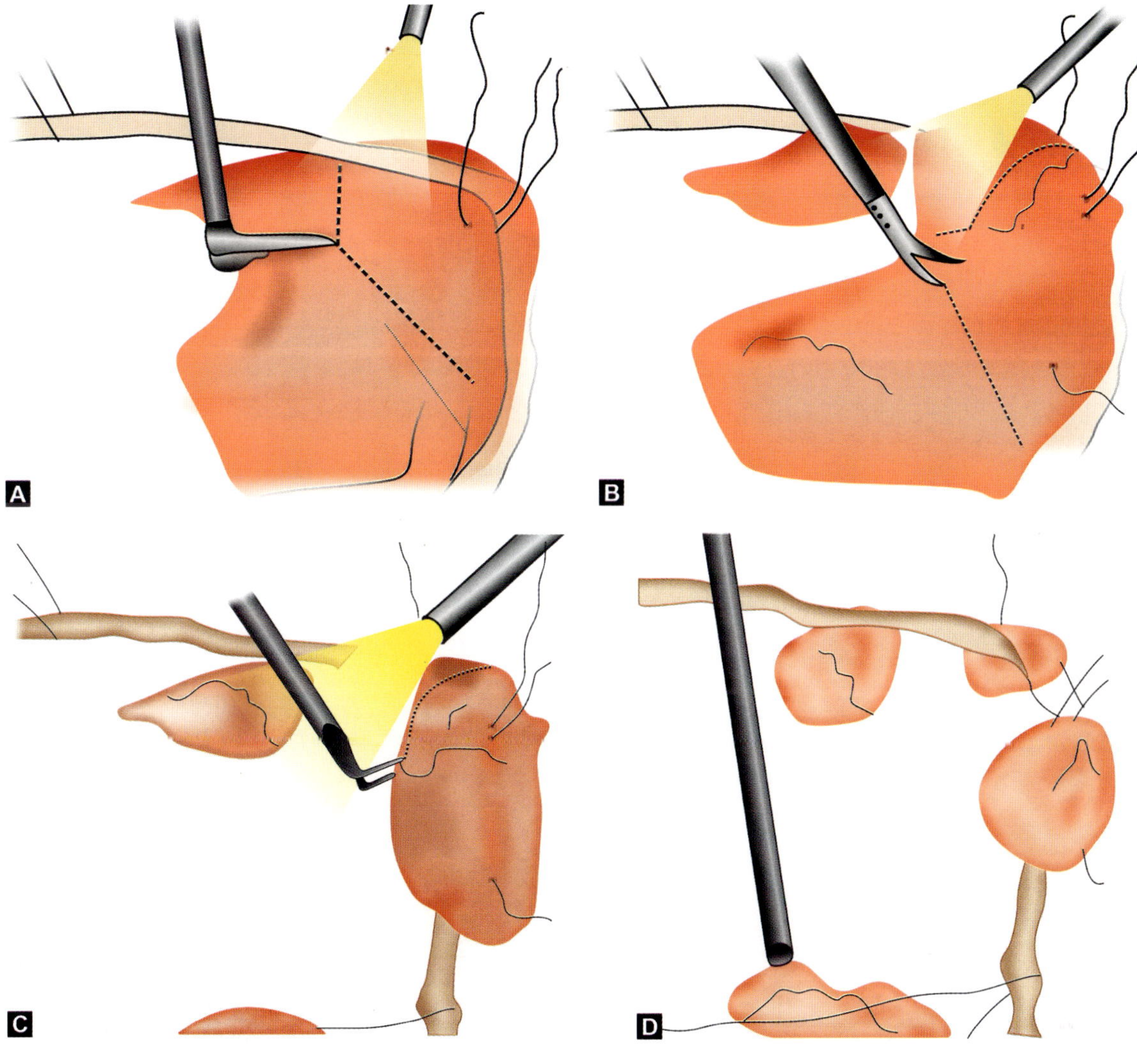

▲ **Figures 17.8A to D**

Membrane surgery. Segmentation resulting in islands of tissue with no residual traction

▶ Intraocular Hemorrhage

Bleeding can occur from sclerotomy sites, neovascularization of the iris, retina and disc and normal vessels of the iris, retina and choroid. Management entails elevating the infusion fluid container to increase the IOP. Lowering the pressure can assist in identifying sites of bleeding. This can be done rapidly by the surgeon through a preset foot pedal. Intraocular diathermy is used to treat the source of the hemorrhage. Thrombin can be mixed with the infusion fluid to reduce bleeding in selected cases.[35] Clotted blood can be adherent to the retina and must be stripped carefully to prevent causing a retinal break.

▶ Retinal Breaks

Retinal breaks can occur in the periphery or posteriorly. Peripheral retinal breaks and dialyses may occur as a result of engaging vitreous with the tip of an instrument inserted through the sclerotomy. Another mechanism of peripheral retinal break formation is extrusion of vitreous through a sclerotomy, in which case a horseshoe-shaped tear may

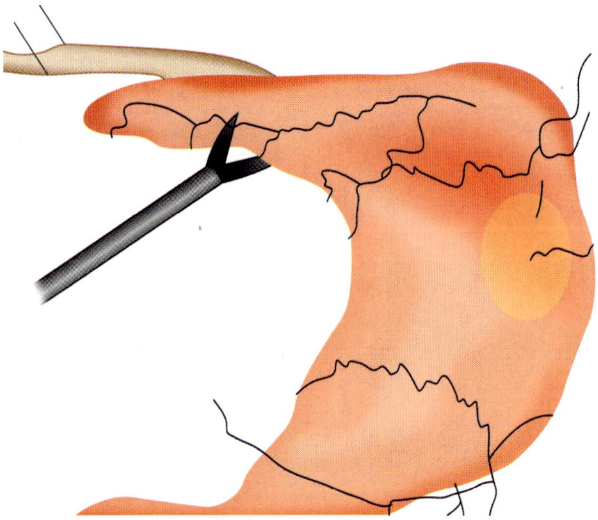

▲ **Figure 17.9**

Membrane surgery. Delamination procedure in progress. Horizontal bladed scissors is used to cut the attachments of fibrovascular tissue

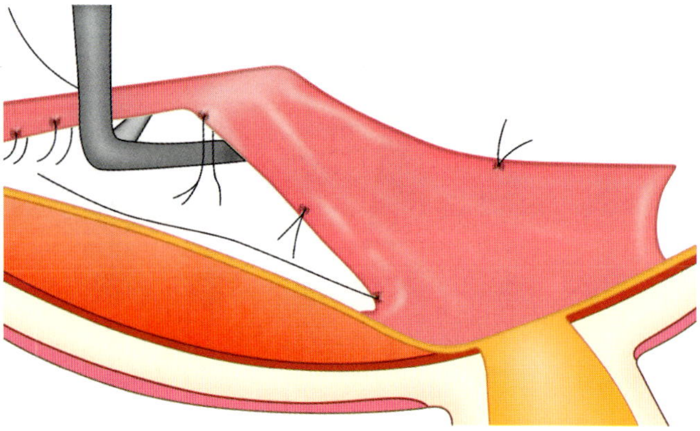

▲ **Figure 17.11**

Membrane surgery. Spreading the blades of scissors can sometimes be used to separate a relatively loose adhesion of fibrovascular tissue

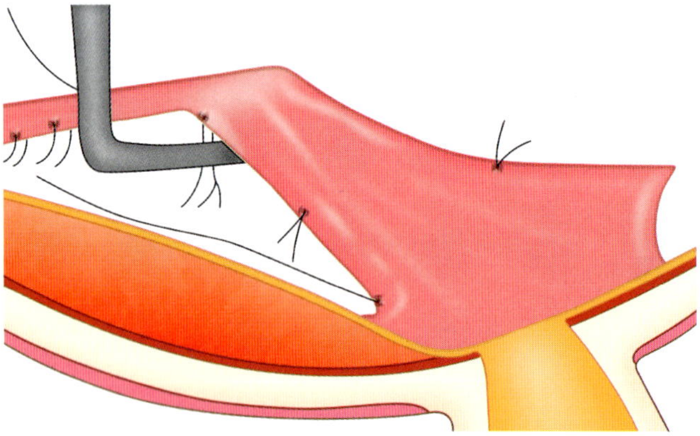

▲ **Figure 17.10**

Membrane surgery. A sharp pic is used to lift the fibrovascular tissue. Loose attachments can be peeled off using a pic-like device

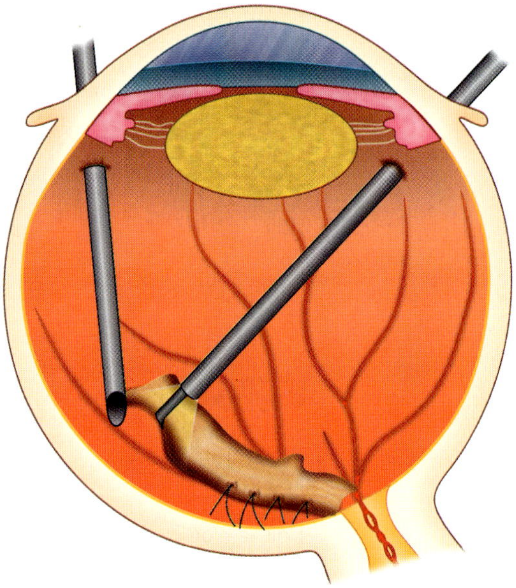

▲ **Figure 17.12**

Membrane surgery. Bimanual dissection using the illuminated pic and cutter

occur at the posterior edge of the vitreous base behind the sclerotomy. The treatment of peripheral retinal breaks typically includes cryotherapy or laser photocoagulation and tamponade with gas or oil. A scleral buckle may be necessary for inferior breaks or in cases of persistent traction.

For posterior retinal breaks, diathermy is used to label the break to facilitate visualization under air. Traction is

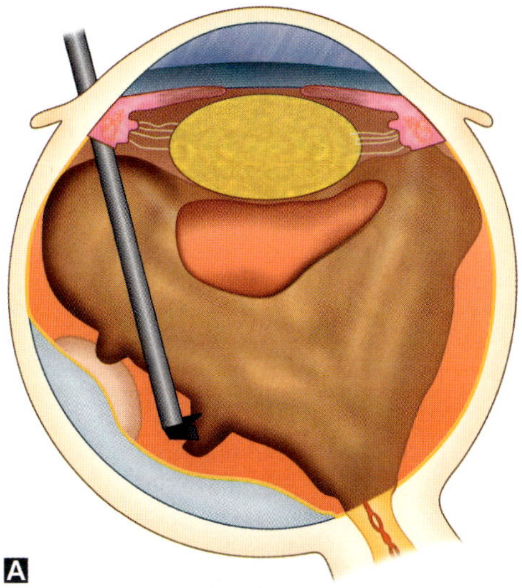

A

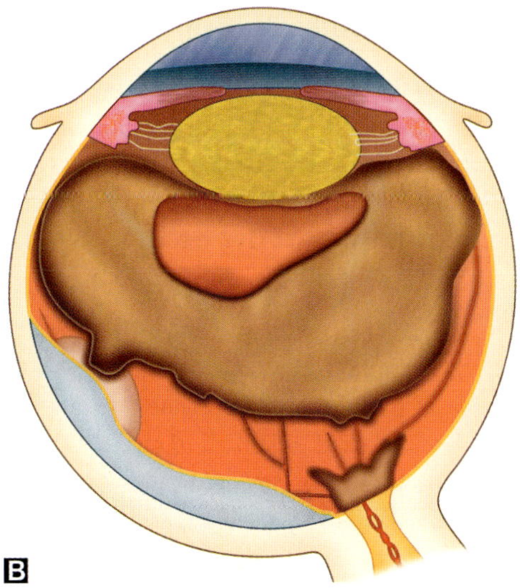

B

▲ Figures 17.13A and B

Membrane surgery. En bloc dissection

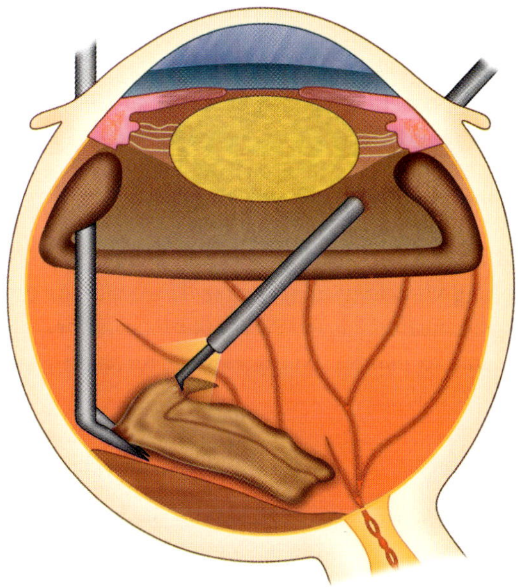

▲ Figure 17.14

Membrane surgery. Bimanual dissection using the illuminated pic and scissors to complete the en bloc dissection

removed and a fluid-air exchange is performed, with subretinal fluid drained through the break.[36]

Postoperative Care

▶ Elevated Intraocular Pressure

Approximately one-third of post-vitrectomy eyes will have IOP >30 mm Hg within the first 2 days.[37] Risk factors include: use of intraocular gas or oil, lensectomy, excessive panretinal photocoagulation and placing a scleral buckle.

Management

Prophylactic topical medications may be given, including a beta-blocker, an alpha-agonist, a carbonic anhydrase inhibitor and a prostaglandin analog. IOP should be measured and followed postoperatively. An anterior chamber tap (or rarely a vitreous tap) can be done for IOP above 40 mm Hg uncontrolled by medications.

Intraocular pressure can be elevated after gas tamponade due to gas expansion or angle closure from forward iris displacement. Keeping the patient face down will position the bubble posteriorly and allow aqueous accumulation in the anterior chamber.[38] Gas can be tapped from the eye. Injection of tissue plasminogen activator (tPA) can relieve pupillary block from fibrin accumulation. Steroids and cycloplegics may help in high IOP cases where choroidal detachments have resulted in angle closure and forward displacement of the iris.[39]

▶ Corneal Epithelial Defects

Persistent epithelial defects in diabetics undergoing eye surgery stem from an abnormal basement membrane that interferes with re-epithelialization.[40] Corneal vascularization can follow endothelial cell damage and may result in irreversible opacification.

Management

Lubricants and patching are first line of treatment. Bandage contact lenses and a temporary tarsorrhaphy can be attempted for nonhealing defects.

Lens Opacification

The incidence of visually significant cataracts in diabetics undergoing vitrectomy ranges from 15–35%.[41] As discussed previously, instrument touch, bubble induced opacities and intraoperative osmotic shifts can all result in significant cataract formation.

Management

Cataract extraction is usually delayed 3–6 months after vitrectomy and the use of silicon intraocular lenses is usually avoided to prevent condensations on the lens if further vitreoretinal surgeries are needed. Furthermore, silicon oil can irreversibly bind to these lenses.[42] In select cases it may be advisable to perform phacoemulsification and intraocular lens implantation prior to vitrectomy surgery.

Rubeosis and Neovascular Glaucoma

Neovascular glaucoma usually develops in eyes with established neovascularization which had little or no PRP preoperatively.[43]

Management

The incidence of this complication has decreased considerably with the development of endolaser and improvements in retinal reattachment techniques. Frequent application of postoperative steroid drops can suppress anterior segment inflammation and lower incidence of postoperative inflammation induced glaucoma. Glaucoma surgery is reserved for refractory cases.

Anterior Hyaloidal Fibrovascular Proliferation

This is a severe complication after diabetic vitrectomy that usually occurs in phakic insulin dependent diabetics with profound retinal ischemia and florid neovascularization but with good renal function and normal blood pressures. Patients who develop this complication tend to be young males with severe retinal neovascularization and extensive retinal ischemia. Risk factors included traction retinal detachment as an indication for surgery, placement of a scleral buckle, postoperative rubeosis irides, recurrent vitreous hemorrhages, retinal detachment and multiple surgeries. Fibrovascular proliferation extends anteriorly to the posterior lens capsule from the ischemic peripheral retina or from a previous sclerotomy site.[44]

Management

This condition requires a high index of suspicion and is managed by aggressive PRP to the anterior retina. In the setting of vitreous hemorrhage and tractional retinal detachment, vitrectomy, lensectomy, careful dissection of anterior membranes and adequate PRP with or without silicone oil are often necessary.

Fibrinoid Syndrome and Intraocular Fibrin Formation

Fibrinoid syndrome describes massive fibrin formation in the vitreous cavity producing pupillary membranes, tractional retinal detachments and neovascular glaucoma.[45] The usual picture is a case that has undergone a scleral buckle placement, lensectomy, extensive retinal surgery and laser.

Management

Subconjunctival dexamethasone can help prevent fibrin formation, but if pupillary block ensues, then intracameral tPA is the current accepted treatment of choice. This is usually injected on the 2 or 3 days postoperatively as it can lead to intraocular hemorrhage. Repeat vitrectomy with injection of silicone oil may be the last resort in severe cases. Those cases usually fair poorly.

Vitreous Hemorrhage

Postoperative vitreous hemorrhage is a very common problem with incidence ranging between 30–75%.[46] Early onset postoperative hemorrhage may result from remnants of fibrovascular membranes, or blood remaining on the retina or within the peripheral vitreous skirt. Weeks to months after surgery, hemorrhage can occur due to neovascularization of the angle, iris or sclerotomy site. Persistent fibrovascular membranes can also re-bleed at this time.[47]

Management

Prevention of this problem starts intraoperatively, with meticulous control of intraoperative bleeding. Postoperative management involves observation with serial B scan ultrasonography. Repeat vitrectomy is indicated for non-clearing vitreous hemorrhage and the waiting period has increasingly become less with advancing techniques. Eyes requiring a second vitrectomy may need extensive laser with extended tamponade and will usually have a less favorable prognosis.[48]

Intravitreal injection of bevacizumab (Avastin) preoperatively may prove a very useful adjunct in the surgical management of severe PDR. Many studies have demonstrated that this helps reduce retinal and iris neovascularization and improve anatomical and surgical outcomes. The best timing of injection may be up to 7 days preoperatively.[49] In most case series, the injection was deemed safe without any observed complications, although increased fibrosis and adhesions were observed in some cases.[50] Some, but not all studies, have reported a decrease in the rate of postoperative vitreous hemorrhage in eyes pretreated with bevacizumab.[51]

Bevacizumab can also be effective if injected after vitrectomy in a silicone-filled eye,[52] and as an adjunct to treat neovascular glaucoma after vitrectomy for PDR. Post vitrectomy injection of bevacizumab has been found to clear postoperative vitreous hemorrhage in PDR patients, but higher incidence of ghost cell glaucoma has been observed in those eyes.[53]

References

1. Eliott D, et al. Proliferative Diabetic Retinopathy: Principles and Techniques of Surgical Treatment. In: Ryan SJ (Ed). Retina, 4th edition. Elsevier Inc; 2006. pp. 2413-49.
2. Machemer R, Buettner H, Norton EW, et al. Vitrectomy: a pars plana approach. Trans Am Acad Ophthalmol Otolaryngol. 1971;75:813-20.
3. Smiddy W, Harry W, Flynn JR. Vitrectomy for diabetic retinopathy. In Diabetes and Ocular disease: Past, Present and Future Therapies. Ophthalmology Monographs 14. 2nd edition. 207-34.
4. Henkind P. Ocular neovascularization. The Krill memorial lecture. Am J Ophthalmol. 1978;85:287-301.
5. Pe'er J, Shweiki D, Itin A, et al. Hypoxia-induced expression of vascular endothelial growth factor (VEGF) by retinal cells is a common factor in neovascularization. Lab Invest. 1995;72:638-45.
6. Amin RH, Frank RN, Kennedy A, et al. Vascular endothelial growth factor is present in glial cells of the retina and optic nerve of human subjects with nonproliferative diabetic retinopathy. Invest Ophthalmol Vis Sci. 1997;38:36-47.
7. Eliott D. Vitreoretinal attachments in proliferative diabetic retinopathy: effect on outcome. In: Vail vitrectomy meeting. Vail, CO: 2004.
8. Fukumoto M, Nakai T, Maeno T, Mano T. Effectiveness of preoperative panretinal photocoagulation in severe proliferative diabetic retinopathy. Nippon Ganka Gakkai Zasshi. 2009;113:901-5.
9. Brucker AJ, Michels RG, Green WR. Pars plana vitrectomy in the management of blood-induced glaucoma with vitreous hemorrhage. Ann Ophthalmol. 1978;10:1427-37.
10. Diabetic Retinopathy Vitrectomy Study Research Group. Two-year course of visual acuity in severe proliferative diabetic retinopathy with conventional management, Diabetic Retinopathy Vitrectomy Study report 1. Ophthalmology. 1985;92: 492-502.
11. Mason JO, Colagross CT, Haleman T, et al. Visual outcome and risk factors for light perception vision after vitrectomy for diabetic retinopathy. Am J Ophthalmol. 2005;140:231-5.
12. Diabetic Retinopathy Vitrectomy Study Research Group. Early vitrectomy for severe proliferative diabetic retinopathy in eyes with useful vision: results of a randomized trial, Diabetic Retinopathy Vitrectomy Study report 3. Ophthalmology. 1988;95:1307-14.
13. Diabetic Retinopathy Vitrectomy Study Research Group. Early vitrectomy for severe proliferative diabetic retinopathy in eyes with useful vision: clinical application of results of a randomized trial, Diabetic Retinopathy Vitrectomy Study report 4. Ophthalmology. 1988;95:1321-34.
14. Kuppermann BD, Thomas EL, de Smet MD, et al. Pooled efficacy results from two multinational randomised controlled clinical trials of a single intravitreous injection of highly purified ovine hyaluronidase (Vitrase) for the management of vitreous hemorrhage. Am J Ophthalmol. 2005;140:573-84.
15. Kuppermann BD, Thomas EL, de Smet MD, et al. Safety results of two phase III trials of an intravitreous injection of highly purified ovine hyaluronidase (Vitrase) for the management of vitreous hemorrhage. Am J Ophthalmol. 2005;140:585-97.
16. Ho T, Smiddy WE, Flynn HW. Vitrectomy in the management of diabetic eye disease. Surv Ophthalmol. 1992;37:190-202.
17. Charles S. Vitrectomy for retinal detachment. Trans Ophthalmol Soc UK. 1980;100:542-9.
18. Charles S, Flinn CE. The natural history of diabetic extramacular traction retinal detachment. Arch Ophthalmol. 1981;99:66-8.
19. Ratner CM, Michels RG, Auer C, et al. Pars plana vitrectomy for complicated retinal detachments. Ophthalmology. 1983;90:1323-7.
20. Blankenship GW. Posterior retinal holes secondary to diabetic retinopathy. Arch Ophthalmol. 1983;101:885-7.
21. Ezra E, Dowler JG, Burgess F, et al. Identifying maculopathy after neodymium:YAG membranotomy for dense diabetic premacular hemorrhage. Ophthalmology. 1996; 103:1568-74.
22. Eliott D. Outcome of vitrectomy for dense, premacular, subhyaloid hemorrhage secondary to proliferative diabetic retinopathy. In: Retina Society/Vitreous Society annual meeting - the combined meeting. San Francisco, CA: 2002.

23. Blankenship GW, Machemer R. Long-term diabetic vitrectomy results: report of 10-year follow-up. Ophthalmology. 1985;92:503-6.
24. Hikichi T, Fujio N, Akiba J, et al. Association between the short-term natural history of diabetic macular edema and the vitreomacular relationship in type II diabetes mellitus. Ophthalmology. 1997;104:473-8.
25. Kaiser PK, Riemann CD, Sears JE, et al. Macular traction detachment and diabetic macular edema associated with posterior hyaloidal traction. Am J Ophthalmol. 2001;131:44-9.
26. Han DP, Lewis H, Lambrou FH, et al. Mechanisms of intraocular pressure elevation after pars plana vitrectomy. Ophthalmology. 1989;96:1357-62.
27. Lloyd MA, Heuer DK, Baerveldt G, et al. Combined molteno implantation and pars plana vitrectomy for neovascular glaucomas. Ophthalmology. 1991;98:140-5.
28. Abrams GW. Dissection methods in vitrectomy for diabetic retinopathy. In: Franklin RM, (Ed), Retina and Vitreous. Amsterdam/New York: Kugler Publication;1993.pp.101-13.
29. Thompson JT, Glaser BM, Michels RG, et al. The use of intravitreal thrombin to control hemorrhageduring vitrectomy. Ophthalmology. 1986;103:279-82.
30. Spaide, RF, Fisher YL. Intravitreal bevacizumab (Avastin) treatment of proliferative diabetic retinopathy complicated by vitreous hemorrhage. Retina. 2006;26:275-8.
31. Bakri SJ, Donaldson MJ, Link TP. Rapid regression of disc neovascularization in a patient with proliferative diabetic retinopathy following adjunctive intravitreal bevacizumab. Eye. 2006;20:1474-5.
32. McCuen BW, Rinkoff JS. Silicon oil for progressiveanterior ocular neovascularization after failed diabetic vitrectomy. Arch Ophthalnol. 1989;107:677-82.
33. Fuller DG, Wilson DL. Translimbal iris hook for pupillary dilation during vitreous surgery. Am J Ophthalmol. 1990;110: 577.
34. Haimann MH, Abrams GW. Prevention of lens opacification during diabetic vitrectomy. Ophthalmology. 1984;91:116-21.
35. De Bustros S, Glaser BM, Johnson MA. Thrombin infusion for the control of intraocular bleeding during vitreous surgery. Arch Ophthalmol. 1985;103:837-9.
36. Abrams GW. En bloc dissection techniques in vitrectomy for diabetic retinopathy. In: Lewis H, Ryan SJ (Eds). Medical and Surgical Retina: advances, controversies, and management. St. Louis: Mosby; 1994. pp. 304-20.
37. Han DP, Lewis H, Lambrou FH, et al. Mechanisms of intraocular pressure elevation after pars plana vitrectomy. Ophthalmology. 1989;96:1357-62.
38. Norton EWD, Fuller DG. The use of intraocular sulfur hexafluoride in vitrectomy. In: Irvine AR, O'Malley C (Eds). Advances in Vitreous Surgery. Springfield, IL: Charles C Thomas; 1976. pp. 535-42.
39. Jaffe GJ, Schwartz D, Han DP, et al. Risk factors for post-vitrectomy fibrin formation. Am J Ophthalmol. 1990;109:66-7.
40. Chung H, Tolentino FI, Cajita VN, et al. Reevaluation of corneal complications after closed vitrectomy. Arch Ophthalmol. 1988;106:916-9.
41. McDermott ML, Puklin JE, Abrams GW, et al. Phacoemulsification for cataract following pars plana vitrectomy. Ophthalm Surg Lasers. 1997;28:558-64.
42. Apple D, Federman J, Krolicki T, et al. Irreversible silicone oil adhesion to silicone intraocular lenses: a clinicopathological analysis. Ophthalmology. 1996;103:1555-61.
43. Lee MS, Eliott D, Rastogi S, et al. Incidence of rubeosis after vitrectomy for proliferative diabetic retinopathy. Invest Ophthalmol Vis Sci. 1998;39:674-6.
44. Lewis H, Abrams GW, Williams GA, et al. Anterior hyaloidal fibrovascular proliferation after diabetic vitrectomy. Am J Ophthalmol. 1987;104:607-13.
45. Sebestyn JG. Fibrinoid syndrome: a severe complication of vitrectomy surgery in diabetics, Ann Ophthalmol. 1982;14:853-6.
46. Blankenship GW. Management of vitreous cavity hemorrhage following pars plana vitrectomy for diabetic retinopathy. Ophthalmology. 1986;93:39-44.
47. McLeod D. Entry site neovascularization after diabetic vitrectomy. Br J Ophthalmol. 2000;84:810-1.
48. Rinkoff JS, de Juan E, McCuen BW. Silicone oil for retinal detachment with advanced proliferative vitreoretinopathy following failed vitrectomy for proliferative diabetic retinopathy. Am J Ophthalmol 1986;101:181-4.
49. di Lauro R, De Ruggiero P, di Lauro R, et al. Bevacizumab for the surgical treatment of severe proliferative diabetic retinopathy. Graefes Arch Clin Exp Ophthalmol. 2010;248: 785-91.
50. Lo WR, Kim SJ, Aaberg TM Sr, et al. Visual outcomes and incidence of recurrent vitreous hemorrhage after vitrectomy in diabetic eyes pretreated with bevacizumab (Avastin). Retina; 2009.pp.926-31.
51. Modarres M, Nazari H, Falavarjani KG, et al. Intravitreal injection of bevacizumab before vitrectomy for proliferative diabetic retinopathy. Eur J Ophthalmol. 2009;19:848-52.
52. Falavarjani K, Modarres M, Nazari H. Theurapeutic effect of bevacizumab injected into the silicone oil in eyes with neovascular glaucoma after vitrectomy for advanced diabetic retinopathy. Eye. 2010;24:717-9.
53. Liu L, Wu WC, Yeung L, et al. Ghost cell glaucoma after intravitreal bevacizumab for postoperative vitreous hemorrhage following vitrectomy for proliferative diabetic retinopathy. Ophthalmic Surg Lasers Imaging. 2010;41: 72-7.

18 Anti-Vascular Endothelial Growth Factor Therapy for Diabetic Macular Edema

David M Wu, Dean Eliott

Introduction

Diabetic macular edema (DME) is the major cause of moderate vision loss in patients with diabetes (Figs 18.1A and B).[1] Hyperglycemia causes microvascular damage, which results in retinal hemorrhages, microaneurysms and capillary closure.[2,3] This results in retinal hypoxia and consequently, high levels of vascular endothelial growth factor (VEGF).[4] While VEGF is a well known and potent stimulus for retinal neovascularization, it also causes vascular permeability and resultant macular edema.[5]

Focal laser photocoagulation has been the gold standard for the treatment of clinically significant DME for over 25 years.[6] However, a new approach is rapidly developing

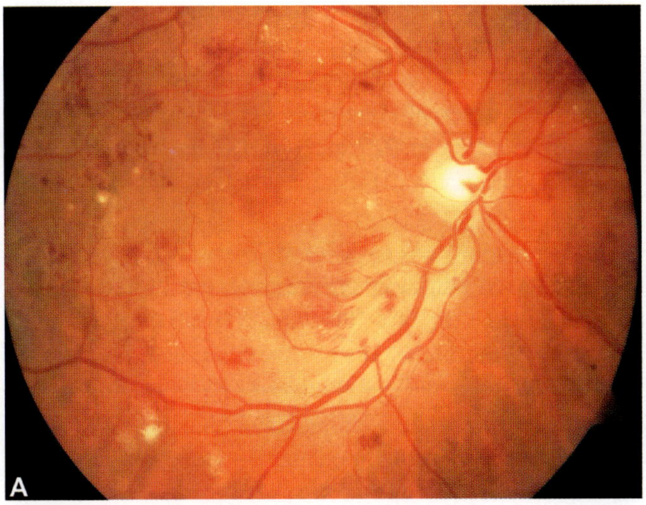

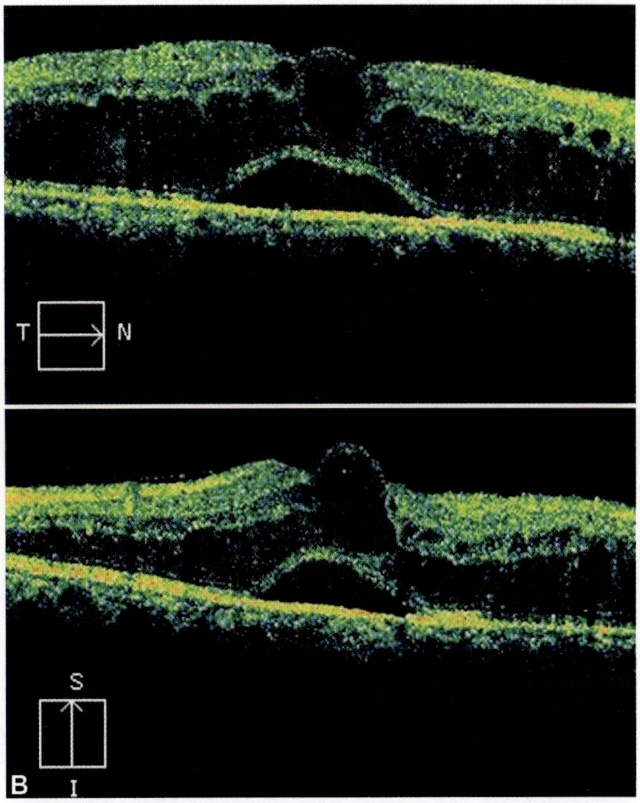

▲ **Figures 18.1A and B**
Color fundus photograph and spectral domain optical coherence tomography show diabetic macular edema

which involves the intravitreal injection of anti-VEGF agents. Below, authors summarize the currently available clinical trials supporting the use of three readily available anti-VEGF agents (Pegaptanib, Bevacizumab and Ranibizumab). Given the promising early data in this area and the explosion of anti-VEGF utilization in ophthalmology, there will no doubt be additional agents available to the clinician in the coming years. Authors briefly discuss one of these agents; VEGF Trap-Eye that has recently completed phase II clinical trials.

Pegaptanib

Pegaptanib sodium (Macugen/Eyetech, New York, USA) is an aptamer, a single-strand of nucleic acid which specifically inhibits the VEGF-165 isomer.[7] Pegaptanib was the first FDA approved anti-VEGF agent for the treatment of choroidal neovascularization (CNV) from age-related macular degeneration (AMD). A phase II study published in 2005 by the Macugen Diabetic Retinopathy Study Group showed encouraging results using pegaptanib for the treatment of DME.[8] A randomized double-masked, multicenter, dose-ranging, controlled clinical trial was carried out consisting of 172 patients with DME. Patients were divided into four groups and received one of the following treatments delivered by intravitreal injection: (1) 0.3 mg pegaptanib, (2) 1 mg pegaptanib, (3) 3 mg pegaptanib, or (4) sham injection at baseline, week 6 and week 12 with additional injections and/or laser grid or focal photocoagulation as needed for another 18 weeks. Final assessments were conducted at 36th week. The sham group had photocoagulation withheld for the first 16 weeks. A larger proportion of those receiving 0.3 mg gained visual acuity of more than or equal to 10 letters (34% vs. 10%) and more than or equal to 15 letters (18% vs. 7%) compared with sham injection. Mean central retinal thickness decreased by 68 mm with 0.3 mg pegaptanib versus an increase of 4 mm in the sham group. Photocoagulation was necessary in fewer subjects in each pegaptanib arm (25% compared to 48% in the sham-treated arm). Endophthalmitis occurred in 1 out of 652 injections and there were no significant differences in rates of cardiac, hemorrhage, thromboembolic, or gastrointestinal disorders. Phase III studies are currently being conducted.

Bevacizumab

Bevacizumab (Avastin/Genentech, South San Francisco, USA) is a full length humanized monoclonal antibody which inhibits all isoforms of VEGF. Bevacizumab was approved in 2005 for the treatment of metastatic colorectal cancer, but given the success of anti-VEGF agents in the eye and its significantly low cost, it has been applied off-label for an ever increasing number of ophthalmologic conditions, including CNV, secondary to age-related macular degeneration and macular edema secondary to retinal vascular disease.[9-11]

Retrospective Studies

Two notable interventional retrospective studies come from the Pan American Collaborative Retina Study Group (PACORES). In 2007, they first reported a retrospective review on 88 consecutive patients (110 eyes) from six study centers in six countries that had undergone treatment with either 1.25 mg (19.2%) or 2.5 mg (80.8%) intravitreal bevacizumab for DME.[12] Excluded in this study were patients with previous laser photocoagulation or intravitreal triamcinolone treatment, as well as those with macular ischemia, epiretinal membrane, or vitreomacular traction. Mean baseline visual acuity was 0.87 logMAR and mean final visual acuity was 0.6 ($p < 0.0001$). Mean central retinal thickness was 387 µm at baseline, decreasing to 276 µm at 6 months ($p < 0.0001$). After the initial injection, 20.5% of eyes required a second injection at the investigator's discretion at a mean of 13.8 weeks and 7.7% required a third injection at a mean of 11.5 weeks. No difference in mean visual acuity or mean central retinal thickness by optical coherence tomography (OCT) was seen when comparing the 1.25 mg versus the 2.5 mg dose.

In a later study by the same group, the group incorporated 38 of the patients from the previous review and expanded their study to 115 consecutive patients from 11 different centers in 8 different countries.[13] These patients received 1.25 mg (53.2%) or 2.5 mg (46.8%) bevacizumab via intravitreal injection for DME. Exclusion criteria were similar to the previous study. Best corrected visual acuity (BCVA) improved from 20/150 to 20/75 at 24 months ($p < 0.0001$). For patients receiving 1.25 mg, mean central retinal thickness decreased from a mean of 466–286 µm ($p < 0.0001$). Patients treated with the higher dose of bevacizumab had similar results and as with the earlier study no significant difference was found between the 1.25 mg and 2.5 mg doses. Multiple injections were allowed throughout the follow-up period and the mean number of injections was 5.8 per eye with a mean interval between injections of 12.2 ± 10.4 weeks.

These studies were limited in that they were non-randomized, uncontrolled and retrospective. There was also no standardized adverse event form for safety data collection. Nevertheless, they suggest a therapeutic benefit of bevacizumab in DME, consistent with the prospective studies discussed below.

Prospective Studies

The first prospective study of bevacizumab was reported by Haritoglou et al.[14] in 2006 and consisted of a consecutive, nonrandomized study of 51 patients with refractory diffuse DME. All patients received 1.25 mg or 0.05 mL injections. Of the 51 patients, 20 had a limited response to the first injection, developed recurrent edema and/or had deterioration of visual acuity during the follow-up period and required a second bevacizumab injection. There were multiple shortcomings to this study. Follow-up time was short (6–12 weeks), there was no control group and the study involved a heterogeneous group of patients that had received a variety of previous treatments (focal laser, panretinal photocoagulation, vitrectomy and/or intravitreal injection of steroids). Nevertheless, significant improvement in mean central retinal thickness was reported [from a baseline mean of 501–425 μm at 2 weeks ($p = 0.002$), 416 μm at 6 weeks ($p = 0.001$) and 377 μm at 12 weeks ($p = 0.001$)]. Changes in visual acuity by Early Treatment Diabetic Retinopathy Study (ETDRS) letters were not significant during this short follow-up period, although there was some slight improvement noted at 6 weeks which was best predicted by a patient's baseline visual acuity. This study demonstrated encouraging short-term results with respect to changes in retinal thickness and a trend toward improvement of visual acuity despite the presence of refractory edema in a patient population who had failed prior treatments.

In 2007, the Diabetic Retinopathy Clinical Research Network (DRCR.net) published results on a phase II study on 121 patients with DME.[15] Patients were randomized into one of five groups: (1) focal photocoagulation at baseline, (2) 1.25 mg bevacizumab at baseline and 6 weeks, (3) 2.5 mg bevacizumab at baseline and 6 weeks, (4) 1.25 mg bevacizumab at baseline and sham injection at 6 weeks, or 1.25 mg bevacizumab at baseline, (5) focal photocoagulation at 3 weeks and 1.25 mg of bevacizumab at 6 weeks. Inherent to the limits of a phase II study and a short 24 week follow-up period, no definitive determination as to a beneficial effect of bevacizumab could be made. However, several interesting observations were made. First, only about half of the eyes injected with bevacizumab were found to have a response. Second, there appeared to be little difference between the low and high dose of the medication. This is consistent with the findings of the retrospective PACORES studies as well as a smaller prospective trial by Lam et al.[16] which also found that 1.25 mg and 2.5 mg bevacizumab doses appeared to have similar efficacy. Third, the reduction in retinal thickness appeared to plateau in most eyes between the 3rd and 6th week visits. Finally, within this short follow-up period, the combination of laser did not appear to add any additional benefit, although the authors acknowledged that the effects of laser may manifest over a longer period of time. A phase III trial has been recommended.

In the same year, Soheilan et al.[17] published initial findings from a three-arm clinical trial comparing the efficacy of bevacizumab, triamcinolone and laser in eyes with clinically significant DME and no previous treatment. The study was expanded to a total of 150 eyes (50 per study arm) and extended to 36 months of follow-up with results reported in 2009.[18] To summarize, eyes were randomized to 1.25 mg of intravitreal bevacizumab, combination of 1.25 mg intravitreal bevacizumab and 2 mg intravitreal triamcinolone, or modified focal or grid laser photocoagulation. Patients were retreated at 12 weeks intervals in the presence of clinically significant macular edema with vision worse than 20/40. At all follow-up visits, patients treated with intravitreal bevacizumab had significant visual acuity improvement in comparison to baseline ($p < 0.001$). For patients treated with the combination of intravitreal bevacizumab and triamcinolone, this was the case only at the 6th and 12th week follow-up visits. Patients treated with laser photocoagulation were not found to have a significant change in visual acuity throughout the study period. In terms of central macular thickness, all groups had a significant decrease from baseline only at the first follow-up visit (6 weeks). The data from these studies must be interpreted with some caution as even with randomization, the baseline visual acuity and central macular thickness of patients in the laser photocoagulation group was significantly better than those treated pharmacologically. Thus, while in this clinical trial pharmacological treatment showed significant gains compared to laser, the injection and laser arms may not have represented equivalent populations. One conclusion that can be taken away from the study was that intravitreal triamcinolone essentially had no additive effect to that of bevacizumab. This corroborates two other trials published in the following year which showed little to no difference with the addition of triamcinolone to bevacizumab therapy.[19,20] Given that triamcinolone is also associated with elevated Intraocular pressure (IOP) and cataract formation, bevacizumab and triamcinolone combination therapy does not appear to be indicated for DME.

In 2010, Michaelides et al.[21] reported the one year findings from their 2 years prospective, randomized, masked single center trial comparing repeated intravitreal bevacizumab to modified ETDRS macular laser therapy (BOLT study). In this study, 80 patients with clinically significant DME and at least one prior focal laser treatment (more than 3 months prior to start of the trial) were randomized to a laser arm or bevacizumab arm. In the laser arm, patients underwent focal laser treatment at baseline and were followed every 4 months, with retreatment if clinically indicated by ETDRS guidelines. In the bevacizumab arm, patients received 3 injections of bevacizumab every 6 weeks for 18 weeks and were then reexamined every 6 weeks. Retreatment was indicated until the central macular thickness was less than 270 μm and stable (stability defined as 3 consecutive visits with central macular thickness within 20 μm of the patients thinnest recorded central macular thickness). In terms of BCVA, the bevacizumab group at 12 months gained a median of 8 ETDRS letters with a mean ETDRS BCVA of 61.3 ± 10.4 whereas the laser arm lost a median of 0.5 ETDRS letters with a median ETDRS of 50 ± 16.6 ($p = 0.0002$). The bevacizumab arm also showed a significant decrease in central macular thickness from 507 ± 145 μm to 378 ± 134 μm whereas over the same time period the laser arm decreased from 481 ± 121 μm to 413 ± 135 μm ($p = 0.02$). The median number of laser treatments in the laser arm was 3, whereas the median number of injections in the bevacizumab group was 9. No serious ocular or systemic safety concerns were identified during the 1 year time point of this study.

Solaiman et al.[22] recently reported results from a 6 month trial in which modified grid laser photocoagulation was compared to intravitreal bevacizumab and a combination of the two treatments. The 62 eyes in this study had not received any prior intravitreal injection, surgery, or laser therapy for diabetic retinopathy. Patients randomized to the intravitreal bevacizumab or laser groups received a single intravitreal injection or a single macular grid or focal photocoagulation treatment at baseline. Those randomized to combination treatment received a single bevacizumab injection at baseline followed by macular photocoagulation 3 weeks afterwards. One month after baseline treatment, both groups receiving bevacizumab showed significant increase in BCVA whereas the patients that had received laser were unchanged (38.09%, $p < 0.05$ and 21.69%, $p < 0.05$ improvement from baseline in bevacizumab and combination treatment groups respectively). Those receiving bevacizumab also showed a significantly improved central macular thickness whereas those receiving laser were relatively unchanged [31.3% reduction in the bevacizumab only group ($p < 0.05$), 23.77% reduction in the combination group ($p < 0.05$) and 10.4% reduction in the laser group ($p > 0.05$)]. Three months after baseline treatment, however, BCVA had regressed in the bevacizumab group such that it was no longer statistically different from baseline. The BCVA improved slightly in the laser group, but not to the point of statistical significance (10.71% $p > 0.05$). In fact, the only group in which the improvement in BCVA remained statistically significant was the combination treatment group (22.89%, $p < 0.05$). Similarly, at 3 months the only patients with sufficiently improved central macular thickness to maintain statistical significance were those receiving the combination of laser and bevacizumab. Patients who had received only laser treatment continued to show a slight improvement in macular thickness, but below the threshold of statistical significance. Those receiving bevacizumab actually had an increase in central macular thickness. Finally, at 6 months, visual acuity gains in those treated with monotherapy (laser or bevacizumab) had regressed to baseline values. Only those with combination treatment held on to visual acuity gains, though these had slipped below the level of statistical significance. While all three groups had somewhat thinner central macular thicknesses 6 months after treatment, only the combination treatment group retained a significantly ($p < 0.05$) decreased macular thickness compared to baseline. This study demonstrated that intravitreal bevacizumab acts rapidly, but may be short-lived, whereas laser has a smaller and more gradual effect, but potentially with more longevity. The combination of laser and bevacizumab may offer the more dramatic initial benefit of bevacizumab treatment with some of the longevity of laser treatment.

Ranibizumab

Ranibizumab (Lucentis/Genentech, South San Francisco) is a monoclonal antibody fragment toward all isoforms of VEGF.[23] Ranibizumab is currently approved by the FDA for the treatment of CNV associated with age-related macular degeneration (AMD).

One of the first reports of the use of ranibizumab as a therapy for DME was a small pilot study by Chun et al.[24] In this study, five patients received 0.3 mg ranibizumab and five received 0.5 mg ranibizumab at day zero, month one and month two. These patients were then observed for 24 months. At month 3, the mean decrease in retinal thickness was 45 μm for the low dose group and 198 μm for the high dose group. In addition, four of ten patients gained more than or equal to 15 letters, five of ten gained more than or equal to 10 letters and eight of ten gained more than or equal to 1 letter. This pilot study demonstrated that ranibizumab had the potential to maintain or improve visual acuity and reduce retinal thickness. The therapy appeared to be well tolerated; while there was mild to moderate ocular inflammation noted in five patients, they were "manageable" and did not lead any patients to withdraw from the study. A second small study involving ten patients with chronic DME was conducted with 0.5 mg ranibizumab given at baseline and then at 1st, 2nd, 4th and 6th months.[25] The primary outcome was a change in foveal thickness at 7 months and secondary outcomes were changes in visual acuity and macular volume. At 7 months (one month after the fifth injection) mean foveal thickness decreased from 503 μm at baseline to 257 μm. Mean visual acuity improved 12.3 letters. These studies helped demonstrate that VEGF is an important therapeutic target for DME and have been followed by larger clinical trials.

One such trial was the Ranibizumab for Edema of the Macular in Diabetes (READ-2).[26] In this study, 126 patients with DME were randomized into three groups (0.5 mg ranibizumab at baseline and months 1, 3 and 5; focal grid laser at baseline and month 3 if needed; or combination 0.5 mg ranibizumab and focal grid laser at baseline and month 3). At 6 months, the mean gain in visual acuity was significantly greater in the group receiving only ranibizumab compared with the laser group and the combination ranibizumab or laser group. It is important to note that the ranibizumab only group received more injections of ranibizumab than the combination group during this period. These patients were then followed out to 2 years and after the 6 months period all study subjects became eligible for ranibizumab treatment as frequently as every 2 months. Ultimately, those in the ranibizumab group had the best overall improvement in BCVA (7.24 letters compared to 5.1 letters in the group initially treated with laser and 6.8 letters in the group initially treated with combination therapy). At the same time, the mean number of ranibizumab injections given was also the highest in the ranibizumab only group (9.3 injections over 2 years; 5.3 in the 18 months follow-up period vs. 4.4 in the 18 months follow-up period for patients in the laser only group and 2.9 in the combination group). Steady ranibizumab treatment over 2 years provided the best visual outcome (especially over the first 6 months), but at the expense of significantly more injections. The effects of laser were much slower to take hold, with little improvement during the initial 6 months of the study. While laser significantly reduced the number of injections required, it remains unclear whether this ultimately sacrifices some degree of visual gain. The authors concluded that aggressive initial treatment with ranibizumab followed by a period of as needed ranibizumab treatment in conjunction with focal laser treatment may provide an optimal balance between visual outcome and reducing the number of intravitreal injections needed.[27]

The DRCR.net also recently published a much larger study utilizing ranibizumab that incorporated 854 eyes with DME.[28] Patients were randomized to 4 groups (sham injection plus prompt laser, 0.5 mg ranibizumab plus prompt laser, 0.5 mg ranibizumab plus deferred laser, or 4 mg triamcinolone plus prompt laser). Compared with the sham plus prompt laser group, the greatest improvement in BCVA at 1 year was observed with ranibizumab plus prompt laser and with ranibizumab plus deferred laser. Patients in the triamcinolone group did not demonstrate significant improvement in visual acuity compared with the control group alone. However, patients receiving either pharmacologic treatment in conjunction with laser had similar significant reductions in mean central subfield thickness. Triamcinolone and ranibizumab also appeared to work equally effective in the subset of eyes that were pseudophakic at baseline, suggesting that cataract formation may have played a role in the lack of visual improvement in the triamcinolone group (59% of patients in the triamcinolone group underwent cataract surgery over the 2 years of follow-up compared to 14% in the ranibizumab and sham groups). At the same time, triamcinolone was also associated with a greater occurrence of increased IOP than either ranibizumab or the sham group (50% of those receiving triamcinolone had an elevation of IOP > 10 mm Hg from baseline, an IOP > 30 mm Hg, or initiation of IOP lowering medications in comparison to only 9% and 11% in ranibizumab and sham plus control groups, respectively). In summary, this recent study affirms the previous discussed study in suggesting intravitreal ranibizumab in combination with focal laser improves upon the gold standard treatment of focal laser alone. Triamcinolone is also effective in reducing macular thickness, but may have more limited use given the adverse effects of IOP and cataract formation.

Finally, Massin et al.[29] recently reported the 12 months results from the European RESOLVE study. In this multicenter, sham controlled, double-masked study, 100 patients with DME were randomized to intravitreal ranibizumab or sham for 3 consecutive months. The initial starting dose of ranibizumab was 0.3 mg or 0.05 mL; however, after the first month the dose could be doubled by the investigators if the change in central retinal thickness was not sufficiently improved. In addition, after 3 months, if the treatment was deemed to be ineffective, "rescue" laser photocoagulation could be performed. In the ranibizumab treatment group, the mean improvement in BCVA was 7.8 letters compared to with sham (-0.1 letters) and mean central retinal thickness decreased 194.2 μm with ranibizumab compared to 48.4 μm with sham. Investigators ordered a "doubling" of the dose in 91.8% of sham treated eyes, compared to 68.6% of the ranibizumab arm. Finally, 85% of patients in the sham treated arm required laser rescue after 3 months compared to only 24.3% of ranibizumab treated eyes. There were no significant differences in the rates of ocular or non-ocular adverse events between sham and ranibizumab eyes.

Vascular Endothelial Growth Factor Trap

Vascular endothelial growth factor Trap-Eye (VEGF Trap-Eye/Regeneron, New York, USA) is a recombinant fusion protein consisting of VEGF binding domains from the human VEGF receptors 1 and 2 fused to the Fc portion of IgG1.[30] This fusion protein has significantly higher binding affinity for VEGF and also binds other VEGF family proteins, including placental growth factors 1 and 2 (PLGF-1 and PLGF-2) that also contribute to neovascularization and vascular permeability.[31] VEGF Trap-Eye may also have a longer duration of action in the eye (10 weeks), which may be advantageous given the frequency of injections with currently available anti-VEGF treatments.[32] Currently, the only published report utilizing VEGF Trap is a small exploratory study in which 5 patients received a single intravitreal injection of 4.0 mg VEGF Trap-Eye and were then followed for 6 weeks.[33] All five patients showed improvement during this time, with a median improvement in BCVA of nine ETRDS letters and median reduction in central foveal thickness of 31% (74 μm).

Although not yet published, in February 2010, results from a larger phase II multicenter, randomized, controlled clinical trial of VEGF Trap-Eye (DA VINCI) were presented at the Angiogenesis 2010 Clinical Trials meeting in Miami, Florida. This study enrolled 219 patients with DME and randomized them to four different dosing protocols of VEGF Trap-Eye (monthly doses of either 0.5 mg or 2 mg for 6 months or 2 mg doses monthly for 3 months followed by either 8 week or as needed dosing through 24 weeks) or control (macular laser at week one followed by potential repeat laser at a minimum of 16 week intervals). At 24 weeks, patients in each of the four groups receiving VEGF Trap-Eye achieved statistically significant greater improvements in visual acuity compared to patients receiving laser. Patients receiving the higher dose VEGF Trap-Eye (2 mg) given monthly were found to perform the best in this study, gaining 11.4 ETDRS letters. Patients on the protocol in which monthly 2 mg injections were administered for 3 months followed by as needed dosing gained 10.3 letters. Those receiving 2 mg VEGF Trap-Eye every other month after 3 initial monthly injections gained 8.5 letters. Patients who received the lower dose VEGF Trap-Eye (0.5 mg) monthly gained 8.6 letters. Finally, patients receiving macular laser therapy gained only 2.5 letters in the same time frame.

The studies reviewed here suggest that anti-VEGF agents will be an important new tool for treating diabetic macular edema. Anti-VEGF therapy appears capable of significantly improving BCVA more rapidly than the current gold standard, macular laser photocoagulation. With the currently available follow-up data, it appears that these gains can be maintained with repeated injections and an acceptable safety profile. Combination therapy with laser may enable a more optimal coupling of the advantageous longevity of laser treatment with the rapid effects of pharmacologic treatment. New anti-VEGF agents under development, such as the VEGF-trap, may eventually allow reduction of the frequency of dosing required by currently available medications.

References

1. Klein R, Klein BE, Moss SE, et al. The Wisconsin epidemiologic study of diabetic retinopathy. II. Prevalence and risk of diabetic retinopathy when age at diagnosis is less than 30 years. Arch Ophthalmol. 1984;102:520-6.
2. Cogan DG, Toussaint D, Kuwabara T. Retinal vascular patterns. IV. Diabetic retinopathy. Arch Ophthalmol. 1961;66:366-78.
3. De Venecia G, Davis M, Engerman R. Clinicopathologic correlations in diabetic retinopathy. I. Histology and fluorescein angiography of microaneurysms. Arch Ophthalmol. 1976;94:1766-73.

4. Kaur C, Sivakumar V, Foulds WS. Early response of neurons and glial cells to hypoxia in the retina. Invest Ophthalmol Vis Sci. 2006;47:1126-41.
5. Antcliff RJ, Marshall J. The pathogenesis of edema in diabetic maculopathy. Semin Ophthalmol. 1999;14:223-32.
6. Photocoagulation for diabetic macular edema. Early Treatment Diabetic Retinopathy Study report number 1. Early Treatment Diabetic Retinopathy Study research group. Arch Ophthalmol. 1985;103:1796-806.
7. Ishida S, Usui T, Yamashiro K, et al. VEGF164 is proinflammatory in the diabetic retina. Invest Ophthalmol Vis Sci. 2003;44:2155-62.
8. Cunningham ET, Adamis AP, Altaweel M, et al. A phase II randomized double-masked trial of pegaptanib, an anti-vascular endothelial growth factor aptamer, for diabetic macular edema. Ophthalmology. 2005;112:1747-57.
9. Rosenfeld PJ. Intravitreal avastin: the low cost alternative to lucentis? Am J Ophthalmol. 2006;142:141-3.
10. Michels S, Rosenfeld PJ, Puliafito CA, et al. Systemic bevacizumab (Avastin) therapy for neovascular age-related macular degeneration twelve-week results of an uncontrolled open-label clinical study. Ophthalmology. 2005;112:1035-47.
11. Rosenfeld PJ, Fung AE, Puliafito CA. Optical coherence tomography findings after an intravitreal injection of bevacizumab (avastin) for macular edema from central retinal vein occlusion. Ophthalmic Surg Lasers Imaging. 2005;36: 336-9.
12. Arevalo JF, Fromow-Guerra J, Quiroz-Mercado H, et al. Primary intravitreal bevacizumab (Avastin) for diabetic macular edema: results from the Pan-American Collaborative Retina Study Group at 6-month follow-up. Ophthalmology. 2007;114:743-50.
13. Arevalo JF, Sanchez JG, Wu L, et al. Primary intravitreal bevacizumab for diffuse diabetic macular edema: the Pan-American Collaborative Retina Study Group at 24 months. Ophthalmology. 2009;116:1488-97.
14. Haritoglou C, Kook D, Neubauer A, et al. Intravitreal bevacizumab (Avastin) therapy for persistent diffuse diabetic macular edema. Retina. 2006;26:999-1005.
15. Scott IU, Edwards AR, Beck RW, et al. A phase II randomized clinical trial of intravitreal bevacizumab for diabetic macular edema. Ophthalmology. 2007;114:1860-7.
16. Lam DS, Lai TY, Lee VY, et al. Efficacy of 1.25 mg versus 2.5 mg intravitreal bevacizumab for diabetic macular edema: six-month results of a randomized controlled trial. Retina. 2009;29:292-9.
17. Soheilian M, Ramezani A, Bijanzadeh B, et al. Intravitreal bevacizumab (avastin) injection alone or combined with triamcinolone versus macular photocoagulation as primary treatment of diabetic macular edema. Retina. 2007;27:1187-95.
18. Soheilian M, Ramezani A, Obudi A, et al. Randomized trial of intravitreal bevacizumab alone or combined with triamcinolone versus macular photocoagulation in diabetic macular edema. Ophthalmology. 2009;116:1142-50.
19. Ahmadieh H, Ramezani A, Shoeibi N, et al. Intravitreal bevacizumab with or without triamcinolone for refractory diabetic macular edema; a placebo-controlled, randomized clinical trial. Graefes Arch Clin Exp Ophthalmol. 2008;246: 483-9.
20. Faghihi H, Roohipoor R, Mohammadi SF, et al. Intravitreal bevacizumab versus combined bevacizumab-triamcinolone versus macular laser photocoagulation in diabetic macular edema. Eur J Ophthalmol. 2008;18:941-8.
21. Michaelides M, Kaines A, Hamilton RD, et al. A prospective randomized trial of intravitreal bevacizumab or laser therapy in the management of diabetic macular edema (BOLT study) 12-month data: report 2. Ophthalmology. 2010;117:1078-86.
22. Solaiman KA, Diab MM, Abo-Elenin M. Intravitreal bevacizumab and/or macular photocoagulation as a primary treatment for diffuse diabetic macular edema. Retina. 2010;30: 1638-45.
23. Presta LG, Chen H, O'Connor SJ, et al. Humanization of an anti-vascular endothelial growth factor monoclonal antibody for the therapy of solid tumors and other disorders. Cancer Res. 1997;57(20):4593-9.
24. Chun DW, Heier JS, Topping TM, et al. A pilot study of multiple intravitreal injections of ranibizumab in patients with center-involving clinically significant diabetic macular edema. Ophthalmology. 2006;113:1706-12.
25. Nguyen QD, Tatlipinar S, Shah SM, et al. Vascular endothelial growth factor is a critical stimulus for diabetic macular edema. Am J Ophthalmol. 2006;142:961-9.
26. Nguyen QD, Shah SM, Heier JS, et al. Primary end point (six months) results of the ranibizumab for edema of the macula in diabetes (READ-2) study. Ophthalmology. 2009;116:2175-81.
27. Nguyen QD, Shah SM, Khwaja AA, et al. Two-year outcomes of the ranibizumab for edema of the macula in diabetes (READ-2) study. Ophthalmology. 2010;117:2146-51.
28. Elman MJ, Aiello LP, Beck RW, et al. Randomized trial evaluating ranibizumab plus prompt or deferred laser or triamcinolone plus prompt laser for diabetic macular edema. Ophthalmology. 2010;117:1064-77.
29. Massin P, Bandello F, Garweg JG, et al. Safety and efficacy of ranibizumab in diabetic macular edema (RESOLVE Study): a 12-month, randomized, controlled, double-masked, multicenter phase II study. Diabetes Care. 2010;33:2399-405.
30. Holash J, Davis S, Papadopoulos N, et al. VEGF-Trap: a VEGF blocker with potent antitumor effects. Proc Natl Acad Sci USA. 2002;99:11393-8.
31. Rakic JM, Lambert V, Devy L, et al. Placental growth factor, a member of the VEGF family, contributes to the development of choroidal neovascularization. Invest Ophthalmol Vis Sci. 2003;44:3186-93.
32. Stewart MW, Rosenfeld PJ. Predicted biological activity of intravitreal VEGF Trap. Br J Ophthalmol. 2008;92:667-8.
33. Do DV, Nguyen QD, Shah SM, et al. An exploratory study of the safety, tolerability and bioactivity of a single intravitreal injection of vascular endothelial growth factor Trap-Eye in patients with diabetic macular oedema. Br J Ophthalmol. 2009;93:144-9.

19 Surgery for Diabetic Macular Edema

Ulrike Stolba, Susanne Binder

Introduction

Worldwide presumably 180 million people suffer from diabetes. Current studies estimate that 50% of those are not diagnosed. The World Health Organization (WHO) predicts that by the year 2030 the number of people suffering from diabetes will increase to 366 million—this being a greater problem in developing countries rather than in developed countries.

The diabetic macular edema is the most frequent cause of visual loss in diabetic patients. It appears in up to 29% of patients with duration of the disease more than 20 years.[1] The type of diabetes as well as the age at onset are decisive factors in the incidence of diabetic macular edema. Type I macular edema is likely to develop in 20–25%, Type II in 14%.[2] Additional factors for the occurrence are panretinal laser coagulation[2] and general factors which point out the severity of the disease (blood pressure, HbA1c, proteinuria).[3]

Pathogenesis

Microvascular changes affecting the entire diabetic organism play a major role in the occurrence of macular edema. In principle, an imbalance of arteriolar filtration and venous absorption develops. The breakdown of the blood-retina barrier leads to an increased transudation of plasma proteins and intraretinal fluid preferably into the inner and outer plexiform layer. Concurrently an increased permeation of growth factors such as vascular endothelial growth factor (VEGF) or interleukin 6 (IL-6) is present.

In recent years the role of the vitreous body became increasingly a center of interest for several reasons.

Basically, different types of collagen (I, II and IV) are present in the vitreous structures. Collagen is chemically a protein and susceptible to non-enzymatic glycation in hyperglycemia due to its special E-amino groups. This makes collagen resistant against proteolytic enzymes leading to an accumulation of collagen fibers in vessel walls, in the vitreous gel and on the vitreous hyaloid. Together these changes result in a premature aging of the vitreous. Anterior-posterior vitreous strands are formed and induce constant traction on the macular area. Thickening of the posterior hyaloid causes a diffusion barrier even for proliferation factors[4] and a tangential traction when shrinking.[5,6] Ageing of the inner limiting membrane (ILM) increases adhesion to the posterior hyaloid due to common collagen fibers type IV especially over the macula. Nasrallah has described a higher incidence of posterior vitreous attachment in diabetic eyes.[7] Additionally, hyper- and hypoglycemia cause permanent changes of the osmolarity in the liquid vitreous with subsequent fluctuation of the volume. These variations also cause traction on the posterior pole.

Non-invasive ocular coherence tomography (OCT) offers detailed information on retinal damages as well as on these vitreoretinal correlations.[8] The impact on the treatment decision is increasing and replacing angiograms more frequently.

The rationales behind vitrectomy are removal of vitreous strands, tangential tractions and a thickened posterior hyaloid. Furthermore, retinal oxygenation is improved by allowing oxygen to be transported in water currents from well oxygenated to ischemic areas of the retina. Stéfansson showed experimentally that the oxygen tension increases over the retina in vitrectomized eyes. This leads to retinal vasoconstriction and a reduction of vascular leakage.[9,10] Additionally, growth factors (VEGF, IL-6) accumulated on the posterior hyaloid or in preretinal membranes in eyes with diabetic edema are eliminated.[3,6]

In the following indications, techniques and outcome of vitrectomy as well as prognostic factors are discussed.

Indications and Outcome

Surgical results after vitrectomy to release traction in diabetic macular edema were published first in 1992.[11] In 1997 Hikichi observed a spontaneous resolution of an edema after posterior vitreous detachment in 55% of the eyes compared to 25% with posterior attachment.[12]

Both reports were followed by numerous papers with retrospective studies. The functional success rate defined as increase of visual acuity (VA) of more than 2 lines was reached in 38–92% of the eyes. The results were much better in smaller studies (85–92%)[11,13,14] than in bigger ones by Tachi,[15] Pendergast,[16] LaHeij,[17] Yamamoto[18] or the Diabetic Retinopathy Clinical Research Network Writing Committee[19] where a visual improvement was found up to 50% of eyes.

In our own prospective study[20] with 65 patients we showed that significantly more patients profit from vitrectomy (52%) compared to a control group (13%) after 6 months. This number corresponds with observations of Hikichi who found a visual improvement in the natural course of diabetic edema without posterior hyaloid detachment in 15%.[12] However, the average VA in the vitrectomy group was not significantly improved and the average VA in the control group showed a negative correlation over time. Furthermore, there was a negative correlation to age (p=0.01) indicating that older patients with long standing edema have a minor change for postoperative improvement. Long-term results show that about 50% of the patients are improved or remain stabilized after a follow-up of 5 years.[21]

The impact of vitrectomy on reading vision was not so marked. The average acuity was not different before and after surgery, but in the control group we found a significant decrease (p=0.01).

OCT measurements of retinal thickness showed a significant decrease after vitrectomy in those studies where they were performed. Usually retinal thickness decreases immediately after surgery and remains stable.[18,20] The anatomic effect is more distinct than the functional outcome indicating that a diabetic edema is a more complex disorder. (Figs 19.1A and B and 19.2A and B).

Surgical Methods

In many studies the question of the necessity of staining and peeling of the inner limiting membrane (ILM) was raised. Gandorfer first reported a 92% rate of resorption of the edema after vitrectomy with ILM-Peeling in a limited number of patients.[22] During postoperative follow-up no recurrent edema was observed for up to 31 months. It is unclear whether this result can be attributed to the method. Comparative studies prove no statistical significant difference between eyes with and without ILM-peeling.[23-27]

The advantage of avoiding recurrences could be redeemed by the potential damage of the physiological function of the Müller cells whose basal membrane forms the ILM. Histological examinations show a swelling of the inner processes after chronic traction.[28] These changes could explain the distinct decrease of retinal thickness without an adequate increase of visual acuity after surgery.[20] Clinically a glistening reflex of the retina after ILM peeling was observed which might be related to a regeneration of the Müller processes.[23]

It is also unclear if a selective staining of the ILM with indocyanine green (ICG) to improve visualization has an impact on the postoperative functional outcome due to toxic effects.[29-31] A modified dilution of the stain reduces potential damages on the ganglion cells[32] but visual field defects have to be considered. A randomized comparative study showed that staining with ICG induces temporary peripheral visual field defects compared to eyes where trypan blue was used for membrane staining. The difference was significant 3 months postoperatively and disappeared after 6 months.[33]

Prognostic Factors

Even though macular traction on diabetic edema is the classic indication for vitrectomy several papers describe morphologic and functional improvements in cases without visible membranes.[15,34-36] In one of Yamamoto studies, tractive membranes were only found in one-third of the included eyes. Intraoperatively, however, membranes could be peeled in the

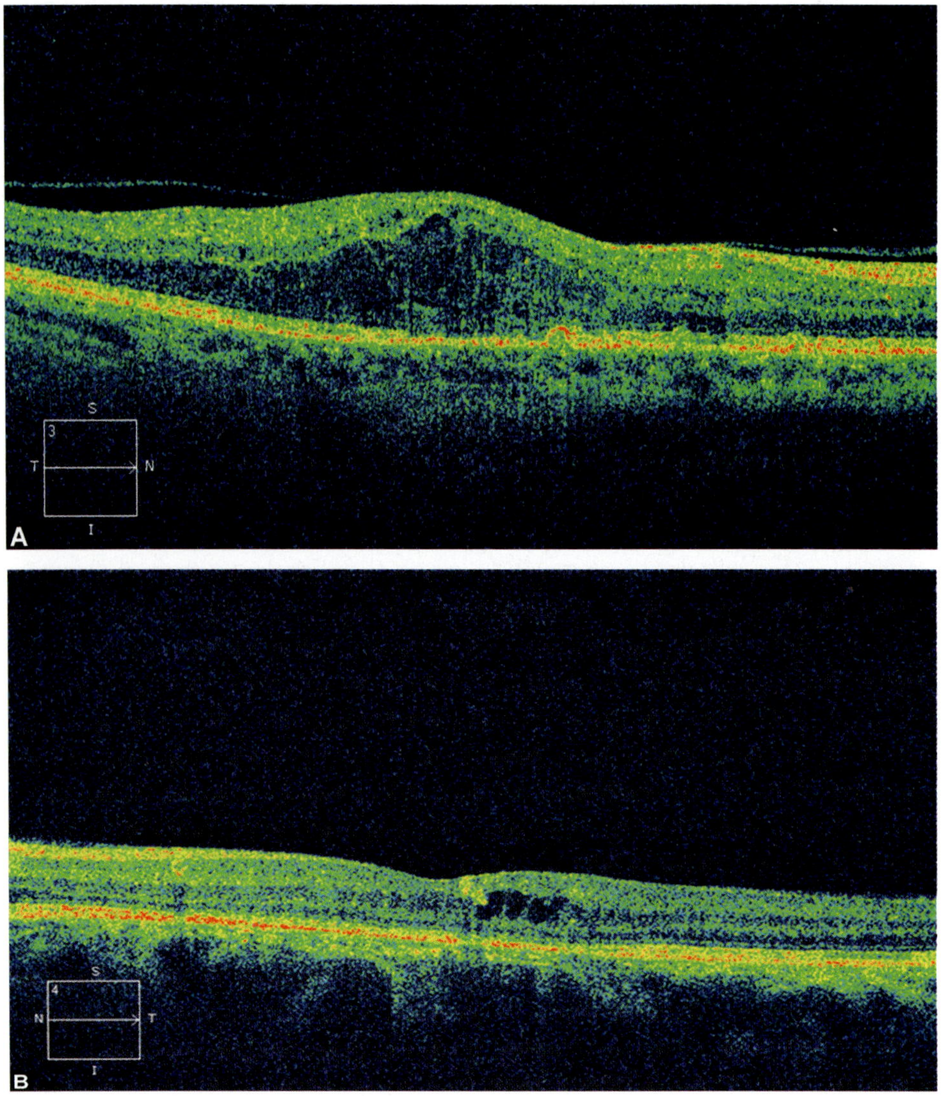

▲ **Figures 19.1A and B**

(A) Preoperative OCT of diabetic macular edema; (B) Postoperative OCT of the same eye shows normal retinal thickness

majority of the eyes. In all eyes independent of posterior hyaloid detachment or tractive membranes significant visual improvements and retinal thickness reductions were achieved.[36] It is suggested that a splitting of the posterior thickened hyaloid might mimic a posterior hyaloid detachment in these eyes[37](Fig. 19.3). During surgery a preretinal membrane is found in many cases which could explain the success rate. Long-term results show an improvement of VA also in more than 50% of these cases after 5 years.[38]

In contrast, in a comparative study Massin described significantly better VA results as well as retinal thickness decreases after vitrectomy only in eyes with macular traction compared to eyes without traction.[39]

The initial VA is another prognostic factor.[19,40,41] In all papers a significant correlation is estimated to postoperative visual improvement (p=0.04-0.00016). The conclusion should be an early vitrectomy in those eyes where the indication is given. Usually eyes are included in studies where several modified grid laser treatments or intravitreal injections with

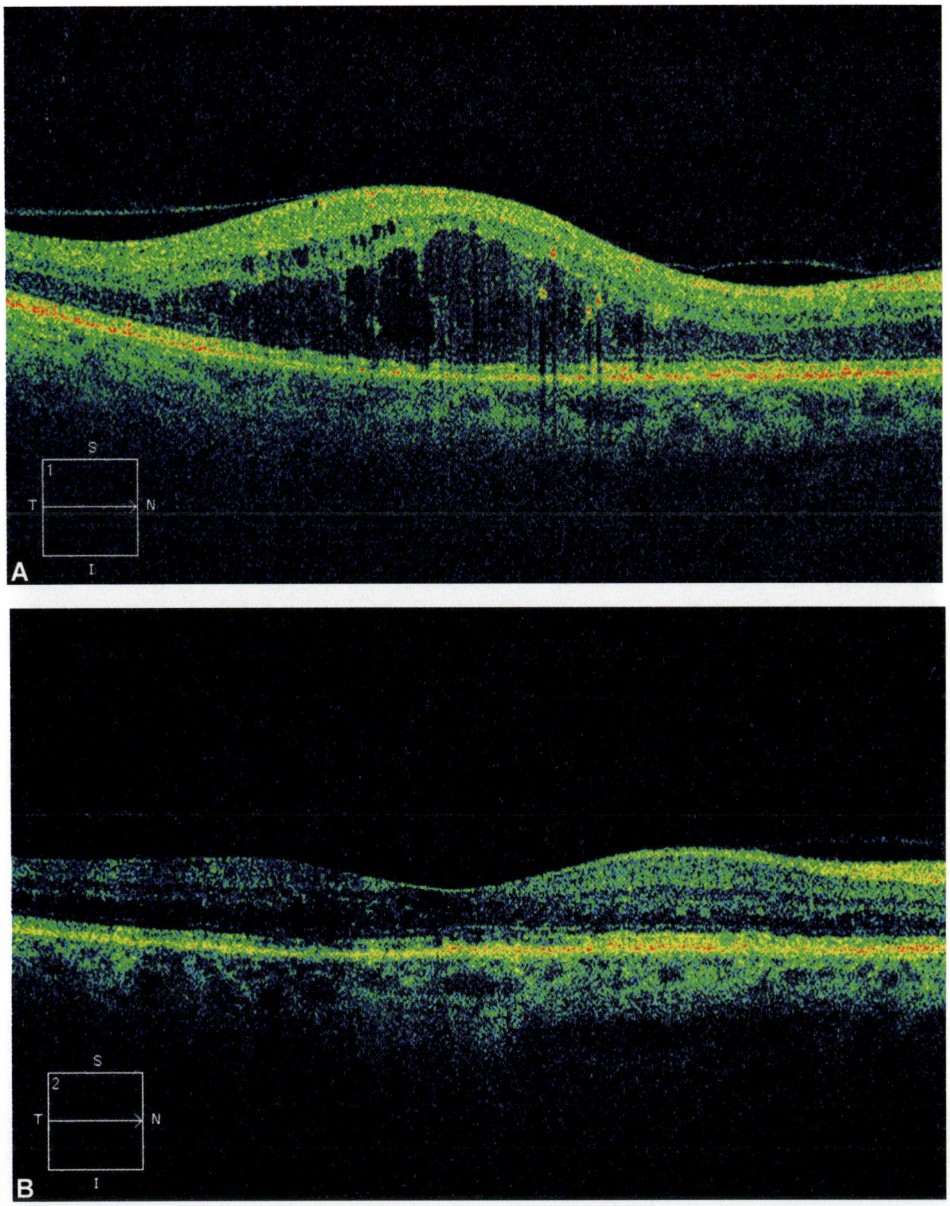

▲ **Figures 19.2A and B**

(A) Preoperative OCT of diabetic macular edema in another study; (B) Postoperative OCT of the same eye shows normal retinal thickness in the same study

triamcinolone acetonide were performed. Comparative studies with grid laser versus vitrectomy show that the decrease of retinal thickness is significantly better,[42] twice better,[43] or at least slightly better after vitrectomy.[44] However, inclusion criteria of those studies are inconsistent concerning pretreatments and vitreoretinal relationship.

New OCT technologies give more evidence of damages within the retinal structure. The presence of subretinal fluid in combination with typical intraretinal fluid accumulation implies a significantly worse prognosis after surgery ($p=0.01$) because the overlying sensory retina is more disordered.[40] The preoperative reflectivity of the inner retinal layers might

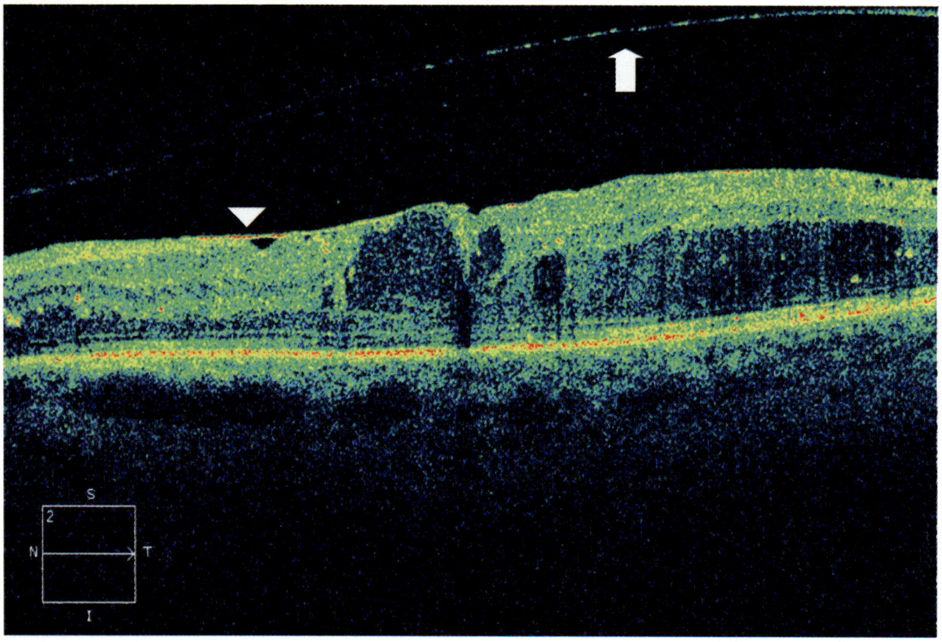

▲ **Figure 19.3**

OCT of a diabetic edema with splitting of the posterior hyaloid (arrow) and a preretinal membrane (arrowhead)

indicate a limited postoperative prognosis. For eyes which were intended for intravitreal triamcinolone acetonide injection a visual increase of more than two ETDRS (early treatment diabetic retinopathy study) lines was reached in 88% with high reflectivity compared to 43% with low reflectivity (p=0.001).[45] Similar observations were done by Forooghian who found a significant negative correlation between length of the photoreceptor outer segment (PROS) and the VA in diabetic edema eyes.[46] One might conclude that all potential treatments including vitrectomy will have a poorer prognosis in these eyes.

Future Aspects

New surgical techniques are developed to remove the posterior hyaloid atraumatically with the help of intravitreal microplasmin as an adjunct to conventional pars plana vitrectomy.[47-49] 0.1–0.2 ml containing 0.8–1.2 IU of autologous plasmin enzyme (APE) is injected 25–15 minutes before vitrectomy leading to a partial or complete posterior hyaloid detachment in the majority of eyes. In all of these eyes surgical peeling of the posterior hyaloid was at least simplified. Recent papers suggest an intravitreal injection of plasmin as a substitute to pars plana vitrectomy.[50]

Modern treatment of diabetic macular edema includes a broader spectrum and is not limited to grid laser coagulation. Careful selection of the cases based on OCT findings will be needed to elaborate new strategies. Classical indications for pars plana vitrectomy are a taut posterior hyaloid or preretinal membranes. A better prognosis might be expected when the preoperative VA is better than 0.05 on Snellen charts, when the height of the edema is moderate showing a high reflectivity of the outer retinal layers and when the photoreceptor layer is intact. Currently a 50% success rate is reported after surgery.

References

1. Klein R, Klein BE, Moss SE, et al. The Wisconsin epidemiologic study of diabetic retinopathy IV. Diabetic macular edema. Ophthalmology. 1984;91:1464-74.
2. Klein R, Moss SE, Klein BE, et al. The Wisconsin epidemiologic study of diabetic retinopathy XI. The incidence of macular edema. Ophthalmology. 1989;96:1501-10.
3. Perkovich BT, Meyers SM. Systemic factors affecting diabetic macular edema. Am J Ophthalmol. 1988;105:211-2.

4. Walton KA, Meyer CH, Harkrider CJ, et al. Age-related changes in vitreous mobility as measured by video B scan ultrasound. Exp Eye Res. 2002;74:173-80.
5. Sebag J, Buckingham B, Charles MA, et al. Biochemical abnormalities of vitreous in humans with proliferative diabetic retinopathy. Arch Ophthalmol. 1992;110:1472-6.
6. Sebag J, Nie S, Reiser K. Raman spectroscopy of human vitreous in proliferative diabetic retinopathy. Invest Ophthalmol Vis Sci. 1994;35:2976-80.
7. Nasrallah FP, Jalkh AE, VanCoppenrolle F, et al. The role of the vitreous in diabetic macular edema. Ophthalmology. 1988;95:1335-9.
8. Campbell RJ, Coupland SG, Buhrmann RR, et al. Optimal optical coherence tomography-based measures in diagnosis of clinically significant macular edema: retinal volume versus foveal thickness. Arch Ophthalmol. 2007;125:619-23.
9. Stéffanson E. The therapeutic effect of retinal laser treatment and vitrectomy. A theory based on oxygen and vascular physiology. Acta Ophthalmol Scand. 2001;79:435-40.
10. Stéfansson E, Landers MB. How does vitrectomy affect diabetic macular edema. Am J Ophthalmol. 2006;141:984.
11. Lewis H, Abrams GW, Blumenkranz MS, et al. Vitrectomy for diabetic macular traction and edema associated with posterior hyaloid traction. Ophthalmology. 1992;99:753-9.
12. Hikichi T, Fujio N, Akiba Y, et al. Association between the short-term natural history of diabetic macular edema and the vitreomacular relationship in type II diabetes mellitus. Ophthalmology. 1997;104:473-8.
13. Yang CM. Surgical treatment for severe diffuse macular edema with massive hard exudates. Retina. 2000;20:121-5.
14. Gandorfer A, Messmer EM, Ulbig MW, et al. Resolution of diabetic macular edema after surgical removal of the posterior hyaloid and the inner limiting membrane. Retina. 2000;20:126-33.
15. Tachi N, Ogino N. Vitrectomy for diffuse macular edema in cases of diabetic retinopathy. Am J Ophthalmol. 1996;122: 258-60.
16. Pendergast SD, Hassan TS, Williams GA, et al. Vitrectomy for diffuse diabetic macular edema associated with a taut premacular posterior hyloid. Am J Ophthalmol. 2000;130:178-86.
17. LaHeij EC, Hendrikse F, Kessels AGH, et al. Vitrectomy results in diabetic macular edema without evident vitreomacular traction. Graefe´s Arch Clin Exp Ophthalmol. 2001;239:264-70.
18. Yamamoto T, Hitani K, Tskukahara I, et al. Early postoperative retinal thickness changes and complications after vitrectomy for diabetic macular edema. Am J Ophthalmol. 2003;135:14-9.
19. Diabetic Retinopathy Clinical Research Network Writing Committee, Haller JA, Qin H, et al. Vitrectomy outcomes in eyes with diabetic macular edema and vitreomacular traction. Ophthalmology. 2010;117:1087-93.
20. Stolba U, Binder S, Gruber D, et al. Vitrectomy for persistent diffuse diabetic macular edema. Am J Ophthalmol. 2005;140: 295-301.
21. Kumagai K, Furukawa M, Ogino N, et al. Long-term follow-up of vitrectomy for diffuse nontractional diabetic macular edema. Retina. 2009;29:464-72.
22. Gandorfer A, Messmer EM, Ulbig MW, et al. Resolution of diabetic macular edema after surgical removal of the posterior hyaloid and the inner limiting membrane. Retina. 2000;20:126-33.
23. Lam RF, Lai WW, Chan WM, et al. Vitrectomy for diabetic macular edema with and without internal limiting membrane removal. Ophthalmologica. 2006;220:206-10.
24. Yamamoto T, Hitani K, Sato Y, et al. Vitrectomy for diabetic macular edema with and without internal limiting membrane removal. Ophthalmologica. 2005;219:206-13.
25. Patel JI, Hykin PG, Schadt M, et al. Pars plana vitrectomy with and without peeling of the inner limiting membrane for diabetic macular edema. Retina. 2006;26:5-13.
26. Kamura Y, Sato Y, Isomae T, et al. Effects of internal limiting membrane peeling in vitrectomy on diabetic cystoid macular edema patients. Jpn J Ophthalmol. 2005;49:297-300.
27. Bardak Y, Cekic O, Tig SU. Comparison of ICG-assisted ILM peeling and triamcinolone-assisted posterior vitreous removal in diffuse diabetic macular oedema. Eye. 2006;20:1357-9.
28. Sebag J, Balazs EA. Pathogenesis of CME: anatomic considerations of vitreoretinal adhesions. Surv Ophthalmol. 1984;29:493-8.
29. Haritoglu C, Gass CA, Gandorfer A, et al. ICG-assisted peeling of the retinal ILM. Ophthalmology. 2002;109:1039.
30. Tsuiki E, Fujikawa A, Miyamura N, et al. Visual field defects after macular hole surgery with indocyanine green-assisted internal limiting membrane peeling. Am J Ophthalmol. 2007;143:704-5.
31. Hillenkamp J, Saikia P, Hermann WA, et al. Surgical removal of idiopathic epiretinal membrane with or without the assistance of indocyanine green: a randomised controlled clinical trial. Graefe´s Arch Clin Exp Ophthalmol. 2007;245: 973-9.
32. Schmidt JC, Rodrigues EB, Meyer CH, et al. A modified technique to stain the internal limiting membrane with indocyanin green. Ophthalmologica. 2004;218:176-9.
33. Schmid-Kubista KE, Lamar PD, Schenk A, et al. Comparison of macular function and visual fields after membrane blue or infracyanine green staining in vitreoretinal surgery. Graefes Arch Clin Exp Ophthalmol. 2010; 248:381-8.
34. Ikeda T, Sato K, Katano T, et al. Improved visual acuity following pars plana vitrectomy for diabetic cystoid macular edema and detached posterior hyaloid. Retina. 2000;20:220-2.
35. Otani T, Kishi S. Tomographic assessment of vitreous surgery for diabetic macular edema. Am J Ophthalmol. 2000;129:487-94.
36. Yamamoto T, Naoko A, Takeuchi S. Vitrectomy for diabetic macular edema: the role of posterior vitreous detachment and epimacular membrane. Am J Ophthalmol. 2001;132;369-77.
37. Sebag J. Anomalous posterior vitreous detachment: a unifying concept in vitreo-retinal disease. Graefe´s Arch Clin Exp Ophthalmol. 2004;242:690-8.

38. Kumagai K, Furukawa M, Ogino N, et al. Long-term follow-up of vitrectomy for diffuse nontractional diabetic macular edema. Retina. 2009;29:464-72.
39. Massin P, Duguid G, Erginay A, et al. Optical coherence tomography for evaluating diabetic macular edema before and after vitrectomy. Am J Ophthalmol. 2003;135:169-77.
40. Shah SP, Patel M, Thomas D, et al. Factors predicting outcome of vitrectomy for diabetic macular edema: results of a prospective study. Br J Ophthalmol. 2006;90:33-6.
41. Song SJ, Sohn JH, Park KH. Evaluation of the efficacy of vitrectomy for persistent diabetic macular edema and associated factors predicting outcome. Korean J Ophthalmol. 2007;21:146-50.
42. Yanyali A, Nohutcu AF, Horozoglu F, et al. Modified grid laser photocoagulation versus pars plana vitrectomy with internal limiting membrane removal in diabetic macular edema. Am J Ophthalmol. 2005;139:795-801.
43. Thomas D, Bunce C, Moorman C, et al. A randomised controlled feasibility trial of vitrectomy versus laser for diabetic macular oedema. Br J Ophthalmol. 2005;89:81-6.
44. Parolini B, Panozzo G, Gusson E, et al. Diode laser, vitrectomy and intravitreal triamcinolone. A comparative study for the treatment of diffuse non tractional diabetic macular edema. Semin Ophthalmol. 2004;19:1-12.
45. Gibran SK, Khan K, Jungkim S, et al. Optical coherence tomography pattern may predict visual outcome after intravitreal triamcinolone for diabetic macular edema. Ophthalmology. 2007;114:890-4.
46. Forooghian F, Stetson PF, Meyer SA, et al. Relationship between photoreceptor outer segment length and visual acuity in diabetic macular edema. Retina. 2010;30:63-70.
47. Azzolini C, D´Angelo A, Maestranzi G, et al. Intrasurgical plasmin enzyme in diabetic macular edema. Am J Ophthalmol. 2004;138:560-6.
48. Asami T, Terasaki H, Kachi S, et al. Ultrastructure of internal limiting membrane removed during plasmin-assisted vitrectomy from eyes with diabetic macular edema. Ophthalmology. 2004;111:231-7.
49. Sakuma T, Tanaka M, Inoue J, et al. Use of autologous plasmin during vitrectomy for diabetic maculopathy. Eur J Ophthalmol. 2006;16:138-40.
50. Diaz-Llopis M, Udaondo P, Arevalo F, et al. Intravitreal plasmin without associated vitrectomy as a treatment for refractory diabetic macular edema. J Ocul Pharmacol Ther. 2009;25:379-84.

Laser in Diabetic Retinopathy

20

Ranjana Mathur

Introduction

The term LASER is derived from Light Amplification by Stimulated Emission of Radiation. Ophthalmic practice has experienced largest application of lasers in past four decades with advent of xenon arc, argon, krypton-argon, diode, tunable dye, Nd:YAG (neodymium-doped yttrium aluminium garnet), excimer laser, photodynamic therapy (PDT), transpupillary thermal (TTT) pattern scan and Femto-second laser.[1] Meyer-Schwickerath and Lttman in conjunction with Zeiss assembled the first xenon arc lamp coagulator in 1956 to produce retinal burn. This system was suboptimal and lacked precision, required long treatment duration and was painful. Clinical applications employing laser-based system replaced xenon lamp in 1970s. These lasers applications employ various properties of laser for therapeutic and diagnostic purposes. In the following sections we will discuss various types of lasers, delivery systems and their clinical applications.

Principles of Laser

Laser radiation is a source of photons (packets of light) with specific properties[2] of

- Monochromatic light (single wavelength): leads to selective absorption by specific ocular target tissue
- Coherent light or "in phase"
- Collimated or non-divergent beam: allows precise focus on ocular tissue to a very small spot of high irradiance.

Light-tissue Interaction

Application of laser to the retina can result in various reactions based on laser wavelength. These tissue interactions are thermal, photochemical and ionizing. It is the thermal mode of reaction that is most commonly employed in retinal pathology.

▶ Thermal Effect

Photocoagulation

Photocoagulation reaction, which is irreversible protein denaturation causing cell damage, occurs when heat rise (moderate temperature of 10º-20º C) is produced as a result of laser absorption by ocular pigments. Although general guidelines of laser settings in treating various retinal conditions, to produce optimal laser burn, are predetermined, these parameters need to be tweaked in different situations. Media opacity, laser wavelength, absorption by target tissues are some of the factors which may influence power density and spot size during laser delivery.

Hyperthermia

Transpupillary thermotherapy (TTT) has been described for its application in choroidal hemangioma, melanoma as well as in occult choroidal neovascularization. Its usefulness in these retinal conditions is still being investigated. Hyperthermia is achieved when tissue temperature rises (42°-52° C) and is maintained for few seconds to minutes, irreversible cellular effect results in membrane alterations but avoids photocoagulation or photovaporization. To facilitate deep penetration into tissue continuous wave laser wavelengths in near-infrared region (88-1064 nm) are employed.

Photovaporization

When laser energy causes tissue temperature to rise above 100° C, biocellular target is photovaporized. If laser wavelength with low penetrance is used in application then this principle can be applied for bloodless incisions—CO_2 laser for photocautery in vitrectomy fibrovascular membranes.

Ionizing Effect

Photodisruption

When tissue temperature exceeds the vaporization threshold (100° C), vapor bubbles are produced and electrons are from molecules in target tissue producing plasma ions. Rapid expansion of the plasma creates acoustic shock waves that have potential to incise or disrupt target tissue regardless of tissue pigmentation and laser absorption. Most common application of this is employing Nd:YAG (1064 nm) for posterior capsulotomy, peripheral iridotomy, vitreolysis, and rarely posterior hyaloidocapsulotomy

Photochemical

Photochemical interactions are based on non-thermal light-induced chemical reaction. Currently photodynamic therapy (PDT) is commonest example of this form of laser therapy.

Prior to PDT special exogenous chromophores, called photosensitizers are injected intravenously. After excitation by laser radiation free radical-induced cytotoxic oxidative damage causing molecular and cellular damage.

Equipment

Laser Source

Thee are many laser sources available to generate laser light. Argon blue-green and krypton red lasers uses ionized gas. Recently Argon green laser is also available in solid state, which uses frequency doubled Nd:YAG (532 nm) system. It has near infrared beam at 1064 nm, but due to property of frequency doubling by a potassium-titanium-phosphate (KTP) crystal it halves the wavelength resulting in green laser. Tunable dye laser (yellow-orange-red) uses liquid solution whereas diode, Nd:YAG, laser are both solid-state lasers that utilize semiconductors and crystals as medium. Solid-state lasers are compact, reliable, portable and have the ability to deliver continuous and pulse mode laser.

The commercially available lasers frequencies for application in retinal conditions include:

- Argon blue: (488 nm)
- Argon blue-green: (518 nm)
- Argon green frequency doubled: (532 nm)
- Krypton red: (647 nm)
- Tunable dye laser: (yellow-orange-red)
- Diode laser: (812 nm)

Laser Delivery Systems

Slit-lamp based laser systems are most commonly used laser delivery system. Binocular indirect ophthalmoscopic delivery system enabled treating anterior retinal pathologies like peripheral retinal tears, retinopathy of prematurity (ROP), FEVR, peripheral neovascularization in presence of media opacity. Endo-fibreoptic system is used during intraocular vitreo-retinal surgery.

Modes of Laser Application

Continuous-wave: Laser is emitted at a sustained energy level for the given period of time (100-200 ms). Major disadvantage of continuous wave system is collateral damage to surrounding retinal tissue secondary to passive thermal diffusion of laser energy beyond intended area of treatment. Delayed enlargement of laser scar size (foveal creep) led to visual morbidity in patients with diabetic maculopathy undergoing focal-grid laser photocoagulation.

Pulsed: Subthreshold micropulse laser mode limits damage to adjacent retinal structures. Ultra-short pulses (microseconds) with laser output source turns on and off induces a temperature rise that is insufficient to cause damage to surrounding tissue. Micropulse diode laser 810 nm in infrared spectrum has been extensively tested in clinical practice for diabetic macular edema (DME). Recently, yellow laser in visible spectrum wavelength is being evaluated with micropulse delivery system.

Q-switched: Pulses are nanosecond and deliver very high peak power due to instant population inversion of stimulated photons as in Nd:YAG laser.

TABLE 20.1: Comparison of various retinal laser contact lenses

	Advantages	*Disadvantages*	*Magnification factor*	*Optical property*
Goldmann 3-mirror	Excellent resolution	Narrow fundus view	0.93	Planoconcave, mirrored lens
Mainster	Higher magnification, better resolution, less distortion	Inverted image, narrower field than quadraspheric lens	1.05	High plus lens
Quadraspheric	High efficiency anti-reflective coating, reduced peripheral aberrations, wide fundus view		0.50	Panfundoscope high plus lens
Rodenstock	Wide fundus view	Inverted image, requires biomicroscope to be pulled away from the patient to focus the image	1.4	-DO-
Area centralis	Excellent macular resolution, non-inverted image	Narrow field	1.0	Double asperic lens

Laser Contact Lens

Retinal laser contact lenses differ in their properties of magnification, field of view, resultant spot size and in quality of image (Table 20.1). These critical parameters aid in selecting right lens for particular clinical situation.[2,3]

Factors Influencing Laser Output

Incident laser light while it travel through the eye to the target tissue, undergoes a series of processes—scattering, reflection and absorption of laser energy by ocular tissues and media opacity.[4] This can affect the final power of laser beam at the target tissue due to scattering, reflection and/or absorption by non-target tissue. Shorter wavelengths (blue-green) scatter more light than longer wavelengths (yellow-red). This explains why in presence of media opacity, more power is required to produce same reaction by blue laser than green-yellow.

Additionally, it is the laser wavelength, ocular pigment, laser power, exposure and spot size that affect laser output on target tissues.

Ocular Pigment

The amount of laser absorbed by ocular tissue is largely dependent on pigment composition within individual target tissue. There are three major ocular pigments—melanin, hemoglobin, and xanthophyll.

- *Melanin:* Absorbs all wavelengths of light (blue-green > red-infrared)
- *Xanthophyll:* Pigment mostly present in the macula, strongly absorbs blue wavelength laser. Hence, blue argon laser are not used in retinal laser therapy to prevent central scotoma.
- *Hemoglobin:* Absorbs blue-green wavelengths and reflects-transmits red-infrared laser (krypton-diode).

Laser Wavelength

Lower wavelengths carry higher energy but are more likely to scatter (blue-green> red-diode). Melanin, a black pigment, absorbs all wavelengths of light (blue-green>>red-diode). Hence, less of krypton red-diode laser is absorbed and more reaches choroid compared to argon green laser. This result in white, superficial burn with argon green and deeper, pale white burns with diode for same energy level. If clinicians increase diode laser power to achieve same white burns as for argon green, it may cause choroidal rupture. Thus, desired endpoint for argon green is milky white, krypton red is pale white and diode is barely visible laser burn.[2]

Red pigment in hemoglobin will absorb non-red wavelengths better, blue-green, particularly yellow laser (twice that of green laser). This principle is useful while treating diabetic microaneurysms, retinal angioma, etc. Hence, yellow laser is considered the best wavelength to treat vascular lesions. In presence of significant subretinal-intraretinal blood, green-yellow laser can be absorbed by the hemorrhage resulting in significant scarring and collateral damage. In this situation it may be advantageous to employ red-diode laser.

Yellow pigment (nuclear sclerosis, xanthophyll) will reflect yellow laser but absorb blue-green. Longer wavelength red-yellow-diode will minimally be absorbed by nuclear sclerotic, which decreases chance of lens damage from laser light absorption and increases laser energy available for treatment.

Blue-green laser is maximally absorbed by macular xanthophyll causing maximum damage. Thus use of blue wavelength is discontinued in photocoagulation. Argon green or frequency doubled green lasers are most widely available and used laser in laser photocoagulation. Although yellow wavelength is optimum laser wavelength for vascular abnormalities, its application is limited due to cost, bulky krypton yellow lasers and tunable dye lasers (Table 20.2).

Modifiable Laser Parameters

Laser power and exposure are inversely related (non-linear) so typically if laser lower is increased then laser duration should be decreased to achieve desired end point. This principle, however, is not strict since other variables like media opacity, amount of melanin in RPE (pigmented vs. blonde fundi). Laser spot size is chosen based on pathology to be treated. For instance, macular work mandates smaller spot size compared to peripheral retinal structure. The spot size is also affected by laser contact lens that is utilized (Table 20.1). Smaller lesions require smaller spot size like central serous retinopathy leak and retinal macroaneurysm.

Complications of Laser Photocoagulation

- Pain, rarely vasovagal attack
- Change in postoperative refraction due to change in accommodative range

TABLE 20.2: Comparison of various laser wavelengths

	Advantages	*Disadvantages*
Blue-green	Very well absorbed by melanin pigment Used for iridotomy	Scatters laser light Increased absorption by cataractous lens Increased foveal damage Photochemical damage to adjacent retinal area
Green	Less damage to xanthophyll than blue-green laser Easily available commercially Well absorbed by vascular abnormal tissue	In presence of significant intraretinal/subretinal blood, Collateral damage to inner retinal layers. Subretinal scarring
Yellow	No absorption by macular xanthophyll Maximum absorption by hemoglobin	In presence of significant intraretinal/subretinal blood, collateral damage to inner retinal layers Subretinal scarring Commercial availability
Red	Deeper penetration to subretinal/ choroidal structures Less collateral damage to inner retinal structures Not absorbed by macular pigments	May cause choroidal bleed with long exposures
Diode	Decreased scatter by cataract Deeper penetration Not absorbed by xanthophyll Not absorbed by preretinal or subretinal bleed	Unpredictable results if used to treat vascular abnormality More pain perceived during laser In blond fundus, difficult to treat subretinal pathology

- Decreased contrast sensitivity
- Reduced peripheral vision
- Corneal abrasion
- Choroidal or subretinal effusion, which may cause acute angle-closure glaucoma (AACG)
- Exacerbate diabetic macular edema after extensive photocoagulation
- Absolute scotoma may develop with overlapping confluent large burns
- Breaks in Bruch's membrane causing secondary choroidal neovascularization (CNV)
- Retinal pigment epithelial rips
- Subretinal fibrosis, retinal pigment epithelium (RPE) metaplasia
- Extension of chorioretinal scar to macular area (laser creep) particularly in myopic patients
- Inadvertent corneal or lenticular burn
- Inadvertent treatment of wrong area (foveal burn).

Pattern Scan Laser Photocoagulation (Pascal Laser)

Thermal damage induced by photocoagulation is influenced by laser wavelength, spot size, power intensity and exposure. By changing these parameters, resultant retinal collateral damage can be minimized.

The pattern scan laser photocoagulation (Opti-Medica Corp, Santa Clara, California, USA) is a semi-automated photocoagulator system that allows delivery of multiple laser burns (1-56) per activation of foot pedal, in a preconfigured pattern array (3X3, 4X4, 5X5, arch, circular, subset grids) produced by a scanner.[5,6] It employs very short duration pulses (10-30 ms) compared to 50-300 ms in conventional lasers. This results in significantly less thermal damage to the surrounding retinal tissue compared to the conventional photocoagulation. Pascal is a 532 nm frequency-doubled neodymium-yttrium aluminium garnet (Nd:YAG) solid-state laser. Also, pascal allows for a large area of retinal ablation in much shorter duration.

It is our experience that higher power intensity is required to achieve therapeutic effect on the retina with short duration burst mode in pascal laser. However, the effective laser energy incident per burn, is much lesser compared to standard laser due to shorter exposure. The main benefits of this expensive laser modality are faster treatment time, greater accuracy, less pain perceived by patient.

Clinical Applications in Diabetic Retinopathy

In contrast to Diabetic Retinopathy Study (DRS), the Early Treatment Diabetic Retinopathy Study (ETDRS) showed that many patients did not develop high-risk retinopathy even after 5 years follow up, so should be followed up closely. However, high-risk retinopathy should be treated with Panretinal photocoagulation (PRP).[7]

Definite Indications

- Neovascularization at the disc (NVD) equal to or greater than 1/4-1/3 disc area, with or without vitreous hemorrhage
- Vitreous or preretinal hemorrhage (VH) with any NVD or neovascularization elsewhere (NVE) greater than ½ disc area.
- Neovascularization of iris (NVI) with NVE/NVD with or without VH.

Probable Indications (Very Severe NPDR 4-2-1 Rule)

If two of the following meet the criteria then PRP can be initiated.

- Microaneurysms and hemorrhages equal to or greater than standard photograph 2A in all four retinal quadrants
- Venous beading equal to or greater than that shown in standard photograph 6A in 2 or more quadrants
- Intraretinal microvascular abnormalities (IRMAs) equal to or greater than that shown in standard photograph 8A in at least one quadrant.

Treatment Protocol

Before initiating PRP, several factors that have been discussed in previous segment need to be considered (type of contact lens for magnification factor, type of wavelength, presence of media opacity, VH, DME, etc.

- Optimal laser burn of medium intensity(gray-white, milky white)
- Effective spot size: 500 µm (Goldmann 500 µm, Volk quadraspheric lens 200 µm, Mainster lens 350 µm)
- Duration or exposure: 100-200 ms
- Power: starting power of 200 mW, increased incrementally till desired endpoint is achieved.
- Laser wavelength: most commonly green or yellow
- Pattern of PRP: Burns are placed in no closer than 1 disc diameter from nasal edge of optic disc and 3 disc

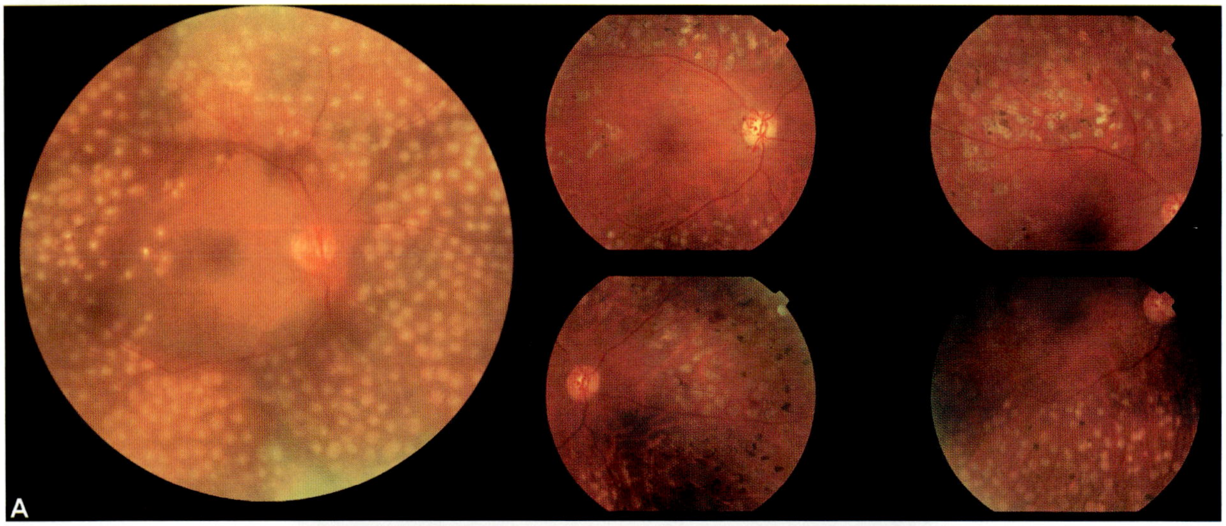

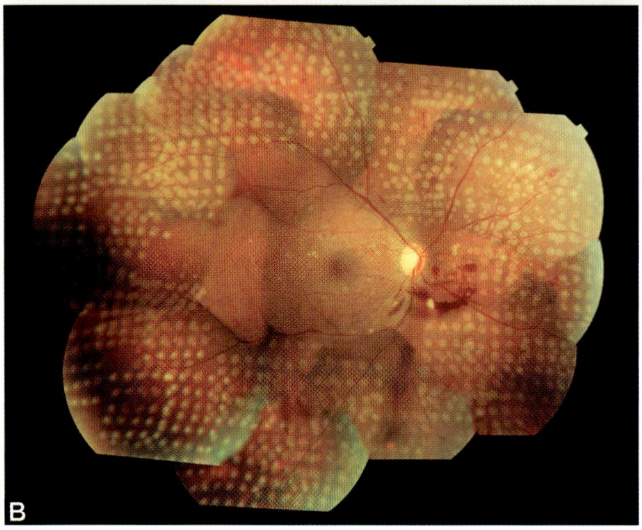

▲ **Figures 20.1A and B**

(A) Panretinal photocoagulation for proliferative diabetic retinopathy (conventional argon green laser); (B) Panretinal photocoagulation for proliferative diabetic retinopathy (Pascal laser)

diameters superior, inferior to macula and 4 disc diameters to temporal edge of macula. These burns extend to the periphery out to vortex vein. Treatment is divided into 1-3 treatment sessions (Figs 20.1A and B).

Special Considerations

- In presence of CSME/CMO, treatment sessions may have to be long apart to avoid exacerbation of DME. DME must be treated at the first session with or without PRP.
- Direct photocoagulation of large NVEs is recommended by some clinicians. However, author prefers to apply homogenous scatter treatment around the NVEs to avoid large areas of retinal atrophy and vitreoretinal traction that may ensue heavy confluent treatment of NVEs.
- NVDs are not treated directly.
- If impending PVD is suspected, inferior retinal quadrant PRP should be attempted first.
- In presence of large area of macular hemorrhage or premacular hemorrhage, diode or red laser may be

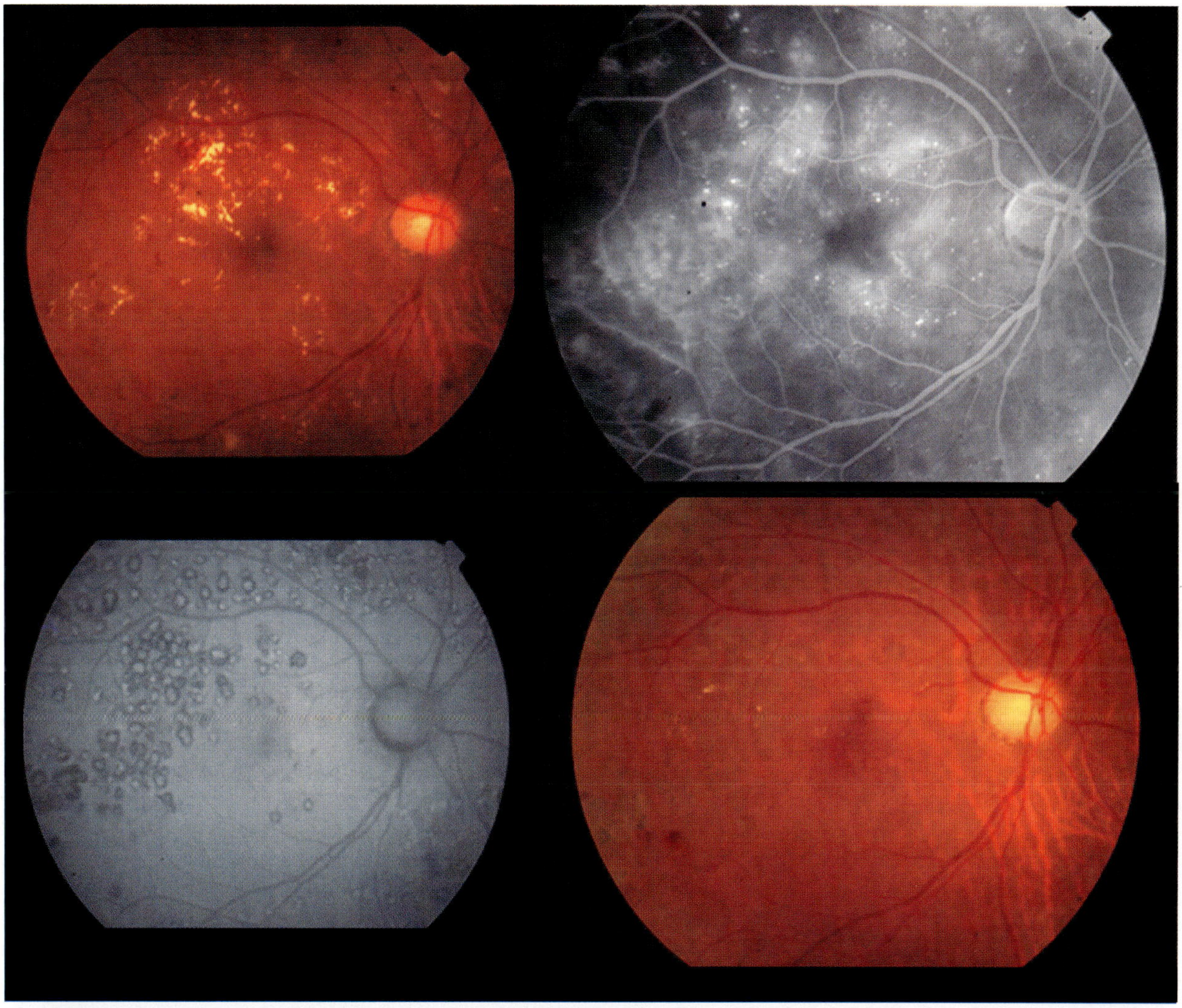

▲ **Figure 20.2**

Focal and diffuse DME treated with focal and grid (modified ETDS)

preferential to avoid excessive scarring and collateral damage from laser absorption.[8]

- It is recommended to tailor the treatment amount and intensity for each patient.

Pascal Photocoagulation

Despite effectiveness of conventional single spot retinal photocoagulation, it induces significant morbidity (pain, contrast sensitivity, worsening of macular edema) mostly due to production of inflammatory cytokines by neighboring tissue damaged by laser heat expansion. Pascal laser addresses some of these issues since reduced laser pulse duration limits damage to surrounding tissue, patterned array of laser spot decreases total laser time, and is less painful (Fig. 20.2).

Our experience shows that despite higher amount of laser power required to induce retinal burns, the shorter pulse duration (0.20-0.30 ms) causes total fluence at each burn to be much lower than in conventional lasers.

Diabetic Macular Edema (DME)

Clinically significant macular edema (CSME) is the most common cause of visual morbidity in diabetic patients. Early

Treatment Diabetic Retinopathy Study (ETDRS) has defined macular edema as (any one of the following):

- Retinal thickening or hard exudates adjacent to thickened retina involving foveal center
- Retinal thickening or hard exudates adjacent to thickened retina extending within 500 μm of foveal center
- Retinal thickening involving 1 disc diameter or more of retina, any part of which is within 1 disc diameter of foveal center.

Types of DME

DME is classified into focal versus diffuse DME. Focal DME is due to discrete points of retinal hyperfluorescence due to leakage from microaneurysms surrounded by hard exudates (circinate ring) and this form of edema can be multifocal. In diffuse edema there are areas of diffuse leakage on FA due to intraretinal leakage from dilated capillary bed and/or from arterioles-venules, and IRMAs without foci of leaking microaneurysms.

The thickened retina is translucent and often shows cystic changes called cystoid macular edema (CMO). Cystoid macular edema results from generalized breakdown of the inner blood retinal barrier with fluid accumulation in the outer plexiform layer.

Hard exudates at the fovea may result in visual loss and are not amenable to laser treatment. The microaneurysms may cause macular edema that is focal, localized to a quadrant of macular or more extensive, involving entire macular area, diffuse macular edema (macular edema involving 2 or more disc diameter of retinal thickening part of which must involve foveal center).

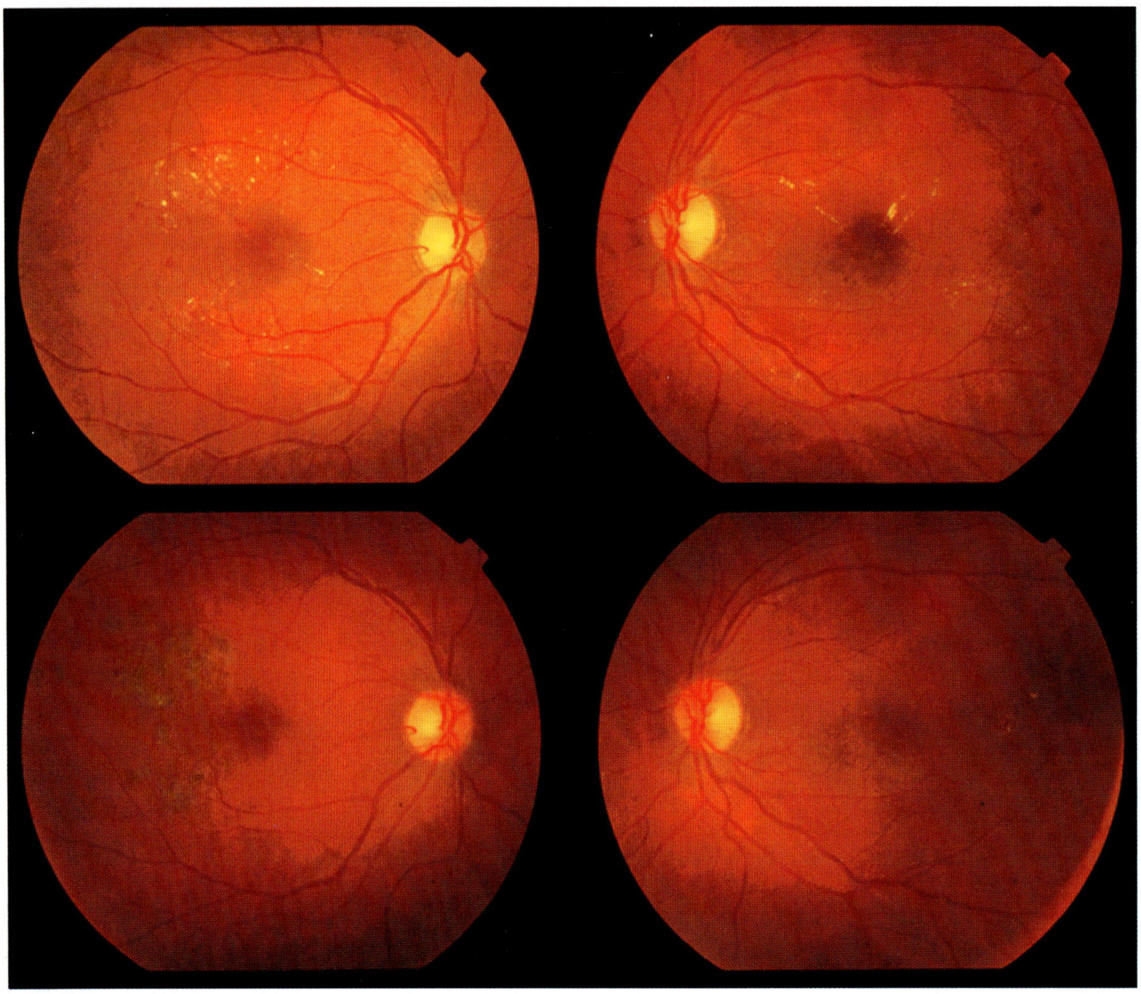

▲ **Figure 20.3**
Diffuse and superior focal DME treated with combination of laser and anti-VEGF therapy

Treatment Protocol

According to ETDRS guidelines, laser treatment reduces macular edema and preserves vision compared to no treatment. Patient received a combination of focal and grid laser with argon green or blue-green laser.[9,10]

It is, however, the *modified ETDRS protocol* which is practiced more commonly. It recommends employing argon green laser, 100 μm effective spot size, 0.1 ms duration and initial power of 80 mW, increased in increments to achieve desired end point of pale white burns to blanch the microaneurysms (Fig. 20.2).

Several studies have documented subthreshold micropulse diode laser photocoagulation to have comparable visual outcomes compared to standard argon laser therapy. However, due to barely visible subthreshold laser burns, optimal power settings are difficult to achieve. This may be one of the reasons that micropulse laser therapy for DME is not widely utilized.

With advent of intravitreal injection of anti-VEGF and steroids, it is often employed as a primary or combination therapy to treat DME. It has been found that long term visual acuity for treatment of DME with intravitreal injections alone or in combination with laser therapy is superior to laser therapy alone or sham treatment[11,12] (Fig. 20.3).

To summarize, based on current evidence, author recommends focal or multifocal DME to be treated with gold standard laser treatment. Whereas, in diffuse DME, a combination of intravitreal anti-VEGF with focal laser therapy, would render best results. You may consider intravitreal triamcinolone or other steroid derivatives to be injected in pseudophakic eyes.

References

1. Folk JC, Pulido JS. Laser Photocoagulation of Retina and Choroid, 3rd edition. CV Mosby, 1983.
2. Ophthalmology Monograph 11 AAO series. Lifelong Education for the Ophthalmologists (LEO)
3. Mainster MA, Crossman JL, Erickson PJ, et al. Retinal laser lenses: magnification, spot size, and field of view. Br J Opthalmol. 1990;74:177-9.
4. Sabates NR, Sabates FN. Applied laser optics. Techniques for retinal laser surger. Duanes Ophthalmology chapter 69A. Lippincott Wlliam and Wilkins.
5. Blumenkranz MS, Yellachich D, Andersen DE, et al. Semiautomated patterned scanning laser for retinal photocoagulation. Retina. 2006;26:370-6.
6. Sanghavi C, McLauchlan R, Delago C, et al. Initial experience with the pascal photocoagulator: a pilot study of 75 procedures. Br J Ophthalmol. 2008;92:1061-4.
7. Early Treatment Diabetic Retinopathy Study Research Group: Early photocoagulation for diabetic retinopathy. ETDRS report number 7. Ophthalmology. 1991;98:741-56.
8. Diabetic Retinopathy Study Group: Photocoagulation treatment of proliferative diabetic retinopathy: relationship of adverse treatment effects to retinopathy severity. Dev Ophthalmol. 1981;2:248-61.
9. Early Treatment Diabetic Retinopathy Study Research Group: Photocoagulation for diabetic macular edema. ETDRS Report Number 1. Arch Ophthalmol 1985;27:265-72.
10. Early Treatment Diabetic Retinopathy Study Research Group: treatment techniques and clinical guidelines for photocoagulation of diabetic macular edema. ETDRS Report Number 2. Ophthalmology 1987;94:761-74.
11. Nguyen QD, Shah SM, Heier JS, Do DV, Lim J, Boyer D, et al. Primary End Point (Six Months) Results of the Ranibizumab for Edema of the macula in diabetes (READ-2) study. Ophthalmology. 2009;116:2175-81.
12. Massin P, Bandello F, Garweg JG, Hansen LL, Harding SP, Larsen M, et al. Safety and efficacy of ranibizumab in diabetic macular edema (RESOLVE Study): a 12-month, randomized, controlled, double-masked, multi-center phase II study. Diabetes Care. 2010;33:2399-2405.

SECTION

4 Other Retinal Vascular Disorders and Inflammation

21

Surgical Management of Retinal Vein Occlusion

Jose Garcia-Arumi, Miguel Zapata, Jose Badal

Central Retinal Vein Occlusion

▶ Introduction

Central retinal vein occlusion (CRVO) is the third most common blinding vascular retinal disorder after diabetic retinopathy and branch retinal vein occlusion.[1,2]

Among patients with CRVO, 34% develop capillary nonperfusion and retinal ischemia (Figs 21.1A and B). Iris neovascularization (INV) and neovascular glaucoma may occur in 45–85% of the eyes affected by ischemic CRVO and only in 5% of the nonischemic eyes.[2,3] The main known risk factors of CRVO are hypertension and open-angle glaucoma.[2-5]

The pathogenesis of CRVO is yet not very well understood. It is thought to be a compartment syndrome, since in a 1.5 mm diameter area, the central retinal artery, the central retinal vein and the optic nerve coexist. Thrombotic occlusion is thought to develop as the result of an increase in the arterial diameter, changes in the scleral ring and the presence of anatomical anomalies and possible systemic factors, which together cause a decrease in the venous lumen, increased turbulence and damage to endothelium and thrombus formation. This is supported by histologic studies that

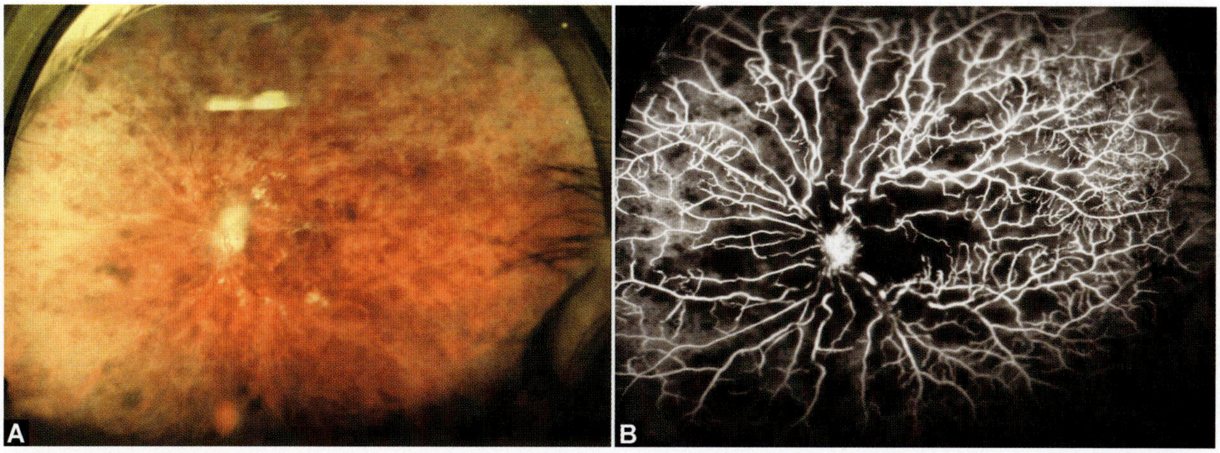

▲ **Figures 21.1A and B**

(A) Central retinal vein occlusion with retinal hemorrhage, diffuse retinal edema, and numerous cotton-wool spots; (B) Fluorescein angiogram reveals marked retinal capillary nonperfusion involving retinal periphery localize the thrombus in the lamina cribrosa in most or all cases.[6,7]

It is clear from the Central Vein Occlusion Study (CVOS)[8] that, when left to follow its natural course, the vision in patients with CRVO will most likely worsen or remain unchanged and that those patients with poor vision initially have little hope of significant spontaneous recovery. There is no known effective treatment for CRVO. Numerous treatments are available, including panretinal laser photocoagulation (PRP), grid macular laser photocoagulation, chorioretinal anastomosis (CRA) via high-intensity laser photocoagulation and intraocular injections of drugs, with varying degrees of effectiveness and complication rates. One surgical procedure that has been developed is termed radial optic neurotomy (RON). Panretinal photocoagulation has only been effective in managing neovascular complications and grid macular laser photocoagulation only decreases macular edema without increasing the final visual acuity (VA).[1,8,9]

The current options for central retinal vein occlusion and their mechanism of action are:

- Intravitreal or endovascular injection
  - Recombinant tissue plasminogen activator: thrombus resolution.
  - Steroids: decrease vascular permeability.
  - Anti-vascular endothelial growth factor (VEGF) drugs: decrease vascular permeability.
- Vitrectomy with or without internal limiting membrane (ILM) peeling: improves vitreoretinal fluid exchange of oxygen, accelerates the clearance of factors that increase vascular permeability as VEGF and cytokines.
- Radial optic neurotomy: release pressure on the central retinal vein or induce CRA.

Pharmacologic Treatment

There are several pharmacologic agents focused on the treatment of central retinal vein occlusion and its complications.

Recombinant Tissue Plasminogen Activator

Thrombolytic agents have been proposed as a treatment against a suspected thrombus in the central retinal vein. Recombinant tissue plasminogen activator (rt-PA) is a synthetic fibrinolytic agent that converts plasminogen to plasmin and destabilizes intravascular thrombi. Reduction in clot size may facilitate dislodging of the entire thrombus or recanalization of the occluded retinal vein. rt-PA, as therapy against CRVO, has been administered by several routes: systemic, intravitreal and by endovascular cannulation of retinal vessels.

Systemic administration of low dose (50 mg) front loaded rt-PA has been attempted in two pilot studies with VA improvement in 30–73% of patients.[10,11] Lahey[12] reported, in a prospective clinical trial of 96 persons with CRVO, a mean improvement of five lines of acuity in 42% of individuals. One person in this study died from an intracranial hemorrhage following rt-PA administration, which has limited enthusiasm for the systemic administration of rt-PA for CRVO.

Intravitreal delivery of rt-PA has potential advantages including less risk of systemic complications, directed delivery to the vitreous cavity and subsequent access to the retinal vessels and low-risk of ocular morbidity from the procedure. Of 47 persons in three studies of intravitreal rt-PA for both ischemic and nonischemic CVO of less than 21 days duration, 28–44% had three lines of VA improvement with 6 months follow-up.[12-14] Administration of rt-PA did not significantly alter final perfusion status, especially in pretreatment ischemic eyes. Although there were no significant treatment related complications, differences in inclusion criteria and dosage of rt-PA used (between 66 and 100 μg) limits generalization from these studies. Ghazi et al.[15] reported using a standard dose of 50 μg of intravitreal rt-PA in 12 eyes with acute CRVO of less than 3 days duration. In all patients, perfusion status remained unchanged at last follow-up, however marked improvement (20/50 or better) was demonstrated in eyes with perfused CRVO. This report suggests prompt use of intravitreal rt-PA, especially in perfused CRVO, may provide significant visual benefit.

Endovascular delivery of rt-PA involves cannulation of retinal vessels, either through a neuroradiologic or a vitreoretinal approach and delivery of minute quantities of rt-PA directly to the occluded vessels to release the suspected thrombus.[16,17] Weiss and Bynoe have reported their technique of pars plana vitrectomy followed by cannulation of a branch vein and with the aid of a stabilization arm, injecting a bolus (average 3.4 ml) of 200 μg/ml rt-PA towards the optic nerve head. Of 28 eyes with CRVO of greater than 1 month duration and worse than 20/400 preoperative acuity, 50% recovered more than three lines of acuity by a mean follow-up of 12 months. There was a trend towards increased perfusion by fluorescein angiography attributed in part to the resolution of intraretinal hemorrhages after the procedure. Complications included vitreous hemorrhage in seven eyes and treated retinal detachment in one eye. This technique has been combined with intravitreal triamcinolone acetonide injection, hypothesized to target retinal edema, following endovascular rt-PA administration in two patients with CRVO under the age of 40 with resultant improvement of 8–11 lines of acuity.[18]

Intraocular Corticosteroids

The role of corticosteroids has been explored in CRVO with particular interest to improve VA by reducing macular edema. The exact mechanism of action of corticosteroids in modulating retinal edema is unknown, but it is believed that a combination of anti-inflammatory effects with modulation of cytokines and growth factors production and stabilization of the blood-retinal barrier with reduction in vascular permeability may be involved. There is little evidence for using oral corticosteroids to treat macular edema from CRVO. Several reports from intravitreal triamcinolone for CRVO macular edema have been published,[19] showing initial improvement but with no longer benefit after one year period. High incidence of cataract (63%) and glaucoma (30%) has also been reported as complications from intravitreal triamcinolone.

The most important study in this area is the SCORE study report 5.[20] The first multicenter, randomized clinical trial with 271 participants. The study compares the efficacy and safety of 1 mg and 4 mg doses of preservative-free intravitreal triamcinolone with observation in eyes with vision loss associated with macular edema secondary to perfused CRVO. Retreatment was done if necessary every 4 months. With a mean of 2.2 injections, at month 12 gain in VA was found in 7%, 27% and 26% of the patients respectively. Rates of adverse events, as elevated intraocular pressure and cataracts, were higher in the 4 mg triamcinolone group. This study concludes that intravitreal triamcinolone is superior to observation for treating vision loss associated with macular edema secondary to CRVO. The 1 mg dose has a safety profile superior to that of the 4 mg dose.

Finally, there is currently a phase III study for intravitreous dexamethasone drug delivery system (DDS-implant) comparing 300 μg, 700 μg and sham injection with 1267 patients involved. Gain in VA is noticed but not significant at 180 days.

Anti-Vascular Endothelial Growth Factor Drugs

Following CRVO subsequent hypoxia leads to upregulation of VEGF, resulting in increased retinal capillary permeability and leakage of fluid and blood into the intraretinal space. In addition, VEGF is a key promoter of angiogenesis, potentially contributing to the development of the neovascularization associated with CRVO. Antiangiogenic drugs may decrease vascular permeability and also the macular edema. Bevacizumab has been the most studied drug in this disease. Good safety and effective in short-term outcomes with this drug have been reported. Main limitations of this treatment modality are its short-term effectiveness and high recurrence rate.[21-23]

Ranibizumab is the other drug studied for CRVO. In a prospective study (CRUISE studies,[24] of 392 participants 3 groups were evaluated (0.3 mg, 0.5 mg or sham injection every month). At 6 months gain in VA was found in 46.2%, 47.9% and 16.9% of the patients respectively. The main problem of these drugs arises from the deal of what will happen when injections get stopped.

▶ Vitrectomy

Pars plana vitrectomy (PPV) techniques are used to address complications of CRVO and, in investigational studies, to attempt to alter the natural course of the disease. Eyes with nonclearing vitreous hemorrhage from secondary retinal neovascularization may require surgical evacuation. At the time of vitrectomy, clearing of the hemorrhage can be combined with removal of epiretinal membranes and removal of fibrovascular proliferations, if present and the placement of complete endolaser PRP.[25] Although this technique may prevent or aid in regression of anterior segment neovascularization, visual outcomes may be limited due to the extent of underlying retinal nonperfusion.[26]

In order to improve oxygenation of the fovea and anatomic and functional outcomes of vitrectomy some authors suggest peeling the ILM.[27]

▶ Radial Optic Neurotomy

Opremcak et al.[28] have proposed combining PPV with transvitreal incision of the nasal scleral ring to release pressure on the central retinal vein at the level of the scleral outlet. The procedure addresses the "compartment syndrome" that may exist in these eyes where the central retinal artery, central retinal vein and optic nerve traverse through a 1.5 mm diameter area. Vascular factors, as well as rigidity of the scleral ring may also decrease venous lumen diameter and incite a thrombotic event. Previous attempts at external decompression of the orbital portion of the optic nerve by optic nerve sheath fenestration and sectioning of the posterior

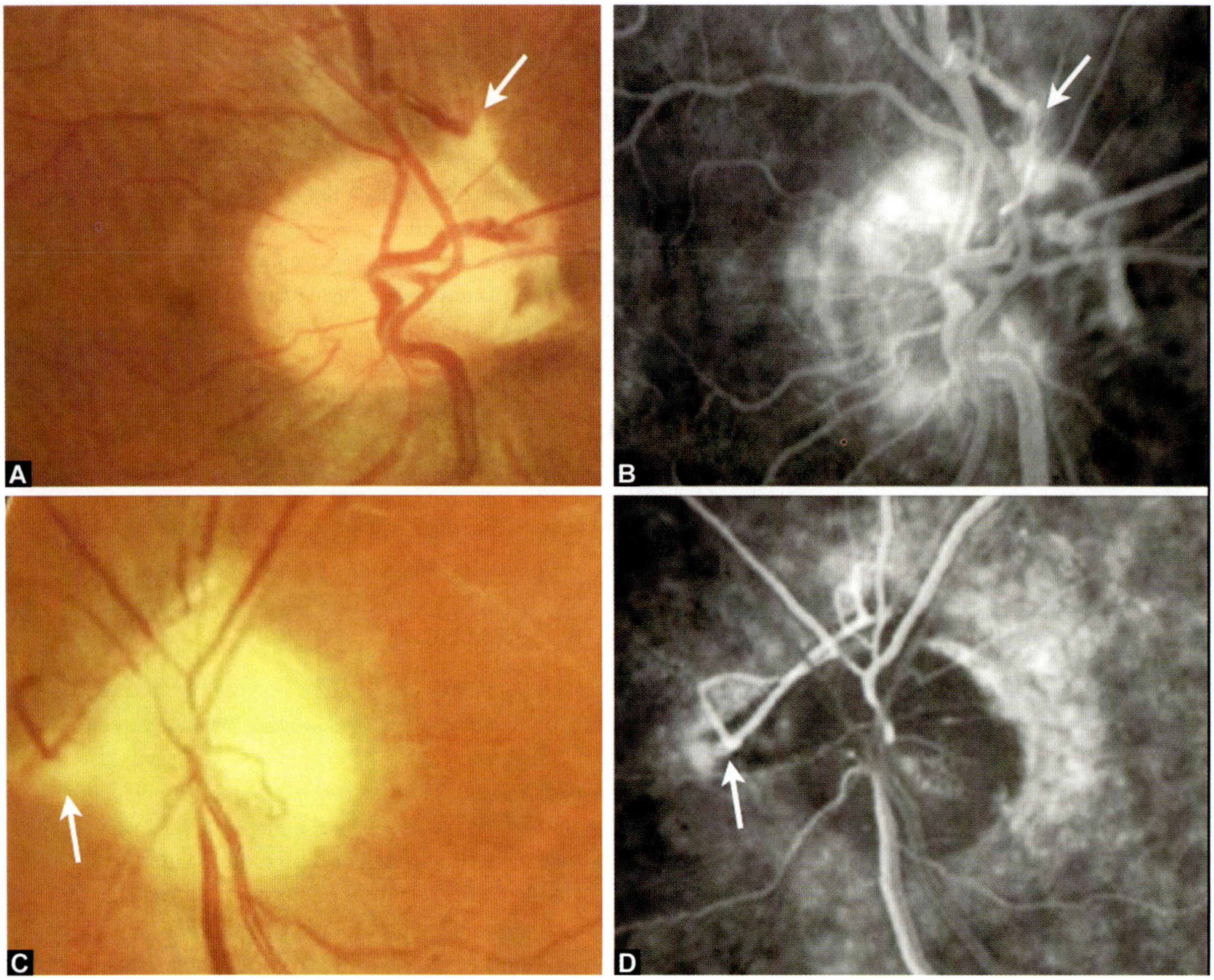

▲ **Figures 21.2A to D**

(A and C) Radial optic neurotomy is done at the nasal side of the optic disc with a radial orientation; (B and D) Fluorescein angiogram shows choroioretinal anastomosis arising from the radial optic neurotomy site

scleral ring have not been validated as effective treatments for CRVO.[29,30] Radial optic neurotomy is performed by PPV followed by use of a 25-gauge microvitreoretinal blade to incise the lamina cribrosa and adjacent retina. Care is taken to avoid major retinal vessels and a radial incision orientation is used to avoid transecting nerve fibers (Figs 21.2A to D). Intraoperative hemorrhage is typically controlled by transient elevation of intraocular pressure. In the initial retrospective report of 11 eyes by Opremcak et al.[28] successful RON was performed with no complications. There was clinical improvement in retinal hemorrhages and venous congestion. With a mean follow-up of 9 months, 73% of patients had improved Snellen acuity; however, two eyes with preoperative iris neovascularization had worsening of acuity associated with the development of neovascular glaucoma. Weizer et al.[31] reported their experience with RON in five eyes (one with hemiretinal vein occlusion). Mean VA improved from 4/200 to 20/400 with 80% demonstrating a rapid resolution of intraretinal hemorrhage and disc congestion as compared to the known natural history of CRVO. Perfusion status was not significantly altered and macular edema significantly improved in one eye. Two eyes developed neovascular complications but responded to PRP. Garcia-Arumí et al.[32] reported, in a prospective interventional trial, successful RON surgery in 14 eyes. Overall, 57% gained one line of distance VA and visual recovery was significantly related to reduction

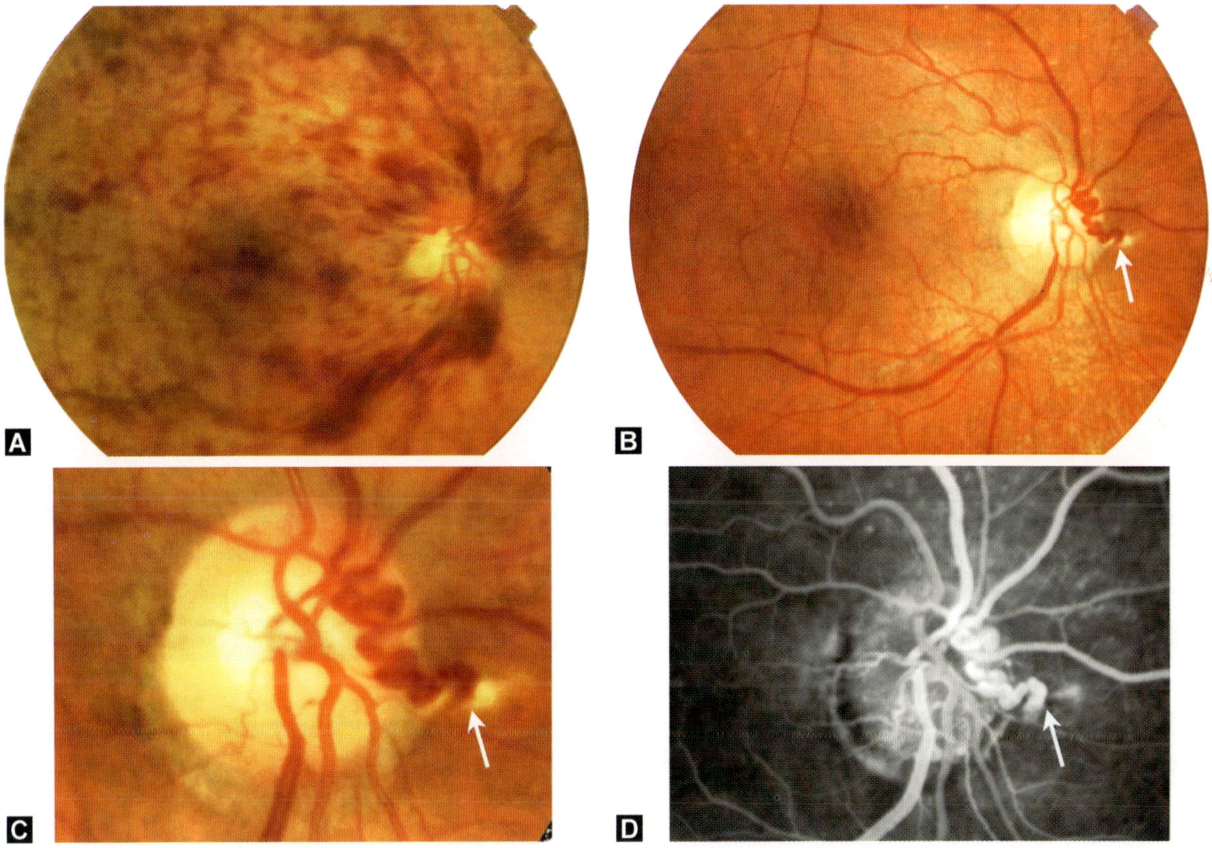

▲ Figures 21.3A to D

(A) Central retinal vein occlusion. Visual acuity was 20/200; (B) 3 months after radial optic neurotomy visual acuity was 20/60 and choroioretinal anastomosis was developed at radial optic neurotomy site (arrow); (C and D) Detailed choroioretinal anastomosis at radial optic neurotomy site allowing choroidal drainage of retinal circulation

in macular edema. Six (43%) developed a postoperative CRA (Figs 21.3A to D and 21.4A and B) at the RON site with a trend towards better final acuity compared to those without anastomosis formation (20/60 vs 20/110). The CRA seen at RON sites may allow for more active drainage of retinal edema and hemorrhage compared to laser-induced CRA. When evaluating the effectiveness of RON for CRVO in patients less than 50 years of age vs those greater than 50 years in 43 patients,[33] better functional results were observed in younger patients (50% vs 30% gained 15 letters), although functional improvement remained limited in those with low baseline VA. In patients with hemicentral retinal vein occlusion RON seems to be a potential treatment in selected patients, probably because of the more rapid appearance of retinochorioretinal collateral vessels, which promote faster resolution of macular edema. In a study of 13 patients, García-Arumí et al.[34] reported gain of 2 or more Snellen lines of vision in 69.2% of patients and in 4 patients (30.8%) VA improved by 4 or more Snellen lines.

In 2006, Opremcak et al.[35] reported in 117 patients with CRVO and severe loss of vision (≤ 20/200) treated with PPV and RON. Anatomic improvement of CRVO was found in 95% of patients. Disc edema improved in 1 week, although most improvements were observed at 2 and 3 months. VA improved in 71% of patients, with an average of 2.5 lines of vision gained. Subgroup analyses suggested that older age, female sex, duration of CRVO, presence of afferent pupillary defect, absence of perfusion by angiography and development of anterior segment neovascularization were associated with poorer visual outcomes.

Finally, a surgical prospective multicentric clinical trial was performed with 90 patients involved evaluating the role

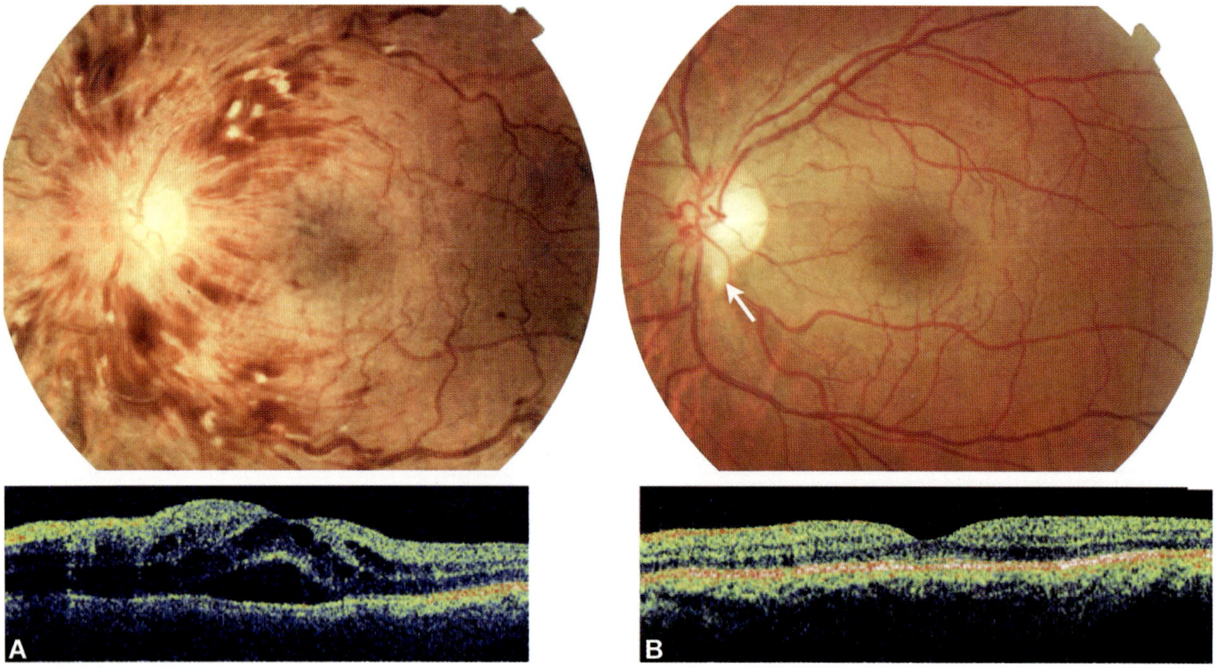

▲ **Figures 21.4A and B**

(A) Central retinal vein occlusion with macular edema. Visual acuity was 20/400; (B) 3 months post radial optic neurotomy (arrow) visual acuity recovered to 20/30 and no macular edema was observed on optical coherence tomography

of RON in CRVO (ROVO study). In international multicentric randomized study intravitreal 4 mg triamcinolone was administered to 25 patients, RON to 38 patients and placebo to 20 patients. Seven patients were excluded. Twelve months after treatment, 48.6% of RON patients improved greater than 3 lines logMAR, 25% of Triamcinolone patients improved greater than 3 lines logMAR and 11.8% of placebo patients improved greater than 3 lines. The Fisher's exact test showed a statistical significant difference comparing RON with placebo [RON vs Placebo (p=0.009)] and with IVT [RON vs IVT (p=0.034)], but it was not significant comparing IVT with placebo. In conclusion, RON appears to be the best option in patients with CRVO, low VA and important cystoid macular edema.

Branch Retinal Vein Occlusion

▶ Introduction

The majority of the venous lesions in branch retinal vein occlusion (BRVO) occur downstream from the arteriovenous crossing site. Changes in rigidity of the artery associated to hypertension induce a vein compression producing turbulence, endothelial cell damage and thrombus formation.[36]

Retinal vein occlusion is the second retinal vascular disorder, until recent years treatment was focused to the vascular proliferative complications and laser photocoagulation was the only treatment proved. The BRVO Study demonstrated that grid photocoagulation improves macular edema and vision in patients with macular edema secondary to BRVO but with preserved foveal vascularization,[37] this improvement was slightly only 1.3 ETDRS lines (early treatment diabetic retinopathy study).

Macular edema is the main cause of decrease in VA in BRVO. The approaches to the management of BRVO are addressed to reperfuse the thrombosed vein, to reduce the permeability of the macular vascular net improving the edema and to increase the vitreoretinal fluid exchange of oxygen and protecting factors.

The current surgical options for BRVO and their mechanism of action are:

- Vitrectomy with or without ILM peeling : improves vitreoretinal fluid exchange of oxygen, accelerates the clearance of factors that increase vascular permeability as VEGF and cytokines.

- Surgical decompression of arteriovenous crossing sheathotomy: mechanic decompression (thrombus release).
- Intravitreal or endovascular injection
  - rt-PA: thrombus resolution
  - Corticosteroids: decrease vascular permeability
  - Anti-VEGF drugs: decreased vascular permeability.

▶ Vitrectomy

There is evidence that PPV and posterior hyaloid dissection may increase oxygenation of the macula and in some cases vitreomacular attachment itself may contribute to the development of macular edema.[38] For this reasons some authors have proposed vitrectomy and posterior hyaloid dissection for BRVO. The few published studies that report outcomes of PPV for complications of BRVO consist only of case reports and small case series, limitations of which include small sample sizes and lack of comparison groups.[39] Despite the lack of large clinical trials, recently PPV has demonstrated to improved perifoveal microcirculation and the visual prognosis in BRVO patients with macular edema.

In order to improve oxygenation of the fovea and anatomic and functional outcomes of vitrectomy some authors proposed the peeling of the ILM. Short series of cases has found good outcomes with this technique.[40] Arai et al.[41] did not find any difference in a non-randomized, comparative study between PPV with and without ILM peeling for BRVO and they concluded that there is no additional benefit in removing the ILM for BRVO associated macular edema.

▶ Sheathotomy

Few years after histological changes in BRVO[42] were described in 1988,[42] Osterloh and Charles published the first report of sheathotomy for BRVO. Authors presented only one case with significant visual improvement after surgery. Despite the success of the technique this treatment was abandoned for nearly 10 years. In 1998 Kumar et al.[43] described again the venous narrowing at the crossing site as the main cause for BRVO and they suggested that removal of the compressive factor by sectioning the adventitial sheath (sheathotomy) may be an effective treatment for BRVO. One year later Opremcak et al.[44] published 15 patients with BRVO treated with sheathotomy.

Surgical technique consists of pars plana vitrectomy with posterior hyaloid dissection (Fig. 21.5). Arteriovenous

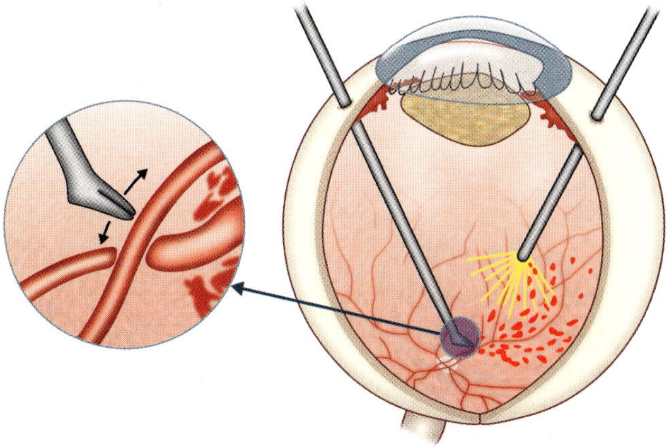

▲ **Figure 21.5**

Sheathotomy. Surgical technique: vitrectomy, posterior hyaloid dissection. Pars plana vitrectomy with posterior hyaliod dissection. Initial dissection of arteriovenous crossing

crossing must be dissected with special forceps and scissors. At this point, the experience of the surgeon plays an important role because small tractions may break the vein (Figs 21.6A and B). Revision of peripheral retina should be performed in order to avoid iatrogenic breaks and no other tamponed than serum is needed.

Potential benefits of sheathotomy include the mechanic decompression of the venule and thrombus release that sometimes we can appreciate during the surgery. Successful decompressive surgery usually is followed by disappearance of collateral vessels at the BRVO blockage site, what is a clinical marker for intravascular reperfusion and resolution of hemorrhages and macular edema.

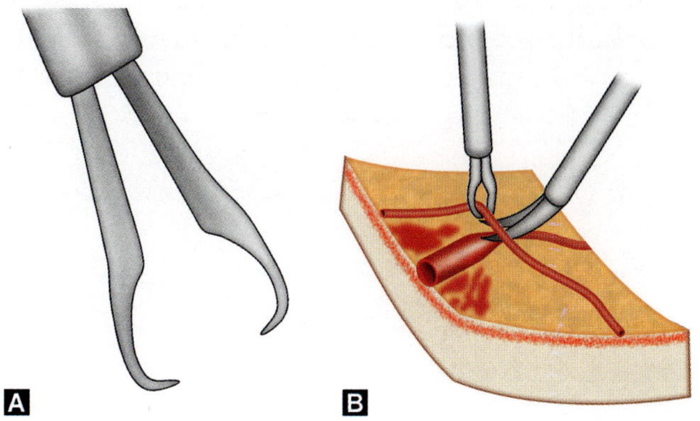

▲ **Figures 21.6A and B**

Sheathotomy. Surgical technique: dissection of arteriovenous crossing with special forceps and scissors

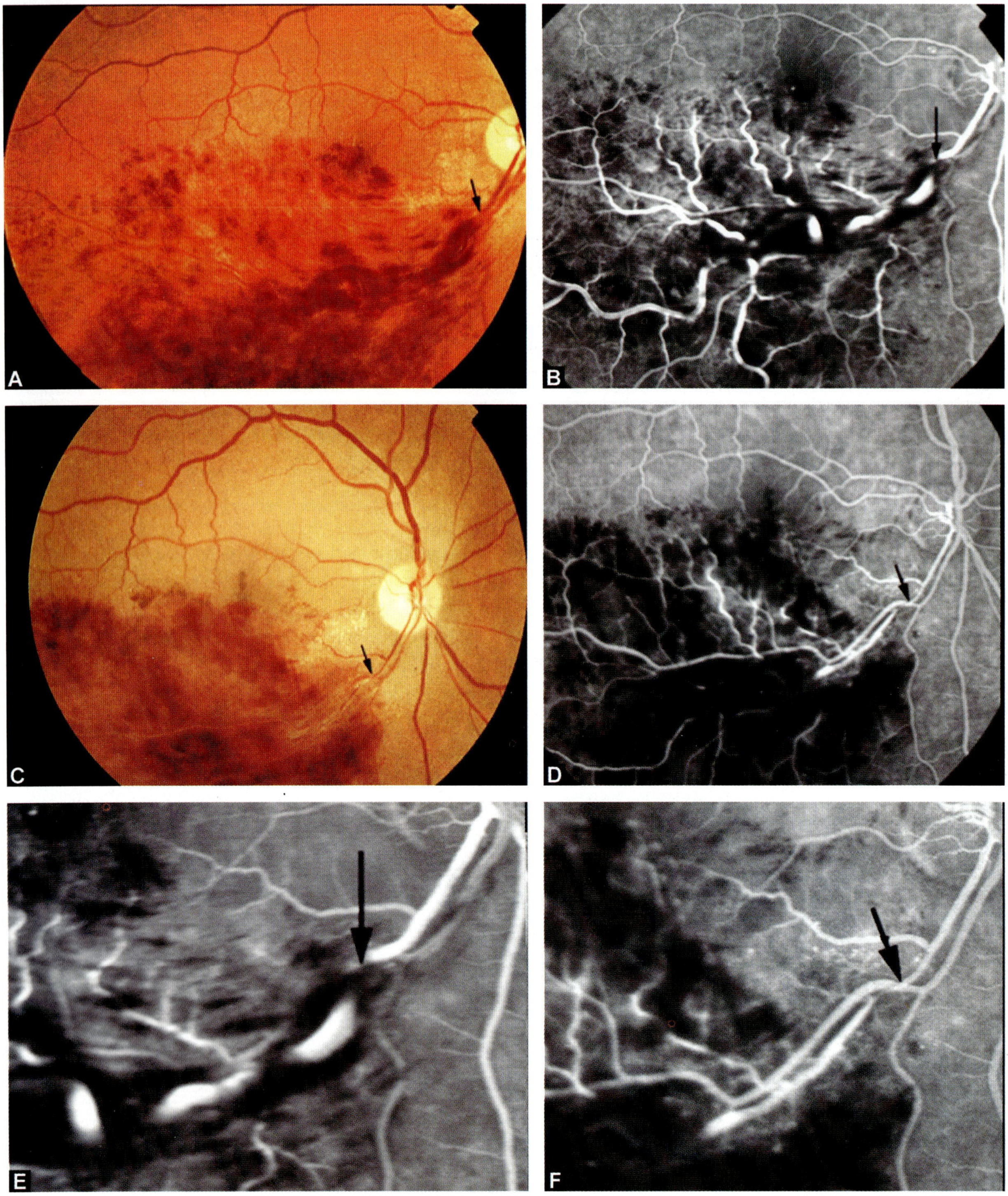

▲ Figures 21.7A to F

Retinography and fluorescein angiography. (A and B) Before the surgery. At the crossing site we observe dilatation of the vein; (C and D) After surgery. Normalization of the vein caliber at the crossing site; (E and F) Details of the crossing site, before and after surgery

With this technique Opremcak et al.[44] reported equal or improved VA in 12 of 15 patients (80%) with less than 1 year of evolution BRVO. Ten of those patients (67%) had improved postoperative visual acuities, with an average gain of four lines of vision. Three patients had a decline in VA, with an average of two lines of vision lost. All patients had marked resolution of the intraretinal hemorrhage and edema. No patient in their series developed worsening edema, ischemia, retinal neovascularization, or secondary vitreous hemorrhage. We can find similar and longer series of sheathotomy reporting good results as Mester[45] with 43 patients, or García-Arumí with 40 patients[46] (Figs 21.7A to F). Kumagai[47] reported good outcomes with vitrectomy but no additional benefit with the arteriovenous sheathotomy in a nonrandomized long-term follow-up series. At the elaboration of this review we can find over 25 references of sheathotomy for BRVO, more than 320 patients. In 18 references sheathotomy was safe and effective and in 7 references this technique has the same result than vitrectomy alone. At this point no randomized, controlled study evaluating the benefit of sheathotomy has been published.

Complications of sheathotomy are related to the experience of the surgeon. Opremcak et al.[44] do not report any vitreous hemorrhage during or after the surgery and their patients did not developed worsening of the edema, ischemia or retinal neovascularization. Other authors have experienced difficulty in separating the artery from the vein at the crossing site.[48] The more frequent complications observed are hemorrhages at the dissection site and vitreous hemorrhage.[49,50] again we think in correlation to surgical experience. Authors also describe retinal holes at the vitreous base and paracentral scotomas in eyes treated by arteriovenous dissection relatively close to the optic disc.[49] We can find also similar complications of vitrectomy as retinal breaks or retinal detachment.[50]

▶ Pharmacologic Treatment

Recombinant Tissue Plasminogen Activator

Intravitreal tissue plasminogen activator has been used alone[51] and in combination with sheathotomy[46] for BRVO. Results are encouraged but actually there are not comparative studies with other treatments. Potential benefits of plasminogen activator include the thrombus resolution.

Intraocular Corticosteroids

The exact mechanism of macular edema development from BRVO has not been elucidated, but breakdown of the blood-retinal barrier is thought to play a role. Potential role of corticosteroids is decrease in vascular permeability and the stabilization of the blood-retinal barrier.

The most important study in this area is the SCORE study.[52] The first multicenter randomized clinical trial with 411 participants. The study compares the efficacy and safety of 1 mg and 4 mg doses of preservative-free intravitreal triamcinolone with standard care (grid photocoagulation in eyes without dense macular hemorrhage and deferral of photocoagulation until hemorrhage clears in eyes with dense macular hemorrhage) for eyes with vision loss associated with macular edema secondary to BRVO. Despite good initial results with triamcinolone conclusions are that there is no difference in VA at 12 months for the standard care group compared with the triamcinolone groups and rates of adverse events, as elevated intraocular pressure and cataracts, were higher in the 4 mg triamcinolone group.

At this point, use of intravitreal triamcinolone is not recommended in macular edema secondary to BRVO.

Anti-VEGF Drugs

Vascular endothelial growth factor is elevated in vitreous of patients with BRVO and plays an important role in the pathogenesis of macular edema secondary to BRVO.[53] At this point antiangiogenic drugs may decrease vascular permeability and also the macular edema. Bevacizumab has been the most studied drug in this disease. We can find short series of cases and retrospective comparative studies concluding good safety and effective in short-term outcomes with this drug. Large and prospective studies report that limitations of this treatment modality are its short-term effectiveness and high recurrence rate.[54]

References

1. The Central Vein Occlusion Study Group. Baseline and early natural history report: the Central Vein Occlusion Study. Arch Ophthalmol. 1993;111:1087-95.
2. The Eye Disease Case-Control Study Group. Risk factors for central retinal vein occlusion. Arch Ophthalmol. 1996;114: 545-54.
3. Rath EZ, Frank RN, Shin DH, et al. Risk factors for central retinal vein occlusions. A case controlled study. Ophthalmology. 1992;99:509-14.
4. Hayreh SS, Zimmerman MB, Podhajsky P. Incidence of various types of retinal vein occlusion and their recurrence and demographic characteristics. Am J Ophthalmol. 1994;117: 429-41.
5. Hayreh SS, Zimmerman MB, McCarthy MJ, et al. Systemic diseases associated with various types of retinal vein occlusion. Am J Ophthalmol. 2001;131:61-77.

6. Green WR, Chan CC, Hutchins GM, et al. Central retinal vein occlusion: a prospective histological study of 29 eyes in 28 cases. Trans Am Ophthalmol Soc. 1981;89:371-422.
7. Hayreh SS. Pathogenesis of occlusion of the central retinal vessels. Am J Ophthalmol. 1971;72:998-1011.
8. The Central Vein Occlusion Study Group. Natural history and clinical management of central retinal vein occlusion. Arch Ophthalmol. 1997;115:486-91.
9. The Central Vein Occlusion Study Group. Evaluation of grid pattern photocoagulation for macular edema in central vein occlusion. The Central Vein Occlusion Study Group M report. Ophthalmology. 1995;102:1425-33.
10. Hattenbach LO, Steinkamp G, Scharrer I, et al. Fibrinolytic therapy with low-dose recombinant tissue plasminogen activator in retinal vein occlusion. Ophthalmologica. 1998; 212:394-8.
11. Hattenbach LO, Wellermann G, Steinkamp GW, et al. Visual outcome after treatment with low-dose recombinant tissue plasminogen activator or hemodilution in ischemic central retinal vein occlusion. Ophthalmologica. 1999;213:360-6.
12. Lahey JM, Fong DS, Kearney J. Intravitreal tissue plasminogen activator for acute central retinal vein occlusion. Ophthal Surg Lasers. 1999;30:427-34.
13. Glacet-Bernard A, Kuhn D, Vine AK, et al. Treatment of recent onset central retinal vein occlusion with intravitreal tissue plasminogen activator: a pilot study. Br J Ophthalmol. 2000;84:609-13.
14. Elman MJ, Raden RZ, Carrigan A. Intravitreal injection of tissue plasminogen activator for central retinal vein occlusion. Trans Am Ophthalmol Soc. 2001;99:219-21.
15. Ghazi NG, Noureddine BN, Haddad RS, et al. Intravitreal tissue plasminogen activator in the management of central retinal vein occlusion. Retina. 2003;23:780-4.
16. Weiss JN. Treatment of central retinal vein occlusion by injection of tissue plasminogen activator into a retinal vein. Am J Ophthalmol. 1998;126:142-4.
17. Paques M, Vallèe JN, Herbreteau D, et al. Superselective ophthalmic artery fibrinolytic therapy for the treatment of central retinal vein occlusion. Br J Ophthalmol. 2000;84:1387-91.
18. Bynoe LA, Weiss JN. Retinal endovascular surgery and intravitreal triamcinolone acetone for central vein occlusion in young adults. Am J Ophthalmol. 2003;135:382-4.
19. Gregori NZ, Rosenfeld PJ, Puliafito CA, et al. One-year safety and efficacy of intravitreal triamcinolone acetonide for the management of macular edema secondary to central retinal vein occlusion. Retina. 2006;26:889-95.
20. Ip MS, Scott IU, Van Veldhuisen PC, et al. A randomized trial comparing the efficacy and safety of intravitreal triamcinolone with observation to treat vision loss associated with macular edema secondary to central retinal vein occlusion: the Standard Care vs Corticosteroid for Retinal Vein Occlusion (SCORE) study report 5. Arch Ophthalmol. 2009;127:1101-14.
21. Rosenfeld PJ, Fung AE, Puliafito CA. Optical coherence tomography findings after an intravitreal injection of bevacizumab (avastin) for macular edema from central retinal vein occlusion. Ophthalmic Surg Lasers Imaging. 2005;36:336-9.
22. Iturralde D, Spaide RF, Meyerle CB. Intravitreal bevacizumab (Avastin) treatment of macular edema in central retinal vein occlusion: a short-term study. Retina. 2006;26:279-84.
23. Wu L, Martínez-Castellanos MA, Quiroz-Mercado H, et al. Twelve-month safety of intravitreal injections of bevacizumab (Avastin): results of the Pan-American Collaborative Retina Study Group (PACORES). Graefes Arch Clin Exp Ophthalmol. 2008;246:81-7.
24. Brown DM, Campochiaro PA, Singh RP, et al. Ranibizumab for macular edema following central retinal vein occlusion: six-month primary end point results of a phase III study. Ophthalmology. 2010;117:1124-33.
25. Lam HD, Blumenkranz MS. Treatment of central retinal vein occlusion by vitrectomy with lysis of vitreopapillary and epipapillary adhesions, subretinal peripapillary tissue plasminogen activator injection, and photocoagulation. Am J Ophthalmol. 2002;134:609-11.
26. Yeshaya A, Treister G. Pars plana vitrectomy for vitreous hemorrhage and retinal vein occlusion. Ann Ophthalmol. 1983;15:615-7.
27. Furino C, Ferrari TM, Boscia F, et al. Combined radial optic neurotomy, internal limiting membrane peeling, and intra-vitreal triamcinolone acetonide for central retinal vein occlusion. Ophthalmic Surg Lasers Imaging. 2005;36: 422-5.
28. Opremcak EM, Bruce RA, Lomeo MD, et al. Radial optic neurotomy for central retinal vein occlusion: a retrospective pilot study of 11 consecutive cases. Retina. 2001;21:408-15.
29. Dev S, Buckley EG. Optic nerve sheath decompression for progressive central retinal vein occlusion. Ophthal Surg Lasers. 1999;30:181-4.
30. Vasco-Posada J. Modification of the circulation in the posterior pole of the eye. Ann Ophthalmol. 1972;4:48-59.
31. Weizer JS, Stinnett SS, Fekrat S. Radial optic neurotomy as treatment for central retinal vein occlusion. Am J Ophthalmol. 2003;136:814-9.
32. Garcia-Arumi J, Boixadera A, Martinez-Castillo V, et al. Chorioretinal anastomosis after radial optic neurotomy for central retinal vein occlusion. Arch Ophthalmol. 2003;121: 1385-91.
33. Garcia-Arumi J, Boixadera A, Martínez-Castillo V, et al. Radial optic neurotomy in central retinal vein occlusion: comparison of outcome in younger vs older patients. Am J Ophthalmol. 2007;143:134-40.
34. Garcia-Arumi J, Boixadera A, Martínez-Castillo V, et al. Radial optic neurotomy for management of hemicentral retinal vein occlusion. Arch Ophthalmol. 2006;124:690-5.
35. Opremcak ME, Rehmar AJ, Ridenour CD, et al. Radial optic neurotomy for central retinal vein occlusion: 117 consecutive cases. Retina. 2006;26:297-305.
36. Frangieh GT, Green WR, Barraquer-Somers E, et al. Histopathologic study of nine branch retinal vein occlusions. Arch Ophthalmol. 1982;100:1132-40.

37. The Branch Vein Occlusion Study Group. Argon laser photocoagulation for macular edema in branch vein occlusion. Am J Ophthalmol. 1984;98:271-82.
38. Takahashi M, Hikichi T, Akiba J, et al. Role of the vitreous and macular edema in branch retinal vein occlusion. Ophthalmic Surg Lasers. 1997;28:294-9.
39. Scott IU. Vitreoretinal surgery for complications of branch retinal vein occlusion. Curr Opin Ophthalmol. 2002;13:161-6.
40. Raszewska-Steglinska M, Gozdek P, Cisiecki S, et al. Pars plana vitrectomy with ILM peeling for macular edema secondary to retinal vein occlusion. Eur J Ophthalmol. 2009;19:1055-62.
41. Arai M, Yamamoto S, Mitamura Y, et al. Efficacy of vitrectomy and internal limiting membrane removal for macular edema associated with branch retinal vein occlusion. Ophthalmologica. 2009;223:172-6.
42. Noma H, Funatsu H, Sakata K, et al. Macular microcirculation before and after vitrectomy for macular edema with branch retinal vein occlusion. Graefes Arch Clin Exp Ophthalmol. 2010;248:443-5.
43. Kumar B, Yu DY, Morgan WH, et al. The distribution of angioarchitectural changes within the vicinity of the arteriovenous crossing in branch retinal vein occlusion. Ophthalmology. 1998;105:424-7.
44. Opremcak EM, Bruce RA. Surgical decompression of branch retinal vein occlusion via arteriovenous crossing sheathotomy: a prospective review of 15 cases. Retina. 1999;19:1-5.
45. Mester U, Dillinger P. Vitrectomy with arteriovenous decompression and internal limiting membrane dissection in branch retinal vein occlusion. Retina. 2002;22:740-6.
46. García-Arumí J, Martinez-Castillo V, Boixadera A, et al. Management of macular edema in branch retinal vein occlusion with sheathotomy and recombinant tissue plasminogen activator. Retina. 2004;24:530-40.
47. Kumagai K, Furukawa M, Ogino N, Uemura A, Larson E. Long-term outcomes of vitrectomy with or without arteriovenous sheathotomy in branch retinal vein occlusion. Retina. 2007;27:49-54.
48. Han DP, Bennett SR, Williams DF, et al. Arteriovenous crossing dissection without separation of the retina vessels for treatment of branch retinal vein occlusion. Retina. 2003;23:145-51.
49. Stoffelns BM, Kramann C, Schoepfer K. Arteriovenous crossing sheathotomy in branch retinal vein occlusion. Klin Monbl Augenheilkd. 2009;226:310-4.
50. Crafoord S, Karlsson N, la Cour M. Sheathotomy in complicated cases of branch retinal vein occlusion. Acta Ophthalmol. 2008;86:146-50.
51. Murakami T, Takagi H, Kita M, et al. Intravitreal tissue plasminogen activator to treat macular edema associated with branch retinal vein occlusion. Am J Ophthalmol. 2006;142:318-20.
52. Scott IU, Ip MS, Van Veldhuisen PC, et al. A randomized trial comparing the efficacy and safety of intravitreal triamcinolone with standard care to treat vision loss associated with macular edema secondary to branch retinal vein occlusion: the Standard Care vs Corticosteroid for Retinal Vein Occlusion (SCORE) study report 6. Arch Ophthalmol. 2009;127:1115-28.
53. Campochiaro PA, Hafiz G, Shah SM, et al. Ranibizumab for macular edema due to retinal vein occlusions: implication of VEGF as a critical stimulator. Mol Ther. 2008;16:791-9.
54. Prager F, Michels S, Kriechbaum K, et al. Intravitreal bevacizumab (Avastin) for macular oedema secondary to retinal vein occlusion: 12-month results of a prospective clinical trial. Br J Ophthalmol. 2009;93:452-6.

22 Vitreoretinal Surgery in Eales' Disease

Sandeep Saxena

Introduction

Eales' disease is an idiopathic retinal periphlebitis that primarily affects the peripheral retina in young adults. Eales' disease was first described by Henry Eales, a British ophthalmologist, in 1880 and 1882.[1,2] Elliot first recognized the inflammation of retinal vein and described it as periphlebitis retinae. Subsequently, several investigators documented both venular and arteriolar inflammation in the disease.[3-8]

Eales' disease most commonly affects healthy young adult males and is an important cause of preventable blindness in young adults. The predominant age of onset of symptoms is 20–30 years. Eales' disease has been reported from UK, USA, Canada, Germany, Greece and Turkey. However, the disease is more commonly seen in the Indian subcontinent.

Eales' disease is characterized by retinal periphlebitis, peripheral retinal ischemia and neovascularization (Figs 22.1 to 22.3). Visual loss is characteristically caused by recurrent vitreous hemorrhage.[9]

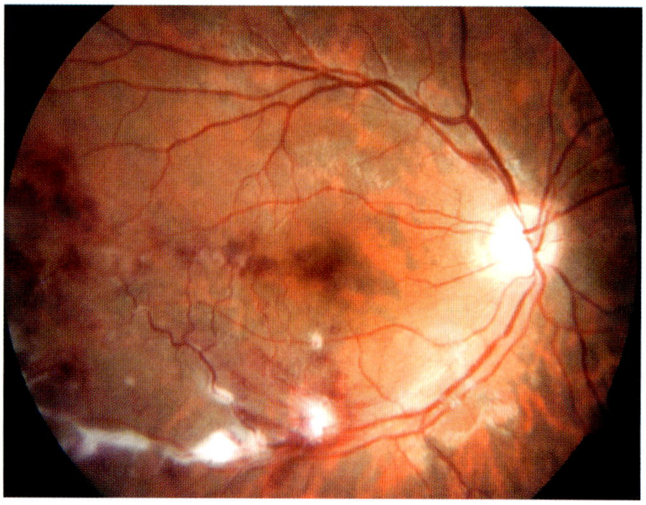

▲ **Figure 22.1**
Color fundus photograph shows retinal periphlebitis along with multiple superficial retinal hemorrhages

Eales' disease appears to be an immunologic reaction that may be triggered by an exogenous exposure. Retinal S-antigen and interphotoreceptor retinoid binding protein play a role in the etiopathogenesis of this condition. An extraneous agent results in the exposure of normally sequestered uveitopathogenic antigens of the immune system, leading to an immune response in the eye that initiates the disease process.[10]

Oxidative stress has been found to play an important role in the etiopathogenesis.[11-18] Elevated lipid peroxides have been found in the proliferative stage, which induce synthesis of cytokines and growth factors in retina during neovascularization.[13]

Cytokines play an important role in the pathogenesis of intraocular inflammation and neovascularization. The cascade of multiple angiogenic cytokines induced by oxidative damage, associated with tissue hypoxia, may interact to promote sustained retinal neovascularization. During the inflammatory and proliferative stages of the disease significant increase in IL-1β, IL-6, IL-10 and TNF-α expression has been observed, highlighting the role of pro-inflammatory and anti-inflammatory cytokines in the pathogenesis. Thus,

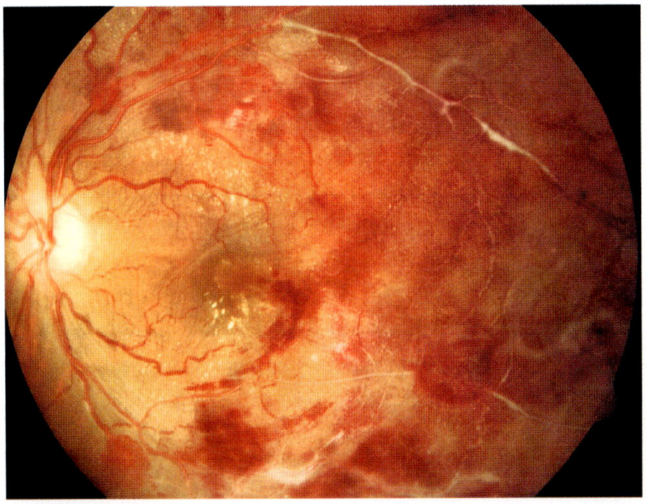

▲ **Figure 22.2**

Color fundus photograph shows sheathing along with superficial retinal hemorrhages, residual vasculitis, neovascularization elsewhere along with hard exudates and macular edema

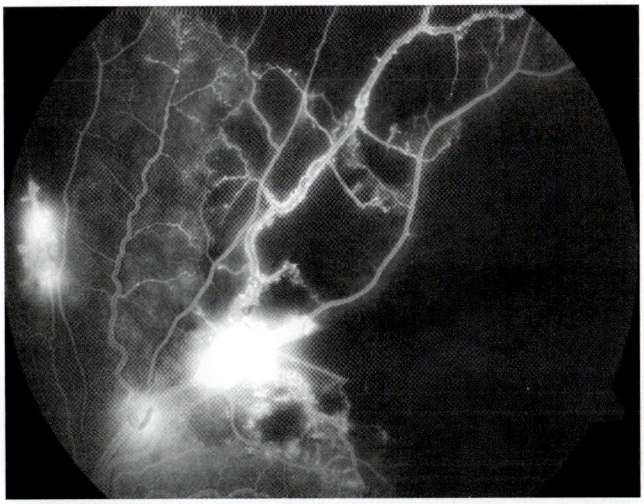

▲ **Figure 22.3**

Fundus fluorescein angiography shows capillary nonperfusion, microaneurysms and leakage of fluorescein dye from retinal neovascularization

the IL-1 system and TNF-α represents a novel target for controlling inflammatory activity and/or the associated long-term sequelae related to angiogenesis in Eales' disease.[19-21]

A close relationship between the prominent neovascular proliferation in Eales' disease and the intense expression of vascular endothelial growth factor (VEGF) has been found. The increased expression of VEGF, when compared to other conditions inducing neovascularization, might explain the severity of neovascular growth and the propensity of repeated vitreous hemorrhage in Eales' disease.[22]

Retinal photoreceptors and platelets have been shown to be an easy target of oxidants because of high proportion of polyunsaturated fatty acids. The decreased membrane fluidity in platelets suggests alterations in the physiological events, which may result in alterations in functioning of retinal photoreceptors.[18]

Clinical Features

Eales' disease with a characteristic clinical picture, fluorescein angiographic findings and natural course is considered a specific disease entity. Recurrent vitreous hemorrhage is the hallmark of this disease. A new classification system has been proposed by the author.[23] This staging system, based on standard terminology and features, provides a simple method to categorize, according to the severity of the disease. This staging system takes into consideration the fundoscopic and fluorescein angiographic variables that have been shown to be prognostic of visual outcome (Table 22.1). Macular involvement is uncommon. Macular ischemia and traction

TABLE 22.1: Classification system for Eales' disease

Stages	*Features*
A. Eales' disease	
Stage 1a	Periphlebitis of small caliber vessels with superficial retinal hemorrhages
Stage 1b	Periphlebitis of large caliber vessels with superficial retinal hemorrhages
Stage 2a	Peripheral capillary nonperfusion
Stage 2b	Neovascularization elsewhere/ Neovascularization of the disc
Stage 3a	Fibrovascular proliferation
Stage 3b	Vitreous hemorrhage
Stage 4a	Traction/combined rhegmatogenous detachment
Stage 4b	Rubeosis iridis, neovascular glaucoma, complicated cataract and optic atrophy
B. Central Eales' disease	

macular detachment are associated with poor visual outcome.[24]

The new classification system is consistent, simple and easy to recall. It can also be used to monitor the effect of medical, laser and/or surgical treatment.

Fluorescein Angiography

Areas of capillary nonperfusion and retinal neovascularization can be easily delineated by fluorescein angiography. Capillary nonperfusion of more than 20 disc area and 60 disc area are associated with neovascularization elsewhere (NVE) and neovascularization of the disc (NVD).[25] Retinal neovascularization sites have been found to cluster around specific anatomic foci. The quadrantic distribution of the sites of NVE in Eales' disease is: superotemporal 46%; inferotemporal 24%; superonasal 16%; and inferonasal 14%.[26]

Management

The management of Eales' disease depends on the severity of the disease. Management strategies can also be defined according to the stage of the disease.

Stage 1: This is the stage of inflammation which is amenable to medical therapy.

Stage 2: This is the stage of ischemia and neovascularization which requires observation or laser photocoagulation.

Stage 3: This is the stage of proliferation which requires laser or pars plana vitrectomy and laser.

Stage 4: This is the stage of complications which requires sophisticated surgical management strategies.[23]

▶ Medical Therapy

Corticosteroids

Anti-inflammatory corticosteroid drugs are potent therapeutic agents for a wide range of ocular and systemic disorders and remain the mainstay of therapy in retinal periphlebitis in Eales' disease (1 mg/kg/day).

Methotrexate

Predominantly T-cell involvement has been demonstrated in the lymphocytic infiltration of epiretinal and subretinal membranes in Eales' disease. Hence, treatment should be directed to the down regulation of the activated T-cells. Search for safer and more specific forms of treatment have led to certain immunosuppressives, like methotrexate, which have found a role in patients with immunologically driven systemic diseases. As opposed to the more "cytostatic" effects of corticosteroids, the "cytotoxic" immunosuppressives exert their beneficial effects by actually killing the rapidly dividing clones of lymphocytes that are responsible for inflammation. Methotrexate, a folic acid antagonist, has anti-inflammatory and immunomodulatory actions. The drug reduces the synthesis of DNA by acting on the enzyme dihydrofolate reductase. Methotrexate is used as a weekly "pulsed" therapy. A "pulse" differs from chronic moderate dose therapy in its ability to "reset" an aberrant immune response. Inhibition of the proliferating lymphocyte clones, the temporary removal of recirculating T-lymphocytes from the blood and eye and the profound suppression of peripheral inflammation, all occur simultaneously. Antigens exposed by viral, bacterial or autoimmune injury are normally perpetuated by the inflammatory response, but in such a system a pulse may abolish the source of antigen at the same time as it suppresses the immune response. When memory T-cells recirculate, the disease falters in the absence of the antigen.[27,28]

▶ Photocoagulation

Photocoagulation is the mainstay of therapy in proliferative stage of the disease. Laser photocoagulation leads to resolution of retinal neovascularization due to its anti-VEGF effect. In cases of gross capillary nonperfusion photocoagulation is suggested. For NVE and NVD, sectoral scatter photocoagulation and panretinal photocoagulation, respectively is suggested (Figs 22.4 and 22.5).

▶ Vitreoretinal Surgery

Vitreous hemorrhage is the primary cause for diminution of vision (Fig. 22.6). The episodes of vitreous hemorrhage do not necessarily correlate with the retinal changes. Vitrectomy is often not required in the first episode of vitreous hemorrhage. The first episode of vitreous hemorrhage usually clears within 6–8 weeks. However, recurrent vitreous hemorrhages may lead to formation of traction bands and membranes in the vitreous and resulting complications. Ultrasonography should always be performed to exclude the presence of an associated retinal detachment.

Vitrectomy alone or combined with other vitreoretinal surgical procedures is often required. Surgical results have

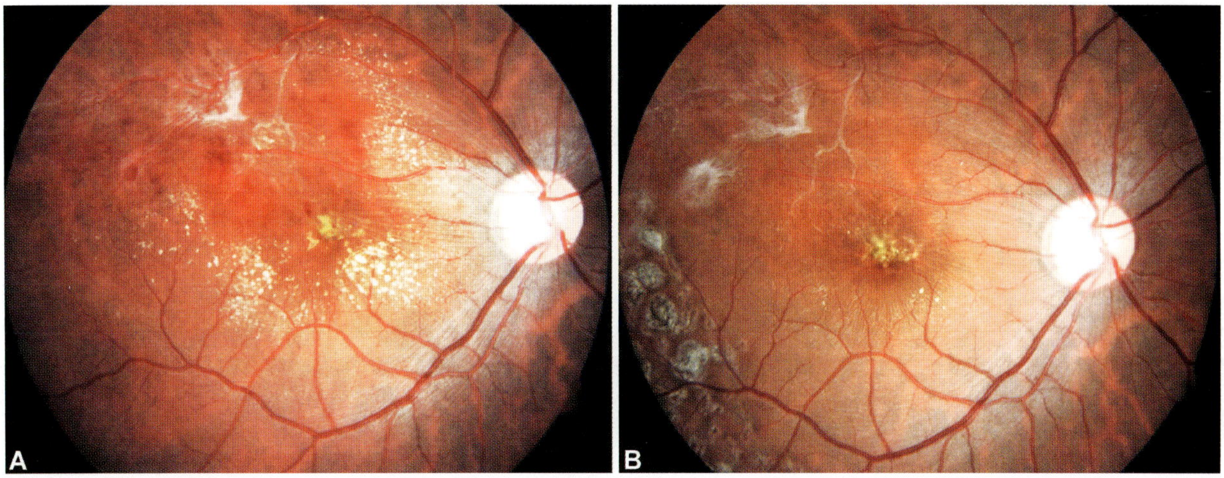

▲ **Figures 22.4A and B**

(A) Color fundus photograph shows neovascularization elsewhere; (B) Color fundus photograph shows regression of retinal neovascularization following laser photocoagulation

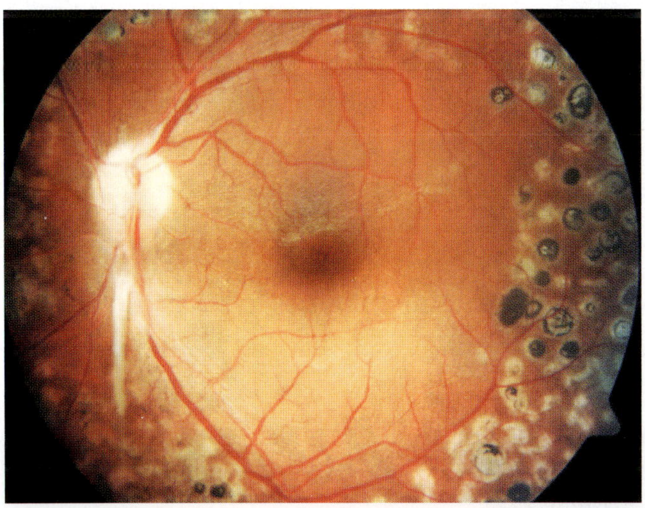

▲ **Figure 22.5**

Color fundus photograph after laser photocoagulation shows residual fibrous proliferation from the disc following resolution of neovascularization at the disc and epiretinal membrane at macula

been variable in the published literature.[29-36] The reported outcomes differ considerably with the surgical indication (vitreous hemorrhage vs tractional complications), the extent of posterior vitreous detachment (PVD) and the surgical techniques employed.[30-35]

Indications

The main indications for vitrectomy include unresolving vitreous hemorrhage, tractional retinal detachment involving the posterior pole, multiple vitreous membranes with or without tractional retinal detachment and combined tractional and rhegmatogenous retinal detachment (Figs 22.7 and 22.8).

Prognosis

The prognosis of vitrectomy in Eales' disease is usually good (Figs 22.9 and 22.10).

Critical Surgical Evaluation and Results

The aim of vitreoretinal surgery is to clear the vitreous opacities and also to critically evaluate the fundus for any retinal neovascularization. In the presence of tractional retinal detachment, extensive vitreous membranes and epiretinal membranes early vitrectomy may be considered.

Vitrectomy in Eales' disease is less complicated than proliferative diabetic retinopathy. A standard three-port pars plana 20-gauge or 23-gauge vitrectomy may be employed for vitreous hemorrhage removal. Excision of posterior hyaloid face and clearing of any subhyaloid hemorrhage is performed. Epimacular membranes are peeled off.

Posterior vitreous usually detaches from the retinal surface early except the attachment at the optic disc and unlike

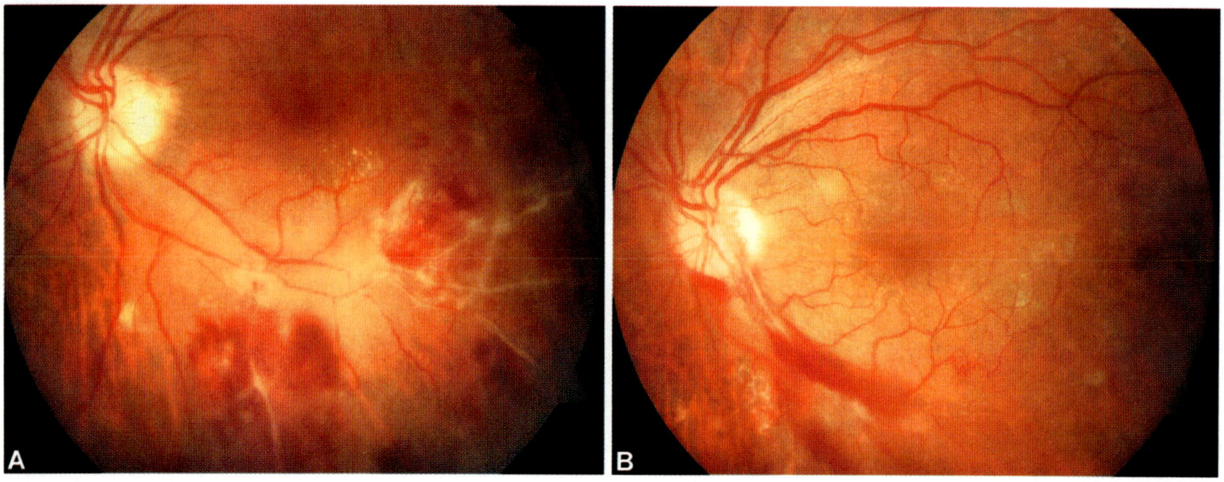

▲ **Figures 22.6A and B**

Color fundus photographs show progression of Eales' disease from inflammatory to proliferative stage with vitreous hemorrhage

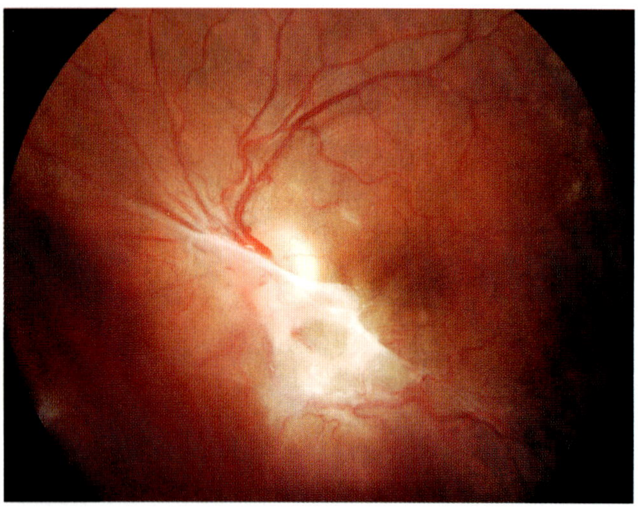

▲ **Figure 22.7**

Color fundus photograph shows vitreous hemorrhage with fibrous proliferation and epimacular membrane

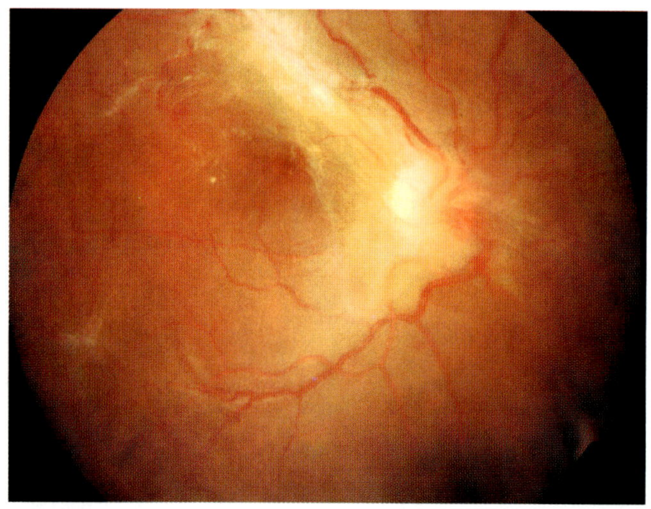

▲ **Figure 22.8**

Color fundus photograph shows vitreous hemorrhage inferiorly along with epiretinal membrane and traction at macula

diabetic retinopathy there are less often multiple retinal attachments and vitreous schisis. The latter helps the surgeon in getting into the correct plane for a safe vitreous surgery. Endolaser application is mandatory at conclusion of vitreous surgery. Additional procedures, such as belt buckling and lensectomy, are occasionally required.

Visual improvement is better with fewer episodes and shorter duration of vitreous hemorrhage. It has also been shown that the patients who had photocoagulation before vitreous surgery had a better prognosis. The indication for surgery, status of PVD and complexity of the surgical procedure performed affects the final outcome. Results of vitrectomy in Eales' disease have been reported for nearly three decades. Vitrectomy was generally performed after long waiting periods. Excellent results have been obtained in the presence of total PVD. Poor outcomes had been reported

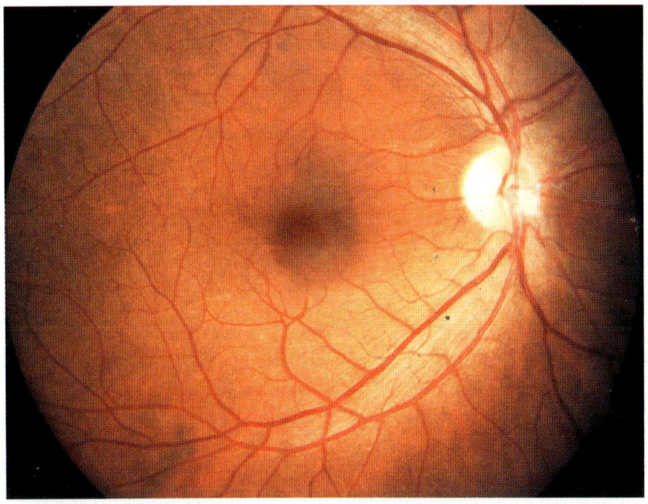

▲ **Figure 22.9**

Postoperative color fundus photograph after pars plana vitrectomy showing residual fibrous stump on the optic nerve head

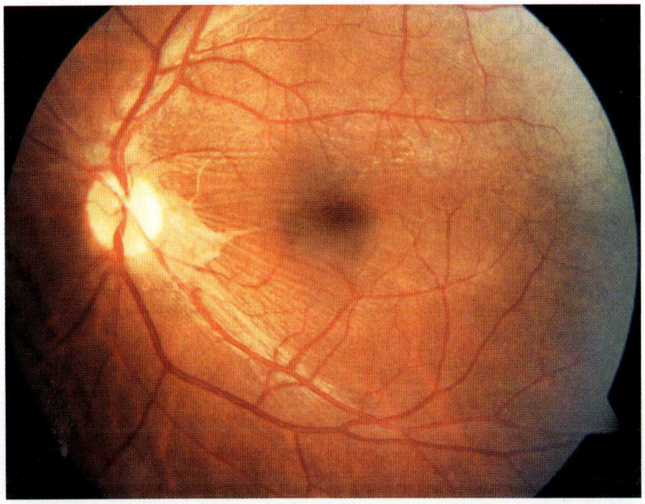

▲ **Figure 22.10**

Postoperative color fundus photograph after pars plana vitrectomy for vitreous hemorrhage shows residual epiretinal membrane in the papillomacular bundle area and internal limiting membrane folds

with preoperative or intraoperative detachments. The overall surgical results had been satisfactory because a majority of cases were operated for vitreous hemorrhage and had complete PVD.[29-39]

Posterior vitreous detachment is not necessarily common in Eales' disease. Badrinath et al.[40] found an incomplete PVD in all the 18 eyes operated for Eales' disease. Fibrous and fibrovascular proliferations were found to have multiple areas of adhesions to the posterior vitreous cortex. The presence of type II collagen in the epiretinal membrane indicated a possible vitreous collagen component to the double-layered membranes (vitreoschisis). Recognition of the double-layered membranes aids in relief of traction during surgery by delamination.[15]

Kumar et al.[31] reported excellent visual outcome in Eales' disease (>20/60 in 92%; PVD: 70–100%),[6] whereas El-Asrar and Al-Kharashi[30] reported acuity more than or equal to 6/12 in a modest 26% (incidence of PVD not reported; preoperative retinal detachment (RD) in 27%). Majji et al.[34] had final acuity more than or equal to 20/50 in 30% cases. Membrane peeling was performed in all, suggesting incomplete PVD. Smiddy et al.[35] reported dismal results with vitrectomy in Eales' disease (functional improvement in only 26.5%). Triester and Machemer[36] reported final acuity of more than or equal to 20/50 in 51%; but 42% presented with the same vision preoperatively. Shukla et al.[41] obtained a final best corrected visual acuity (BCVA) more than or equal to 6/12 in 60% eyes, notwithstanding an incomplete PVD in 60% eyes; only three (4%) of their cases had BCVA more than or equal to 20/40 preoperatively. The presence of preoperative RD in only a third of eyes probably improved the prognosis. But absence of RD did not necessarily mean a simple surgery. Adjunctive procedures, such as sclera buckling or C_3F_8 or silicone oil, were required in 43% cases.

The major postoperative complications are recurrent vitreous hemorrhage, rubeosis iridis, neovascular glaucoma and early development of cataract.

Preoperative panretinal photocoagulation does affect the surgical outcome.[29-32] Additional surgical procedures (scleral buckling/C_3F_8/silicone oil) have a relatively high incidence of postoperative cataract formation.

Surgical failure rate is mostly related to the difficulty of peeling tractional membranes in the peripheral retina. Peripheral tears or retinotomies may be observed in all the persistent or inoperable detachments.[41] Encirclage helps in neutralizing the peripheral traction from fibrovascular membranes.

Vitrectomy with removal of persistent vitreous hemorrhage and focal neovascular membranes and endolaser photocoagulation may lead to improved visual acuity in the majority of eyes with Eales' disease. However, extensive fibrovascular membranes and long-standing retinal detachment result in poor visual outcome. Earlier surgery can be considered to prevent visual loss in the patients.[42]

Although surgical outcomes in Eales' disease depend on preoperative PVD or RD to some extent; good results are possible in the presence of incomplete PVD and tractional sequelae.

Role of Preoperative Intravitreal Bevacizumab

Intravitreal bevacizumab has been found to be effective as an adjunctive treatment of retinal neovascularization in patients with Eales' disease.[43] However, repeated intravitreal bevacizumab in patients with Eales' disease with dense vitreous hemorrhage may not hasten the resolution of vitreous hemorrhage or reduce the need for vitrectomy. Moreover, tractional retinal detachment may be a serious complication of therapy and hence should be closely monitored because it entails a poor visual prognosis.[44] Intravitreal bevacizumab, 5–7 days before surgery, is a useful adjunct. It reduces intra-operative bleeding thereby decreasing the surgical time and improving the visual outcome.

References

1. Eales H. Retinal haemorrhage associated with epistaxis and constipation. Brim Med Rev. 1880;9:262.
2. Eales H. Primary retinal haemorrhage in young men. Ophthalmic Rev. 1882;1:41.
3. Duke-Elder S, Dobree JH. Primary perivasculitis of the retina: Eales disease, In: Duke Elder, Perkins EJ (Eds). System of Ophthalmology. London: Henry Kimpton; 1967. pp. 222-36.
4. Elliot AJ. 30-year observation of patients with Eales disease. Am J Ophthalmol. 1975;80:404-8.
5. Kimura SJ, Carriker FR, Hogen MJ. Retinal vasculitis with intraocular hemorrhage. Classification and results of special studies. Arch Ophthalmol. 1956;56:361-5.
6. Cross AG. Vasculitis retinae. Trans Ophthalmol Soc UK. 1963;83:133.
7. Keith-Lyle T, Wybark A. Retinal vasculitis. Br J Ophthalmol. 1961;45:77-8.
8. Gilbert TW. Periphlebitis and endovasculitis of retinal vessels. Klin Monatsbl Augenheilkd. 1935;94:335-49.
9. Kumar D, Saxena RC, Saxena S. Vitreous hemorrhage in Eales' disease. Afro-Asian J Ophthalmol. 1995;13:109-12.
10. Saxena S, Rajasingh J, Biswas S, et al. Cellular response to Retinal S-antigen and Inter photoreceptor retinoid binding protein fragments in patients with Eales' disease. Pathobiology. 1999;67:37-44.
11. Saxena S, Khanna VK, Kumar D, et al. Enhanced oxidative stress in Eales' disease. Ann Ophthalmol. 2001;33:40-2.
12. Saxena S, Kumar D, Srivastava P, et al. Low levels of platelet glutathione in Eales' disease. Med Sci Res. 1999;42:125-6.
13. Srivastava P, Saxena S, Khanna VK, et al. Raised platelet thiobarbituric acid reacting substances in proliferative Eales' disease. Indian J Ophthalmol. 2000;48:307-10.
14. Saxena S, Khanna VK, Kumar D, et al. Impaired antioxidant defense mechanism in central Eales' disease. Ann Ophthalmol. 2004;36:29-31.
15. Bhooma V, Sulochana KN, Biswas J, et al. Eales' disease: accumulation of reactive oxygen intermediates and lipid peroxides and decrease of antioxidants causing inflammation, neovascularization and retinal damage. Curr Eye Res. 1997;16:91-5.
16. Sulochana KN, Biswas J, Ramakrishnan S. Eales' disease: increased oxidation and peroxidation products of membrane constituents chiefly lipids and antioxidant enzymes and reduced glutathione in vitreous. Curr Eye Res. 1999;19: 254-9.
17. Swamy-Mruthinti S, Miriam KC, Kumar SK, et al. Immuno-localization and quantification of advanced glycation end products in retinal neovascular membranes and serum: a possible role in ocular neovascularization. Curr Eye Res. 2002;25:139-45.
18. Saxena S, Srivastava P, Kumar D, et al. Decreased platelet membrane fluidity in retinal periphlebitis in Eales' disease. Ocul Immunol Inflamm. 2006;14:113-6.
19. Saxena S, Pant AB, Khanna VK, et al. Interleukin-1 and tumor necrosis factor- alpha: novel targets for immunotherapy in Eales' disease. Ocul Immunol Inflamm. 2009;17:201-6.
20. Saxena S, Pant AB, Khanna VK, et al. Tumor necrosis factor-α-mediated severity of idiopathic retinal periphlebitis in young adults (Eales' disease): implication for anti-TNF-α therapy. J Ocul Biol Dis Inform. 2010;3:35-8.
21. Saxena S, Khanna VK, Pant AB, et al. Elevated tumor necrosis factor-α in serum is associated with increased retinal ischemia in proliferative Eales' disease. Pathobiology. (in press).
22. Perentes Y, Chan CC, Bovey E, et al. Massive vascular endothelium growth factor (VEGF) expression in Eales' disease. Klin Monatsbl Augenheilkd. 2002;219:311-4.
23. Saxena S, Kumar D. A new staging system of idiopathic retinal periphlebitis. Eur J Ophthalmol. 2004;14:236-9.
24. Saxena S, Kumar D. Macular involvement in Eales' disease. Ann Ophthalmol. 2000;32:98-100.
25. Saxena S, Kumar D, Maitreya A, et al. Retinal neovascularization in Eales' disease. Ann Ophthalmol. 2003;35:25-7.
26. Saxena S, Kumar D. Topographic distribution of retinal neovascularisation in Eales' disease. 2005;37:273-5.
27. Saxena S, Kumar D, Kapoor S. The efficacy of oral methotrexate pulsed therapy in Eales' disease. Ann Ophthalmol. 2000;32:60-2.
28. Bali T, Saxena S, Kumar D, et al. Response time and efficacy of oral methotrexate pulsed therapy in idiopathic retinal periphlebitis. Eur J Ophthalmol. 2005;15:374-8.
29. Biswas J, Sharma T, Gopal L, et al. Eales disease—an update. Surv Ophthalmol. 2002;47:197-214.
30. El-Asrar AM, Al-Kharashi SA. Full panretinal photocoagulation and early vitrectomy improve prognosis of retinal vasculitis associated with tuberculoprotein hypersensitivity (Eales' disease). Br J Opthalmol. 2002;86:1248-51.

31. Kumar A, Tiwari HK, Singh RP, et al. Comparative evaluation of early vs deferred vitrectomy in Eales' Disease. Acta Ophthalmol Scand. 2000;78:77-8.
32. Shanmugam MP, Badrinath SS, Gopal L, et al. Long-term visual results of vitrectomy for Eales disease complications. Int Ophthalmol. 1998;22:61-4.
33. Atmaca LS, Nagpal PN. Eales' disease: medical, laser, and surgical treatments. Ophthalmol Clin North Am. 1998;11:619-6.
34. Majji AB, Vemuganti GK, Shah VA, et al. A comparative study of epiretinal membranes associated with Eales' disease: a clinicopathologic evaluation. Eye. 2006;20:46-54.
35. Smiddy WE, Isernhagen RD, Michels RG, et al. Vitrectomy for nondiabetic vitreous hemorrhage: retinal and choroidal vascular disorders. Retina. 1988;8:88-95.
36. Treister G, Machemer R. Results of vitrectomy for rare proliferative and hemorrhagic disease. Am J Ophthalmol. 1977;84:394-412.
37. Mason JO, Colagross CT, Haleman T, et al. Visual outcome and risk factors for light perception and no light perception vision after vitrectomy for diabetic retinopathy. Am J Ophthalmol. 2005;140:231-5.
38. Atmaca LS, Batioglu F, Sonmez PA. A long-term follow-up of Eales' disease. Ocul Immunol Inflam. 2002;10:213-21.
39. Dehghan MH, Ahmadieh H, Soheilian M. Therapeutic effects of laser photocoagulation and/or vitrectomy in Eales' disease. Eur J Ophthalmol. 2005;15:379-83.
40. Badrinath SS, Gopal L, Sharma T, et al. Vitreoschisis in Eales' disease: pathogenic role and significance in surgery. Retina. 1999;19:51-4.
41. Shukla D, Kanungo S, Prasad NM, et al. Surgical outcomes for vitrectomy in Eales' disease. Eye. 2008;22:900-4.
42. Hui Y, Wang L, Cao X. Vitrectomy for complicated Eales disease. Yan Ke Xue Bao. 1997;13:25-8.
43. Küçükerdönmez C, Akova YA, Yilmaz G. Intravitreal injection of bevacizumab in Eales disease. Ocul Immunol Inflamm. 2008;16:63-5.
44. Patwardhan SD, Azad R, Shah BM, et al. Role of intravitreal bevacizumab in Eales disease with dense vitreous hemorrhage. A Prospective Randomized Control Study. Retina; 2011;31: 866-70.

23

Vitrectomy in Uveitis

Ozay Oz, Ebru Nevin Cetin, Levent Akduman

Introduction

Vitreoretinal surgery can be employed for diagnostic and therapeutic purposes in patients with uveitis. Technological advancements in vitrectomy techniques and implementation of scientific developments in diagnostic and therapeutic methods have influenced surgical interventions. This section will cover the diagnostic and therapeutic value of vitrectomy and the value of combined procedures in patients with uveitis.

Vitreous surgeries are performed in patients with uveitis for two primary reasons: diagnostic and therapeutic.

Vitrectomy in Patients with Uveitis for Diagnostic Purposes

Patients with uveitis that may require diagnostic vitrectomy (Table 23.1).

TABLE 23.1: Uveitis that may require diagnostic vitrectomy

- Diagnostic/therapeutic challenge (uveitis that could not be diagnosed with uveitis workup and not responding to the treatment)
- Cases where definite diagnosis require biopsy (i.e. intraocular lymphoma)

▶ Diagnostic or Therapeutic Challenge

Diagnostic vitrectomy is useful when etiology of the disease is in question. If the diagnosis can be established clinically or with diagnostic workup with a favorable treatment response, diagnostic vitreous sample is not necessary. Retinal and choroidal biopsies through vitrectomy may also be obtained for pathological examination or polymerase chain reaction (PCR) testing for malignancy, inflammatory and infectious conditions.[1,2]

Uveitis falls into two categories: (1) infectious and (2) noninfectious. Infectious uveitis can be bacterial, viral, fungal, or parasitic. These agents may be identified through serologic tests, cultures, PCR, or pathologic examinations from vitreous samples obtained with vitreous tap or vitrectomy.

Vitreous biopsy is also beneficial in assessing uveitis in patients with immunodeficiency. Diseases that follow a typical clinical course may follow a different clinical course in immunodeficient patients. For example, ocular toxoplasmosis can be caused by a focus adjacent to the typical chorioretinal scar in an immunocompetent patient; it may present as a primary lesion, vitritis instead of a reactivation from the area adjacent to the old scar, or without any chorioretinal lesions in a patient with AIDS.[3,4]

Technique

Sampling for the detection of infectious agents can be done with paracentesis, vitreous biopsy, or retina-choroid biopsy. Vitreous biopsy can be performed in two ways: (1) vitreous aspiration or (2) pars plana vitrectomy. There are also two methods for performing vitreous aspiration; that is, aspiration without vitrectomy, which can be accomplished in an office setting, or aspiration during vitrectomy in the operating room.

Aspiration without vitrectomy is performed by withdrawing the vitreous humor with a syringe using a short (3/8–5/8 inch) needle, 23-gauge or thinner, inserted through the pars plana. The rate of success in obtaining fluid with this procedure in eyes without prior vitrectomy or vitreous liquefaction is quite low. It is essential that the tip of the needle penetrate the liquefied vitreous humor to obtain a sample in a nonvitrectomized eye and this is not always accomplished.

Another office-based aspiration procedure employs a vitreous biopsy device (Visitec Cutter, Visitec, Sarasota, FL). Vitreous is manually aspirated with this device by penetrating the vitreous through the pars plana with a 23-gauge needle through the conjunctiva. The motorized device provides a cutting like a vitrector as the vitreous is being manually aspirated so that larger amount of vitreous sample can be obtained.

The most reliable and established vitreous biopsy method utilizes a vitrectomy device in an operating room setting. This can be accomplished in two ways. One method involves aspiration of vitreous with vitrectomy without infusing liquid into the eye. The aspiration is provided with a syringe, very short tubing of only a few centimeters connected to the aspiration port of the vitrectomy probe (Fig. 23.1). This technique ensures easy, low-risk removal of approximately a 0.5 cc sample. Immediately after the specimen is obtained, balanced salt solution (BSS) is flown into the vitreous cavity through the infusion cannula. In cases where samples larger than 0.5 cc are desired, air is used at the start of the vitrectomy instead of the infusion fluid. This ensures the sample is not diluted and larger samples can be obtained without collapsing the globe. After obtaining a sufficient sample, the infusion is switched from air to BSS and vitrectomy is continued.

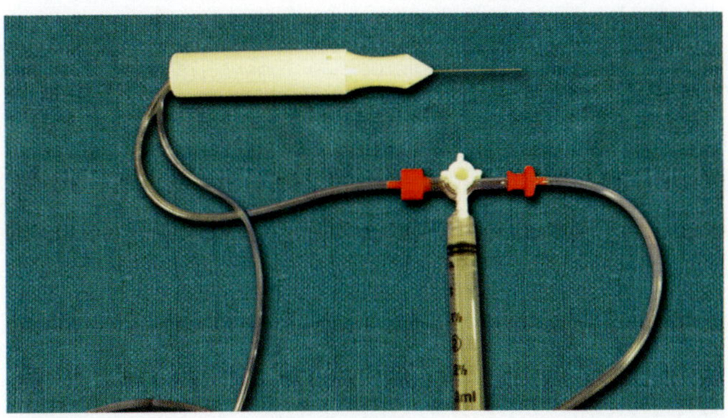

▲ **Figure 23.1**

Setting for vitreous tap using the vitrectomy probe. A syringe is attached to the aspiration tubing of the vitrectomy probe using a stopcock

Another sampling method in the operating room setting involves pars plana vitrectomy utilizing the liquid in the vitrectomy cassette as the sample. Since the liquid is diluted with this technique, it is less effective in aiding identification of infectious agents with direct staining, culture and serologic tests. If the sample is centrifuged, detection by direct staining and cytological testing can be facilitated.

▶ Testing the Specimen

Samples obtained with any of the vitreous biopsy methods outlined above can be assessed in various ways. The suspected disease is a primary consideration in determining how to assay the vitreous sample. The possibilities include microbiological tests such as gram staining or culture, serologic tests such as antibody titration, cytological testing, cytopathologic analysis, flow cytometry, immunohistochemical stains, or polymerase chain reaction (PCR).[5,6] Cytological and immunochemical tests prove useful in the differential diagnosis of masquerading syndromes and neoplastic cases. Local antibody production can be detected with serologic tests and it is particularly valuable as an adjunct to systemic serologic testing when the infection is mostly limited to the eye.

Even if the amount of sample for PCR is very low, it is a method that can rapidly reproduce genetic material and lead to the detection of DNA or RNA genetic material within a very short period. The most common application is for human leukocyte antigen (HLA) typing. It is a diagnostic technique especially useful for diagnosis of viral uveitis.[6-8] The amount of genetic material detectable using PCR is constantly increasing. Some of the agents that cause uveitis and can be detected with PCR are listed in Table 23.2. A

TABLE 23.2: Some of the organisms that can be detected with polymerase chain reaction in patients with uveitis

Bacteria	*Protozoa or parasites*	*Viruses*
1. *P. Acnes*	1. *Toxoplasma*	1. *CMV*
2. *Mycobacterium*	2. *Onchocerca*	2. *VZV-HSV*
3. *Borrelia*		3. *EBV*
4. *Leptospira*		4. *HTLV-I*
5. *T. whippelii*		

possible diagnosis should be considered prior to review of PCR and PCR should only be used for supportive purposes. Positive PCR results are more likely in cases with vascular inflammation, optic nerve involvement, common retinitis, or in immunocompromised patients. PCR testing for the purpose of detecting various agents, but without a possible diagnosis would be excessive and unreasonably costly.

▶ Cases Where Definite Diagnosis Requires Biopsy

Vitreous biopsy may increase survival in cases of intraocular lymphoma by contributing to early diagnosis. In a case that raises suspicion of intraocular lymphoma, but presents as panuveitis and deep retinal yellow spotted lesions, treatment would differ completely from that for uveitis.[9-12] Margolis et al.[13] reported a diagnostic vitrectomy sensitivity of 63.6% in 45 eyes suspected of having intraocular infection or malignancy. Wittenberg et al.[14] on the other hand, observed 76 cases of chronic nonspecific inflammation, 41 cases of granulomatous inflammation and 14 cases of primary intraocular lymphoma in the vitreous cytology among 278 patients with vitritis that could not be clinically diagnosed.

Retinal detachment (RD), intraocular foreign body, phaco-anaphylactic glaucoma, vitreous hemorrhage, melanoma and multiple myeloma are pathologies that merit consideration in the differential diagnosis of vitritis.[15-17]

Vitrectomy for Therapeutic Purposes in Patients with Uveitis

Patients with uveitis that may require therapeutic vitrectomy (Table 23.3).

TABLE 23.3: Indications for therapeutic vitrectomy in uveitis patients

1. Media opacity (i.e. inflammatory vitreous debris, vitreous hemorrhage)
2. Better control of intraocular inflammation
3. Chronic uveitic hypotony
4. Sequelae of uveitis and cases that require lensectomy
5. Intraocular implants
6. Retinal detachment
7. Choroidal neovascularization (CNV)
8. Intraocular parasites.

▶ Media Opacity

Diagnostic vitrectomy may sometimes be therapeutic since it also clears media opacity. It has been suggested that vitrectomy can reduce inflammation in patients with uveitis by removing inflammatory cells.[13,18-20] It should be noted, however, that surgical trauma to an inflamed eye may increase inflammation, therefore nondiagnostic therapeutic vitrectomy should be used in an inflamed eye only in cases of emergency.

After the inflammation is controlled in eyes with uveitis, vision may be decreased due to media opacity. Debris that accumulates in the vitreous after inflammation may cause visual impairment, may make the observation of the retina difficult or impossible and may obscure accurate assessment of the status of the retina. Pars plana vitrectomy in this setting can improve vision and facilitate identification of findings in the retina.

In addition to inflammatory debris, media opacity may be the result of vitreous hemorrhage. Vitreous hemorrhage in patients with uveitis can be caused by retinal neovascularization secondary to retinal ischemia or angiogenic factors released from inflammatory cells. One example of the former is vein branch occlusions, common in patients with Behçet's disease.[21-22] Another well-known etiology is hemorrhage secondary to peripheral retinal neovascularization commonly observed in patients with pars planitis.[23-24] Eales' disease can also cause retinal neovascularization leading to vitreous hemorrhage.

▶ Better Control of Intraocular Inflammation

Pars plana vitrectomy can be considered along with peripheral cryopexy and immunomodulatory therapy in cases where intermediate uveitis does not respond to immunosuppressives treatment.[25-26] Vitrectomy has proven useful in treatment of intermediate uveitis refractory to long-term immunosuppressive treatment and with accompanying vitreoretinal complications, including severe vitreous condensation, tractional RD, vitreous hemorrhage, refractory cystoid macular edema, epimacular membrane and peripheral neovascularization. It has also been reported to improve visual prognosis and may reduce the need for long-term immunosuppressive treatment.

▶ Chronic Uveitic Hypotony

Hypotony in eyes with uveitis can be acute or chronic. Acute hypotony is usually accompanied by active inflammation and is reversible when the inflammation is controlled. However, if the ciliary body has gone into atrophy, the intraocular pressure (IOP) does not improve due to insufficient aqueous release and hypotony may become chronic. If chronic hypotony is secondary to cyclitic membranes or thickened anterior cortical hyaloid, pars plana vitrectomy can relieve traction on the ciliary body and reduce secondary hypotony. However, if there is already permanent damage to the ciliary body in an eye with pre-existing hypotony, IOP may not ever achieve desired values.

If IOP at 4–6 mm Hg persists, disc edema, maculopathy and finally phthisis bulbi may develop. Chronic uveitic hypotony usually presents with decreased visual acuity, low IOP, posterior synechia, often times with lack of iris bombe despite extensive posterior synechia and band keratopathy. Exudative RD and retinal folds may be observed.

Pars plana vitrectomy, lensectomy (by cleaning ciliary processes and membranes) and silicone oil injection may be attempted in an effort to improve IOP and prevent phthisis bulbi.[27,28] Interestingly, several patients in these reported cases continued to have gradual decrease of IOP despite the injection of silicone oil.

Sequelae of Uveitis and Cases that Require Lensectomy

Pars plana vitrectomy can be combined with pars plana lensectomy in the presence of severe cataract. Lensectomy may be preferred over cataract surgery in pediatric patients with juvenile rheumatoid arthritis. It has also been reported that pars plana vitrectomy and phacoemulsification used in combination in patients with chronic uveitis often yield significant improvement in visual acuity.[29,30] Pars plana vitrectomy may also be employed for sequelae of chronic ocular inflammation such as cystoid macular edema, retinal detachment, or epiretinal membrane. It has also been noted to reduce the amount of systemic medication needed to control inflammation in children.[31-33]

Pars plana vitrectomy has been reported to help reduce persistent macular edema in posterior uveitis where periocular or systemic corticosteroid treatment has not satisfactorily controlled macular edema.[34] While the regression mechanism in cystoid macular edema after vitrectomy is not clear, removal of cytokines from the vitreous may contribute to regression of the edema. Pars plana vitrectomy and intra-operative intravitreal triamcinolone injection have been found to improve cystoid macular edema, as well as visual acuity.[35,36] However, this would accelerate cataract formation in phakic eyes and might increase IOP.

Intravitreal bevacizumab injections have been reported to help improve macular edema in uveitic eyes.[37-40] Studies have revealed that bevacizumab leads to a significant decrease in central foveal thickness in optical coherence tomography (OCT) and stabilizes or improves visual acuity, although this effect is temporary and repeat injections are needed and the interval between injections may vary.

The efficacy of intravitreal triamcinolone and bevacizumab in the treatment of refractory uveitic macular edema was compared and the results appear to favor triamcinolone.[41] However, better results were obtained when triamcinolone was combined with bevacizumab. Preservative free triamcinolone 40 mg/ml (Triesence® triamcinolone acetonide injectable suspension - Alcon Laboratories, Inc, Fort Worth, TX), has been approved for use in sympathetic ophthalmia and temporal arteritis.[42]

Intraocular Implants

It is very difficult to maintain an effective drug level in the vitreous and the retina when the medication is administered systemically or topically. Intraocular drug release systems have been developed to establish longer-acting effects and to require less frequent administration.[43-47] These implants for uveitis can be classified in two groups:

Non-biodegradable

Vitrasert® (ganciclovir—for cytomegalovirus retinitis), Retisert® (fluocinolone— for noninfectious posterior uveitis).

Biodegradable

Ozurdex® (dexamethasone for noninfectious posterior uveitis) (Figs 23.2 and 23.3).

Both Retisert® (fluocinolone acetonide, 0.59 mg) (Bausch and Lomb, Rochester, New York, USA) and Ozurdex® (Allergan, Irvine, CA, USA) are approved by the FDA. They have been evaluated in multicenter studies and found to be

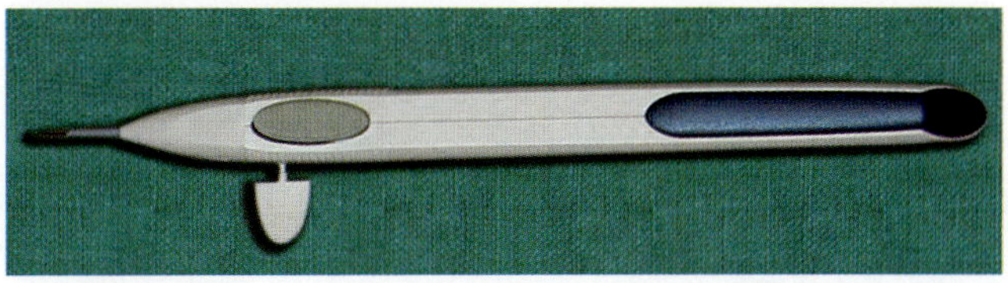

Figure 23.2
Ozurdex® injector. The procedure is usually performed in the office setting using the preloaded 23-gauge injector

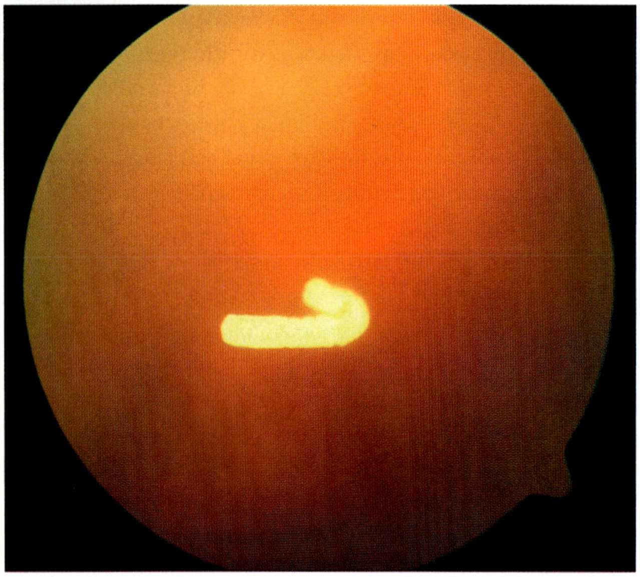

▲ **Figure 23.3**

Ozurdex® implant in the vitreous. The implant in this patient has already began degrading in 6 weeks (Stephen S Feman, MD)

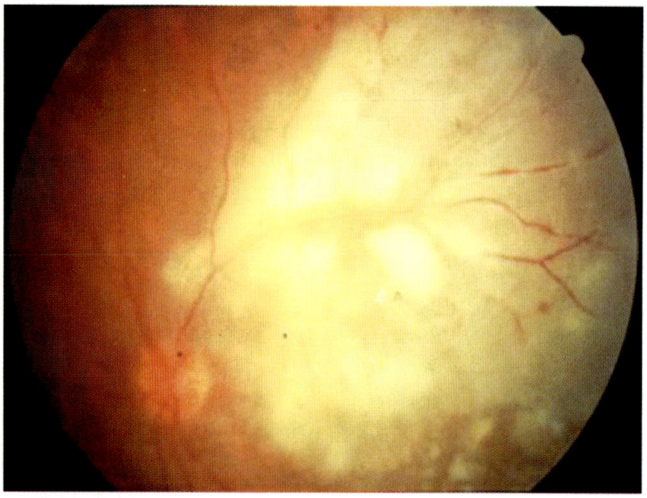

▲ **Figure 23.4**

Retinal detachment in an AIDS patient with CMV retinitis

effective and reasonably safe.[47,48] Studies revealed that Retisert® significantly decreased inflammation for approximately 3 years, eliminated or reduced the need for systemic corticosteroids or immunosuppressive treatment and improved visual acuity.[49] Ozurdex® effect lasts approximately six months.

Retisert® implantation is performed by making a scleral cut in the pars plana. The device is inserted into the eye with its top surface and release orifice facing anteriorly and then sutured to the sclera with 8-0 Prolene.

Common adverse effects of Retisert® and Ozurdex® are cataract development and increase in IOP. In cases of moderate cataract in patients for whom implantations are planned, combined implantation and phacoemulsification are recommended.[50-52] Topical medical treatment has been tried as first line therapy for IOP increase and most patients have required filtration surgeries (trabeculectomy or glaucoma drainage devices). Cyclodestructive procedures, such as viscocanalostomy and deep sclerectomy, are not recommended due to the possible subsequent development of hypotony.

▶ Retinal Detachment

Retinal detachment in patients with uveitis can occur with a serous rhegmatogenous, tractional, or combined (tractional and rhegmatogenous) mechanism. It may be necessary to eliminate the traction in tractional and combined detachments with pars plana vitrectomy. In patients with uveitis, rhegmatogenous retinal detachment may develop after severe viral infections of the retina, cytomegalovirus (CMV) retinitis (Fig. 23.4), or acute retinal necrosis.[3,53-55] Even though the incidence of CMV retinitis decreased after the use of new protease inhibitors in combination with anti-HIV drugs, resistance to these drugs develops and it is possible for CMV retinitis and related RD to recur. Retinal detachment in connection with CMV retinitis is observed in ratios of 25–50% among AIDS patients and treatment is possible by filling the vitreous space with silicone oil after pars plana vitrectomy.

Acute retinal necrosis is another form of uveitis treated with vitrectomy and silicone oil. Retinal detachment is observed in up to 80% of patients with acute retinal necrosis. Scleral buckling is not recommended in an effort to avoid increase in peripheral retinal ischemia, which is thought to play a role in the etiopathogenesis of multiple holes in the peripheral retina. Pars plana vitrectomy, silicone oil and laser barrier are recommended for repair of RD in acute retinal necrosis. Serous RD develops secondary to the inflammation of choroid or sclera and does not require vitrectomy.

▶ Choroidal Neovascularization

When serous detachment develops secondary to choroidal neovascular membrane, removal of the membrane via submacular surgery has been successful in vitrectomy

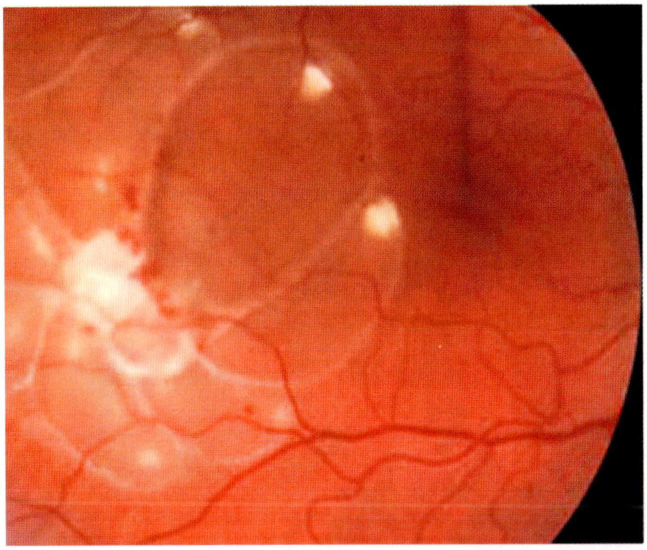

▲ Figure 23.5

Subretinal Tinea crassiceps cysts, preoperative fundus photo

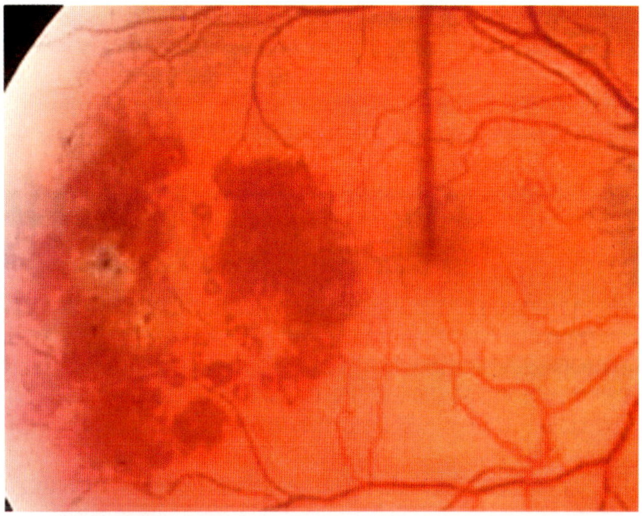

▲ Figure 23.6

Postoperative fundus photo of the same eye in Figure 23.5 after subretinal surgery

surgeries where the membrane is subfoveal.[56] While CNV can be seen in all diseases that damage Bruch's membrane, it is most commonly observed in types of uveitis, such as multifocal choroiditis, punctate inner choroidopathy, serpiginous choroidopathy and toxoplasmosis. Intravitreal bevacizumab injections have also been tried in the treatment of CNV related to inflammatory diseases. Bevacizumab has been shown to be an effective treatment for CNV when inflammation is controlled, as intravitreal bevacizumab causes significant foveal flattening and increases visual acuity.[57-60]

▶ Intraocular Parasites

Pars plana vitrectomy has been reported for extractions of intraocular parasites. It is not uncommon for onchocerciasis to cause intraocular larvae and there are several reports of removal of these larvae with vitrectomy. Authors have extracted subretinal Tinea crassiceps cysts by means of vitrectomy and subretinal surgery[61] (Figs 23.5 and 23.6). Table 23.3 outlines the therapeutic indications for use of vitrectomy.

References

1. Lim LL, Suhler EB, Rosenbaum JT, et al. The role of choroidal and retinal biopsies in the diagnosis and management of atypical presentations of uveitis. Trans Am Ophthalmol Soc. 2005;103:84-91.
2. Johnston RL, Tufail A, Lightman S, et al. Retinal and choroidal biopsies are helpful in unclear uveitis of suspected infectious or malignant origin. Ophthalmology. 2004;111:522-8.
3. Jabs DA, Enger C, Barlett JG. Cytomegalovirus retinitis and acquired immunodeficiency syndrome. Arch Ophthalmol. 1989;107:75-80.
4. Holland GN, Pepose JS, Pettit TH, et al. Acquired immune deficiency syndrome: ocular manifestations. Ophthalmology. 1983;90:859-73.
5. Short G, Margolis T, Kuppermann B, et al. A polymerase chain reaction-based assay for diagnosing varicella-zoster virus retinitis in patients with acquired immunodeficiency syndrome. Am J Ophthalmol. 1997;123:157-64.
6. BenEzra D. Diagnostic intraocular interventions. In: BenEzra D (Ed). Ocular Inflammations. Basic and Clinical Concepts. USA: Martin Dunitz; 1999. pp. 83-90.
7. Van Gelder RN, Kaplan HJ. Diagnostic and therapeutic vitrectomy for uveitis. In: Ryan SJ (Ed). Retina, 3rd edition. St. Louis, MO: MosbyYear Book Inc; 2001. pp. 2264-71.
8. Van Gelder RN, Kaplan HJ. Application of the polymerase chain reaction to the diagnosis of uveitis. Ocular immunology and inflammation. 1998;6:129-34.
9. Freeman LN, Schachat AP, Knox DL, et al. Clinical features, laboratory investigations, and survival in reticulum cell sarcoma. Ophthalmology. 1987;94:1631-9.
10. Muhaya M, Calder VL, Towler HM, et al. Characterization of phenotype and cytokine profiles of T cell lines derived from vitreous humour in ocular inflammation in man. Clin Exp Immunol. 1999;116:410-4.
11. Wilson DJ, Braziel R, Rosenbaum JT. Intraocular lymphoma. Immunopathologic analysis of vitreous biopsy specimens. Arch Ophthalmol. 1992;110:1455-8.

12. Karma A, von Willebrand EO, Tommila PV, et al. Primary intraocular lymphoma: improving the diagnostic procedure. Ophthalmology. 2008;114:1372-7.
13. Margolis R, Brasil OF, Lowder CY, et al. Vitrectomy for the diagnosis and management of uveitis of unknown cause. Ophthalmology. 2007;114:1893-7.
14. Wittenberg LA, Maberley DA, Ma PE, et al. Contribution of vitreous cytology to final clinical diagnosis fifteen-year review of vitreous cytology specimens from one institution. Ophthalmology. 2008;115:1944-50.
15. Akduman L, M Hasanreisoglu B, Kurtar K. A case of ocular brucellosis: importance of vitreous specimen. Acta Ophthalmol. 1993;71:130-2.
16. Biswas JB, Madhavan HN, Gopal L, et al. Intraocular tuberculosis. Clinicopathologic study offive cases. Retina. 1995;15: 461-8.
17. Davis JL, Miller DM, Ruia P. Diagnostic testing of vitrectomy specimens. Am J Ophthalmol. 2005;140:822-9.
18. Algvere P, Alanko H, Dickhoff K, et al. Pars plana vitrectomy in the management of intraocular inflammation. Acta Ophthalmol. 1981;59:727-36.
19. Heiligenhaus A, Bomfeld N, Foerster MH, et al. Long-term results of pars plana vitrectomy in the management of the complicated uveitis. Br J Ophthalmol. 1994;78:549-54.
20. Becker M, Davis J. Vitrectomy in the treatment of uveitis. Am J Ophthalmol. 2005;140:1096-105.
21. Mochizuki M, Akduman L, Nussenblatt RB. Behcet Disease. In: Pepose JS, Holland GN, Wilhelmus KR (Eds). Ocular Infection and Immunity. St. Louis, MO: Mosby-Year Book Inc; 1996. pp. 663-75.
22. Sullu Y, Alotaiby H, Beden U, et al. Pars plana vitrectomy for ocular complications of Behçet's disease. Ophthalmic Surg Lasers Imaging. 2005;36:292-7.
23. Potter MJ, Myckatyn SO, Maberley AL, et al. Vitrectomy for pars planitis complicated by vitreous hemorrhage: Visual outcome and long-term follow-up. Am J Ophthalmol. 2001;131:514-5.
24. Mieler WF, Will BR, Lewis H, et al. Vitrectomy in the management of peripheral uveitis. Ophthalmology. 1988;95: 859-64.
25. Stavrou P, Bahatzis S, Letko E, et al. Pars plana vitrectomy in patients with intermediate uveitis. Ocular Immunol Inflamm. 2001;9:141-51.
26. Leki Y, Kiryu J, Kita M, et al. Pars plana vitrectomy for vitreous opacity associated with ocular sarcoidosis resistant to medical treatment. Ocul Immunol Inflamm. 2004;12:35-43.
27. Gupta P, Gupta A, Gupta V, et al. Successful outcome of pars plana vitreous surgery in chronic hypotony due to uveitis. Retina. 2009;29:638-43.
28. Kapur R, Birnbaum AD, Goldstein DA, et al. Treating uveitis-associated hypotony with pars plana vitrectomy and silicone oil injection. Retina. 2010;30:140-5.
29. Diamond JG, Kaplan HJ. Lensectomy and vitrectomy for complicated cataract secondary to uveitis. Arch Ophthalmol. 1978;96:1798-804.
30. Androudi S, Ahmed M, Fiore T, et al. Combined pars plana vitrectomy and phacoemulsification to restore visual acuity in patients with chronic uveitis. J Cataract Refract Surg. 2005;31:472-8.
31. Flynn HW, Davis JL, Culbertson WW. Pars plana lensectomy and vitrectomy for complicated cataracts in juvenile rheumatoid arthritis. Ophthalmology. 1988;95:1114-9.
32. Giuliari GP, Chang PY, Thakuria P, et al. Pars plana vitrectomy in the management of paediatric uveitis: the Massachusetts eye research and surgery institution experience. Eye. 2010;24: 7-13.
33. Trittibach P, Koerner F, Sarra GM, et al. Vitrectomy for juvenile uveitis: prognostic factors for the long-term functional outcome. Eye. 2006;20:184-90.
34. Dugel PU, Rao NA, Ozler S, et al. Pars plana vitrectomy for intraocular inflammation-related cystoid macular edema unresponsive to corticosteroids. A Preliminary study. Ophthalmology. 1992;99:1535-41.
35. Tranos P, Scott R, Zambarakji H, et al. The effect of pars plana vitrectomy on cystoid macular oedema associated with chronic uveitis: a randomised, controlled pilot study. Br J Ophthalmol. 2006;90:1107-10.
36. Gutfleisch M, Spital G, Mingels A, et al. Pars plana vitrectomy with intravitreal triamcinolone: effect on uveitic cystoid macular oedema and treatment limitations. Br J Ophthalmol. 2007;91:345-8.
37. Cordero, Coma M, Sobrin L, et al. Intravitreal bevacizumab for treatment of uveitic macular edema. Ophthalmology. 2007;114:1574-9.
38. Mackensen F, Heinz C, Becker MD, et al. Intravitreal bevacizumab (avastin) as a treatment for refractory macular edema in patients with uveitis: a pilot study. Retina. 2008;28: 41-5.
39. Lott MN, Schiffman JC, Davis JL. Bevacizumab in inflammatory eye disease. Am J Ophthalmol. 2009;148:711-7.
40. Kurup S, Lew J, Byrnes G, et al. Therapeutic efficacy of intravitreal bevacizumab on posterior uveitis complicated by neovascularization. Acta Ophthalmol. 2009;87:349-52.
41. Lasave AF, Zeballos DG, El-Haig WM, et al. Short-term results of a single intravitreal bevacizumab (avastin) injection versus a single intravitreal triamcinolone acetonide (kenacort) injection for the management of refractory noninfectious uveitic cystoid macular edema. Ocul Immunol Inflamm. 2009;17:423-30.
42. Dyer D, Callanan D, Bochow T, et al. Clinical evaluation of the safety and efficacy of preservative-free triamcinolone triesence triamcinolone acetonide injectable suspension 40 mg/ml for visualization during pars plana vitrectomy. Retina. 2009;29:38-45.
43. Jaffe GJ, Ben-nun J, Guo Hong, et al. Fluocinolone acetonide sustained drug delivery device to treat severe uveitis. Ophthalmology. 2000;107:2024-33.
44. Jaffe GJ, Pearson PA, Ashton P. Dexamethasone sustained drug delivery implant for the treatment of severe uveitis. Retina. 2000;20:402-3

45. Kuno N, Fujii S. Biodegradable intraocular therapies for retinal disorders: progress to date. Drugs Aging. 2010;27:117-34.
46. Nguyen QD, Callanan D, Dugel P, et al. Treating chronic noninfectious posterior segment uveitis: the impact of cumulative damage. Proceedings of an expert panel roundtable discussion. Retina; 2006.pp.1-16.
47. Jaffe GJ, Martin D, Callanan D, et al. Fluocinolone Acetonide Uveitis Study Group. Fluocinolone acetonide implant (Retisert) for noninfectious posterior uveitis: thirty-four-week results of a multicenter randomized clinical study. Ophthalmology. 2006;113:1020-7.
48. Mohammad DA, Sweet BV, Elner SG. Retisert: is the new advance in treatment of uveitis a good one? Ann Pharmacother. 2007;41:449-54.
49. Callanan DG, Jaffe GJ, Martin DF, et al. Treatment of posterior uveitis with a fluocinolone acetonide implant: three-year clinical trial results. Arch Ophthalmol. 2008;126:1191-201.
50. Taban M, Lowder CY, Kaiser PK. Outcome of fluocinolone acetonide implant (Retisert) reimplantation for chronic noninfectious posterior uveitis. Retina. 2008;28:1280-8.
51. Mahajan VB, Gehrs KM, Goldstein DA, et al. Management of sympathetic ophthalmia with the fluocinolone acetonide implant. Ophthalmology. 2009;116:552-7.
52. Pavesio C, Zierhut M, Bairi K, et al. Fluocinolone Acetonide Study Group. Evaluation of an Intravitreal Fluocinolone Acetonide Implant versus Standard Systemic Therapy in Noninfectious Posterior Uveitis. Ophthalmology. 2010;117: 567-75.
53. Culbertson WW, Dix RD. Variella-Zoster virus diseases: posterior segment of the eye. In: Pepose JS, Holland GN, wilhelmus KR (Eds). Ocular Infection and Immunity. St. Louis, MO: Mosby-year BookInc; 1996. pp. 1131-54.
54. Freeman WR, Friedberg DN, Berry C, et al. Risk factors for development of rhegmatogenous retinal detachment in patients with cytomegalovirus retinitis. Am J Ophthalmol. 1993;116: 713-20.
55. Culbertson WW, Blumenkranz MS, Pepose JS, et al. Vaicella zoster virus is a cause of the acute retinal necrosis syndrome. Ophthalmology. 1986;93:559-69.
56. Thomas MA, Dickinson JD, Melberg NS, et al. Visual results after surgical removal of subfoveal choroidal neovascular membranes. Ophthalmology. 1994;101:1384-96.
57. Martidis A,Duker JS, Puliahto CA. Intravitreal triamcinolone for refractory cystoid macular edema secondary to Birdshot Retinochoroidopathy. Arch Ophthalmol. 2001; 119:1380-3.
58. Halperin LS, Akduman L, Olk RJ. Ocular histoplasmosis syndrome. In: Albert DM, Jakobiec FA (Eds). Principles and Practice of Ophthalmology, 2nd edition. Philadelphia: W.B. Saunders,1994.
59. Fitzgerald CR. Pars plana vitrectomy for vitreous opacity secondary to presumed toxoplasmosis. Arch Ophthalmol. 1980;98:321-3.
60. Akduman L, Del Priore LV, Desai V, et al. Perfusion of the subfoveal choriocapillaris affects visual recovery after submacular surgery in presumed ocular histoplasmosis syndrome. Am J Ophthalmol. 1997;123:90-6.
61. Chuck RS, Olk RJ, Weil GJ, et al. Surgical removal of a subretinal proliferating cysticercus of Taenia crassiceps. Arch Ophthalmol. 1997;115:562-3.

SECTION

5

Macular Surgery

Macular Epiretinal Membrane Removal

24

Paolo Lanzetta, Daniele Veritti, Gloria Dal Mas, Valentina Sarao

Introduction

Epiretinal membrane (ERM) is caused by a glial proliferation on the retinal surface. It usually presents as a translucent sheet on the retinal surface. Contraction of the ERM may occur and produce various degrees of retinal distortion. This condition may be idiopathic or secondary to different ocular pathologies (such as retinal vascular diseases, ocular trauma, intraocular inflammation) or associated with retinal procedures.

Epidemiology

The majority of patients who develop ERM are older than 50 years of age.[1] Few population-based studies regarding the prevalence of ERM have been reported.[2-11] The prevalence of primary ERM in Asians seems to be higher than that in Caucasians;[3] the Singapore Malay Eye Study reported a prevalence of 15.7% while the Blue Mountains Eye Study showed a prevalence of 7%. It has been accounted that there is an increased prevalence of ERM in urban population with respect to rural population.[4] Age standardized prevalence was higher for secondary (16.4%) compared to idiopathic (5.4%) ERM, reflecting the presence of underlying ocular pathology associated with aging. In the Blue Mountains Eye Study the incidence of ERM was 5.3% over a 5 year follow-up. Over this period, the incidence was 3.7% among patients younger than 60 years of age, 6.6% in patients from 60–69 years of age, 6.1% between 70 to 79 years and 1.1% in those older than 80.[4] The lower rate found for older age group was supposed to be due to lens opacity, making difficult to obtain a clear image of the retina. ERMs are present in 3.5–5.5% of autopsied eyes.[5] No statistically significant gender difference has been reported. Refractive error, such as increasing myopia, was significantly associated with the development of ERMs.[10] Differently, the Blue Mountains Eye Study reported an important association with hyperopia.[4] Idiopathic ERMs are bilateral in 20–30% of cases and the second eye involvement has been reported in 13.5% of patients after 5 years of follow-up. Diabetes in the absence of retinopathy has been associated with idiopathic ERM. Smoking seems to have a moderate protective role in the development of ERM.[10,11] ERM occurred in 3–8.5% of cases after retinal detachment surgery and were found in 9% of patients undergoing cataract surgery.[12] Patients with the preoperative presence of rolled retinal edge, star pattern retinal folds and equatorial ridges have the greatest risk of developing these membranes. ERMs have been found in association with retinal vascular diseases, retinal breaks and detachments, ocular trauma, uveitis and following retinal cryopexy, laser photocoagulation and intraocular surgery.

Etiology

Epiretinal membrane is a relatively common finding in older persons and they may be secondary to different ocular pathologies, such as retinal vascular diseases, ocular inflammation, post-trauma and postsurgical conditions, intraocular tumors and inherited retinal dystrophies.[13] Retinal vascular diseases include vascular occlusions, angiomas,[14,15] telangectasias, arteriolar macroaneurysms, sickle cell retinopathy[16] and diabetic retinopathy.[17] Sarcoidosis, pars planitis and Takayasu's disease are ocular inflammation conditions that can be related to ERMs formation. Any trauma associated with vitreous hemorrhage and all types of ocular surgery (including cataract extraction, retinal detachment surgery and laser therapy) are known to be associated with ERMs development.[18,19] Other possible associations are retinal angiomas and hamartomas as well as intraocular tumors and retinal dystrophies, such as retinitis pigmentosa.[20] However, ERMs can occur in healthy eyes, in absence of associated disease or without any ocular anomaly other than posterior vitreous detachment. In this case the membranes are classified as idiopathic.[20-23]

Pathogenesis

Epiretinal membranes derive from fibrocellular proliferation on the inner surface of the internal limiting membrane and are characterized by cell-mediated contraction that occurs idiopathically or as a secondary process of the disease.[21-24] The pathogenesis of ERMs is not completely understood. A first explanation of the pathological mechanism involved in idiopathic ERM formation was described by Roth and Foos.[5,25] The development of posterior vitreous detachment appears to be pivotal to the formation of idiopathic ERMs. Since a posterior vitreous detachment is present in approximately 90% of eyes with idiopathic membranes.[26] The vitreoretinal traction that occurs during the development of posterior vitreous detachment may create defects in the internal limiting membrane that allow migration of retinal glial cells and subsequent proliferation and contraction on the inner retinal surface.[27] An alternative hypothesis for idiopathic ERM formation involves proliferation, fibrous metaplasia and contraction of hyalocytes that persist on the inner retinal surface after posterior vitreous detachment.[18,28] ERMs are composed of two main components: extracellular matrix (collagen, laminin, tenascin, fibronectin, vitronectin, thrombospondin) and cells of retinal and extraretinal origin. A wide variety of cell types characterize ERMs: glial cells (including microglia, Müller cells and fibrous astrocytes), epithelial cells from the retinal pigment epithelium and ciliary body, immune cells (macrophages, lymphocytes, neutrophils), fibrocytes and myofibrocytes.[29] Microglial cells play an important role in host defense against invading microorganisms, initiation of inflammatory process and tissue repair. Astrocytes are activated and proliferate especially under conditions of vascular injury and retinal neovascularization. Müller cells may act as modulators of immune and inflammatory responses producing proinflammatory cytokines. Müller cells are also capable of phagocytosing cellular fragments and foreign substances. The development of Müller cells' process into the vitreal surface of the retina has been suggested to represent the initial event of ERM formation. Within the membranes, glial and pigment epithelial cells may transdifferentiate into contractile myofibrocytes. This process can create a scar like tissue and increase the capacity of glial cells to generate tractional forces that distort the anatomic profile of the retina.[30] Secondary ERMs are often observed in eyes with proliferative vitreoretinal disorders such as proliferative diabetic retinopathy or proliferative vitreoretinopathy. Cellular proliferation stimulated by vitreous inflammation or breakdown of blood retinal barriers can be a plausible pathogenic mechanism for secondary ERMs.[31] Many recent studies have shown a strong correlation between development of ERMs and the expression of growth factors and their receptors in the proliferative vitreoretinal diseases. Multiple factors may induce proliferation and translocation of Müller cells toward the retinal surface.[32] Among these factors, HGF (hepatocyte growth factor) and PDGF (platelet-derived growth factor) stimulate the scattering and migration or proliferation of retinal cells such as glial and pigmented cells. The contraction of ERMs is stimulated by vitreal factors, in particular IGF (insulin-like growth factor) and PDGF. The production and the deposition of extracellular matrix components is stimulated by TGF-β (transforming growth factor beta).[33-35] Other growth factors related to the formation of secondary ERMs are: VEGF (vascular endothelial growth factor), EGF (endothelial growth factor), FGF (fibroblast growth factor) and CTGF (connective tissue growth factor).[36,37] In addition, several cytokines can be found in the vitreous and in ERMs and these include IL-1, IL-6, monocyte chemotactic protein and macrophage-colony stimulating factor.[38] To determine the relative contribution of the various growth factors present in the vitreous remains a pressing question. In fact those growth factors and cytokines can be possible therapeutic targets for future treatments.

Classification

Gass[39] proposed a classification system based on the appearance of the membrane and the underlying retinal tissue and vessels.

- *Grade 0 (cellophane maculopathy):* A translucent ERM is not associated with distortion of the inner retina. It is seen ophthalmoscopically as a irregular light reflex, like a "cellophane". Patients are usually asymptomatic and the membrane may be discovered by chance (Figs 24.1A to D).
- *Grade I (crinkled cellophane maculopathy):* The inner retinal surface is distorted following contraction of the ERM. The gathering of the inner retinal layers into folds gives to the retina a crinkled cellophane appearance. Ophthalmoscopically fine retinal folds, radiating outward from the center of the ERM, can be seen. The wrinkling of the inner retinal surface may be sufficient to produce tortuosity of the paramacular vessels pulling them toward the fovea. In these patients, cystoid macula edema, retinal hemorrhage, exudates and RPE disturbance are usually not present. In this stage of the disease patients may be still asymptomatic with normal visual acuity or have mild visual disturbance (Figs 24.2A to D).
- *Grade II (macular pucker):* The membrane is thicker and opaque, with grayish appearance. It partly obscures the underlying vessels and causes marked distortion of the retina. Usually a full-thickness puckering of the macula is present. In "macular pucker", macular edema, retinal hemorrhage and cotton-wools spots are often present. Usually, in this stage of the disease, vision is markedly reduced, and patients experience central photopsia and metamorphopsia (Figs 24.3A to D).

Another classification has been proposed by Joondeph[40]

- *Grade 1:* A transparent ERM alters the light reflex without retinal distortion.
- *Grade 2:* An ERM obscures part of the underlying retina, with a moderate retinal distortion.
- *Grade 3:* An opaque ERM causes marked distortion of the underlying retina. Retinal striae, radiating from the center of the epiretinal membrane are present.
- *Grade 4:* An ERM causes marked distortion of the retina.

Symptoms

The spectrum of clinical manifestation may vary from no symptoms at all to severe visual dysfunction. ERM may be discovered by chance during a physical examination, in this case the patients may be asymptomatic and have normal visual acuity. Clinical manifestation, according to the degree of disease severity, is linked with the thickness of the membrane, wrinkling location and retinal distortion degree. At the beginning, visual disturbances are minor, like mild distortion or blurred vision. Moderate and severe forms can be characterized by different degrees of metamorphopsia, visual loss and, less commonly, diplopia, central photopsia, micropsia and macropsia. Visual acuity is commonly in the range of 20/30–20/70 and relatively few patients have vision worse than 20/200.[22,41] Macropsia is probably caused by crowding of the photoreceptors. Diplopia may be caused by foveal ectopia in the case of lateral displacement of the fovea.

Diagnosis

Diagnosis of ERM is based on fundus examination. Membrane may be discovered by chance during a physical examination in asymptomatic patients. It appears as a glinting, irregular light reflex. The cellophane maculopathy has no distinct edges. Sometime it can be useful to examine the fundus with a contact lens, especially in case of subtle membranes. Over time, ERM may undergo contraction, causing distortion of the inner retinal surface and tortuosity and straightening of paramacular vessel. Opthalmoscopically it is seen as a wrinkling of the retinal surface, often associated with superficial radiating retinal folds extended outward from the margins of the contracted membrane (Figs 24.4A to C). Initially this contraction involves only the inner layers of the retina, but with thicker membranes there is a marked distortion also of the underlying retina. In such cases the membrane may appear opaque, with grayish appearance and it produces a tangential traction throughout the thickness of the retina. This traction on the retina may cause macular edema, preretinal or intraretinal hemorrhage and tractional macular detachment. Pseudohole may be seen in association with ERM. It represents a defect in the central portion of the membrane overlying the fovea and appears at the ophthalmoscopic examination as an altered darker red light reflex (Figs 24.5A to C). Watzke-Allen test (at the slit lamp) is useful to distinguish a pseudohole from full-thickness hole. In this test, a narrow vertical slit beam is projected in the fovea: when patients detect a break in the bar of light that they perceive, the test is considered positive meaning that there is a full-thickness hole. Fluorescein angiography usually does not contribute significantly to the diagnosis. Though, it

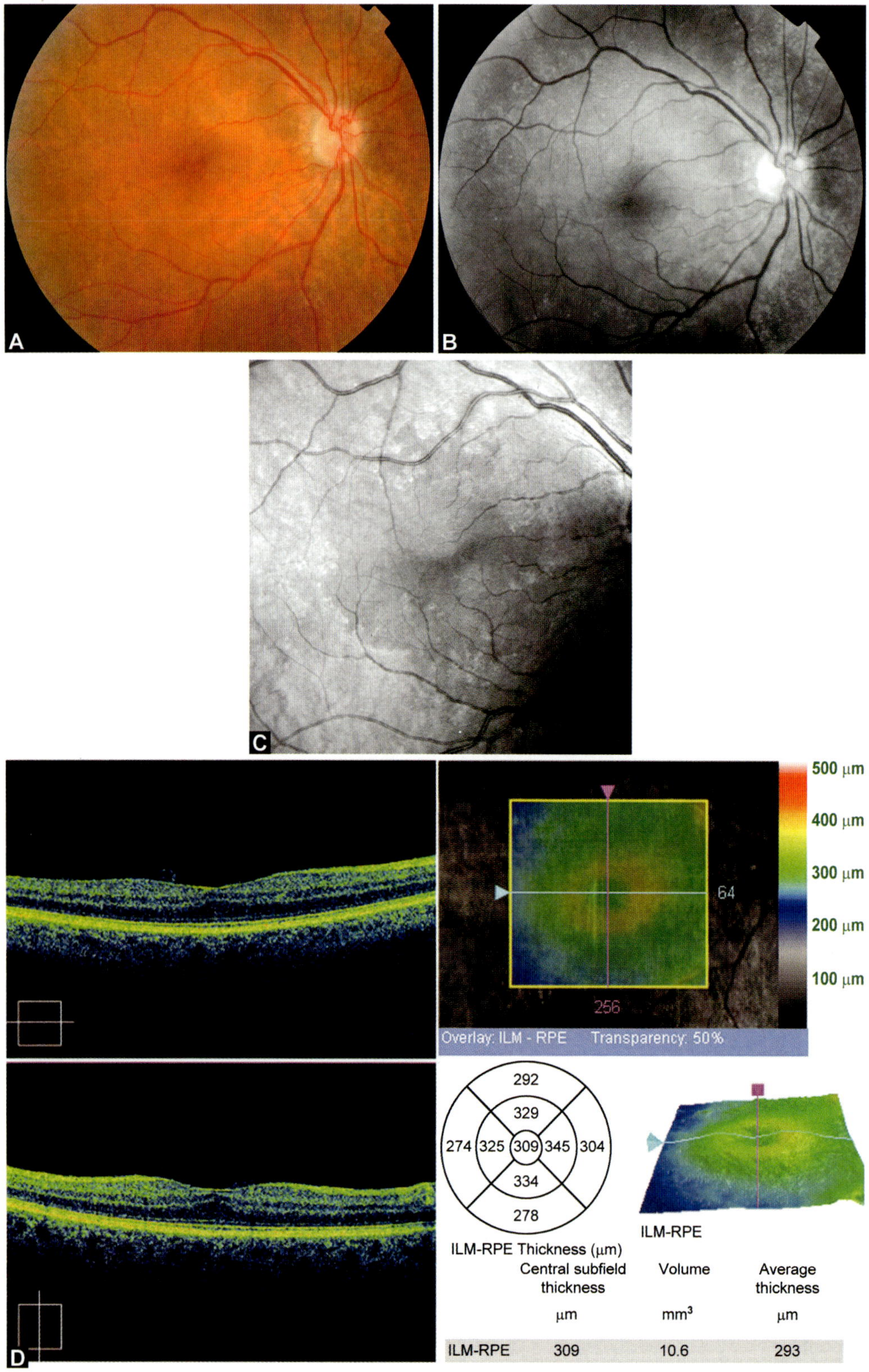

▲ **Figures 24.1A to D**

(A) Color photograph of grade 0 epiretinal membrane showing irregular light reflex; (B) Red-free; (C) Infrared imaging of the same eye; (D) Optical coherence tomography illustrating an inner layer of increased reflectance and thickening of the foveal area

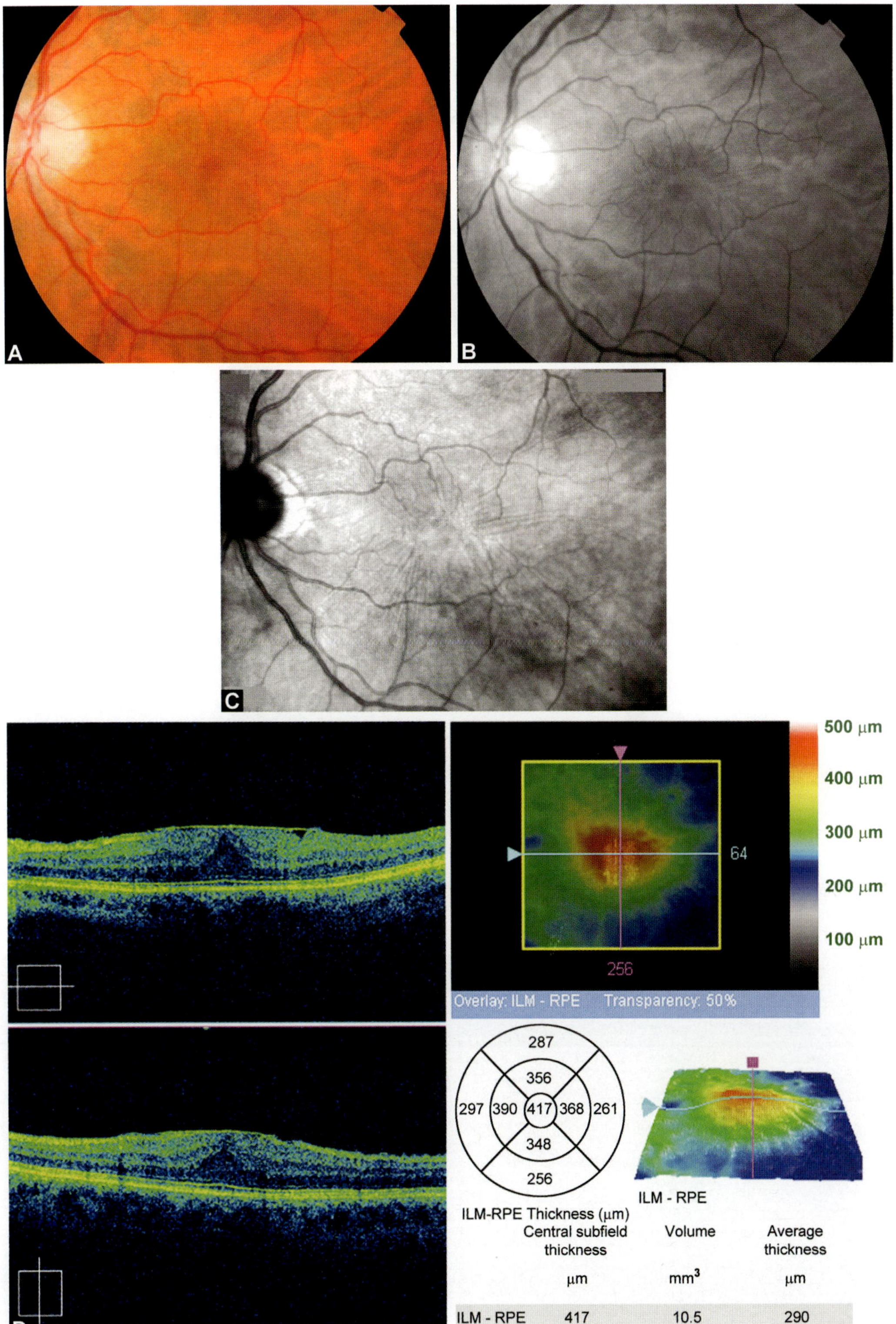

▲ **Figures 24.2A to D**

(A) Color photograph of grade I epiretinal membrane revealing subtle radiating striae in the macula. Note the tortuosity of small vessels in this region; (B) Red-free; (C) Infrared imaging permit improved visualization of retinal surface abnormalities; (D) Optical coherence tomography illustrating increased retinal thickening, with the epiretinal membrane distorting the retinal surface

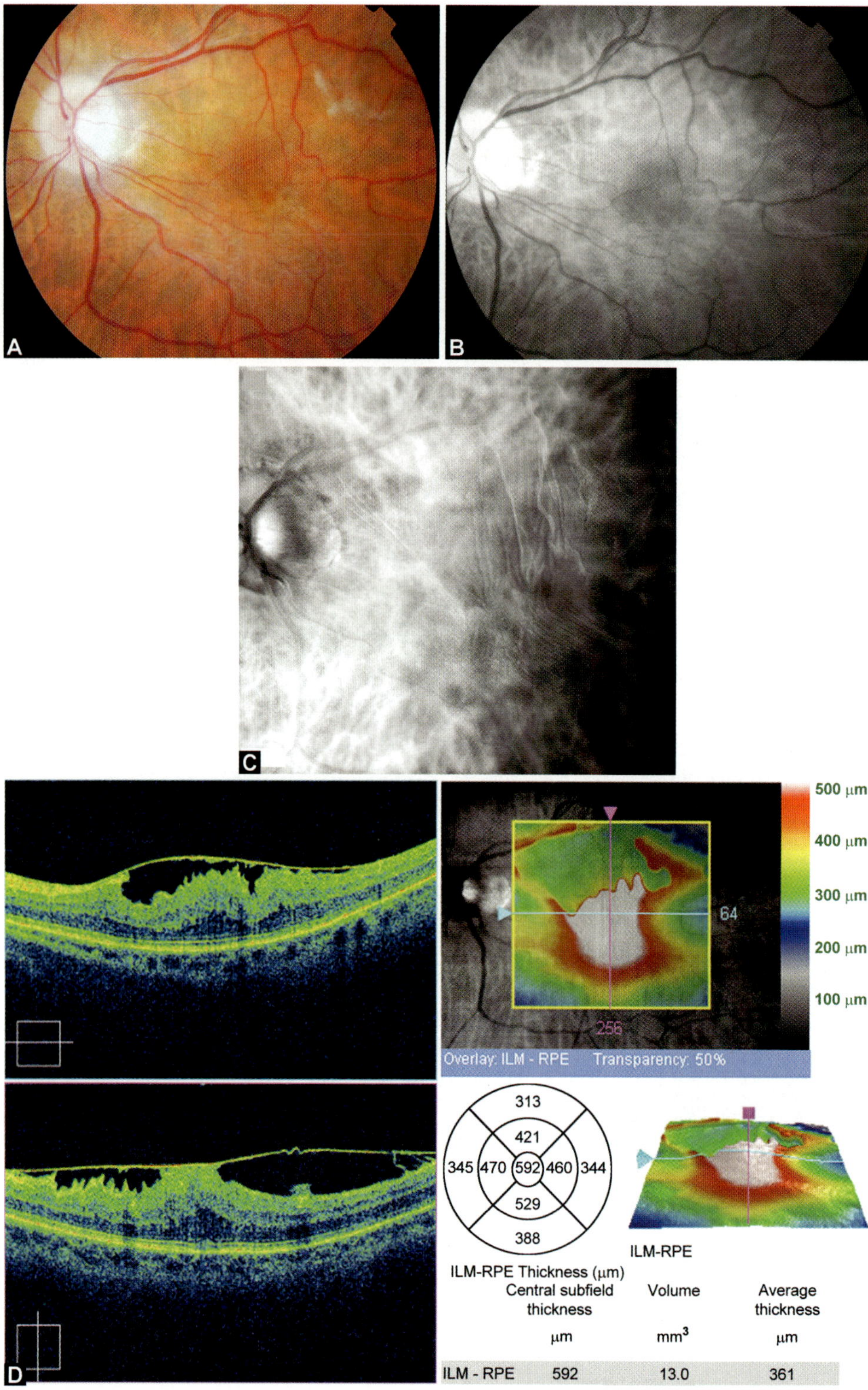

▲ **Figures 24.3A to D**

(A and B) Color photograph and red-free image illustrating eccentric grade II epiretinal membrane creating foveal ectopia and significant vascular tortuosity; (C) Retro-mode image of the same eye obtained with F-10 Nidek camera. It uses infrared laser and an aperture deviated laterally from the confocal light path to form a pseudo tridimensional image to detect anomalies in the deeper retinal layers; (D) Optical coherence tomography showing increased retinal thickness with epiretinal membrane exerting traction

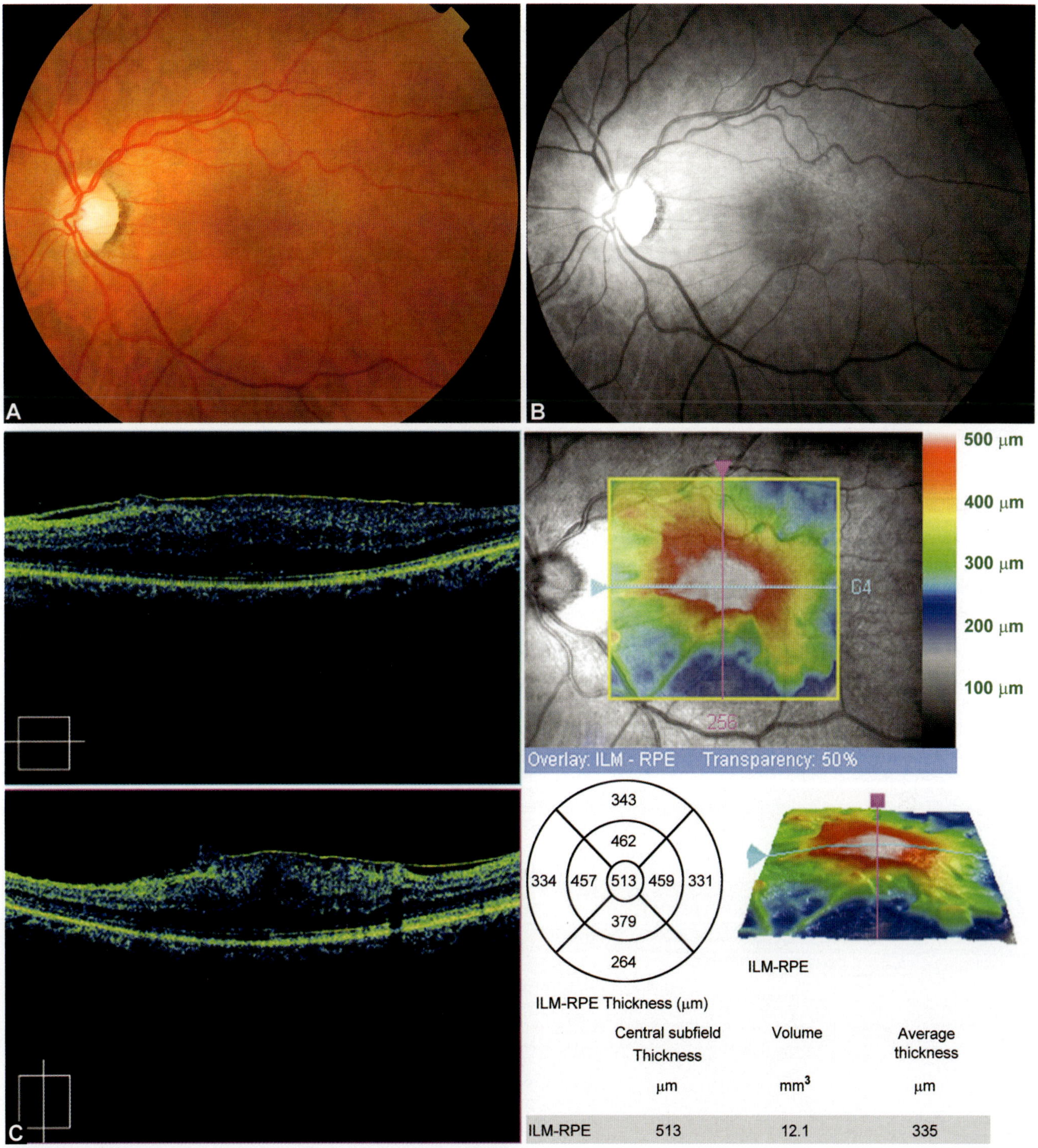

▲ **Figures 24.4A to C**

(A and B) Color photograph and red-free image showing wrinkled retinal surface associated with superficial radiating retinal folds; (C) Optical coherence tomography reveals the presence of an epiretinal membrane associated with distortion of the inner retinal layers and increased retinal thickness

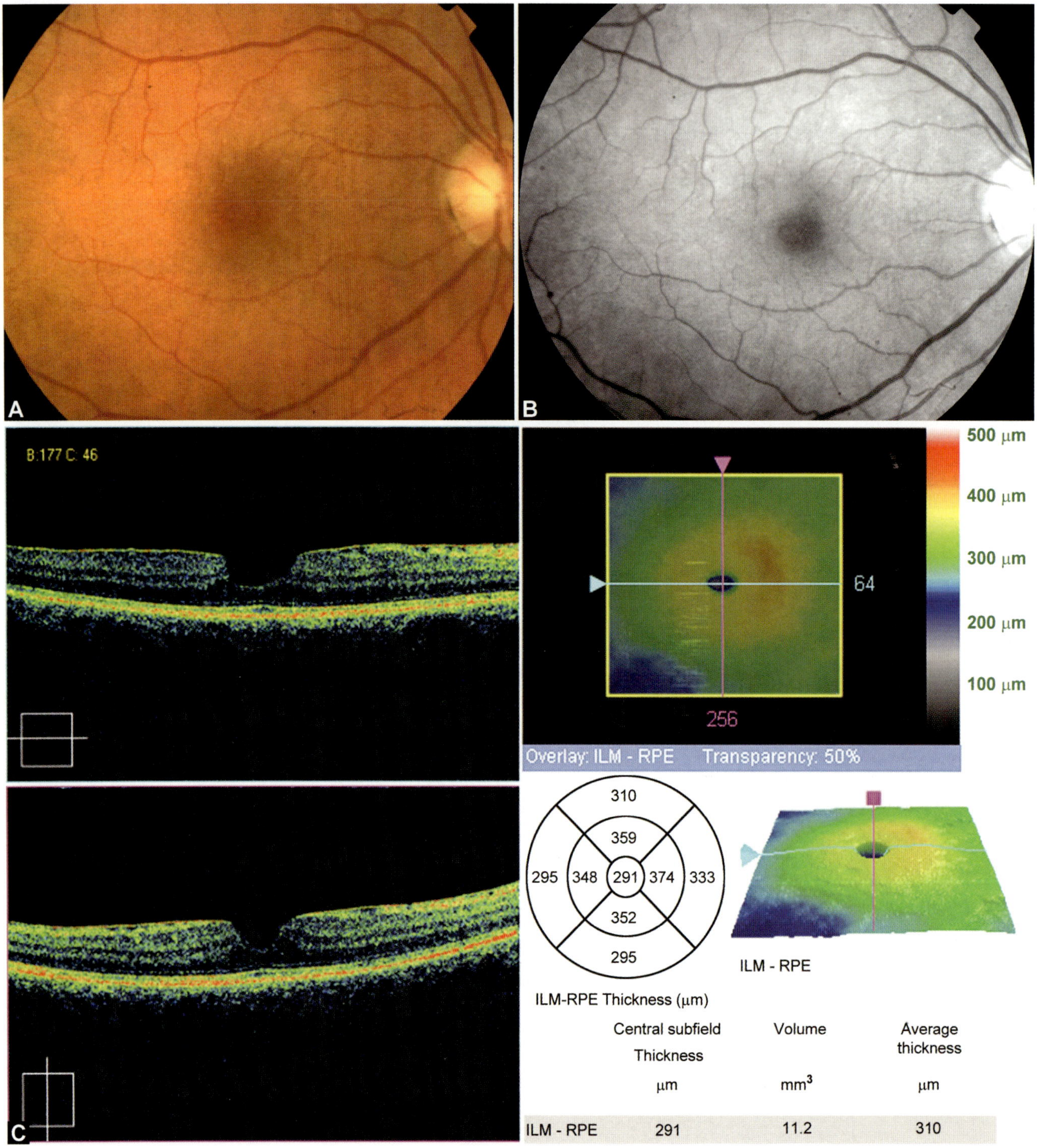

▲ **Figures 24.5A to C**

(A and B) Color photograph and red-free image revealing altered light reflex and darker appearance of the fovea in association with epiretinal membrane; (C) Optical coherence tomography appearance of macular pseudohole. Note the epiretinal membrane which causes wrinkling of the retina

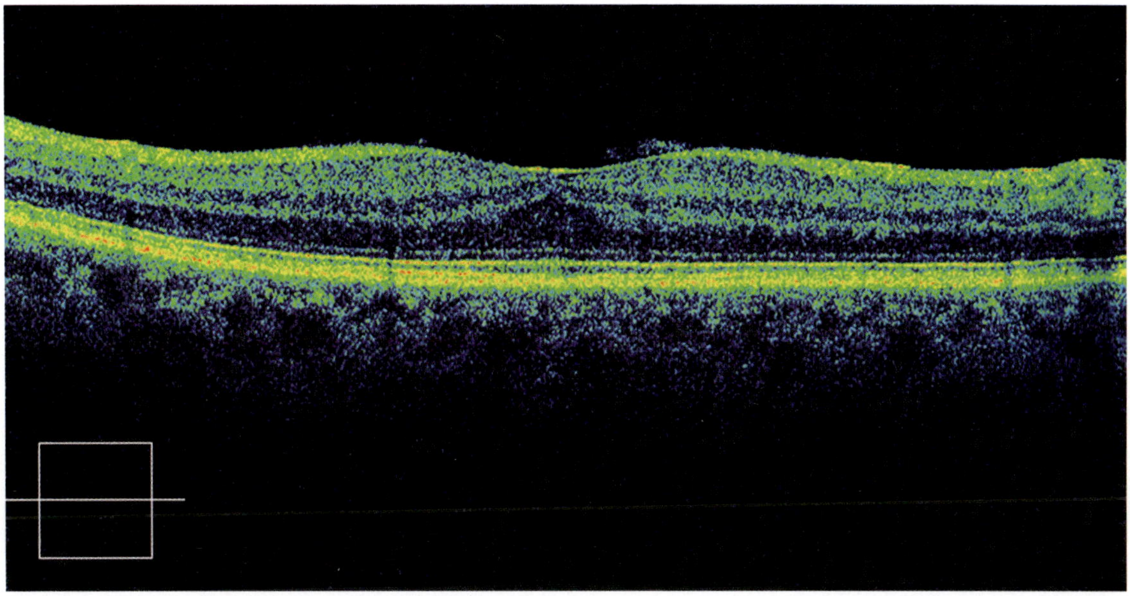

▲ Figure 24.6

A highly reflective layer on the inner surface of the retina without alterations of the foveal profile can be seen on optical coherence tomography in early cases of macular epiretinal membrane

may be useful to evaluate the degree of retinal vessel tortuosity, to highlight the vascular tortuosity and to show hyperfluorescence areas if leakage is present. Fluorescein angiography can be helpful in distinguishing macular edema caused by ERM from edema of different origin. Optical coherence tomography (OCT) is indicated to confirm the diagnosis. It provides qualitative and quantitative information of the retinal architecture and its anatomical relationship with the vitreous. In mild cases OCT shows only a highly reflective layer on the surface of the retina without alterations of foveal profile (corresponding to the cellular proliferation on the retinal surface) (Fig. 24.6). In moderate and severe cases OCT can show different degrees of macular thickening and alterations of the retinal architecture (Fig. 24.4C). Moreover, OCT highlights the presence of macular edema and any associated vitreous traction on the retina. Amsler grid, is useful to investigate and evaluate the presence and progression of metamorphopsia. However, this test does not provide objective data: metamorphopsia is detected as a subjective symptom and can be influenced by visual acuity disturbances such as severe cataract or corneal opacity. In a recently published study, the correlation between the degree of metamorphopsia using an Amsler chart and the thickness of the inner retinal layers based on 3-dimensional (3D) spectral-domain optical coherence tomography (SD-OCT) was assessed. Nineteen eyes were examined and classified in three groups based on Amsler chart results: no metamorphopsia, local metamorphopsia (defined as metamorphopsia involving less than two-third of Amsler chart) and broad metamorphopsia (defined as metamorphopsia involving more than two-third of Amsler chart). Furthermore, the thickness of inner nuclear layer (INL), outer plexiform layer (OPL) and outer nuclear layer (ONL) were measured on 5 horizontal cross-sections using the SD-OCT system. Metamorphopsia was found in almost the same position as the edematous areas of INL, especially areas that were more than 50 μm thick. The ONL and OPL also tended to be edematous in the area of metamorphopsia, but these changes were not significantly related to the area of metamorphopsia.[42]

Differential Diagnosis

The differential diagnosis of ERM includes vitreomacular tractions, combined hamartoma of the retina and retinal pigment epithelium, a particularly apparent foveal reflex in young subjects, postoperative cystoid macular edema, full-thickness macular hole. The patient affected by combined hamartoma of the retina and retinal pigment epithelium may have similar symptoms of a patient with ERM, especially metamorphopsia. This happens because in this condition there is a membrane on the retinal surface that can determine a traction involving the adjacent tissue. Clinical appearance of these lesions allows differentiation from ERM. Combined hamartoma of the retina and retinal pigment epithelium is typically elevated and variably pigmented and it may show leakage of dye on fluorescein angiography.[43] Pseudoholes are commonly seen in association with macular pucker (grade 2 epiretinal membrane) and may be confused with full-thickness macular holes.

Treatment

Clinical Criteria for Surgery

ERM may infrequently separate spontaneously from the retina, but the great majority of membranes remain quite stable after an initial period of growth. Vision rarely improves or worsens dramatically. Vitreoretinal surgery may be performed to remove those ERMs that cause significant visual loss.[44] The goal of surgery is to relieve the traction caused by the ERM. The appropriate criteria for surgery vary by patient and represent a multifactorial process based on symptoms, extent of visual loss, visual needs, status of the other eye, age, duration, medical status and the presence of other ocular diseases.[45] Surgery is usually reserved for patients in which vision has decreased at least to 20/60. However, eyes with a preoperative vision higher than 20/50 are occasionally considered for surgery if the patient is significantly symptomatic, in good health, relatively young and requires better vision to achieve his life's tasks.[46] A shorter disease duration is usually associated with better visual outcomes. However, even patients with a ten year's disease duration may experience visual improvement after surgery.[47,48] A careful preoperative evaluation is mandatory in all eyes candidate for ERM stripping to determine whether the visual loss is caused strictly by the membrane or by other retinal pathologic conditions that may mimic the presence of ERM: macular hole, choroidal neovascularization, Irvine-Gass syndrome, macular telangiectasias, retinal vascular occlusion, retinal vascular abnormalities, vasoproliferative tumors.[49,50] Contraindications to surgery are represented by reduced vision before membrane formation, hereditary photoreceptor degeneration and previous central retinal artery occlusion.[51,52] Surgery involves pars plana vitrectomy, removal of ERM with or without peeling of the internal limiting membrane (ILM).

Pars Plana Vitrectomy

Machemer first developed the concept of membrane peeling in 1972, using pars plana vitrectomy techniques.[44] A three port vitrectomy is the routine approach. Sclerotomies are usually located 3.5–4 mm posterior to the limbus in phakic eyes and approximately 0.5 mm more anteriorly in aphakic or pseudophakic eyes. An infusion cannula is typically placed in the inferotemporal site, to allow balanced saline solution to replace the excised tissue and thereby maintain the intraocular pressure (IOP). The remaining ports are used to introduce the instrumentation into the vitreous cavity, to illuminate the posterior segment and manipulate intraocular tissues. The 20-gauge vitrectomy system has been considered the gold standard since 1974.[53] However recent advancements in vitreous surgery consisted in the development of minimally invasive transconjunctival vitrectomy systems: 25-gauge and 23-gauge systems. The recent spread of 25-gauge instrumentation for vitreous surgery has promoted great interest in the transconjunctival sutureless vitrectomy systems.[54] In fact, smaller incisions with self-sealing wounds might decrease surgical trauma and operating time, possibly resulting in a surgical outcome superior to conventional 20-gauge vitrectomy.[55,56] Some surgeons believe that the significant time saved by the reduced opening and closing time makes 25-gauge vitrectomy more efficient.[57] On the other hand, others assert that efficiency is decreased because the smaller gauge has significantly lower flow rate, which may result in increased vitrectomy time for removal of an equal volume of vitreous.[58] However, the nature of sutureless small-gauge vitrectomy leads to less traumatic conjunctival and scleral manipulation, less surgically-related astigmatism and less postoperative patient discomfort and facilitates early visual improvement.[59] Therefore, 25-gauge vitrectomy seems a good solution for the management of macular surgery and in particular ERM removal. In spite of its essentially positive aspects, certain limitations to the 25-gauge system persist to date. For instance, the higher flexibility and delicateness that is associated with the 25-gauge instruments, versus the considerably more stable 20-gauge instruments, make specific surgeon training a prerequisite.[60] Moreover, high instrument flexibility renders certain procedures impossible or subject to limitations. While the 20-gauge instrument may be used to rotate eye for a better view of the periphery, this is hardly possible with the 25-gauge system and it represents a serious restriction for the removal peripheral vitreous.[61] Hypotony and endophthalmitis seem to be more frequent in 25-gauge vitrectomy than in 20-gauge vitrectomy, depending on the type of scleral incision, straight or angled. This may be, at least in part, due to the incision construction technique.

Epiretinal Membrane Removal

When the membrane is thick and fibrotic, it may be possible to grasp the membrane directly with intraocular end-grasping forceps and strip it away from the macular surface. However, in same cases a barbed microvitreoretinal (MVR) blade may used to engage the membrane at its edge and lift it up from the retinal surface. The blade is then employed to strip away connections with the retina. During this procedure it is important not to fragment the ERM by pulling too hard or too long in any direction. Once a broad edge of membrane has been elevated, a blunt-tripped pick may also be used. This tool can provide less chance of tearing the membrane and a better capacity to find a new edge to restart the surgical process. When a complete side of the membrane has been elevated, fine-tripped intraocular forceps are used to continue the dissection, elevating the membrane at multiple sites along the advancing edge of residual adhesion. Once the advancing edge comes close to the fovea, the membrane should be grasped near the fovea and peeled over. The distal portions of the membrane are wheeled centrally after the membrane has been stripped away from the macula. The membrane can then be entirely stripped away from the retina and removed from the eye. Normally, smooth traction force is applied with unhurried movement of forceps. During the dissection of the ERM, care should always be given to any distortion of the retinal surface or tiny retinal bleeding, in order to avoid possible iatrogenic retinal tear or large retinal hemorrhage. Commonly, no clearly identifiable edges can be seen in idiopathic ERMs. The barbed MVR blade can be used to develop an edge by dragging its downwardly curved edge along the membrane surface. This dissection should be started over the thickest part of the membrane or the most highly refractile portion. The membrane is then engaged and gently elevated. During this procedure, it is often difficult to recognize what tissue has been engaged and the surgeon must interpret what tissue has been elevated recognizing the stiffness of the dissected tissue. ERM come-up away from the retina in smooth and uniform sheets, the ILM appears sticky and more adherent. Nerve fiber layer appears fluffy and is often associated with small hemorrhages.

Some surgeons have suggested using a soft-tipped extrusion needle to aspirate the membrane and start the dissection.[62] Others believe that the membrane can be grasped on its surface by a pair of fine-tipped forceps, bypassing the need for finding or developing an edge. Obviously, there are potential problems with this technique, including retinal pigment epithelial and retinal break formation. Finally, an instrument in use by many surgeons is the Tano diamond-dusted membrane scraper, a silicone-tipped device coated with diamond particles that can be helpful in initiating the removal of the ERM.[63,64] When an ERM is too fragile or too thin, a diamond-dusted membrane scraper may be useful to give firm grip on the tissue.[65] If a thin layer of residual cortical vitreous is present, it can be lifted either with diamond dusted membrane scraper or by gentle aspiration from a silicone-brushed aspirating needle.

Internal Limiting Membrane Peeling

Some studies have shown that the removal of the ILM improves the anatomic success rate and visual outcomes in several macular conditions, such as ERM.[66,67] The peeling of ILM may ensure not only the complete removal of the ERM but also a lower rate of recurrence of ERM after its removal. Recurrences after combined ERM and ILM removal have been observed in less than 9% of cases, while they have been reported between 7.5% and 56% following surgical removal of ERM alone.[49,68] Some case control studies and case series have shown good visual results following combined ERM removal and ILM peeling.[69] ILM is a very thin and semitransparent basement membrane 2.5 µm thick. The presence of the ILM can be interpreted by shiny reflection of the retina, but such delicate structure may be difficult to identify during vitreoretinal surgery. Many different instruments such as forceps, sharp disposable needle or MVR blade can be used to grasp or puncture and peel a small area of the ILM 3–5 mm from the fovea. Alternatively, a diamond-dusted membrane scraper can be employed to create the initial ILM flapped tear. The peeled edge can be lifted up using an ILM elevator or grasped using ILM forceps. Finally, ILM forceps are used for ILM maculorrhexis. There is no general agreement regarding the extent of the area of ILM to be peeled. Some reports have described peeling an area of about one disk diameter centered at the fovea. Others reported on surgical results following peeling of areas two, three or four disk diameters large. It has been suggested that extensive ILM peeling up to the vascular arcade may prevent recurrences of symptomatic ERM.[70] It can be technically difficult to peel the nearly invisible ILM, even to experienced vitreoretinal surgeons. Difficulties can be encountered to start and to complete the peeling of the ILM if the edge of flap is lost or even to determine the total extent of the peeled area. In order to facilitate this procedure, chromovitrectomy was introduced.[71,72] Chromovitrectomy is a surgical technique that uses vital dyes or crystals to improve the visualization and the removal of the ILM. Staining of the ILM has made the peeling procedure easier and has reduced the operating time and the mechanical trauma to the retina.[73] Safety issues still exists on the use of different dyes.

Indocyanine Green Staining

Indocyanine green is a tricarbocyanine dye, first used in ophthalmology in 1970 for choroidal angiography. It is a hydrophilic dye with a great affinity for the matrix components of the ILM, such as collagen type 4 and laminin. The collagen of the ILM is stained positively, the cellular component of the ERM is stained negatively.[74] The intravitreal injection of indocyanine green facilitates the visualization and complete removal of the ILM and it may help to distinguish ERM.[75] Indocyanine green is supplied as a powder, which contains iodine to increase its solubility. There is no standard method for its preparation. It can be dissolved in water or in a mixture of glucose solution and water prior to the addiction of balanced salt solution to prevent its precipitation, which may reduce its staining properties. Various concentrations of indocyanine green have been used to stain the ILM, ranging from 0.6 mg/ml to 5 mg/ml. Some authors found that the 1.25% concentration stained the ILM consistently well with no need for re-staining.[76] Indocyanine green-guided chromovitrectomy initially gained worldwide popularity and large studies showed an easier and less traumatic peeling procedure with the achievement of good visual outcomes.[77] However, subsequent studies revealed the risk of indocyanine green toxicity to the retina. After 12 months of follow-up, several studies have shown clinical postoperative side effects of indocyanine green-guided chromovitrectomy, such as RPE damages, visual field defects and possible optic nerve atrophy.[78] It has been postulated that the use of indocyanine green at low concentrations for ILM peeling could be a safer alternative. Lower rates of RPE abnormalities have been observed with indocyanine green staining with a concentration of 0.5 mg/ml or less and an osmolarity of approximately 290 mOsm. Various hypothesis are involved to explain the mechanism of retinal damage induced by the use of indocyanine green. It has been shown that indocyanine green may change the osmolarity in the vitreous cavity, thereby damaging either the neurosensory retina or the RPE cells directly.[79] In addition, harmful effect of hypo-osmotic indocyanine green solutions could be increased by intraoperative light exposure. Moreover, indocyanine green causes direct retinal damage, especially when applied over the neuroretina or into the subretinal space at either moderate and high doses (2.5 mg/ml and 25 mg/ml). An impairment of retinal function was described even at low doses of indocyanine green (0.025 mg/ml). Retinal damage may also be caused by 5% iodine contained in the indocyanine green molecules, by the self-sensitized decomposition product or by a potentiated photodynamic effect due to the light exposure.[80]

Infracyanine Green Staining

Infracyanine green is a green dye with the same chemical formula and similar pharmacologic properties as indocyanine green. However, infracyanine green dye has two pharmacologic differences when compared to indocyanine green. First, infracyanine green contains no sodium iodine in its formulation either as free ion or as a part of dye molecule. For this reason, infracyanine green is believed to have less potential for RPE toxicity, in contrast with indocyanine green solution. Second, the iodine-free infracyanine green, diluted in 5% glucose, generates an iso-osmotic solution of 294–314 mmol/kg. This is advantageous when using infracyanine green dye for ILM peeling, because the iso-osmolar solution helps to decrease the risks of adverse effects.[81,82]

Trypan Blue Staining

Trypan blue is a vital dye used in ophthalmology to stain corneal endothelial cells and the lens capsule. In vitreoretinal surgery, trypan blue has been used to stain the ERM. It is a dye that binds to intraocular tissues with high rates of cellular proliferation.[83] For this reason, it has high affinity for epiretinal glial tissues such as ERM. Trypan blue staining of the ERM may minimize mechanical trauma to the retina during removal and can allow a good recognition of the entire extension of the ERM. A dose of 0.1 ml of trypan blue may be injected into the vitreous cavity after fluid-air exchange or it may be mixed with glucose 10%, obtaining a solution of 1 mg/ml and 300 mOsm.[84] The result is a dense solution that may be used without fluid-air exchange. No RPE defects or signs of retinal toxicity have been reported in most reports, even if larger studies are needed to determine its safety.[85-87]

Patent Blue Staining

Patent blue is a suitable vital dye for staining the glial ERM. However, several preliminary clinical studies have demonstrated poor affinity for the ILM, similarly to trypan blue. There is conflicting data regarding the retinal toxicity of patent blue.[88] Further studies are needed in order to determine its safety and efficacy.

Brilliant Blue G Staining

Brilliant blue G is a blue dye that selectively stains ILM in an iso-osmolar solution of 0.25 mg/ml (0.025%) with good clinical results and no signs of toxicity. Brilliant blue G can become a good alternative to indocyanine green and infracyanine green in chromovitrectomy, thanks to its remarkable affinity for the ILM. However, limited toxicity data are available.[89] Further clinical and experimental studies are needed to evaluate the safety and efficacy of this dye in the staining of the ILM.

Triamcinolone Acetonide

Triamcinolone acetonide is a relatively water insoluble steroid that can be used in vitreoretinal surgery to improve the identification of ILM. Triamcinolone acetonide facilitates the visualization of the ILM by being deposited as white flecks on the remnants of the vitreous still adherent to the ILM or over the ILM itself.[90] The intravitreal dose of triamcinolone acetonide commonly used to stain ILM is 4 mg. Several reports have concluded that triamcinolone acetonide-guided ILM peeling is a safe and effective procedure. In fact, possible adverse effects of intravitreal injection of triamcinolone acetonide, which are reported using triamcinolone acetonide for different purposes (rise of intraocular pressure, endophthalmitis and cataract progression), have not been described following triamcinolone acetonide-assisted ILM peeling.[91]

Double Staining

The double staining technique is an elegant procedure that may facilitate the identification of the ERM as well as the ILM. In this technique, the initial step consists in the injection of a dye with high affinity for ERM, followed by a second dye to stain and peel ILM. In alternative, two different vital dyes may be injected simultaneously before initiating peeling procedures.[92]

In conclusion there is a wide consensus that the application of vital dyes facilitates the fine removal of intraocular membranes during vitreoretinal surgery. It is important to decrease the potential of dyes toxicity, therefore, the use of an iso-osmolar solution, with low dye concentrations (0.25–0.5 mg/ml, 0.025–0.05%) is advocated. In addition, in case of dye application, the light pipe should be kept far away from the retina and turned off when possible to minimize dye decomposition and thermal or photodynamic damage.

Management of Coexisting Cataract

Progressive nuclear sclerosis of the lens is a very common complication after vitreoretinal surgery and pre-existing lens opacities can make retinal repair difficult to achieve.[93] ERM surgery requires excellent visualization and should not be attempted if significant nuclear sclerosis or posterior subcapsular cataract are present. Combining phacoemulsification and vitrectomy improves the operative view in patients with significant lens opacity, reduces the need for a second procedure and enhance postoperative visual rehabilitation, increasing patient satisfaction.[94] Moreover, lens removal allows a more complete vitrectomy and removal of the anterior vitreous without risking lens injury. In addition, phacoemulsification in postvitrectomized eyes may present a higher risk of complication due to the possible instability of the Zinn's zonules, possible damage to the posterior capsule during the previous vitrectomy and increased frequency of posterior capsular rupture. Delayed phacoemulsification may also be difficult due to small pupil size, posterior synechiae or abnormal fluctuations in anterior chamber depth, caused by zonular laxity and reduction of vitreous volume.

Outcome

The majority of eyes experience visual acuity improvement, 60–87% of eyes gain 2 or more Snellen lines (Figs 24.7A to F). Mean time to achieve best final vision is about 1 year.[95] Sometimes, however, metamorphopsia may persist despite improvement in visual acuity, especially in cases with an

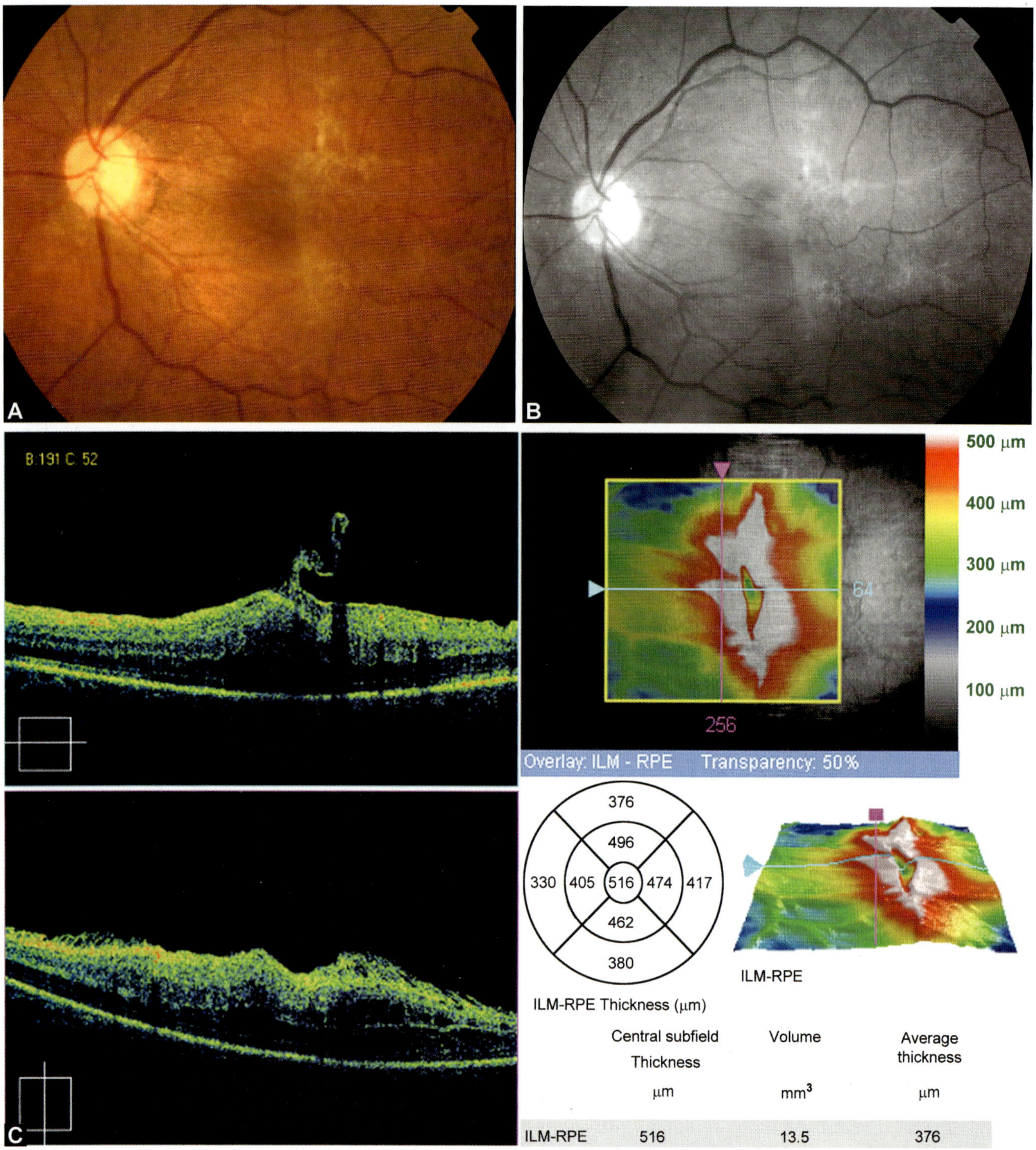
A
B
B:191 C 52
500 µm
400 µm
300 µm
200 µm
100 µm
64
256
Overlay: ILM - RPE Transparency: 50%
376
496
330 405 516 474 417
462
380
ILM-RPE Thickness (µm)
ILM-RPE
Central subfield Thickness µm
Volume mm³
Average thickness µm
ILM-RPE 516 13.5 376
C

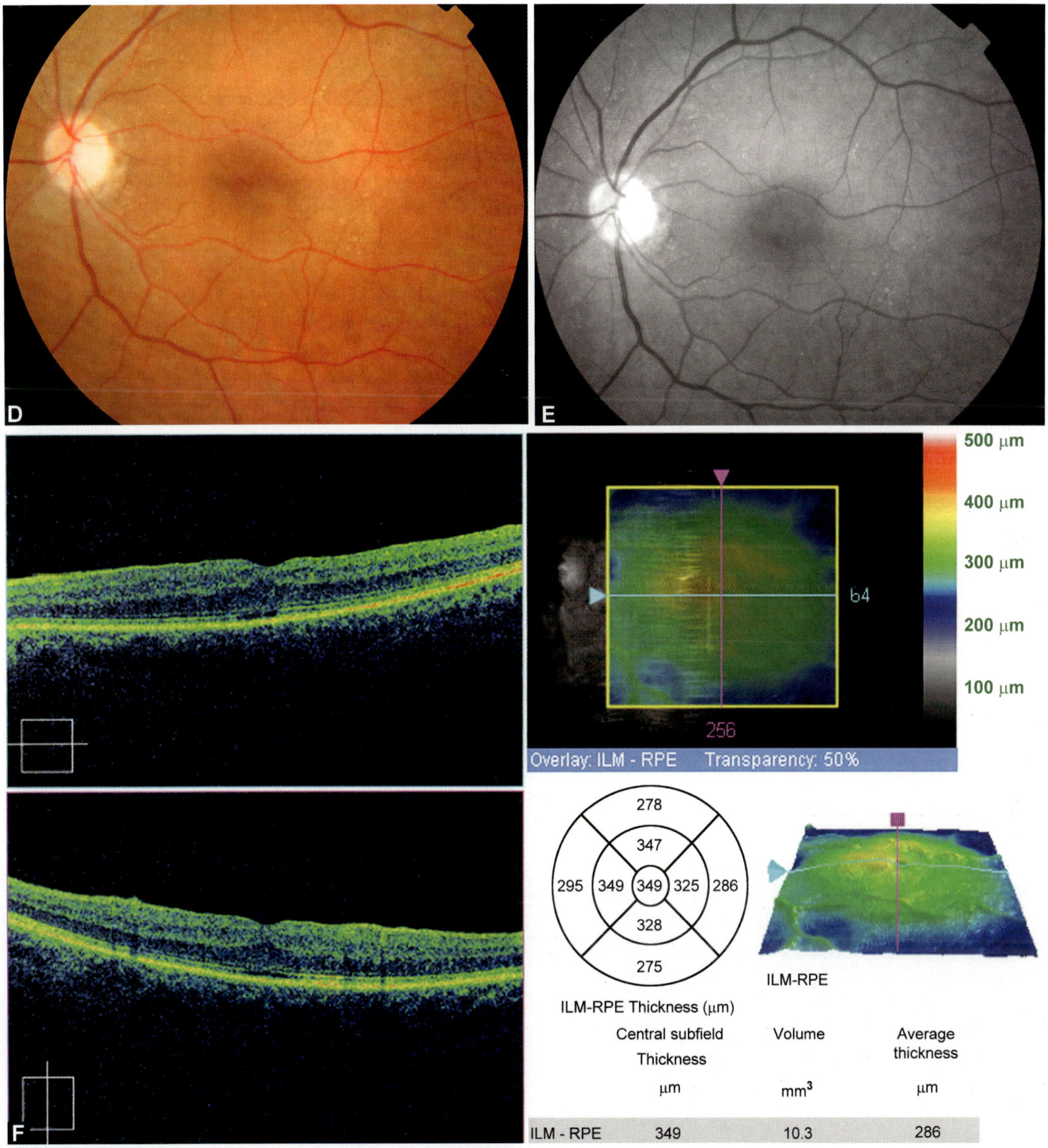

▲ Figures 24.7A to F

(A) Color photograph; (B) Red-free image (C) Optical coherence tomography appearance of epiretinal membrane puckering macula and reducing vision to 20/400. Six months after surgical removal of the membrane visual acuity improved to 20/50; (D) Color photograph; (E) Red-free image; (F) Optical coherence tomography reveal released traction and diminished vascular tortuosity incomplete peeling of the membrane. Although ERM stripping usually results in significant visual improvement, few eyes gain a 20/20 vision. Prognostic factors associated with visual outcome include preoperative visual acuity, duration of symptoms prior to surgery, preoperative lens status, intraoperative complications, etiology and patient's age.[96] Unsurprisingly, eyes with poorer preoperative visual acuity usually have inferior final vision compared with those with better preoperative visual function. Eyes with a long history of symptoms usually have less improvement in vision. This may be due to the longer tractional damage to the retina. Patients with good vision of the unaffected eye have a better functional outcome and higher subjective satisfaction. The etiology of the ERM influences the surgical outcome.[97] Patients with secondary ERMs report a worse improvement of visual acuity than those with idiopathic membrane. Young patients and those with secondary ERM usually experience higher recurrence rate, thus final outcome may be less satisfactory.

Complications

ERM peeling is generally a safe operation. Intraoperative complications include vitreoretinal hemorrhages, retinal bleeding and iatrogenic retinal breaks. The incidence of intraoperative posterior pole breaks ranges from 0–15%, while that of peripheral breaks ranges from 5–6%.[98] Posterior pole tears usually result from poor visualization during surgery and they are treated with fluid-air exchange and postoperative prone positioning. Peripheral breaks may be created by inserting instruments through vitreous base or by stripping posterior hyaloid out toward the vitreous base insertion in cases with incomplete vitreous detachment. Peripheral tears are treated with cryotherapy or endolaser photocoagulation followed by air or gas exchange. In case of idiopathic ERM where complete posterior vitreous detachment is present, the incidence of peripheral retinal breaks is reduced. Postoperative complications include endophthalmitis, rhegmatogenous retinal detachment, recurrence of epiretinal proliferation, proliferative vitreoretinopathy, retinal whitening, intraocular pressure abnormalities and cataract progression.[98] Several studies have shown an increased risk of endophthalmitis using the 25-gauge system. The literature reports an average incidence of 0.7% compared to a rate of 0.018% after 20-gauge surgery. This issue may be related to the trocar inserting procedure previously described in this chapter.[99] Retinal detachment is perhaps the most common serious complication of vitrectomy surgery. This complication is related to inadvertent force application on the vitreous base during vitreous removal and instrument introduction or it may be related to the incarceration of vitreous in the sclerotomy's site. Several studies have reported postoperative intraocular pressure abnormalities after 25-gauge vitrectomy. It appears that 25-gauge technology is associated with a higher rate of hypotony (2.3–27.6%) than 20-gauge surgery.[56,100] Low postoperative intraocular pressures are associated with an increased risk of serous and hemorrhagic choroidal detachment. Cataract progression is a common event after vitrectomy. Reported rate of cataract development ranges from 12.5–80% after 20-gauge surgery and from 2–79% after 25-gauge vitrectomy.[101,102] Recently nonvitrectomizing vitreous surgery has been proposed to prevent cataract progression in case of epiretinal membrane removal.[103,104] Typically, a 27-gauge chandelier illuminator is inserted superonasally and a 25-gauge trans-scleral microcannula is set at the superotemporal quadrant for the insertion of membrane-peeling forceps. With these instruments, the epiretinal membrane can be directly grasped by the membrane forceps without performing a vitrectomy. After peeling the membrane from the retinal surface, the membrane remnant, along with attaching vitreous, is removed through the trans-scleral cannula and excised at the sclerotomy site.

Epiretinal membrane is a macular condition that affects a large proportion of subjects and may cause significant visual dysfunction. The surgical removal of the membrane is the gold standard therapy and it has been validated by several clinical trials. The ongoing technological innovation in surgical instrumentation and the use of intraoperative tools to help identification of ocular tissues have permitted less invasive procedures with minimal patient discomfort and faster visual recovery. Considering the complexity of ERM pathogenesis it is also possible that in near future pharmacologic therapies targeted to ERM-inducing cytokines and the surgical approach may be combined to obtain an optimal retinal anatomy restoration.

References

1. Pearlstone AD. The incidence of idiopathic preretinal macular gliosis. Ann Ophthalmol. 1985;17:378-80.
2. Klein R, Klein BE, Wang Q, et al. The epidemiology of epiretinal membranes. Trans Am Ophthalmol Soc. 1994;92: 403-25.

3. Kawasaki R, Wang JJ, Mitchell P, et al. Racial difference in the prevalence of epiretinal membrane between Caucasians and Asians. Br J Ophthalmol. 2008;92:1320-4.
4. Mitchell P, Smith W, Chey T, et al. Prevalence and associations of epiretinal membranes. The Blue Mountains Eye Study, Australia. Ophthalmology. 1997;104:1033-40.
5. Roth AM, Foos RY. Surface wrinkling retinopathy in eyes enucleated at autopsy. Trans Am Acad Ophthalmol Otolaryngol. 1971;75:1047-58.
6. Miyazaki M, Nakamura H, Kubo M, et al. Prevalence and risk factors for epiretinal membranes in a Japanese population: the Hisayama study. Graefes Arch Clin Exp Ophthalmol. 2003;241:642-6.
7. Fraser-Bell S, Guzowski M, Rochtchina E, et al. Five-year cumulative incidence and progression of epiretinal membranes: the Blue Mountains Eye Study. Ophthalmology. 2003;110:34-40.
8. Fraser-Bell S, Ying-Lai M, Klein R, et al. Prevalence and associations of epiretinal membranes in latinos: the Los Angeles Latino Eye Study. Invest Ophthalmol Vis Sci. 2004;45:1732-6.
9. Livingston PM, Carson CA, Stanislavsky YL, et al. Methods for a population-based study of eye disease: the Melbourne Visual Impairment Project. Ophthalmic Epidemiol. 1994;1:139-48.
10. McCarty DJ, Mukesh BN, Chikani V, et al. Prevalence and associations of epiretinal membranes in the visual impairment project. Am J Ophthalmol. 2005;140:288-94.
11. Duan XR, Liang YB, Friedman DS, et al. Prevalence and associations of epiretinal membranes in a rural Chinese adult population: the Handan Eye Study. Invest Ophthalmol Vis Sci. 2009;50:2018-23.
12. Contreras I, Noval S, Tejedor J. Use of optical coherence tomography to measure prevalence of epiretinal membranes in patients referred for cataract surgery. Arch Soc Esp Oftalmol. 2008;83:89-94.
13. Appiah AP, Hirose T. Secondary causes of premacular fibrosis. Ophthalmology. 1989;96:389-92.
14. Laatikainen L, Immonen I, Summanen P. Peripheral retinal angiomalike lesion and macular pucker. Am J Ophthalmol. 1989;108:563-6.
15. McDonald HR, Schatz H, Johnson RN, et al. Vitrectomy in eyes with peripheral retinal angioma associated with traction macular detachment. Ophthalmology. 1996;103:329-35.
16. Carney MD, Jampol LM. Epiretinal membranes in sickle cell retinopathy. Arch Ophthalmol. 1987;105:214-7.
17. Nicoletti VG, Nicoletti R, Ferrara N, et al. Diabetic patients and retinal proliferation: an evaluation of the role of vascular endothelial growth factor (VEGF). Exp Clin Endocrinol Diabetes. 2003;111:209-14.
18. Hagler WS, Aturaliya U. Macular puckers after retinal detachment surgery. Br J Ophthalmol. 1971;55:451-7.
19. Lobes LA, Burton TC. The incidence of macular pucker after retinal detachment surgery. Am J Ophthalmol. 1978;85:72-7.
20. Wiznia RA. Posterior vitreous detachment and idiopathic preretinal macular gliosis. Am J Ophthalmol. 1986;102:196-8.
21. Noble KG, Carr RE. Idiopathic preretinal gliosis. Ophthalmology. 1982;89:521-3.
22. Hirokawa H, Jalkh AE, Takahashi M, et al. Role of the vitreous in idiopathic preretinal macular fibrosis. Am J Ophthalmol. 1986;101:166-9.
23. McDonald HR, Aaberg TM. Idiopathic epiretinal membranes. Semin Ophthalmol. 1986;1:189-95.
24. Sidd RJ, Fine SL, Owens SL, et al. Idiopathic preretinal gliosis. Am J Ophthalmol. 1982;94:44-8.
25. Foos RY. Vitreoretinal juncture; epiretinal membranes and vitreous. Invest Ophthalmol Vis Sci. 1977;16:416-22.
26. Machemer R, van Horn D, Aaberg TM. Pigment epithelial proliferation in human retinal detachment with massive periretinal proliferation. Am J Ophthalmol. 1978;85:181-91.
27. Heilskov TW, Massicotte SJ, Folk JC. Epiretinal macular membranes in eyes with attached posterior cortical vitreous. Retina. 1996;16:279-84.
28. Cherfan GM, Smiddy WE, Michels RG, et al. Clinicopathologic correlation of pigmented epiretinal membranes. Am J Ophthalmol. 1988;106:536-45.
29. Kampik A, Green WR, Michels RG, et al. Ultrastructural features of progressive idiopathic epiretinal membrane removed by vitreous surgery. Am J Ophthalmol. 1980;90:797-809.
30. Bringmann A, Wiedemann P. Involvement of Muller glial cells in epiretinal membrane formation. Graefes Arch Clin Exp Ophthalmol. 2009;247:865-83.
31. Kenyon KR, Michels RG. Ultrastructure of epiretinal membrane removed by pars plana vitreoretinal surgery. Am J Ophthalmol. 1977;83:815-23.
32. Campochiaro PA, Hackett SF, Vinores SA. Growth factors in the retina and retinal pigmented epithelium. Progr Retin Eye Res. 1996;15:547-67.
33. Cui J, Lei H, Samad A, et al. PDGF receptors are activated in human epiretinal membranes. Exp Eye Res. 2009;88:438-44.
34. Lei H, Hovland P, Velez G, et al. A potential role for PDGF-C in experimental and clinical proliferative vitreoretinopathy. Invest Ophthalmol Vis Sci. 2007;48:2335-42.
35. Lashkari K, Rahimi N, Kazlauskas A. Hepatocyte growth factor receptor in human RPE cells: implications in proliferative vitreoretinopathy. Invest Ophthalmol Vis Sci. 1999;40:149-56.
36. Minchiotti S, Stampachiacchiere B, Micera A, et al. Human idiopathic epiretinal membranes express NGF and NGF receptors. Retina. 2008;28:628-37.
37. Hinton DR, He S, Jin ML, et al. Novel growth factors involved in the pathogenesis of proliferative vitreoretinopathy. Eye. 2002;16:422-8.
38. Harada C, Mitamura Y, Harada T. The role of cytokines and trophic factors in epiretinal membranes: involvement of signal

transduction in glial cells. Prog Retin Eye Res. 2006;25:149-64.
39. Gass JDM. Macular dysfunction caused by epiretinal membrane contraction. Stereoscopic Atlas of Macular Diseases: Diagnosis and Treatment. St. Louis: Mo: Mosby; 1997. pp. 938-50.
40. Joondeph HC. The incidence of epiretinal membrane with retinal breaks and detachments. In: Fine SL, Owens SL (Eds). Management of Retinal Vascular and Macular Disorders. Baltimore, MD: Williams and Wilkins; 1983. pp. 100-1.
41. Wise GN. Preretinal macular fibrosis. (An analysis of 90 cases). Trans Ophthalmol Soc UK. 1972;92:131-40.
42. Watanabe A, Arimoto S, Nishi O. Correlation between metamorphopsia and epiretinal membrane optical coherence tomography findings. Ophthalmology. 2009;116:1788-93.
43. Gass JDM. Differential diagnosis of intraocular tumors: a stereoscopic presentation. St Louis: MO: Mosby; 1974. p. 241.
44. Machemer R. A new concept for vitreous surgery: 7. Two instrument techniques in pars plana vitrectomy. Arch Ophthalmol. 1974;92:407-12.
45. de Bustros S, Thompson JT, Michels RG, et al. Vitrectomy for idiopathic epiretinal membranes causing macular pucker. Br J Ophthalmol. 1988;72:692-5.
46. Shea M. The surgical management of macular pucker in rhegmatogenous retinal detachment. Ophthalmology. 1980;87:70-4.
47. Okamoto F, Okamoto Y, Fukuda S, et al. Vision-related quality of life and visual function after vitrectomy for various vitreoretinal disorders. Invest Ophthalmol Vis Sci. 2010;51: 744-51.
48. Kwon SI, Ko SJ, Park IW. The clinical course of the idiopathic epiretinal membrane after surgery. Korean J Ophthalmol. 2009;23:249-52.
49. Margherio RR, Cox MS, Trese MT, et al. Removal of epimacular membranes. Ophthalmology. 1985;92:1075-83.
50. McDonald HR, Verre WP, Aaberg TM. Surgical management of idiopathic epiretinal membranes. Ophthalmology. 1986;93:978-83.
51. Poliner LS, Olk RJ, Grand MG, et al. Surgical management of premacular fibroplasia. Arch Ophthalmol. 1988;106:761-4.
52. Michels RG. Vitreous surgery for macular pucker. Am J Ophthalmol. 1981;92:628-39.
53. O'Malley C, Heintz RM. Vitrectomy via the pars plana—a new instrument system. Trans Pac Coast Otoophthalmol Soc Annu Meet. 1972;53:121-37.
54. Rizzo S, Genovesi-Ebert F, Murri S, et al. 25-gauge, sutureless vitrectomy and standard 20-gauge pars plana vitrectomy in idiopathic epiretinal membrane surgery: a comparative pilot study. Graefes Arch Clin Exp Ophthalmol. 2006;244:472-9.
55. Fujii GY, De Juan E, Humayun MS, et al. Initial experience using the transconjunctival sutureless vitrectomy system for vitreoretinal surgery. Ophthalmology. 2002;109:1814-20.
56. Fujii GY, De Juan E, Humayun MS, et al. A new 25-gauge instrument system for transconjunctival sutureless vitrectomy surgery. Ophthalmology. 2002;109:1807-12.
57. Ibarra MS, Hermel M, Prenner JL, et al. Longer-term outcomes of transconjunctival sutureless 25-gauge vitrectomy. Am J Ophthalmol. 2005;139:831-6.
58. Kadonosono K, Yamakawa T, Uchio E, et al. Comparison of visual function after epiretinal membrane removal by 20-gauge and 25-gauge vitrectomy. Am J Ophthalmol. 2006;142:513-5.
59. Lakhanpal RR, Humayun MS, de Juan E, et al. Outcomes of 140 consecutive cases of 25-gauge transconjunctival surgery for posterior segment disease. Ophthalmology. 2005;112:817-24.
60. Charles S. Tips and tricks for 25-gauge sutureless vitrectomy. Rev Ophthalmol. 2005;12:82-4.
61. Lam DS, Yuen CY, Tam BS, et al. Sutureless vitrectomy surgery. Ophthalmology. 2003;110:2428-9.
62. Garretson BR, de Bustros S, Packo KH. Suction elevation of epiretinal membranes. Arch Ophthalmol. 1992;110:449.
63. Kuhn F, Mester V, Berta A. The Tano Diamond Dusted Membrane Scraper: indications and contraindications. Acta Ophthalmol Scand. 1998;76:754-5.
64. Lewis JM, Park I, Ohji M, et al. Diamond-dusted silicone cannula for epiretinal membrane separation during vitreous surgery. Am J Ophthalmol. 1997;124:552-4.
65. Johnston RL. Modification of the Tano Diamond Dusted Scraper. Retina. 2000;20:427.
66. Bovey EH, Uffer S, Achache F. Surgery for epimacular membrane: impact of retinal internal limiting membrane removal on functional outcome. Retina. 2004;24:728-35.
67. Hasegawa T, Emi K, Ikeda T, et al. Long-term prognosis of internal limiting membrane peeling for idiopathic epiretinal membrane. Nippon Ganka Gakkai Zasshi. 2004;108:150-6.
68. Abdelkader E, Lois N. Internal limiting membrane peeling in vitreo-retinal surgery. Surv Ophthalmol. 2008;53:368-96.
69. Park DW, Dugel PU, Garda J, et al. Macular pucker removal with and without internal limiting membrane peeling: pilot study. Ophthalmology. 2003;110:62-4.
70. Kwok A, Lai TY, Yuen KS. Epiretinal membrane surgery with or without internal limiting membrane peeling. Clin Experiment Ophthalmol. 2005;33:379-85.
71. Rodrigues EB, Maia M, Meyer CH, et al. Vital dyes for chromovitrectomy. Curr Opin Ophthalmol. 2007;18:179-87.
72. Farah ME, Maia M, Rodrigues EB. Dyes in ocular surgery: principles for use in chromovitrectomy. Am J Ophthalmol. 2009;148:332-40.
73. Hiebl W, Gunther B, Meinert H. Substances for staining biological tissues: use of dyes in ophthalmology. Klin Monbl Augenheilkd. 2005;222:309-11.
74. Kwok AK, Lai TY, Li WW, et al. Indocyanine green-assisted internal limiting membrane removal in epiretinal membrane surgery: a clinical and histologic study. Am J Ophthalmol. 2004;138:194-9.

75. Haritoglou C, Gandorfer A, Gass CA, et al. The effect of indocyanine-green on functional outcome of macular pucker surgery. Am J Ophthalmol. 2003;135:328-37.
76. Sakamoto H, Yamanaka I, Kubota T, et al. Indocyanine green-assisted peeling of the epiretinal membrane in proliferative vitreoretinopathy. Graefes Arch Clin Exp Ophthalmol. 2003;241:204-7.
77. Sorcinelli R. Surgical management of epiretinal membrane with indocyanine-green-assisted peeling. Ophthalmologica. 2003;217:107-10.
78. Maia M, Haller JA, Pieramici DJ, et al. Retinal pigment epithelial abnormalities after internal limiting membrane peeling guided by indocyanine green staining. Retina. 2004;24:157-60.
79. Engel E, Schraml R, Maisch T, et al. Light-induced decomposition of indocyanine green. Invest Ophthalmol Vis Sci. 2008;49:1777-83.
80. Stalmans P, Van Aken EH, Veckeneer M, et al. Toxic effect of indocyanine green on retinal pigment epithelium related to osmotic effects of the solvent. Am J Ophthalmol. 2002;134:282-5.
81. Ullern M, Roman S, Dhalluin JF, et al. Contribution of intravitreal infracyanine green to macular hole and epimacular membrane surgery: preliminary study. J Fr Ophtalmol. 2002;25:915-20.
82. Lanzetta P, Polito A, Del Borrello M, et al. Idiopathic macular hole surgery with low-concentration infracyanine green-assisted peeling of the internal limiting membrane. Am J Ophthalmol. 2006;142:771-6.
83. Haritoglou C, Eibl K, Schaumberger M, et al. Functional outcome after trypan blue-assisted vitrectomy for macular pucker: a prospective, randomized, comparative trial. Am J Ophthalmol. 2004;138:1-5.
84. Haritoglou C, Gandorfer A, Schaumberger M, et al. Trypan blue in macular pucker surgery: an evaluation of histology and functional outcome. Retina. 2004;24:582-90.
85. Feron EJ, Veckeneer M, Parys-Van Ginderdeuren R, et al. Trypan blue staining of epiretinal membranes in proliferative vitreoretinopathy. Arch Ophthalmol. 2002;120:141-4.
86. Perrier M, Sebag M. Epiretinal membrane surgery assisted by trypan blue. Am J Ophthalmol. 2003;135:909-11.
87. Teba FA, Mohr A, Eckardt C, et al. Trypan blue staining in vitreoretinal surgery. Ophthalmology. 2003;110:2409-12.
88. Luke C, Luke M, Sickel W, Schneider T. Effects of patent blue on human retinal function. Graefes Arch Clin Exp Ophthalmol. 2006;244:1188-90.
89. Maia M, Farah ME, Rodrigues EB, et al. Subretinal brilliant blue G migration during internal limiting membrane peeling. Br J Ophthalmol. 2009;93:1687.
90. Maia M, Farah ME, Belfort RN, et al. Effects of intravitreal triamcinolone acetonide injection with and without preservative. Br J Ophthalmol. 2007;91:1122-4.
91. Peyman GA, Cheema R, Conway MD, et al. Triamcinolone acetonide as an aid to visualization of the vitreous and the posterior hyaloid during pars plana vitrectomy. Retina. 2000;20:554-5.
92. Stalmans P, Feron EJ, Parys-Van Ginderdeuren R, et al. Double vital staining using trypan blue and infracyanine green in macular pucker surgery. Br J Ophthalmol. 2003;87:713-6.
93. de Bustros S, Thompson JT, Michels RG, et al. Nuclear sclerosis after vitrectomy for idiopathic epiretinal membranes. Am J Ophthalmol. 1988;105:160-4.
94. Cherfan GM, Michels RG, de Bustros S, et al. Nuclear sclerotic cataract after vitrectomy for idiopathic epiretinal membranes causing macular pucker. Am J Ophthalmol. 1991;111:434-8.
95. Scott IU, Smiddy WE, Feuer W, et al. Vitreoretinal surgery outcomes: results of a patient satisfaction/functional status survey. Ophthalmology. 1998;105:795-803.
96. Rice TA, De Bustros S, Michels RG, et al. Prognostic factors in vitrectomy for epiretinal membranes of the macula. Ophthalmology. 1986;93:602-10.
97. Patelli F, Radice P, Zumbo G, et al. 25-gauge macular surgery: results and complications. Retina. 2007;27:750-4.
98. Amato JE, Akduman L. Incidence of complications in 25-gauge transconjunctival sutureless vitrectomy based on the surgical indications. Ophthalmic Surg Lasers Imaging. 2007;38:100-2.
99. Kunimoto DY, Kaiser RS. Incidence of endophthalmitis after 20- and 25-gauge vitrectomy. Ophthalmology. 2007;114:2133-7.
100. Hsu J, Chen E, Gupta O, et al. Hypotony after 25-gauge vitrectomy using oblique versus direct cannula insertions in fluid-filled eyes. Retina. 2008;28:937-40.
101. Holekamp NM, Shui YB, Beebe DC. Vitrectomy surgery increases oxygen exposure to the lens: a possible mechanism for nuclear cataract formation. Am J Ophthalmol. 2005;139:302-10.
102. Saito Y, Lewis JM, Park I, et al. Nonvitrectomizing vitreous surgery: a strategy to prevent postoperative nuclear sclerosis. Ophthalmology. 1999;106:1541-5.
103. Sawa M, Saito Y, Hayashi A, et al. Assessment of nuclear sclerosis after nonvitrectomizing vitreous surgery. Am J Ophthalmol. 2001;132:356-62.
104. Sawa M, Ohji M, Kusaka S, et al. Nonvitrectomizing vitreous surgery for epiretinal membrane long-term follow-up. Ophthalmology. 2005;112:1402-8.

25

Vitrectomy for Macular Hole

Alain Gaudric, Ramin Tadayoni

Introduction

Today, surgery for macular hole (MH) is usually very successful. Routinely, it results in hole closure in more than 85% of cases and in significant visual improvement at least once the subsequent cataract has been operated on. In the first report on MH surgery by Kelly and Wendel[1] published in 1991, the rate of hole closure was only 58%. Exactly how it improved so greatly is unclear. The surgical technique is still based on extensive vitrectomy with posterior vitreous detachment (PVD), peeling of any epimacular membrane (EMM), thorough fluid-gas exchange, and postoperative face-down positioning of the patient.

Optical Coherence Tomography of Macular Hole

The diagnosis and understanding of the formation of MHs has greatly benefited from examination by optical coherence tomography (OCT), which indeed allows easy differentiation between a full-thickness MH and a pseudohole or lamellar hole.[2,3] OCT also makes it easy to measure the diameter of the hole, which is an important prognostic factor of surgical closure. Lastly, the increasing use of OCT allows the recording of data concerning the early stages of MH formation, which were not hitherto detectable on biomicroscopy.

Impending Macular Hole

In most cases, MHs in the early stages are foveal cysts.[4,5] The earliest detectable changes in eyes, which are at risk of evolving into MHs, are the elevation of the foveal floor and the formation of intrafoveal cystic spaces, combined with incomplete separation of the posterior hyaloid (PH) from the foveola.

However, before any change occurs in the foveal structure, it is possible to detect, at least among fellow eyes, those, which are at risk of developing a MH. It has indeed been shown that idiopathic MHs occur during the process of PH detachment from the macular surface. Therefore, fellow eyes whose PH is already detached from this surface do not risk developing a MH, even if the hyaloid remains attached to the optic disc (OD) and the periphery of the posterior pole.[6] OCT makes it possible to diagnose such premacular PVD, which cannot be done by biomicroscopy alone (Figs 25.1A to C).

When, on the other hand, part of the PH remains attached to the foveal center, the risk of MH cannot be ruled out, at least for patients presenting with a hole in the fellow eye. This partial detachment of the PH from the posterior pole but not from the foveal center is quite common after the age of 50 years, and is the first sign of PVD.[7] However, in some cases, spectral domain (SD) OCT has been able to show very subtle changes in the shape of the foveal pit at the junction between the PH and the internal limiting membrane (ILM), due to vitreous traction. Except in individuals whose fellow

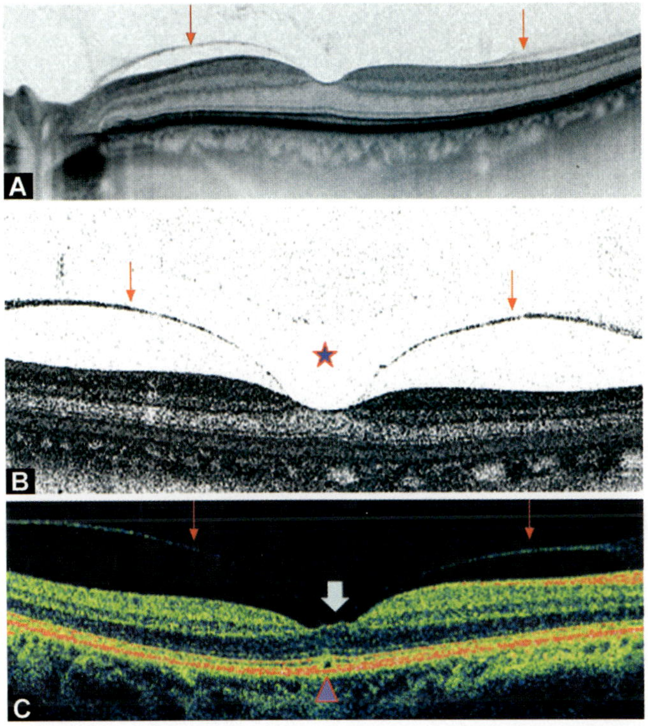

▲ **Figures 25.1A to C**

Partial PVD in the fellow eyes of eyes with MHs, on OCT scans. (A) Early stage of partial PVD. The PH (arrows) is more detached on the nasal side of the fovea than on the temporal side; (B) Partial PVD with visibility of the bursa premacularis (star). The PH (arrows) is equally detached temporally and nasally; (C) Partial PVD (red arrows) exerting traction on the foveal center. Note the slight deformation of the foveal floor (large arrow), and minor disruption of the inner segment/outer segment photoreceptor line (arrowhead)

eyes already exhibit a MH, it is difficult to predict whether these small tractions on the foveal floor constitute a significant risk of MH.

Stage 1A: Impending Macular Hole

The macula may look normal on fundus biomicroscopy, or else an outer central yellow spot may be present combined with a flattened foveal pit and foveolar radial striae.[8] In both cases, OCT image is the same. A central hyporeflective cyst develops in the inner portion of the foveal center, resulting in the elevation of the foveal floor. The outer retinal layer remains intact.[4,5,9,10] The foveal cyst often extends laterally, cleaving the inner retinal layer from the outer layer at the edge of the fovea (Figs 25.2A to C and 25.3A to E).

At this stage, the PH is variously detached from the macular surface, exhibiting a biconvex appearance on scan profiles. It adheres to the top of the foveal cyst.

In about half of the cases, the PH detaches itself from the retinal surface of the fovea and the foveal cyst collapses with the improvement of vision. Normalization of the macular profile may take some weeks, and during this period, intrafoveal cleavage may coexist with a detached PH.

Stage 1B: Impending Macular Hole or Outer Macular Hole

On fundus biomicroscopy, the foveola has a cystic appearance with radial striae. An outer yellow ring is present.[8] OCT shows a central hyporeflective cyst in the foveal center, which opens the outer retinal layer. This foveal cyst also extends laterally, causing a split between the inner and outer retina.[5,11] By then, vision has often already deteriorated, due to the disruption of the photoreceptor layer, and Stage 1B should therefore be considered as occult MH[10] (Figs 25.4A to C).

The PH is still attached to the roof of the foveal cyst. Some Stage 1B holes may close spontaneously, but usually the roof of the cyst tends to open due to the traction exerted by the PH and the impending hole is transformed into a full-thickness hole (Figs 25.5A to D).

▶ Full-Thickness Macular Hole

Stage 2 Macular Hole

Stage 2 is the early stage of the full-thickness MH. It is characterized by the presence of an incompletely detached operculum and persistent adherence of the PH to this operculum.[8] The macular profile depends on the direction of the scan. The typical image of the partially detached operculum attached to the PH is only seen on scans which cross both the operculum and its attachment to the edge of the hole[4,11,12] (Figs 25.6A to D). The diameter of the Stage 2 hole is usually small, less than 400 μm at its smallest. Stage 2 hole sometimes expand, while retaining an incompletely detached operculum. Although generally small, the Stage 2 hole cannot be exclusively associated with a diameter smaller than 400 μm (Figs 25.7A and B).

Stage 3 Macular Hole

The Stage 3 hole is a full-thickness MH characterized by complete separation of the PH from the macular surface, although the hole remains attached to the OD (the Weiss ring

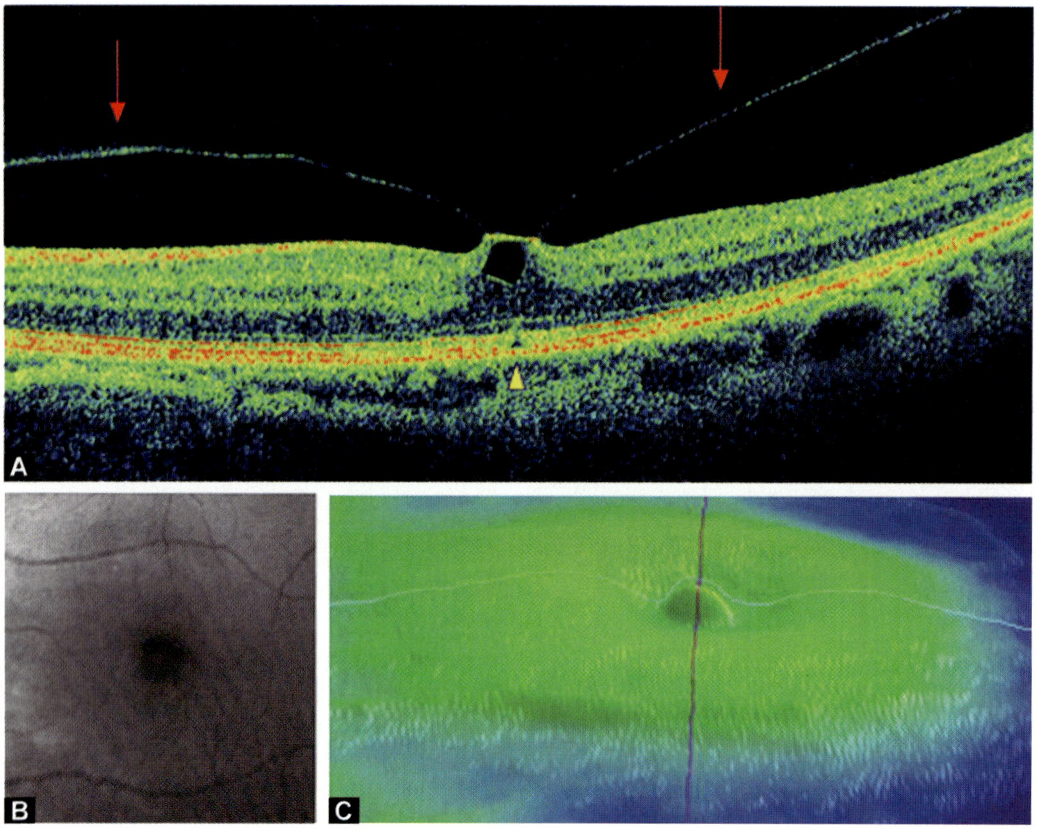

▲ Figures 25.2A to C

Impending MH, Stage 1A: foveal cyst. (A) OCT scan showing an inner foveal cyst due to the traction exerted by the PH (arrows) on the foveal floor, and minor disruption of the IS/OS photoreceptor line (arrowhead); (B) Blue filter photograph of the fovea showing discrete loss of xanthophyll pigment in the center of the foveola; (C) View of the foveal surface showing slight elevation of the roof of the foveal cyst in the middle of the foveal pit

is not detached) and to the circumference of the posterior pole (Figs 25.8A to G). Thus, the PH is only slightly detached from the retinal surface and remains visible on the scan profile. Note that SD OCT has a field depth of 2 mm. When the retinal scan is centered in the box, the PH is still visible if it is detached less than 1 mm above the inner boundary of the macula. When the PH is not visible even though it is not detached from the OD, the retinal scan in the box can be lowered, leaving more room above for the PH. Therefore, in Stage 3 holes, the PH no longer exerts traction on the hole edge.

It is important to note that when the PH is not visible on the OCT scan profile, MHs cannot be correctly staged by OCT alone. In such cases it is essential to examine the fundus by biomicroscopy, in order to ascertain whether or not the Weiss ring remains attached.

The edge of the Stage 3 MH is usually thicker than in Stage 2. It is often rounded, exhibits intraretinal cysts, and is slightly elevated. The contour of the hole edge may differ from one case to another, depending on the thickening of the edge and its degree of elevation. The size of the hole is generally larger than in Stage 2. However, some Stage 3 holes have an aperture diameter of less than 400 µm.

Ultra high resolution OCT has shown that the elevated portion of the hole edge contained altered, but detectable photoreceptors.[11] White dots on the bare retinal pigment epithelium (RPE) at the center of the hole may be seen as small hyper-reflective deposits on some scan profiles.

Sometimes, the reflectivity of an epiretinal membrane (ERM) is visible next to the hole edge as an additional layer upon the ILM.

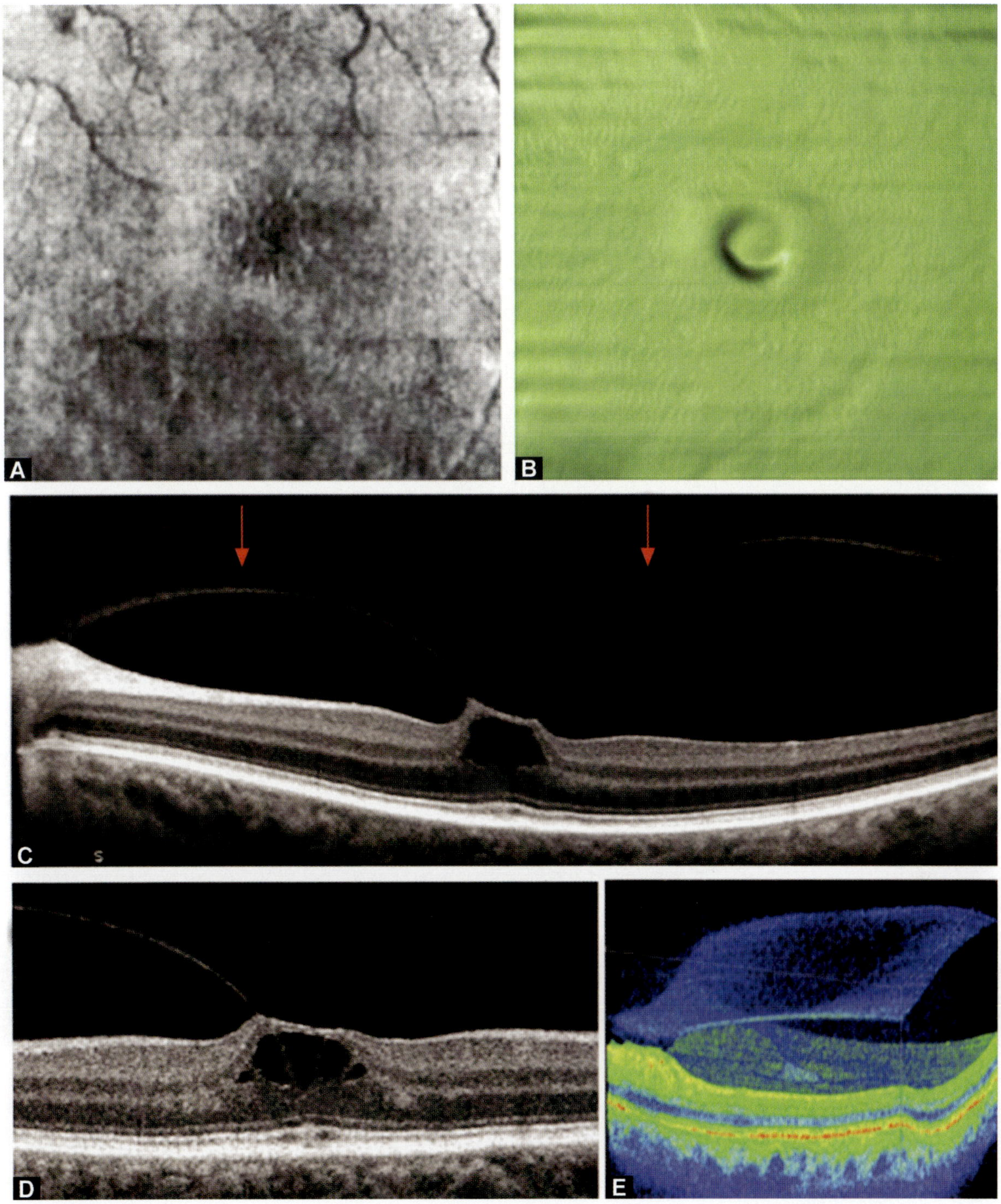

▲ **Figures 25.3A to E**

Impending MH, Stage 1A: foveal cyst. (A) Scanning laser ophthalmoscopy image of the macula showing radial striae around the fovea corresponding to the foveal cystic spaces due to vitreofoveal traction; (B) View of the foveal surface on OCT, showing slight elevation of the roof of the foveal cyst in the middle of the foveal pit; (C) OCT scan (9 mm long) showing an inner foveal cyst due to traction exerted by the PH (arrows) on the foveal floor; (D) OCT scan (3 mm long) giving a detailed view of the radial elongated structures within the foveal cyst. These structures probably correspond to Henle fibers; (E) Three-dimensional appearance of the PH attached to the top of the foveal cyst

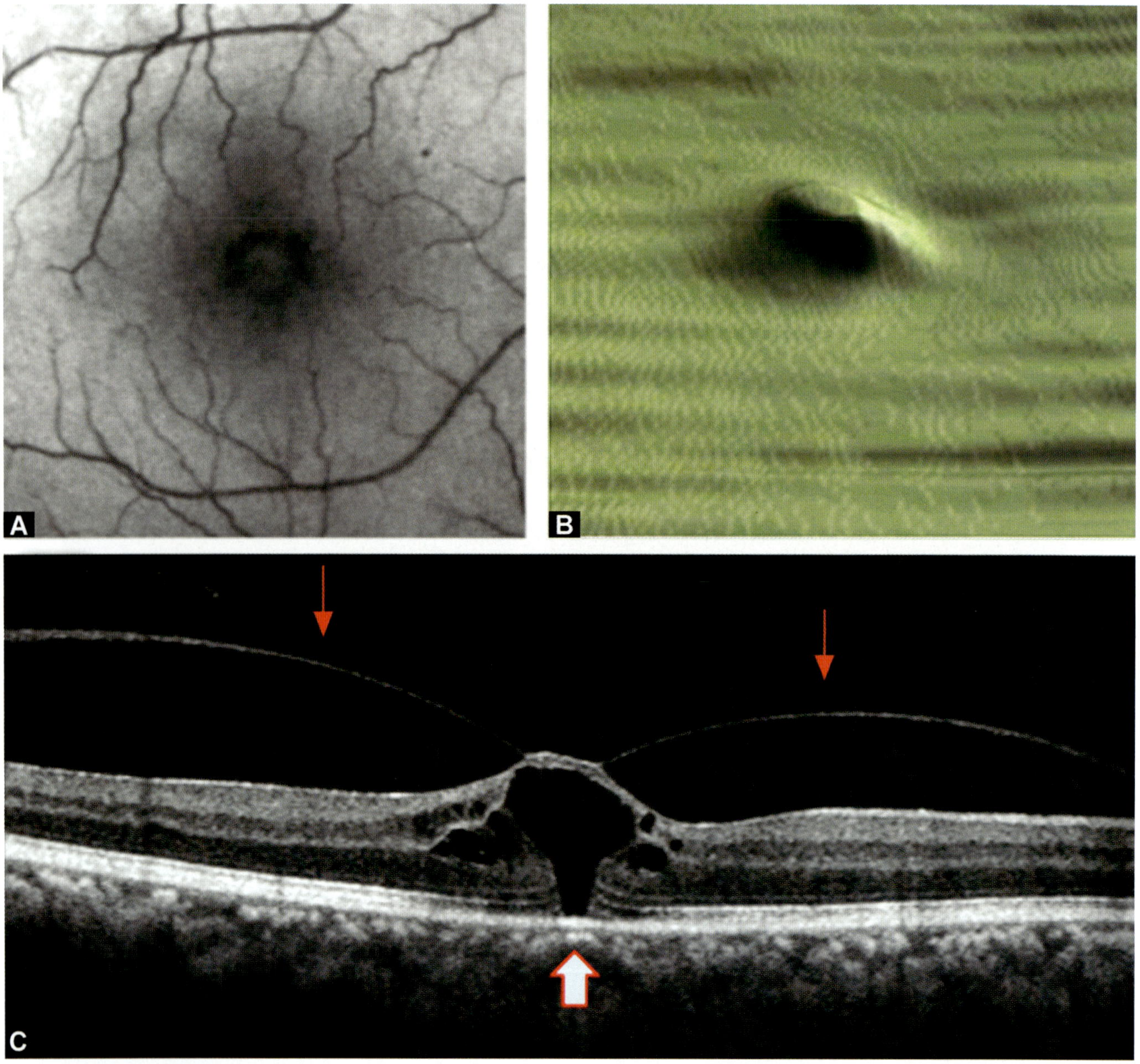

▲ **Figures 25.4A to C**

Impending MH, Stage 1B. (A) Blue filter photograph showing a central lacuna in the macular pigment corresponding to the central foveal cyst; (B) View of the foveal surface on OCT, showing the elevation of the foveal floor, which constitutes the roof of the cyst; (C) High-definition horizontal OCT scan (6 mm), showing the partially detached PH, still attached to the roof of the foveal cyst (small arrows). The inner foveal cyst communicates with a break in the outer retina (large arrow). Stage 1B impending MH can be considered as an occult full-thickness MH

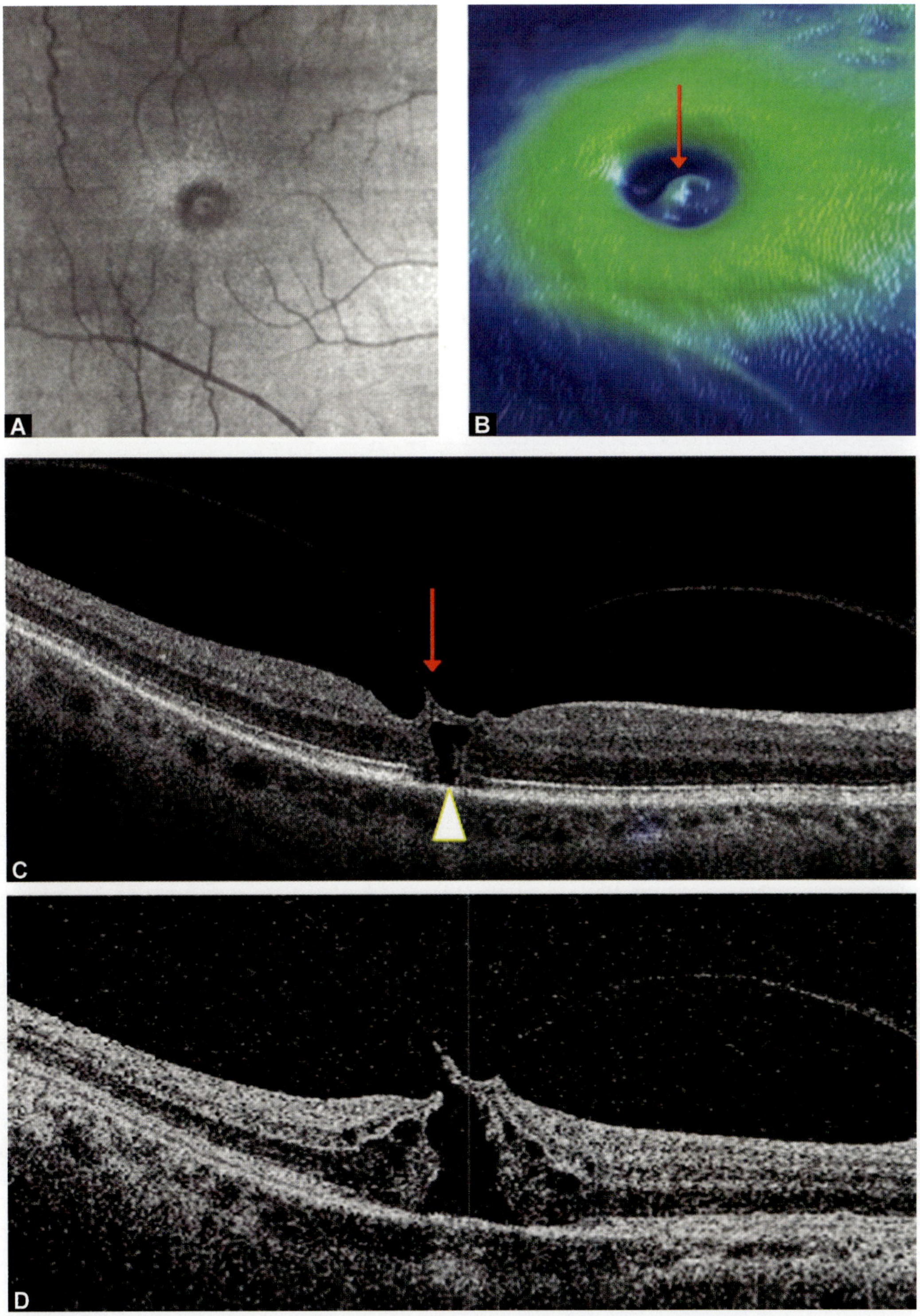

▲ **Figures 25.5A to D**

Evolution of a Stage 1B impending MH to a stage 2 hole. (A) Fundus image showing a small defect in the foveola; (B) View of the foveal surface on OCT, showing the elevation of the foveal floor in the center of the foveal pit (arrow). This elevation corresponds to the traction exerted by the PH shown on the OCT scan profile in C (arrow); (C) OCT scan showing a foveal cyst involving the entire foveal thickness, although the foveal floor remains intact (Stage 1B impending MH); (D) 5 weeks later, evolution to a Stage 2 full-thickness MH, due to the opening of the foveal floor. The edge of the hole has now thickened and is microcystic

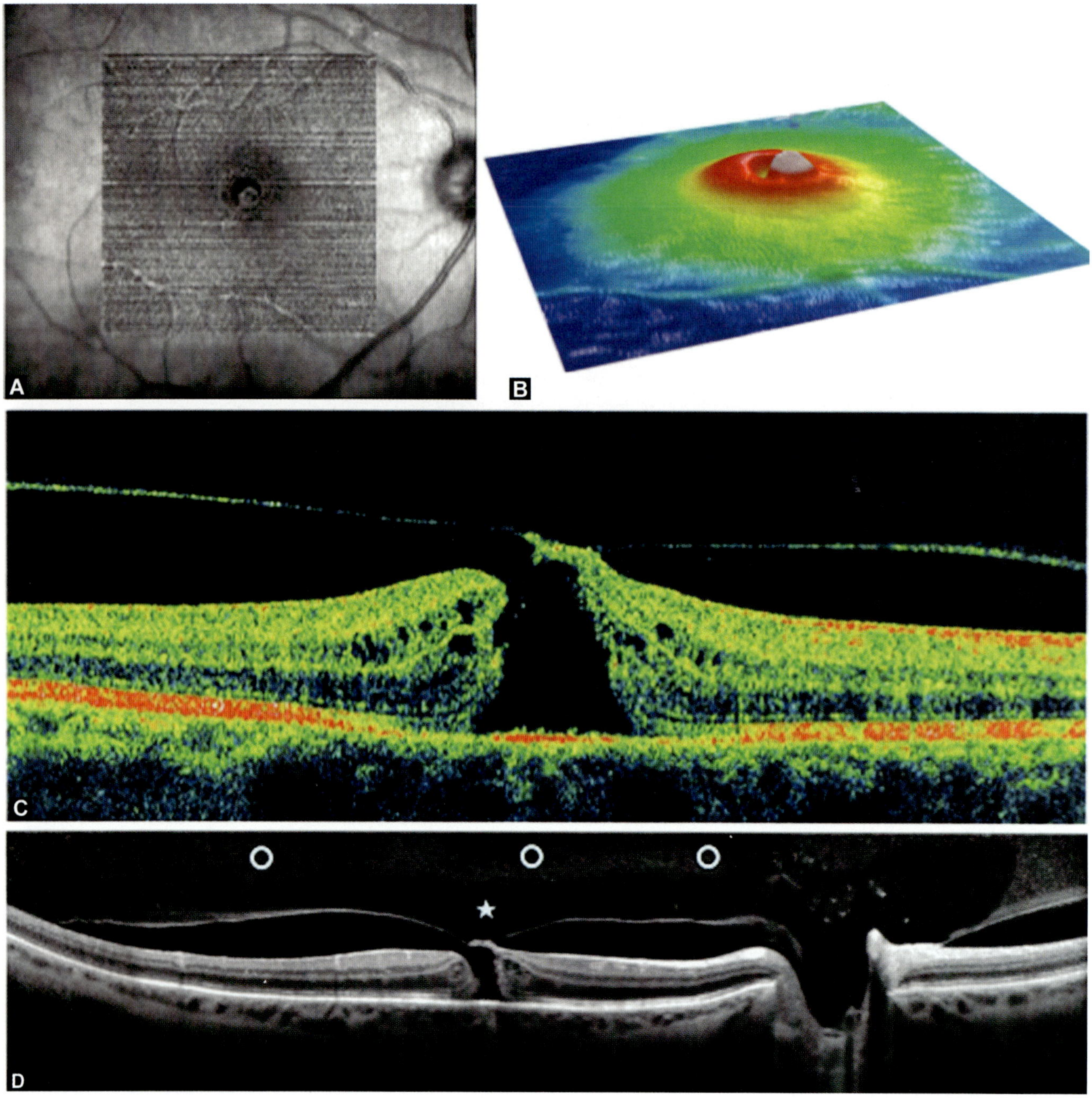

▲ **Figures 25.6A to D**

Stage 2 MH. (A) OCT/Scanning laser ophthalmoscopy fundus photograph showing the MH (arrow); (B) View of the macular surface showing the elevation of the hole edge and the operculum (arrow); (C) OCT scan profile (3 mm) showing the partially detached PH, still attached to the operculum (arrow); (D) Long OCT scan (9 mm) showing the PH attached to the operculum and OD (arrows), bursa premacularis (star), and vitreous body (circles)

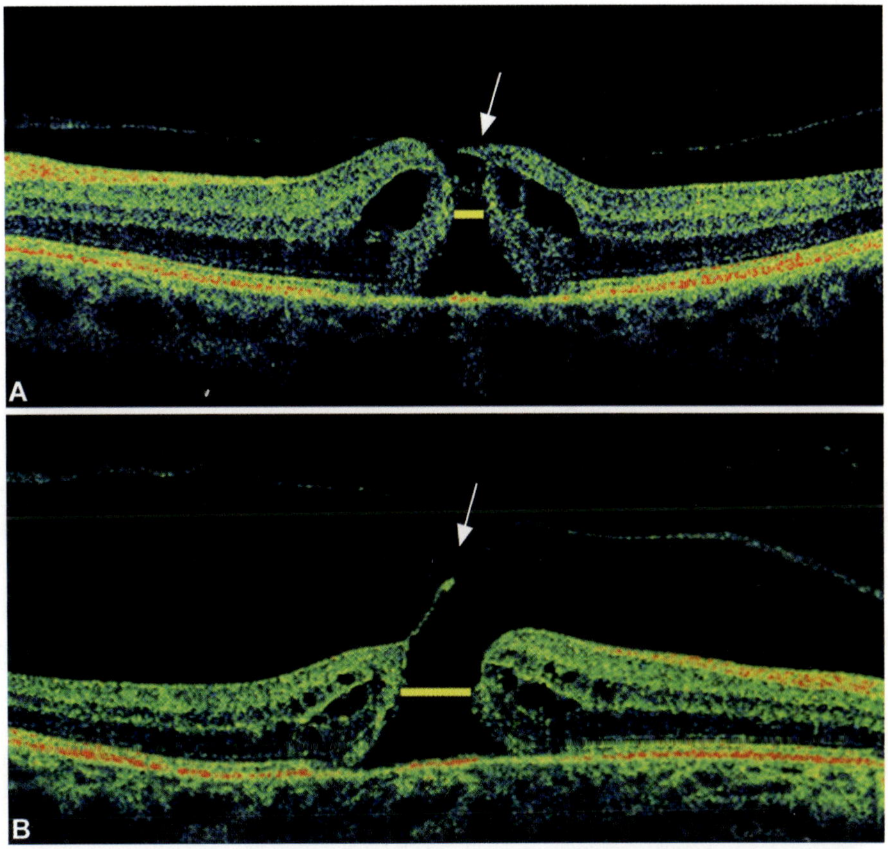

▶ **Figures 25.7A and B**

Various types of Stage 2 MHs. (A) Small Stage 2 MH. The PH still adheres to the operculum, which is not detached from the hole edge (arrow). The hole is less than 400 µm in diameter (bar); (B) Large Stage 2 MH. The PH pulls up the operculum, which is not detached from the hole edge (arrow). The hole is more than 400 µm in diameter (bar)

Stage 4 Macular Hole

There are a few differences on OCT between Stage 3 and Stage 4 MHs. The main difference is the absence of visibility of the PH and operculum on the scan profile. This is because the PVD is complete, with a Weiss ring that is mobile in the vitreous cavity, a feature that is only visible on biomicroscopy. The PH will then be out of focus for OCT. The diagnosis must be confirmed by biomicroscopy. The evolution from impending MH to Stage 4 MH is illustrated in Figure 25.9.

Differential Diagnosis

▶ Macular Pseudohole

Lamellar Macular Hole

Lamellar macular holes (LMHs) are characterized by a thinning of the base of the foveal center combined with a cleft between the inner and outer retina on the edge of the fovea. The thickness of the foveal edge is normal. The LMH could be considered as an aborted process of MH formation.[13,14]

Lamellar Macular Hole: Evolution of an Impending Hole

When the LMH results from the evolution of an impending MH, it is due to the avulsion of the roof of the foveal cyst in a Stage 1A impending MH. The torn inner wall of the cyst is then often visible as an operculum in front of the fovea, which adheres to the incompletely detached PHs.[13] The size of the opening of the inner retina and thickness of the remaining outer retina both vary, and this variability probably accounts for the different degrees of visual acuity (VA) impairment in such cases. The foveal profile is, however, characteristic on an OCT scan. The foveal floor is thinner than normal and irregular, and a cleft between inner and outer retina is visible in the foveal edge (Figs 25.10A to C).

Lamellar Macular Hole of Various Origins

However, LMHs are not always the result of a process of MH formation, but may occur as the ultimate evolution of a cystoid macular edema, or the complication of a vitreomacular traction syndrome (VMTS).[15-18]

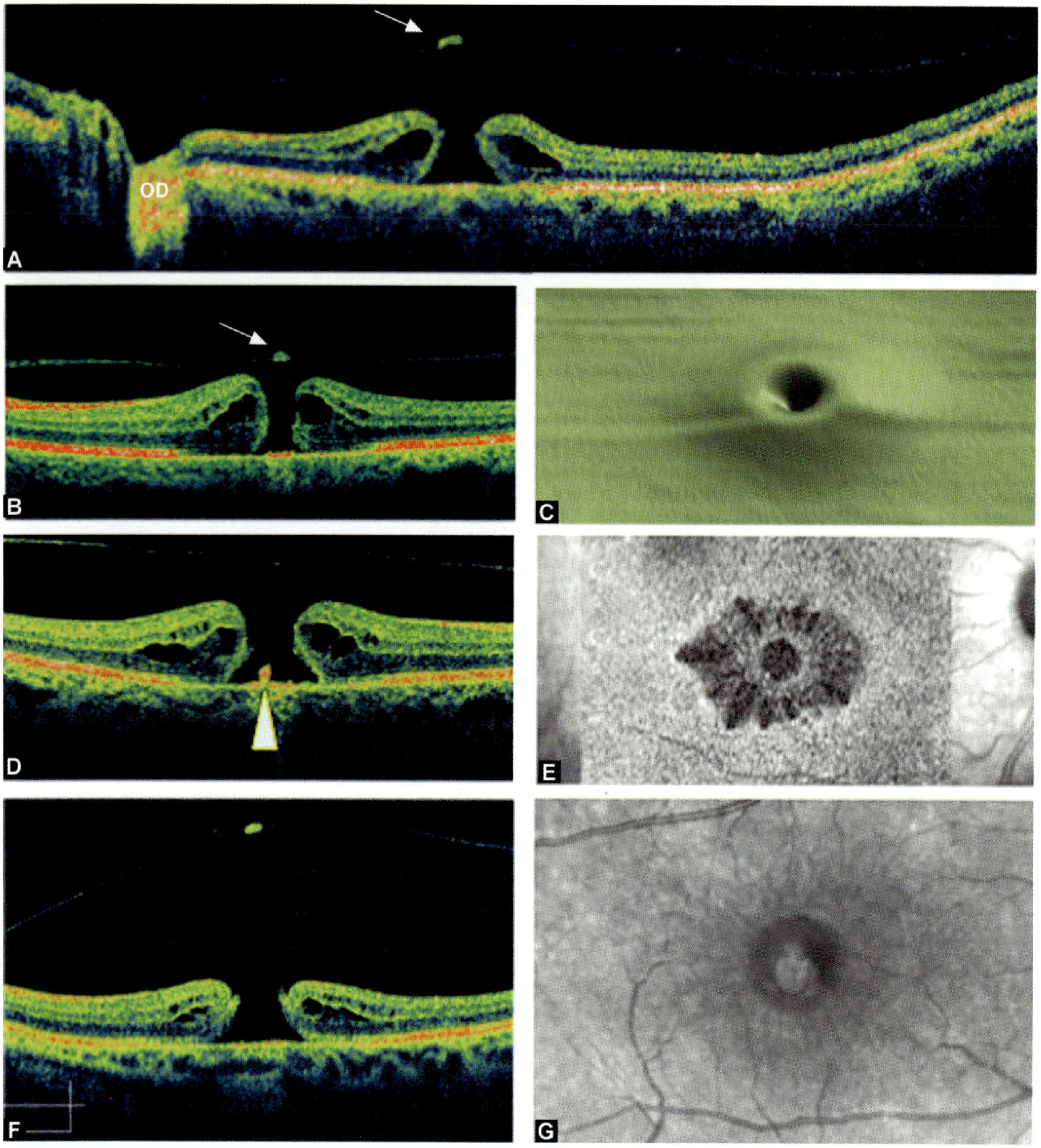

▲ **Figures 25.8A to G**

Various features of Stage 3 MHs. (A) Montage of 2 linear OCT scans showing a MH with a premacular operculum in the plane of the PH (arrow), which is detached from the retinal surface but not from the OD; (B) Small MH, less than 400 μm in diameter. The PH is detached from the retinal surface and contains an operculum (arrow); (C) Macular surface of the same eye showing the elevation of the hole edge; (D) MH, medium size, with proliferation of the retinal pigment epithelial cells in its center (arrowhead); (E) Coronal scan of the same eye showing the petaloid aspect of the cystic cavities within the hole edge; (F) Large MH, more than 400 μm in diameter. Most of the PH is detached; (G) Scanning laser ophthalmoscopy view of the hole showing characteristic radial striae around the hole

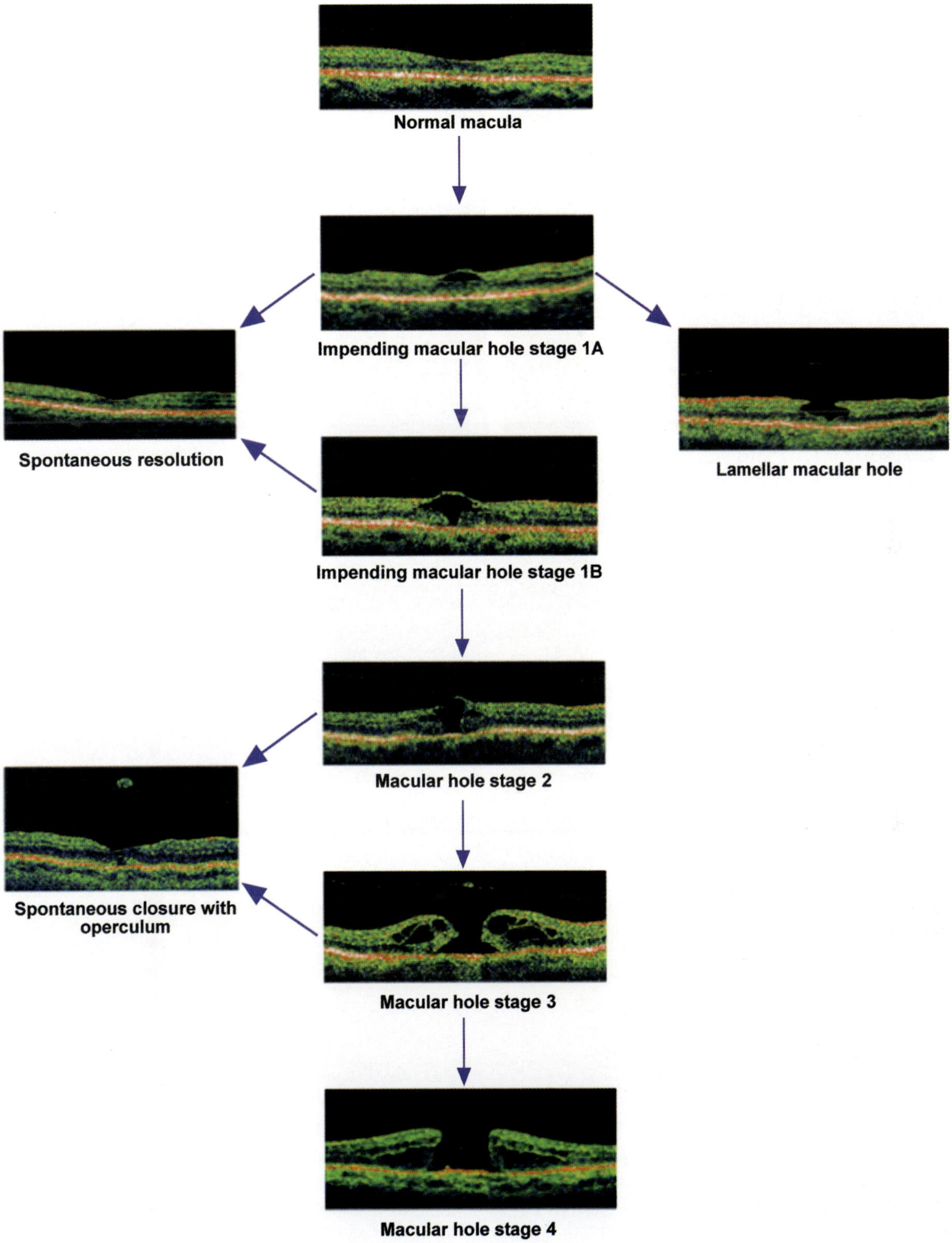

▲ **Figure 25.9**

Schematic representation of the evolution of MHs on OCT. Source: Gaudric A. Arch.Ophthalmol. 1999.

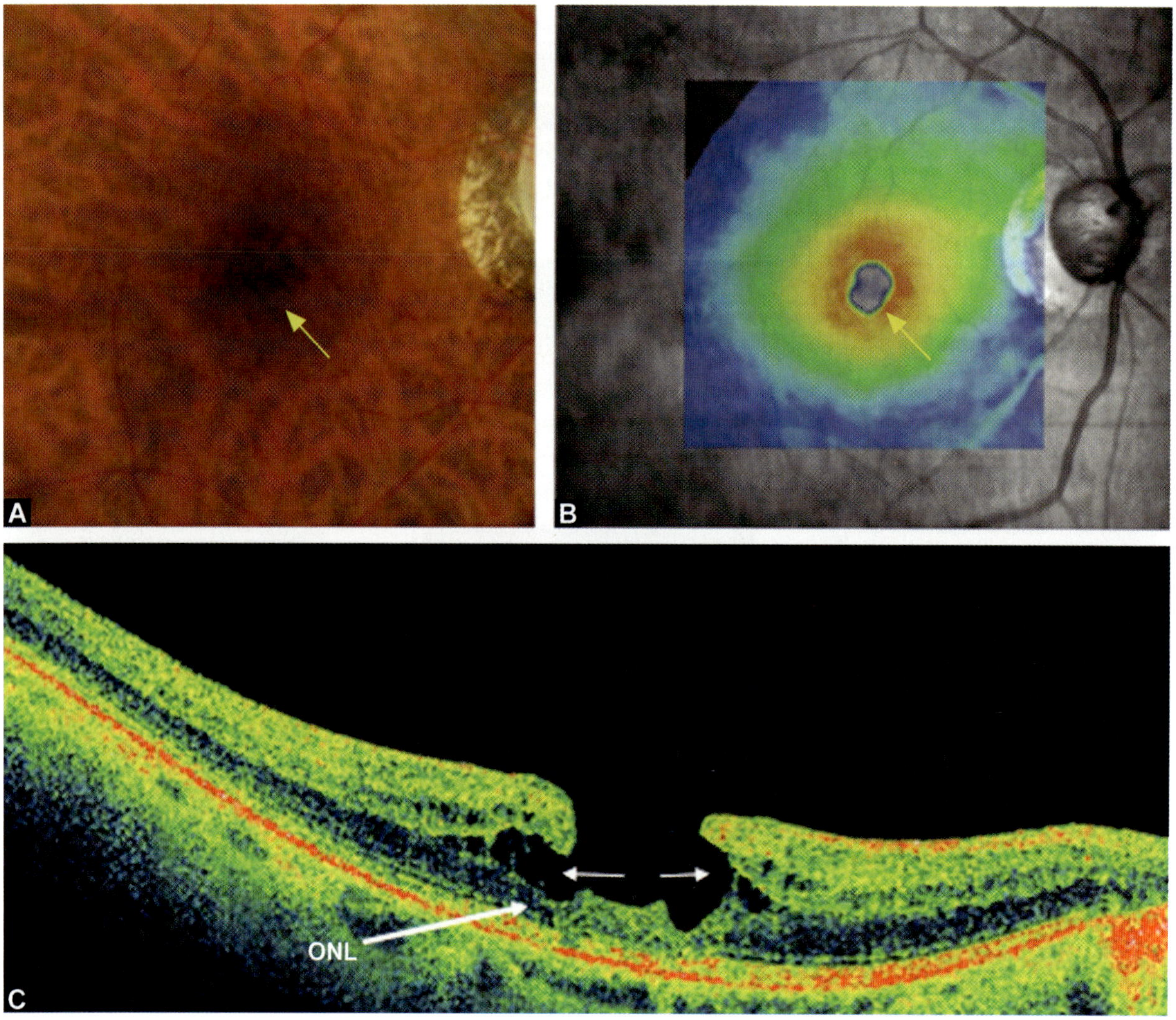

▲ **Figures 25.10A to C**

Lamellar MH. (A) Color fundus photograph showing the typical reddish polycyclic appearance of the fovea (arrow); (B) OCT map showing the contour of the foveal thinning (arrow); (C) OCT scan showing a cleft in the hole edge (arrows) between the inner and outer retina. Note the irregular thinning of the outer nuclear layer

Secondary Macular Holes

▶ Traumatic

Post-traumatic MHs mostly occur in young males and are due to ocular contusion by balls while practicing sports. They are variously associated with other contusive lesions of the eyeball. The MH may be isolated or associated with an area of RPE atrophy at the posterior pole, which on OCT scans corresponds to retinal thinning and to a deep scotoma in the visual field. If the RPE atrophy involves the foveal center, there is a risk that vision will not improve, even if the hole is closed (Figs 25.11A to C). In other cases, a break in Bruch's membrane passing through the foveal center may prevent vision from improving.

Traumatic MH is due to a violent deformation of the eyeball, which results in rupture of the fovea.[19,20] The vitreous remains completely attached to the retinal surface and is therefore not visible on OCT. The profile of the traumatic hole is not different from that of the idiopathic hole, except in cases in which the retina is thinner than normal at the hole edge due to post-traumatic atrophy of the RPE.

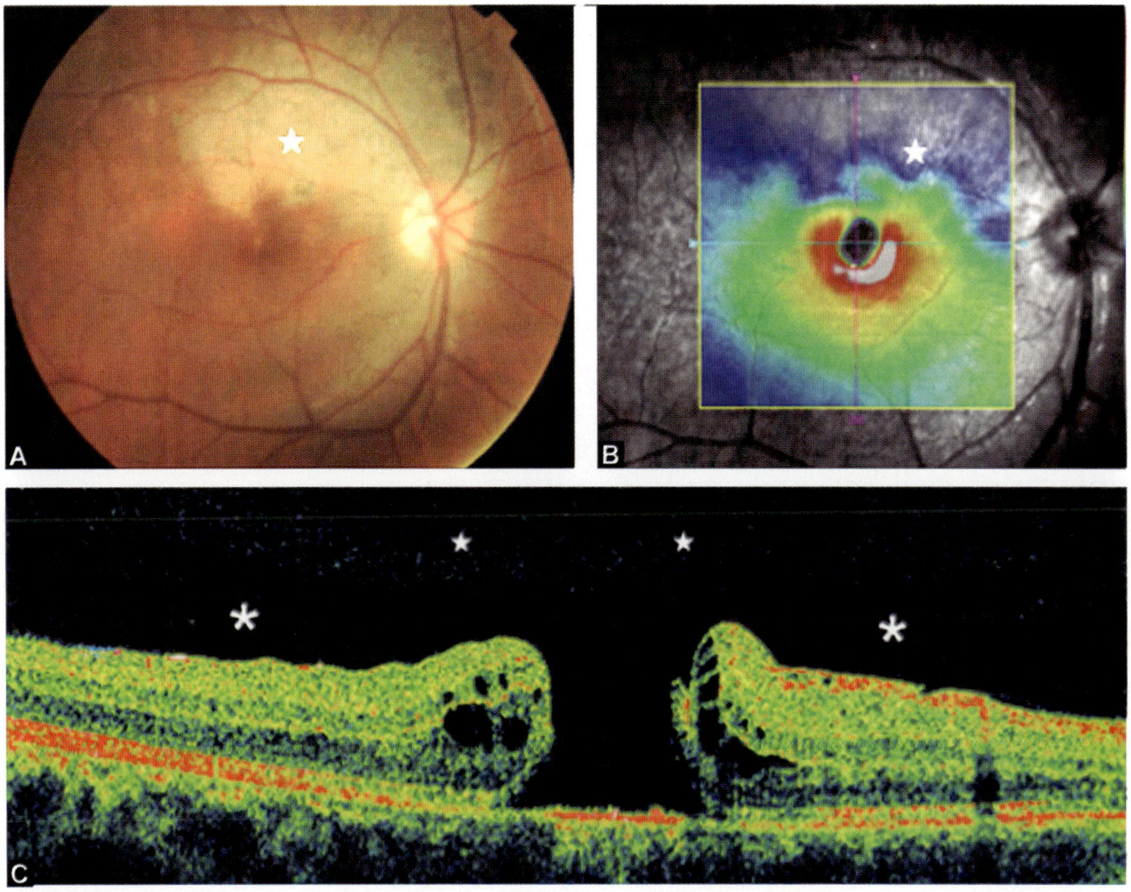

▲ **Figures 25.11A to C**

Contusive MH. (A) Color fundus photograph showing a sus-macular whitish area of the outer retina, and RPE atrophy secondary to ocular blunt trauma (star); (B) OCT map, showing the retinal thinning corresponding to the contusive retinal atrophy (star). The MH is spared by this atrophy and surgery may be recommended; (C) OCT scan showing a typical aspect of MH with thickened edges. Note that the vitreous is not detached at all; the vitreous gel (stars), is normally separated from the macular surface by the bursa premacularis (asterisks)

High Myopia

OCT is the best method of diagnosing MH in highly myopic eyes with a staphyloma. In about 10% of cases, OCT reveals the presence of a MH in the staphyloma, which causes moderate loss of vision and is not seen on biomicroscopy. In eyes with high myopia, a MH may occur after a long evolution of a myopic foveoschisis, especially when it is complicated by foveal detachment.[21-23]

Vitreomacular Traction Syndrome

On OCT, VMTS is characterized by a PH that is incompletely detached from the posterior pole, remains attached to the OD and foveal center, and exerts traction on the foveal tissue (see below). The PH is usually thicker than normal and hyper-reflective on OCT. Traction on the fovea results in cystic changes, sometimes combined with photoreceptor detachment. This condition may worsen and lead to a MH. The frontier between these cases and an impending MH is not clear-cut. The main difference is that in impending holes, the PH has normal reflectivity and is not thickened.

Other Causes of Secondary Macular Holes

Adult-Onset Pseudovitelliform Dystrophy

It may, in some cases, result in significant thinning of the foveal center in front of the subretinal deposit. In rare cases, this thinning evolves into an atrophic MH, an evolution that coincides with the disappearance of the subretinal deposit. MHs may also occur in Best's disease.

Group 2 Macular Telangiectasis

It is characterized by retinal capillary dilation temporal to the fovea, whitening of the inner retina mainly in the temporal part of the macula, inconstant intraretinal crystalline deposits, and cystic cavitations in the fovea without retinal thickening. The foveal center tends to become more atrophic with time. In some cases the process may result in a MH.

Principles and Technique of Macular Hole Surgery

Since the technique introduced by Kelly and Wendel, MH surgery has been, and still is, based on extensive vitrectomy with PVD, peeling of any EMM, thorough fluid-gas exchange, and postoperative face-down positioning of the patient. Many variants of Kelly and Wendel's technique have been tried, such as the use of an adjuvant (TGFß,[24] autologous serum,[25] or autologous platelets[26]), but have all been abandoned. Different types of gas tamponade have also been used (C_3F_8, C_2F_6, SF_6, or air), but the ideal duration of a tamponade ensuring hole closure has never been clear. Peeling off the ILM around the hole has become easier, thanks to various vital dyes, but its usefulness in all cases is questionable. Lastly, the dogmatic application of face-down positioning could perhaps be avoided, at least for small holes.

▶ Vitrectomy

It is often thought that the reason for posterior vitreous cortex removal is to release the vitreous traction on the edge of the hole, even though OCT shows that this cortex is completely detached from the macular surface and hole edge in Stage 3 and 4 MHs, i.e. in most cases. The role of extensive vitrectomy should rather be to make room for a gas bubble as large as possible, because it is clear that a gas bubble's ability to cover the macula depends on the volume of gas mixture injected into the eye, combined with appropriate head positioning.

Sclerotomy Size

Macular hole surgery is a correct indication for small transconjunctival sutureless vitrectomy, as well as for other kinds of macular surgery. The use of 23-gauge probes has recently become popular, because vitreous removal with these probes is quite as fast as with 20-gauge probes, especially with the new machines that combine an ultra-high speed cut rate with flow control. However, 25-gauge probes have also been improved and are stiffer and faster than they were previously, thus competing with the standard 23-gauge probe. One advantage of the oblique 25G probe incisions is their excellent tightness in most cases.

Core Vitrectomy

For Stage 4 MHs, vitrectomy is easily completed. To make the maximum amount of room for the gas bubble, care must be taken to shave off as much of the vitreous base as possible (see below).

In Stage 2 and 3 MHs, the vitreous is not detached from either the retina or the OD, but only from the macular area. Vitrectomy will, therefore, be done in two steps; core vitrectomy, and then vitreous cortex removal. After the core vitrectomy, the vitreous cortex is detached from the OD and retinal surface up to the equator.

Vitreous Cortex Separation and Vitrectomy Completion

The easiest way to peel off the vitreous cortex from the retinal surface is to start by detaching the Weiss ring from the OD. Different instruments may be used, including a soft-tipped cannula with active aspiration, aspirating forceps, or the vitreous probe itself. The new 23/25G probe, with the aspirating port close to the tip, is especially effective for exerting traction on the vitreous and detaching it from the OD. The tip of the probe can be efficiently positioned in the disc cup, with the aspirating port turned toward, or directly placed on the nasal side of the OD, because the attachment of the vitreous cortex is stronger on that side. Once this attachment has been broken, the entire Weiss ring will have been detached, and it will be easy to lift up the entire vitreous cortex, often containing the prefoveolar operculum. During this maneuver, one can easily follow the progression of the vitreous cortex detachment, which extends centrifugally up to the equator. Some surgeons also use triamcinolone to better visualize the PH during its detachment.

The vitrectomy is then completed and it may be wise to shave off as much of the vitreous base as possible in the inferior periphery, which is only possible with scleral indentation to avoid touching the lens. The main reason why vitrectomy should be very complete is to make room for the largest possible gas bubble. Another reason is to prevent the

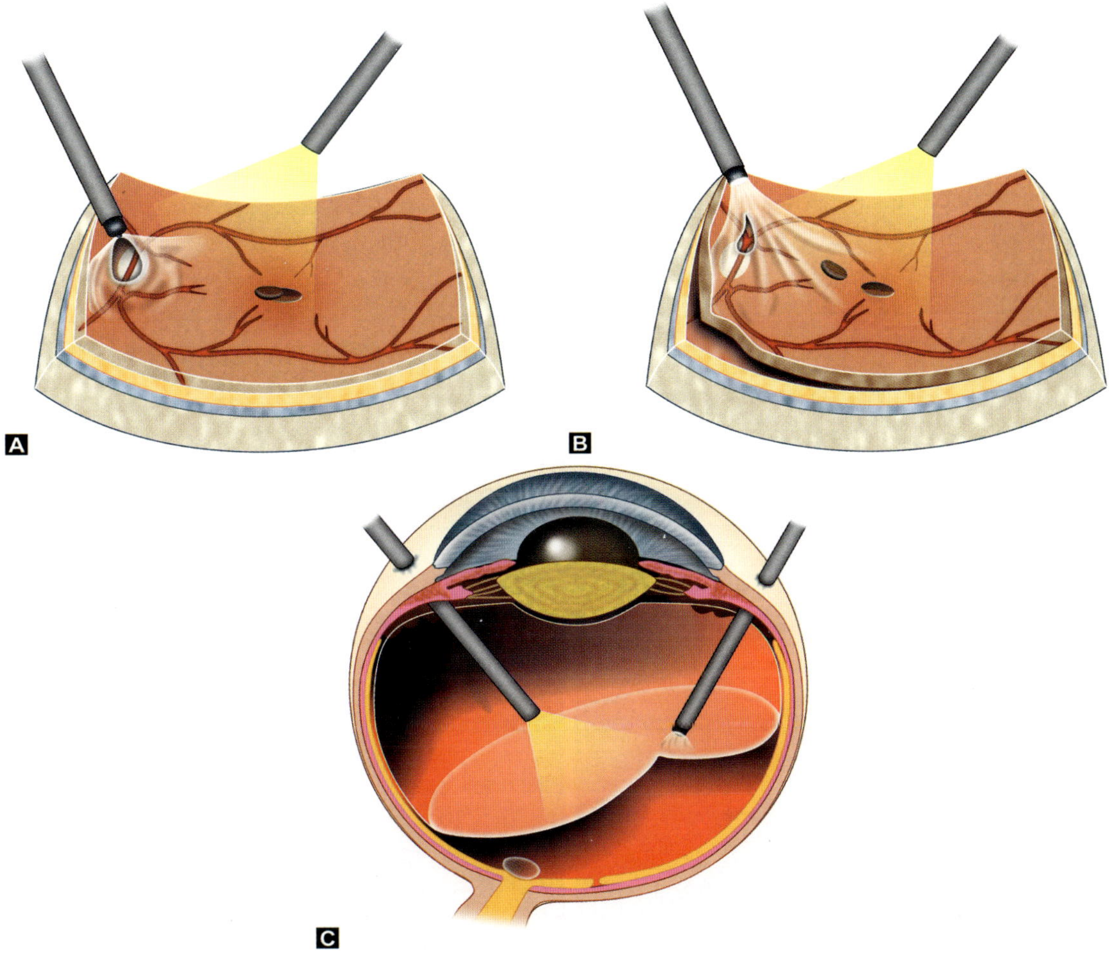

▲ **Figures 25.12A to C**

MH surgery, detachment of the PH. (A) The prepapillary vitreous gel is engaged in the vitreous probe by aspiration and pulled up until the Weiss ring is gradually lifted; (B) Once the Weiss ring is detached, the operculum is also elevated above the retinal plane together with the PH; (C) By gently pulling on the PH with the aspiration of the vitreous probe, the hyaloid is progressively detached from the retina up to the equator

gas from exerting traction on the inferior retina via the vitreous remnants, thus reducing the risk of postoperative inferior retinal breaks and detachment (Figs 25.12A to C).

▶ Epiretinal Membrane Removal

In about 30% of cases, there is an ERM around the MH. Membranes are more frequent in Stage 4 and 3 holes than in Stage 2 holes.[27,28] Unlike idiopathic ERMs, they are not contractile, and their consistency, which is soft and friable is also different. Rather than trying to remove the ERM with forceps, it is easier to remove it by gently brushing the retinal surface from the outside to the MH edge, with either the soft tip of a back-flush cannula or a soft retinal scraper. These membranes often adhere firmly to the hole edge and have to be cut with the vitreous probe. They consist of vitreous collagen and a few cellular elements, especially fibroblasts (Figs 25.13A to D).[29-34]

▶ Internal Limiting Membrane Peeling

Although the rationale for ILM peeling is unclear, it is currently performed in MH surgery. The ILM is probably not involved in the pathogenesis of MHs, but its peeling may

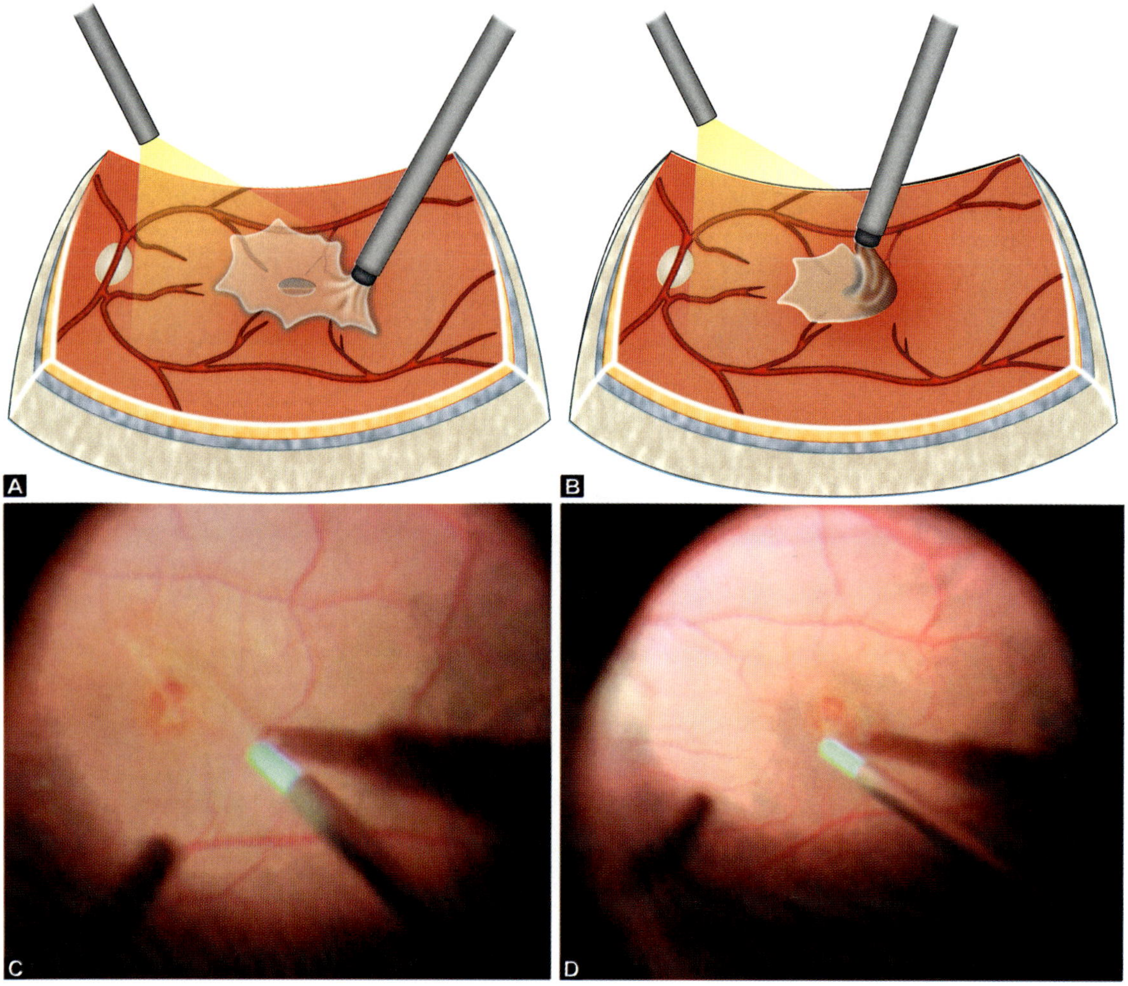

▲ Figures 25.13A to D

MH surgery: detachment of an ERM around the hole. (A) The ERM is gently brushed off the retinal surface by a soft-tipped extrusion cannula until it is detached; (B and C) The yellowish soft and friable membrane is progressively detached around the hole; (D) In the end, the membrane only adheres to the hole edge and often has to be cut with the vitreous probe

favor hole shrinking and healing by removing all the remnants of vitreous cortex or ERM around the hole. It might also act as a stimulus to glial proliferation, and thus promote hole healing. However, one should bear in mind that at least 80% of all MHs and about 95% of small MHs close without ILM peeling.

Since 1997, many studies have been published in the literature concerning the surgery of MHs with ILM peeling,[35-42] but very few were randomized. The conclusions of our randomized study[43] indicate that ILM peeling is mainly useful for large MH, i.e. with a diameter of 400 µm or more. ILM peeling may perhaps also reduce the rate of MH reopening (Figs 25.14A and B).[38,44,45]

However, ILM removal is not without side effects, due either to the peeling itself or to the use of dyes for ILM staining.[46-54]

Internal limiting membrane peeling has been greatly facilitated by the use of dyes. Indocyanine green (ICG) was the first to be applied, initially at the concentration of 0.5%,[55] but it involved a risk of toxicity for the RPE.[56] The affinity of ICG for RPE cells is indeed well known, and at certain concentration, its use may result in RPE cell death.[57,58] Thus, RPE atrophy in the area of the MH has been described.[56,59-67] Moreover, infrared photographs of the fundus, taken weeks or months after the application of ICG still showed abnormal fluorescence of the foveal RPE, as

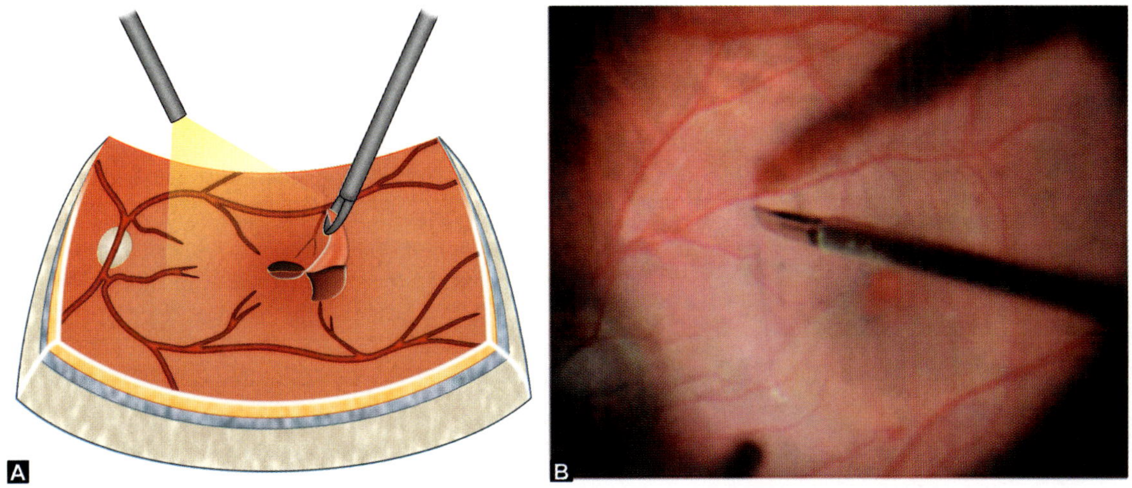

▲ **Figures 25.14A and B**

MH surgery, ablation of the ILM. (A) The ILM is grasped by an end-gripping forceps and torn away; (B) After staining by Brilliant Blue G, the ILM is torn off and progressively detached around the hole (fundus photograph)

well as staining of the optic nerve fibers in the retina and OD. Animal experiments have shown that the optic nerve fibers are stained up to the cuniculus.[65,68] Several authors have pointed out that the use of ICG carries the risk of obtaining less good visual results or increased visual field disturbances,[69,70] as also indicated by Gandorfer and Kampik.[71]

However, by reducing the ICG concentration and the duration of ICG contact with the fundus, such harmful effects may be avoided,[72,73] and in general, the authors of most publications believe that when ICG is used in macular surgery to facilitate ILM peeling, it is harmless if its application is brief.[73]

In any case, other dyes assumed to be less or not at all toxic for retinal cells are now available. Trypan blue provides faint but sufficient staining of the ILM at the concentration of 0.15%. It can be injected after a partial fluid-air exchange, or directly in front of the posterior pole after mixing with 10% glucose, which makes the mixture heavier and also minimizes its concentration at 0.075% without decreasing its staining property.[74] Trypan blue appears to be less toxic than ICG when used in dye assisted peeling of ILM during MH repair as reflected by the better visual results in the trypan blue group of patients and the higher rate of persistent central scotoma in the ICG group.[75,76]

Brilliant Blue G specifically stains the ILM and not the ERM. Its innocuousness for retinal cells has been shown both on cell cultures and *in vivo*.[77-79] It is used at the concentration of 0.25% and is left in contact with the retinal surface for 1 minute. It is preferable to inject Brilliant Blue G after a partial fluid-air exchange.

Triamcinolone can also be used, but only to help delineate the area of ILM already peeled off, and for easier detection of edge of the ILM that remains to be peeled off.[80-84]

▶ Gas Filling

The role of gas tamponade is to create the necessary conditions for MH healing, which is achieved by glial cell proliferation resulting in a central foveal scar whose diameter is very much smaller than that of the original hole. The contact of the gas bubble with the macula rapidly results in the flattening of the edematous hole edge and in mechanical narrowing of the foveal defect. It does not matter whether the patient's head is in the face down or vertical position, as the bubble gas acts more by its superficial tension, which isolates the retina from liquid intrusion than by its buoyancy. The desirable duration of the tamponade on the hole edge depends on the duration of the healing process, which probably differs from one eye to another and may require 3–7 days or more. By using different air-gas mixtures, it is possible to act on the duration of the contact of the gas bubble with the fovea in both the face down and upright positions.

Air alone has been used,[85-88] but resorbs too quickly to be effective enough in all cases. Twenty percent SF_6-air may

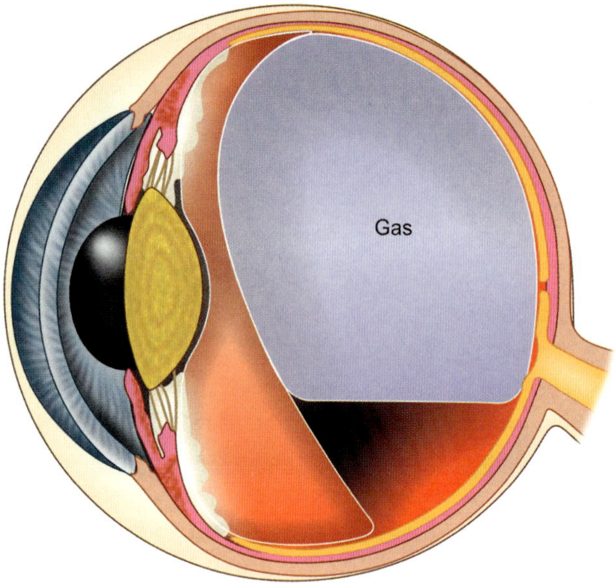

▲ Figure 25.15

Schematic representation of the vitreous cavity filled with 17% C_2F_6-air, 1 week after surgery, with the patient in the upright position. The gas bubble still amply covers the posterior pole

be a good option, but probably does not cover the macula in the upright position for more than 5 days, which is not long enough in some cases. Seventeen percent C_2F_6-air isolates the macula from liquid infiltration for more than a week, even when the head is upright (Fig. 25.15), and is completely resorbed in 4–5 weeks. Fifteen percent C_3F_8 has the same macular tamponade properties, but lasts in the eye for 6–8 weeks.

These estimations of the duration of the effectiveness of different gas mixtures of course depend on different parameters, such as the extent of vitrectomy, the attention given to maximizing intraocular fluid in the fluid-gas exchange, and the tightness of sclerotomies. The amount of vitreous base left in place probably varies from one patient to another, depending on the width of the base, and will leave less or more room for the gas bubble. The volume of air (and, therefore, of gas mixture) injected will be also larger if care is taken to wait for 10 minutes after the end of fluid-air exchange before collecting the residual fluid that comes from the vitreous base. Lastly, with the sutureless transconjunctivoscleral incisions, the tightness of the sclerotomies may be an issue and special care must be taken to avoid gas leakage.

▶ Postoperative Positioning

Postoperative positioning of the head depends on the desired duration of the tamponade on the macula, the volume of gas introduced into the vitreous cavity and the kind of gas mixture used. The reclining position must be ruled out for the entire period necessary for hole healing. For all other positions, various options can be considered. The most common rule is to encourage the patient to remain face down as much as possible (for instance, for 20 hours out of 24) for 7–10 days. However, during the first postoperative days, face down positioning is in fact not really necessary, whatever the gas mixture used, as the gas bubble covers the macula when the head is in the upright position and only the reclining position should be avoided.

Another option is to vary the recommended positioning on the basis of estimated duration of hole healing, which depends on hole diameter.

Two randomized series connected with this option have been studied to date. One showed a significant reduction in the success rate without face-down positioning, but a post hoc analysis suggested that this reduction was only significant for MH greater than 400 μm and not for smaller holes.[89] The other series concerned idiopathic MHs less than equal to 400 μm in diameter and demonstrated that without face-down positioning, the results were just as good as with it (confidence interval for closure rate reduction: 0–14.88%, with a 5% risk of error).[90] In this study, a large bubble of C_2F_6 (> 90%) was used and patients were instructed to avoid the supine position for 10 days, thus ensuring that at least during that period the posterior pole remained in continuous contact with the gas bubble. These results may not apply to patients treated with a small volume of short duration postoperative bubble gases, or to patients with full freedom of positioning including the supine position.

In summary, no face-down positioning may be indicated for small holes less than 400 μm in diameter, which probably heal in 3–5 days, provided that in the upright position, the volume of the gas bubble is enough to continue to cover the macula throughout this entire period. In these cases the indication will, therefore, be to keep the head in the upright position during the day, and avoid the reclining position during the night. It is for larger holes that face down positioning should be recommended for 7–10 days. In fact, as stated above, various positions may be recommended depending on the size of the hole, the type of gas used, the extent of vitrectomy and the tightness of the incisions.

Process of Macular Hole Closure and Prognostic Factors

Histology

Three histologic reports have described the characteristics of MH that closed after surgery in eyes obtained post-mortem.[91-93] In all three cases, the hole was sealed by the proliferation of Müller cells, although a small defect persisted in the photoreceptor layer. Retinal healing has also been reproduced experimentally in rabbit eyes[94] and was shown to be due to the proliferation of glial cells, which sealed the hole in less than 7 days.

Optical Coherence Tomography Findings

Early MH closure after surgery has been documented by several publications[86,95-97] including intraoperative observations by the use of handled OCT.[98] These publications show that reapproximation of the hole edge is obtained quite soon after surgery and that closure of the hole may occur as soon as the 3rd postoperative day.

At gas resorption, OCT shows various foveal profiles as well as a small central break in the IS/OS photoreceptor layer (Figs 25.16A to C). The size of this break varies from one case to another, tends to decrease with time, and more or less correlates with VA.[99-102]

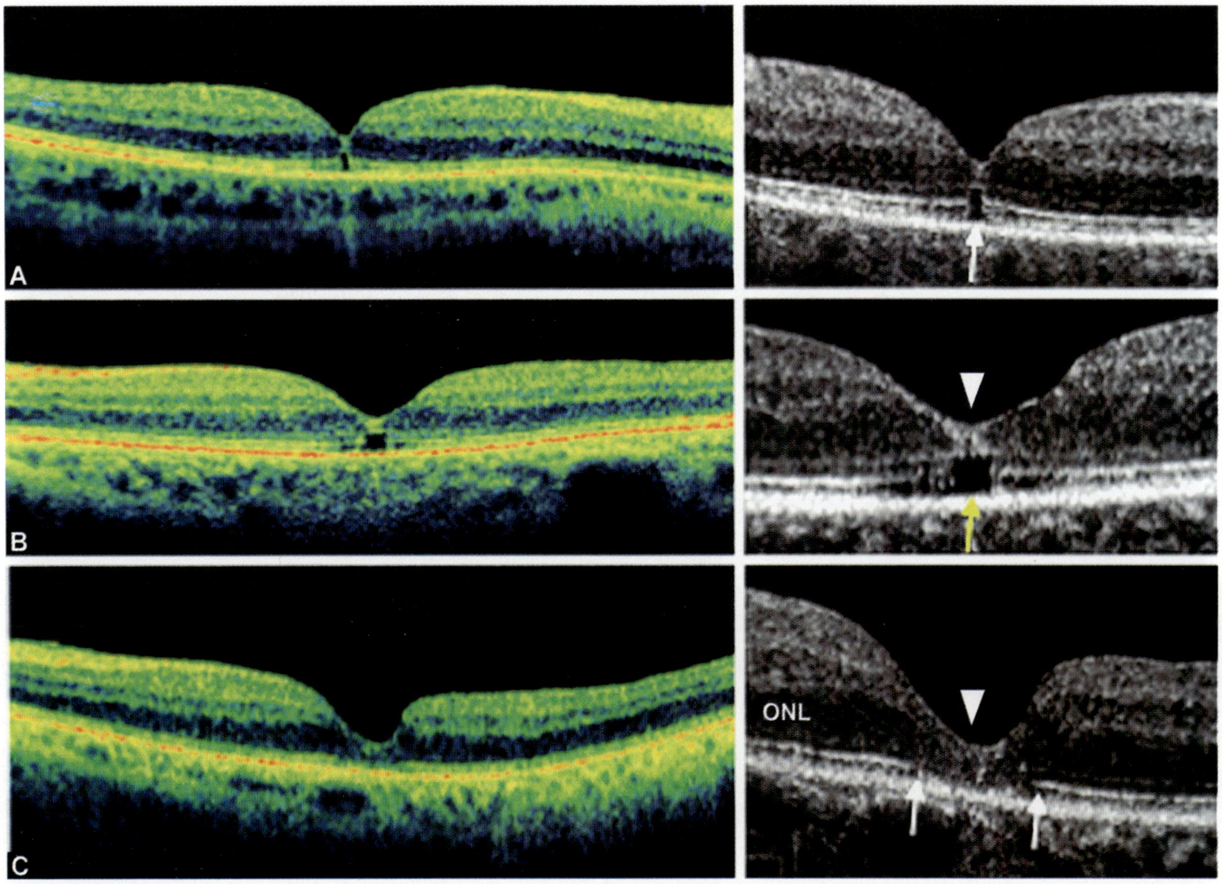

▲ **Figures 25.16A to C**

Various aspects of MHs that closed after surgery. (A) Narrow foveal pit, with a very small break in the IS/OS photoreceptor junction (arrow); (B) Wider foveal pit, with a larger break in the IS/OS photoreceptor junction (arrow). Note also the hyper-reflectivity of the glial scar closing the hole (arrowhead); (C) Wide deep abnormal foveal pit, with a large break in the inner/outer segment photoreceptor junction (arrows). Note also the hyper-reflectivity of the glial scar closing the hole (arrowhead), and the disappearance of the outer nuclear layer at the foveal center

Prognostic Factors

Different parameters have been studied as possible indicators of the success of MH surgery including preoperative VA[103] and MH size. Different methods of measuring MH size have been proposed,[41,104-106] but in all cases the conclusion reached was that a small hole has more chance of closing than a large one, at least with conventional surgery that does not include ILM peeling. Measuring the opening of the hole on OCT scans has shown that there is a significant difference in the postoperative diagnosis, depending on whether the MH diameter is more or less than 400 μm.[41,106] The visual prognosis may also depend on the size of the hole, the initial VA and the age of the patient.[107]

Functional Results

In most cases, VA improves once the hole has closed. When the eye is phakic, visual improvement may be reduced by the progression of a nuclear cataract as soon as the 3rd postoperative month. In pseudophakic eyes, or in eyes that become rendered pseudophakic at the time of MH surgery, VA continues to improve at least during the first 6 months.[108] In recent publications, significant visual improvement was reported to vary from 77%[108] to 95%.[44] MH closed after surgery and made pseudophakic, had a median VA of 20/40 in two recent series[108,109] and in two others their mean VA varied from 20/60 to 20/40.[44,110] It also appears that final VA is mainly affected by the extent of IS/OS photoreceptor breakdown on OCT.[109] However, despite the frequent persistence of microscotomas in eyes with closed MH, these eyes keep to derive long-term benefit from surgery and their maximum ready speed is comparable to that of healthy eye.[111]

Complications of Macular Hole Surgery

The most serious postoperative complication is retinal detachment, which may occur within days or weeks of the operation. Its frequency has been reported to vary from 1 to 14% of cases.[44,112-115] Most of the retinal tears causing such detachments seem to be located in the inferior periphery.[113] Today, with improved fluidics and surgical precautions, the rate of retinal detachment should remain below 2%.

The occurrence of a cataract after MH surgery is common[108,116,117] and patients should be aware that in most cases, cataract surgery becomes necessary 6 months to 1 year after MH surgery. This has favored a tendency to operate the lens during the MH procedure.[118,119]

A MH may reopen even 6 years or more after surgery.[113,114,120,121] However, most cases occur during the first 2 years (approximately the mean and median value for the time elapsing from surgery to reopening).[122] The rate of reopening reported in the literature vary considerably, from 0 to 25%, with a mean about 6%. The real reason for reopening is not yet known. Recently, its incidence seems to have decreased, concomitantly with the rise in the success rate of MH surgery. Some authors believe this is connected with the optimization of surgery that includes ILM peeling.[44,45,122]

Conclusion

Macular hole surgery has achieved a significant success rate with hole closure in more than 90% of cases and concomitant visual improvement. The size of the hole emerges as one of the most relevant prognostic factors of postoperative closure. Large MHs probably require more aggressive surgery, and in particular ILM peeling, to reach the same success rate as smaller ones. The complications of MH surgery have decreased with fewer cases of retinal detachment and MH reopening. The eye can be made pseudophakic at the time of MH surgery to avoid subsequent cataract operations.

References

1. Kelly NE, Wendel RT. Vitreous surgery for idiopathic macular holes. Results of a pilot study. Arch Ophthalmol. 1991;109:654-9.
2. Hee MR, Puliafito CA, Wong C, et al. Optical coherence tomography of macular holes. Ophthalmology. 1995;102:748-56.
3. Puliafito CA, Hee MR, Lin CP, et al. Imaging of macular diseases with optical coherence tomography. Ophthalmology. 1995;102:217-29.
4. Gaudric A, Haouchine B, Massin P, et al. Macular hole formation: new data provided by optical coherence tomography. Arch Ophthalmol. 1999;117:744-51.
5. Haouchine B, Massin P, Gaudric A. Foveal pseudocyst as the first step in macular hole formation: a prospective study by optical coherence tomography. Ophthalmology. 2001;108:15-22.
6. Chan A, Duker JS, Schuman JS, et al. Stage 0 macular holes: observations by optical coherence tomography. Ophthalmology. 2004;111:2027-32.

7. Uchino E, Uemura A, Ohba N. Initial stages of posterior vitreous detachment in healthy eyes of older persons evaluated by optical coherence tomography. Arch Ophthalmol. 2001;119:1475-9.
8. Gass JD. Reappraisal of biomicroscopic classification of stages of development of a macular hole. Am J Ophthalmol. 1995;119:752-9.
9. Spaide RF, Wong D, Fisher Y, et al. Correlation of vitreous attachment and foveal deformation in early macular hole states. Am J Ophthalmol. 2002;133:226-9.
10. Takahashi A, Nagaoka T, Ishiko S, et al. Foveal anatomic changes in a progressing Stage 1 macular hole documented by spectral-domain optical coherence tomography. Ophthalmology. 2010;117:806-10.
11. Ko TH, Fujimoto JG, Duker JS, et al. Comparison of ultrahigh- and standard-resolution optical coherence tomography for imaging macular hole pathology and repair. Ophthalmology. 2004;111:2033-43.
12. Johnson MW, Van Newkirk MR, Meyer KA. Perifoveal vitreous detachment is the primary pathogenic event in idiopathic MH formation. Arch Ophthalmol. 2001;119:215-22.
13. Haouchine B, Massin P, Tadayoni R, et al. Diagnosis of macular pseudoholes and lamellar macular holes by optical coherence tomography. Am J Ophthalmol. 2004;138:732-9.
14. Gass JD. Idiopathic senile macular hole. Its early stages and pathogenesis. Arch Ophthalmol. 1988;106:629-39.
15. Unoki N, Nishijima K, Kita M, et al. Lamellar macular hole formation in patients with diabetic cystoid macular edema. Retina. 2009;29:1128-33.
16. Shimada N, Ohno-Matsui K, Yoshida T, et al. Progression from macular retinoschisis to retinal detachment in highly myopic eyes is associated with outer lamellar hole formation. Br J Ophthalmol. 2008;92:762-4.
17. Chen JC, Lee LR. Clinical spectrum of lamellar macular defects including pseudoholes and pseudocysts defined by optical coherence tomography. Br J Ophthalmol. 2008;92:1342-6.
18. Ioannidis AS, Liasis A, Sheldrick J, et al. Lamellar macular hole as the presenting feature in a child with Coats' disease. J Pediatr Ophthalmol Strabismus. 2005;42:378-9.
19. Oehrens AM, Stalmans P. Optical coherence tomographic documentation of the formation of a traumatic macular hole. Am J Ophthalmol. 2006;142:866-9.
20. Johnson RN, McDonald HR, Lewis H, et al. Traumatic macular hole: observations, pathogenesis, and results of vitrectomy surgery. Ophthalmology. 2001;108:853-7.
21. Coppe AM, Ripandelli G, Parisi V, et al. Prevalence of asymptomatic macular holes in highly myopic eyes. Ophthalmology. 2005;112:2103-9.
22. Ripandelli G, Parisi V, Friberg TR, et al. Retinal detachment associated with macular hole in high myopia: using the vitreous anatomy to optimize the surgical approach. Ophthalmology. 2004;111:726-31.
23. Baba T, Ohno-Matsui K, Futagami S, et al. Prevalence and characteristics of foveal retinal detachment without macular hole in high myopia. Am J Ophthalmol. 2003;135:338-42.
24. Thompson JT, Smiddy WE, Williams GA, et al. Comparison of recombinant transforming growth factor-beta-2 and placebo as an adjunctive agent for macular hole surgery. Ophthalmology. 1998;105:700-6.
25. Ezra E, Gregor ZJ. Surgery for idiopathic full-thickness macular hole: two-year results of a randomized clinical trial comparing natural history, vitrectomy, and vitrectomy plus autologous serum: Morfields Macular Hole Study Group Report no. 1. Arch Ophthalmol. 2004;122:224-36.
26. Paques M, Chastang C, Mathis A, et al. Effect of autologous platelet concentrate in surgery for idiopathic macular hole: results of a multicenter, double-masked, randomized trial. Platelets in Macular Hole Surgery Group. Ophthalmology. 1999;106:932-8.
27. Kurihara K, Ishibashi T, Oshima K. The residual epiretinal membrane after vitrectomy for macular hole. Graefes Arch Clin Exp Ophthalmol. 1999;237:648-53.
28. Blain P, Paques M, Massin P, et al. Epiretinal membranes surrounding idiopathic macular holes. Retina. 1998;18:316-21.
29. Heidenkummer HP, Kampik A. Morphologic analysis of epiretinal membranes in surgically treated idiopathic macular foramina. Results of light and electron microscopy. Ophthalmologe 1996;93:675-9.
30. Gandorfer A, Scheler R, Haritoglou C, et al. Pathology of the macular hole rim in flat-mounted internal limiting membrane specimens. Retina. 2009;29:1097-105.
31. Mackenzie SE, Gandorfer A, Rohleder M, et al. Ultrastructure and retinal imaging of internal limiting membrane: a clinicopathologic correlation of trypan blue stain in macular hole surgery. Retina. 2010;30:648-54.
32. Schumann RG, Remy M, Grueterich M, et al. How it appears: electron microscopic evaluation of internal limiting membrane specimens obtained during brilliant blue G assisted macular hole surgery. Br J Ophthalmol. 2008;92:330-1.
33. Green WR. The macular hole: histopathologic studies. Arch Ophthalmol. 2006;124:317-21.
34. Haritoglou C, Gandorfer A, Kampik A. Results of a retrospective analysis of patients with a macular hole. Retina. 2005;25:545.
35. Eckardt C, Eckardt U, Groos S, et al. Removal of the internal limiting membrane in macular holes. Clinical and morphological findings. Ophthalmologe. 1997;94:545-51.
36. Olsen TW, Sternberg P, Capone A, et al. Macular hole surgery using thrombin-activated fibrinogen and selective removal of the internal limiting membrane. Retina. 1998;18:322-9.
37. Park DW, Lee JH, Min WK. The use of internal limiting membrane maculorrhexis in treatment of idiopathic macular holes. Korean J Ophthalmol. 1998;12:92-7.
38. Brooks HLJ. Macular hole surgery with and without internal limiting membrane peeling. Ophthalmology. 2000;107:1939-48.

39. Al-Abdulla NA, Thompson JT, Sjaarda RN. Results of macular hole surgery with and without epiretinal dissection or internal limiting membrane removal. Ophthalmology. 2004;111:142-9.
40. Kumagai K, Furukawa M, Ogino N, et al. Vitreous surgery with and without internal limiting membrane peeling for macular hole repair. Retina. 2004;24:721-7.
41. Tadayoni R, Gaudric A, Haouchine B, et al. Relationship between macular hole size and the potential benefit of internal limiting membrane peeling. Br J Ophthalmol. 2006;90:1239-41.
42. Tognetto D, Grandin R, Sanguinetti G, et al. Internal limiting membrane removal during macular hole surgery: results of a multicenter retrospective study. Ophthalmology. 2006;113:1401-10.
43. Tadayoni R, Creuzot-Garcher C, Korobelnik JF, et al. Internal limiting membrane peeling for large macular holes: a randomized, multicentric, and controlled clinical trial. Invest Ophthalmol Vis Sci. 2009;50:E-Abstract 5206.
44. Passemard M, Yakoubi Y, Muselier A, et al. Long-term outcome of idiopathic macular hole surgery. Am J Ophthalmol. 2010;149:120-6.
45. Yoshida M, Kishi S. Pathogenesis of macular hole recurrence and its prevention by internal limiting membrane peeling. Retina. 2007;27:169-73.
46. Haritoglou C, Gass CA, Schaumberger M, et al. Macular changes after peeling of the internal limiting membrane in macular hole surgery. Am J Ophthalmol. 2001;132:363-8.
47. Tadayoni R, Paques M, Massin P, et al. Dissociated optic nerve fiber layer appearance of the fundus after idiopathic epiretinal membrane removal. Ophthalmology. 2001;108:2279-83.
48. Terasaki H, Miyake Y, Nomura R, et al. Focal macular ERGs in eyes after removal of macular ILM during macular hole surgery. Invest Ophthalmol Vis Sci. 2001;42:229-34.
49. Karacorlu M, Karacorlu S, Ozdemir H. Iatrogenic punctate chorioretinopathy after internal limiting membrane peeling. Am J Ophthalmol. 2003;135:178-82.
50. Nakata K, Ohji M, Ikuno Y, et al. Sub-retinal hemorrhage during internal limiting membrane peeling for a macular hole. Graefes Arch Clin Exp Ophthalmol. 2003;241:582-4.
51. Mitamura Y, Ohtsuka K. Relationship of dissociated optic nerve fiber layer appearance to internal limiting membrane peeling. Ophthalmology. 2005;112:1766-70.
52. Miura M, Elsner AE, Osako M, et al. Spectral imaging of the area of internal limiting membrane peeling. Retina. 2005;25:468-72.
53. Rubinstein A, Bates R, Benjamin L, et al. Iatrogenic eccentric full thickness macular holes following vitrectomy with ILM peeling for idiopathic macular holes. Eye. 2005;19:1333-5.
54. Mason JO, Feist RM, Albert MA. Eccentric macular holes after vitrectomy with peeling of epimacular proliferation. Retina. 2007;27:45-8.
55. Kadonosono K, Itoh N, Uchio E, et al. Staining of internal limiting membrane in macular hole surgery. Arch Ophthalmol. 2000;118:1116-8.
56. Gandorfer A, Haritoglou C, Gass CA, et al. Indocyanine green-assisted peeling of the internal limiting membrane may cause retinal damage. Am J Ophthalmol. 2001;132:431-3.
57. Ho JD, Tsai RJ, Chen SN, et al. Cytotoxicity of indocyanine green on retinal pigment epithelium: implications for macular hole surgery. Arch Ophthalmol. 2003;121:1423-9.
58. Lee JE, Yoon TJ, Oum BS, et al. Toxicity of indocyanine green injected into the subretinal space: subretinal toxicity of indocyanine green. Retina. 2003;23:675-81.
59. Sippy BD, Engelbrecht NE, Hubbard GB, et al. Indocyanine green effect on cultured human retinal pigment epithelial cells: implication for macular hole surgery. Am J Ophthalmol. 2001;132:433-5.
60. Weinberger AW, Kirchhof B, Mazinani BE, et al. Persistent indocyanine green (ICG) fluorescence 6 weeks after intraocular ICG administration for macular hole surgery. Graefes Arch Clin Exp Ophthalmol. 2001;239:388-90.
61. Yonemura N, Hirata A, Hasumura T, et al. Fundus changes corresponding to visual field defects after vitrectomy for macular hole. Ophthalmology. 2001;108:1638-43.
62. Engelbrecht NE, Freeman J, Sternberg P, et al. Retinal pigment epithelial changes after macular hole surgery with indocyanine green-assisted internal limiting membrane peeling. Am J Ophthalmol. 2002;133:89-94.
63. Haritoglou C, Gandorfer A, Gass CA, et al. Indocyanine green-assisted peeling of the internal limiting membrane in macular hole surgery affects visual outcome: a clinicopathologic correlation. Am J Ophthalmol. 2002;134:836-41.
64. Hirata A, Inomata Y, Kawaji T, et al. Persistent subretinal indocyanine green induces retinal pigment epithelium atrophy. Am J Ophthalmol. 2003;136:353-5.
65. Tadayoni R, Paques M, Girmens JF, et al. Persistence of fundus fluorescence after use of indocyanine green for macular surgery. Ophthalmology. 2003;110:604-8.
66. Ikagawa H, Yoneda M, Iwaki M, et al. Chemical toxicity of indocyanine green damages retinal pigment epithelium. Invest Ophthalmol Vis Sci. 2005;46:2531-9.
67. Uemoto R, Yamamoto S, Takeuchi S. Changes in retinal pigment epithelium after indocyanine green-assisted internal limiting lamina peeling during macular hole surgery. Am J Ophthalmol. 2005;140:752-5.
68. Paques M. Nonaxoplasmic transfer of indocyanine green into the optic nerve after intravitreal application. Retina. 2005;25:544.
69. Ferencz M, Somfai GM, Farkas A, et al. Functional assessment of the possible toxicity of indocyanine green dye in macular hole surgery. Am J Ophthalmol. 2006;142:765-70.
70. Rodrigues EB, Meyer CH. Meta-analysis of chromovitrectomy with indocyanine green in macular hole surgery. Ophthalmologica. 2008;222:123-9.
71. Gandorfer A, Haritoglou C, Kampik A. Toxicity of indocyanine green in vitreoretinal surgery. Dev Ophthalmol. 2008;42:69-81.
72. Lai MM, Williams GA. Anatomical and visual outcomes of idiopathic macular hole surgery with internal limiting

membrane removal using low-concentration indocyanine green. Retina. 2007;27:477-82.

73. Thompson JT, Haritoglu C, Kampik A, et al. Should indocyanine green be used to facilitate removal of the internal limiting membrane in macular hole surgery. Surv Ophthalmol. 2009;54:135-8.
74. Lesnik Oberstein SY, de Smet MD. Use of heavy trypan blue in macular hole surgery. Eye. 2010;24:1177-81.
75. Beutel J, Dahmen G, Ziegler A, et al. Internal limiting membrane peeling with indocyanine green or trypan blue in macular hole surgery: a randomized trial. Arch Ophthalmol. 2007;125:326-32.
76. Lee KL, Dean S, Guest S. A comparison of outcomes after indocyanine green and trypan blue assisted internal limiting membrane peeling during macular hole surgery. Br J Ophthalmol. 2005;89:420-4.
77. Enaida H, Hisatomi T, Goto Y, et al. Preclinical investigation of internal limiting membrane staining and peeling using intravitreal brilliant blue G. Retina. 2006;26:623-30.
78. Enaida H, Hisatomi T, Hata Y, et al. Brilliant blue G selectively stains the internal limiting membrane/brilliant blue G-assisted membrane peeling. Retina. 2006;26:631-6.
79. Remy M, Thaler S, Schumann RG, et al. An in vivo evaluation of Brilliant Blue G in animals and humans. Br J Ophthalmol. 2008;92:1142-7.
80. Kimura H, Kuroda S, Nagata M. Triamcinolone acetonide-assisted peeling of the internal limiting membrane. Am J Ophthalmol. 2004;137:172-3.
81. Karacorlu M, Ozdemir H, Arf Karacorlu S. Does intravitreal triamcinolone acetonide-assisted peeling of the internal limiting membrane effect the outcome of macular hole surgery? Graefes Arch Clin Exp Ophthalmol. 2005;243:754-7.
82. Shah GK, Rosenblatt BJ, Blinder KJ, et al. Triamcinolone-assisted internal limiting membrane peeling. Retina. 2005;25: 972-5.
83. Kampougeris G, Cheema R, McPherson R, et al. Safety of Triamcinolone acetonide (TA)-assisted pars plana vitrectomy in macular hole surgery. Eye. 2007;21:591-4.
84. Nomoto H, Shiraga F, Yamaji H, et al. Macular hole surgery with triamcinolone acetonide-assisted internal limiting membrane peeling: one-year results. Retina. 2008;28:427-32.
85. Sato Y, Isomae T. Macular hole surgery with internal limiting membrane removal, air tamponade, and 1-day prone positioning. Jpn J Ophthalmol. 2003;47:503-6.
86. Hasler PW, Prunte C. Early foveal recovery after macular hole surgery. Br J Ophthalmol. 2008;92:645-9.
87. Eckardt C, Eckert T, Eckardt U, et al. Macular hole surgery with air tamponade and optical coherence tomography-based duration of face-down positioning. Retina. 2008;28:1087-96.
88. Hasegawa Y, Hata Y, Mochizuki Y, et al. Equivalent tamponade by room air as compared with SF_6 after macular hole surgery. Graefes Arch Clin Exp Ophthalmol. 2009;247: 1455-9.
89. Guillaubey A, Malvitte L, Lafontaine PO, et al. Comparison of face-down and seated position after idiopathic macular hole surgery: a randomized clinical trial. Am J Ophthalmol. 2008;146:128-34.
90. Tadayoni R, Vicaut E, Devin F, et al. A randomized controlled trial of alleviated positioning after small macular hole surgery. Ophthalmology. 2011;118:150-5.
91. Rosa RH, Glaser BM, de la Cruz Z, et al. Clinicopathologic correlation of an untreated macular hole and a macular hole treated by vitrectomy, transforming growth factor-beta 2, and gas tamponade. Am J Ophthalmol. 1996;122:853-63.
92. Madreperla SA, Geiger GL, Funata M, et al. Clinicopathologic correlation of a macular hole treated by cortical vitreous peeling and gas tamponade. Ophthalmology. 1994;101:682-6.
93. Funata M, Wendel RT, de lCZ, et al. Clinicopathologic study of bilateral macular holes treated with pars plana vitrectomy and gas tamponade. Retina. 1992;12:289-98.
94. Yamana T, Kita M, Ozaki S, et al. The process of closure of experimental retinal holes in rabbit eyes. Graefes Arch Clin Exp Ophthalmol. 2000;238:81-7.
95. Sato H, Kawasaki R, Yamashita H. Observation of idiopathic full-thickness macular hole closure in early postoperative period as evaluated by optical coherence tomography. Am J Ophthalmol. 2003;136:185-7.
96. Kasuga Y, Arai J, Akimoto M, et al. Optical coherence tomograghy to confirm early closure of macular holes. Am J Ophthalmol. 2000;130:675-6.
97. Jumper JM, Gallemore RP, McCuen BWn, et al. Features of macular hole closure in the early postoperative period using optical coherence tomography. Retina. 2000;20:232-7.
98. Dayani PN, Maldonado R, Farsiu S, et al. Intraoperative use of handheld spectral domain optical coherence tomography imaging in macular surgery. Retina. 2009;29:1457-68.
99. Sano M, Shimoda Y, Hashimoto H, et al. Restored photoreceptor outer segment and visual recovery after macular hole closure. Am J Ophthalmol. 2009;147:313-8 e1.
100. Chang LK, Koizumi H, Spaide RF. Disruption of the photoreceptor inner segment-outer segment junction in eyes with macular holes. Retina. 2008;28:969-75.
101. Ko TH, Witkin AJ, Fujimoto JG, et al. Ultrahigh-resolution optical coherence tomography of surgically closed macular holes. Arch Ophthalmol. 2006;124:827-36.
102. Villate N, Lee JE, Venkatraman A, et al. Photoreceptor layer features in eyes with closed macular holes: optical coherence tomography findings and correlation with visual outcomes. Am J Ophthalmol. 2005;139:280-9.
103. Larsson J, Holm K, Lovestam-Adrian M. The presence of an operculum verified by optical coherence tomography and other prognostic factors in macular hole surgery. Acta Ophthalmol Scand. 2006;84:301-4.
104. Ruiz-Moreno JM, Staicu C, Pinero DP, et al. Optical coherence tomography predictive factors for macular hole surgery outcome. Br J Ophthalmol. 2008;92:640-4.
105. Ullrich S, Haritoglou C, Gass C, et al. Macular hole size as a prognostic factor in macular hole surgery. Br J Ophthalmol. 2002;86:390-3.

106. Ip MS, Baker BJ, Duker JS, et al. Anatomical outcomes of surgery for idiopathic macular hole as determined by optical coherence tomography. Arch Ophthalmol. 2002;120:29-35.
107. Gupta B, Laidlaw DA, Williamson TH, et al. Predicting visual success in macular hole surgery. Br J Ophthalmol. 2009;93:1488-91.
108. Scott IU, Moraczewski AL, Smiddy WE, et al. Long-term anatomic and visual acuity outcomes after initial anatomic success with macular hole surgery. Am J Ophthalmol. 2003;135:633-40.
109. Oh J, Smiddy W, Flynn H, et al. Photoreceptor inner/outer segment defect imaging by spectral domain OCT and visual prognosis after macular hole surgery. Invest Ophthalmol Vis Sci. 2010;51:1651-8.
110. Christensen UC, Kroyer K, Sander B, et al. Macular morphology and visual acuity after macular hole surgery with or without internal limiting membrane peeling. Br J Ophthalmol. 2010;94:41-7.
111. Richter-Mueksch S, Sacu S, Osarovsky-Sasin E, et al. Visual performance 3 years after successful macular hole surgery. Br J Ophthalmol. 2009;93:660-3.
112. Wendel RT, Patel AC, Kelly NE, et al. Vitreous surgery for macular holes. Ophthalmology. 1993;100:1671-6.
113. Park SS, Marcus DM, Duker JS, et al. Posterior segment complications after vitrectomy for macular hole. Ophthalmology. 1995;102:775-81.
114. Paques M, Massin P, Blain P, et al. Long-term incidence of reopening of macular holes. Ophthalmology. 2000;107:760-5.
115. Guillaubey A, Malvitte L, Lafontaine PO, et al. Incidence of retinal detachment after macular surgery: a retrospective study of 634 cases. Br J Ophthalmol. 2007;91:1327-30.
116. Thompson JT, Glaser BM, Sjaarda RN, et al. Progression of nuclear sclerosis and long-term visual results of vitrectomy with transforming growth factor beta-2 for macular holes. Am J Ophthalmol. 1995;119:48-54.
117. Sjaarda JT, Coll E. Improvement in visual acuity following cataract extraction after successfull macular hole surgery. ARVO; 1996.
118. Miller JH, Googe JM, Hoskins JC. Combined macular hole and cataract surgery. Am J Ophthalmol. 1997;123:705-7.
119. Demetriades AM, Gottsch JD, Thomsen R, et al. Combined phacoemulsification, intraocular lens implantation, and vitrectomy for eyes with coexisting cataract and vitreoretinal pathology. Am J Ophthalmol. 2003;135:291-6.
120. Paques M, Massin P, Santiago PY, et al. Late reopening of successfully treated macular holes. Br J Ophthalmol. 1997;81:658-62.
121. Christmas NJ, Smiddy WE, Flynn HW. Reopening of macular holes after initially successful repair. Ophthalmology. 1998;105:1835-8.
122. Kumagai K, Furukawa M, Ogino N, et al. Incidence and factors related to macular hole reopening. Am J Ophthalmol. 2010;149:127-32.

Vitreoretinal Surgery for Myopic Foveoschisis

26

Yasushi Ikuno

Introduction

Myopic foveoschisis is characterized by retinoschisis and sometimes localized retinal detachment. The retina normally is only elevated slightly and it is challenging to make an accurate diagnosis using simply fundus microscopy. Optical coherence tomography (OCT) has demonstrated the microstructural changes in myopic foveoschisis, but before the advent of OCT, the retinal pathologies were not well understood. For instance, in the 1950s, Phillips described a case of a localized retinal detachment without a macular hole,[1] which was presumed to be a subtype of myopic foveoschisis. In addition, the textbook by Duke-Elder contains a picture of a histologic section of a highly myopic case showing retinoschisis.[2] However, it was extremely difficult to make a real-time diagnosis of foveoschisis without OCT *in vivo* and it was not a curable disease. OCT has enabled imaging of the micropathologies of myopic foveoschisis and the disease is now curable.

Clinical Manifestations of Myopic Foveoschisis

Incidence

High myopia, normally defined as a refractive error exceeding -6 diopters, is a major cause of visual loss in many ethnic groups and countries. Excessive elongation of the axial length is a hallmark of several specific macular diseases due to dimensional changes such as choroidal neovascularization, macular holes with retinal detachment and myopic chorioretinal atrophies.[3] Myopic foveoschisis is a major vision threatening condition in highly myopic eyes. It is more commonly observed in eyes with posterior staphyloma, reportedly with an incidence of about 9%.[4]

Clinical Features

Myopic foveoschisis typically causes metamorphopsia when only retinoschisis is present. A relative central scotoma may be seen when foveal detachment occurs. An absolute scotoma can be recognized if a macular hole is developed. Retinoschisis is sometimes very shallow and difficult to find using only slit-lamp-based fundus microscopy (Figs 26.1A and B). With disease progression, the retinal elevation increases and is more distinguishable on fundus examination. However, OCT is still critical to confirm the extent of the retinal detachment and the presence or absence of small macular holes.

Optical Coherence Tomography Findings

In 1999, the details of the micropathology of myopic foveoschisis were seen first using OCT.[5] In that study, macular retinoschisis or retinal detachment was observed in 12 of 32 highly myopic eyes, indicating that those pathologies

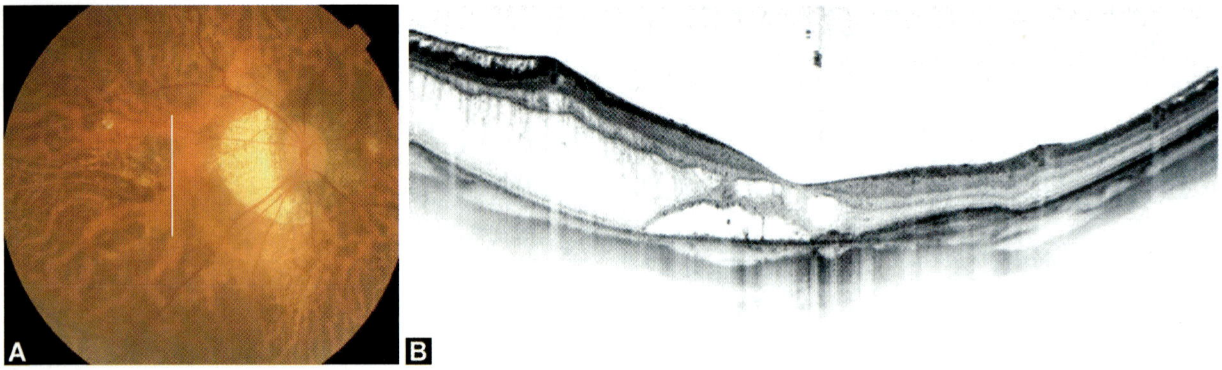

▲ **Figures 26.1A and B**

Typical appearance of myopic foveoschisis. (A) Fundus photograph shows a slight but not prominent retinal elevation involving the macula; (B) OCT shows a foveal retinal detachment and retinoschisis around

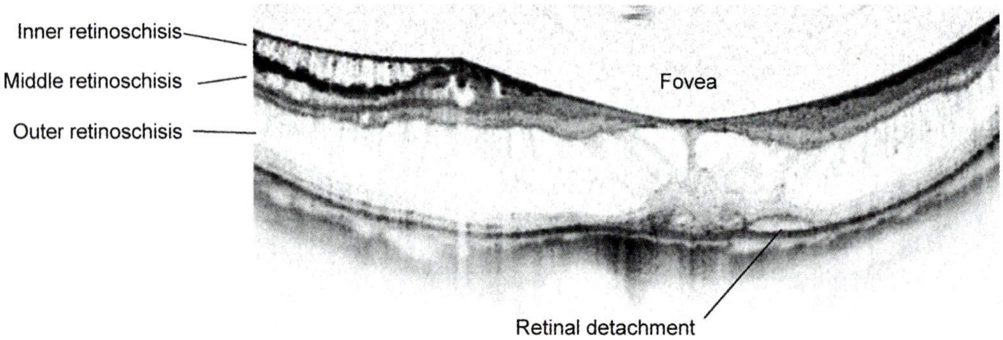

▲ **Figure 26.2**

Microstructure of myopic foveoschisis. Optical coherence tomography shows multiple retinoschisis at various layers. An ILM detachment (or inner retinoschisis) is a separation between the ILM and retinal nerve fiber layer, middle retinoschisis between the inner nuclear layer and ganglion cell layer, and outer retinoschisis between the inner and outer nuclear layers

are common in highly myopic eyes. A typical OCT finding is retinoschisis (a split in the retina) at the posterior pole. Retinoschisis typically is located at the outer plexiform layer (outer retinoschisis), inner plexiform layer (middle retinoschisis), or beneath the internal limiting membrane (ILM) (inner retinoschisis or ILM detachment) (Fig. 26.2). Foveal detachment, a separation from the retinal pigment epithelium (RPE), is sometimes seen and is an important decision making sign for vitreous surgery. Not only retinoschisis but also many other structural changes are observed. For instance, cystic changes and a lamellar hole might be observed together with retinoschisis.[6]

Pathogenesis

The tractional force at the inner retinal layer along with growth of posterior staphyloma is considered a main cause of myopic foveoschisis. Besides vitreous cortex adhering to the retinal surface, several factors have been identified, including epiretinal membranes, ILM rigidity and retinal vascular sclerotic changes.[7-9] For instance, epiretinal membranes are seen more frequently in histologic sections from excised ILMs during surgery.[10] Retinal vascular microfolds, which often are visualized in vertical OCT images of foveoschisis, seem to elevate the retina locally along the vessels.[8,11] Those factors make the inner retina inflexible compared to the outer retina within an area of posterior staphyloma, resulting in inward tractional force at the inner retina. Thus, the goal of surgical intervention is to remove these factors to reattach the retina.

Management of Myopic Foveoschisis

Natural Course

The natural course of myopic foveoschisis is not fully understood; however, it is generally agreed that the initial event is development of retinoschisis at the posterior staphyloma. An eye with only retinoschisis but not foveal detachment or macular hole is referred to as "the retinoschisis type" and it can sometimes be stable for many years. Patients can be asymptomatic if the retinoschisis is present only outside of the fovea. However, once the macula is involved, patients complain of metamorphopsia. If the tractional force is sufficient to lift the full thickness retina from the RPE, the retinal detachment starts and progresses to a foveal detachment. Retinal detachment mostly begins around or at the fovea and becomes more extensive with time. If the fovea is torn, a macular hole is generated and the extent of the retinal detachment is accelerated.

Myopic foveoschisis is also an important preclinical condition for macular holes with retinal detachment in highly myopic eyes, which has a very poor prognosis despite vitreous surgery. Once a macular hole and retinal detachment occur, the mean postoperative Visual acuity (VA) is about 20/200.[12] It has not been well investigated; however, 20–50% of cases of myopic foveoschisis develop a macular hole and/or a retinal detachment in 2–3 years.[13,14]

Treatment

Scleral Buckling

Few reports have described successful foveal reattachment by macular buckling.[15] However, the results from the large case series have not been well investigated. Therefore, the safety and efficacy of this procedure have not been confirmed.

Vitrectomy

Vitrectomy is the most commonly accepted procedure for treating myopic foveoschisis. A Japanese group first described the efficacy of surgical intervention for myopic foveoschisis.[16] Several subsequent reports including ours confirmed this.[17-20] The efficacy of vitrectomy currently is accepted; however, the timing and the detailed intraoperative procedure is still controversial.

When deciding to perform surgery, the patient must be symptomatic. There is no consensus about the level of the preoperative VAs; however, author normally performs surgeries on patients with VA of 20/40 or worse, after considering risks and benefits. Only retinoschisis with no foveal detachment (retinoschisis type) sometimes causes metamorphopsia, which patients complain about; however, the rate of substantial visual improvement is as low as 50% (Figs 26.3A and B).[21] As discussed, the advanced stage, the foveal detachment type, is associated with a higher rate of visual improvement. Therefore, the retinoschisis type is not the best stage to perform surgery in terms of patient satisfaction.

It is recommended to wait for the foveal detachment sign and follow-up on the OCT findings because of the higher visual improvement rate. We reported that up to 80% of patients had a substantial visual improvement (Fig. 26.3).[21] At this stage, the VA is usually worse than 20/40 and patients are mostly symptomatic.

A macular hole sometimes develops soon after foveal detachment. Once that happens, there is little chance for visual improvement and good vision even with anatomic success. In addition, the macular hole is unlikely to close with surgery if accompanied by foveoschisis.[22] It is critical to rule out the presence of a macular hole preoperatively. However, a macular hole can be very small and hard to detect even with careful observation with OCT.[23] It is difficult to predict how soon the macular hole occurs. Sometimes it takes years, but sometimes just weeks. We recommend making a surgical decision immediately and performing surgery without delay in this stage.

Surgical Procedures

Macular surgery in highly myopic eyes is sometimes difficult, because the multiple layers of the membrane must be removed. The membrane must be identified with adjuncts and accurately and safely removed with maximum care. The pearls for this procedure have been described previously.[24]

First, core vitrectomy must be performed to make room to create a posterior vitreous detachment. The vitreous cortex then is separated from the inner retinal surface. Triamcinolone is useful for visualization since the vitreous cortex is typically

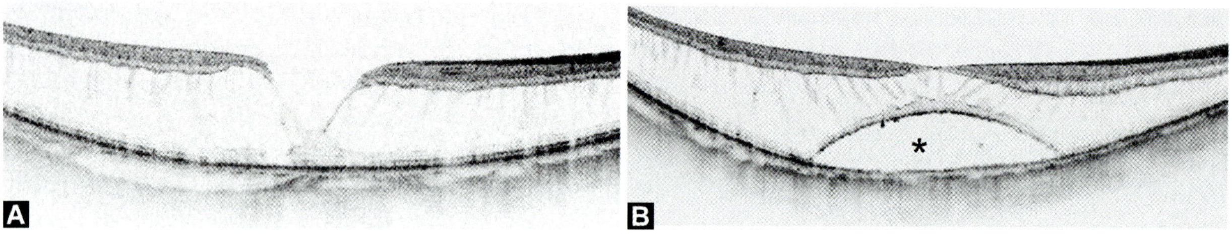

▲ **Figures 26.3A and B**

The OCT subtypes of myopic foveoschisis. (A) Retinoschisis type is simple retinoschisis with no retinal detachment; (B) Foveal detachment type is a more advanced subtype with a foveal detachment (asterisk) with surrounding retinoschisis

thin and adheres tightly to the retina. If the cortex is sufficiently thick, a vitreous cutter with active suction can be used. However, if the cortex is very thin, using a vitreous cutter increases the risk of retinal breaks. Author uses the Tano diamond-dusted membrane scraper (DDMS), which facilitates gentle separation of the cortex from the retina. Vitreous separation must be started at the posterior pole, where there is sometimes space between the cortex and the retina. Once a small vitreous detachment is created, it can be extended towards the periphery using the DDMS or vitreous cutter. If the cortex is membrane-like, the intravitreal forceps can be used to grasp the membrane. The vitreous sometimes adheres tightly to the retina in the midperiphery. Author does not extend the vitreous separation beyond it because of the high risk of a retinal break. A paravascular microhole is sometimes recognized and any traction must be removed from around the hole. Vitreous or any epiretinal membrane must be removed.

The necessity for ILM peeling is still controversial; however, at our institution peeling is routine, because ILM separation is often observed in OCT images of myopic foveoschisis,[25] indicating that the ILM is causative in most patients. Triamcinolone can be used in patients with mild chorioretinal atrophy. However, authors experience is that triamcinolone has not worked appropriately in more than half of patients, because it does not contrast adequately with the whitish atrophy. The highly myopic retina is often extremely thin and grasping the outer retina easily causes retinal tears. In those cases, we normally use 0.25% indocyanine green for safety. ILM is normally peeled for two to three disc diameters.

The requirement for gas tamponade is also controversial, since this is basically caused by tractional component and releasing only the retina is supposedly sufficient to cause reattachment. However, it often takes more than 1 year to attain foveal reattachment and delayed reattachment may damage the photoreceptors more, resulting in unfavorable macular function. Gas tamponade and prone positioning for a couple of days push the fovea back onto the RPE promptly and it may accelerate photoreceptor recovery. Application of just air or 20% sulfur fluororide tamponade is routinely performed at our institution.

Complications

Besides the general complication of vitreous surgery, such as infectious endophthalmitis, cataract progression and retinal detachment, postoperative macular hole formation occurs in less than 5% of patients. The causes have been poorly described and the relation to ILM peeling or gas tamponade is unclear. Extreme stretching of the retina after reattachment is thought to cause a retinal break at the fovea.

Myopic foveoschisis results basically from traction by several mechanical factors. The rationale for vitreous surgery is to eliminate those factors and a favorable surgical outcome is provided in the foveal detachment type. The optimal surgical procedure is still under investigation; however, surgery must be planned without delay before a macular hole develops.

References

1. Phillips CI. Retinal detachment at the posterior pole. Br J Ophthalmol. 1958;42:749-53.
2. Duke-Elder S, Abrams D. Pathological myopia. Duke-Elder's system of ophthalmology vol. V, Refractive Optics and Refraction. London: Henry Kimpton; 1970. p. 308.

3. Soubrane G, Coscas GJ. Choroidal neovascular membrane in degenerative myopia. In: Ryan SJ (Ed). Retina, 4th edition. St. Louis: Mosby; 2005. pp. 1136-52.
4. Baba T, Ohno-Matsui K, Futagami S, et al. Prevalence and characteristics of foveal retinal detachment without macular hole in high myopia. Am J Ophthalmol. 2003;135:338-42.
5. Takano M, Kishi S. Foveal retinoschisis and retinal detachment in severely myopic eyes with posterior staphyloma. Am J Ophthalmol. 1999;128:472-6.
6. Benhamou N, Massin P, Haouchine B, et al. Macular retinoschisis in highly myopic eyes. Am J Ophthalmol. 2002;133:794-800.
7. Panozzo G, Mercanti A. Optical coherence tomography findings in myopic traction maculopathy. Arch Ophthalmol. 2004;122:1455-60.
8. Ikuno Y, Gomi F, Tano Y. Potent retinal arteriolar traction as a possible cause of myopic foveoschisis. Am J Ophthalmol. 2005;139:462-7.
9. Sayanagi K, Ikuno Y, Tano Y. Tractional internal limiting membrane detachment in highly myopic eyes. Am J Ophthalmol. 2006;142:850-2.
10. Bando H, Ikuno Y, Choi JS, et al. Ultrastructure of internal limiting membrane in myopic foveoschisis. Am J Ophthalmol. 2005;139:197-9.
11. Sayanagi K, Ikuno Y, Gomi F, Tano Y. Retinal vascular microfolds in highly myopic eyes. Am J Ophthalmol. 2005;139:658-63.
12. Nakanishi H, Kuriyama S, Saito I, et al. Prognostic factor analysis in pars plana vitrectomy for retinal detachment attributable to macular hole in high myopia: a multicenter study. Am J Ophthalmol. 2008;146:198-204.
13. Gaucher D, Haouchine B, Tadayoni R, et al. Long-term follow-up of high myopic foveoschisis: natural course and surgical outcome. Am J Ophthalmol. 2007;143:455-62.
14. Shimada N, Ohno-Matsui K, Baba T, et al. Natural course of macular retinoschisis in highly myopic eyes without macular hole or retinal detachment. Am J Ophthalmol. 2006;142:497-500.
15. Baba T, Tanaka S, Maesawa A, et al. Scleral buckling with macular plombe for eyes with myopic macular retinoschisis and retinal detachment without macular hole. Am J Ophthalmol. 2006;142:483-7.
16. Ishikawa F, Ogino N, Okita K, et al. Vitrectomy for macular detachment without macular hole in highly myopic eyes. Journal of the Eye (Atarashii Ganka). 2001;18:953-6.
17. Kobayashi H, Kishi S. Vitreous surgery for highly myopic eyes with foveal detachment and retinoschisis. Ophthalmology. 2003;110:1702-7.
18. Ikuno Y, Sayanagi K, Ohji M, et al. Vitrectomy and internal limiting membrane peeling for myopic foveoschisis. Am J Ophthalmol. 2004;137:719-24.
19. Hirakata A, Hida T. Vitrectomy for myopic posterior retinoschisis or foveal detachment. Jpn J Ophthalmol. 2006;50:53-61.
20. Kwok AK, Lai TY, Yip WW. Vitrectomy and gas tamponade without internal limiting membrane peeling for myopic foveoschisis. Br J Ophthalmol. 2005;89:1180-3.
21. Ikuno Y, Sayanagi K, Soga K, et al. Foveal anatomical status and surgical results in vitrectomy for myopic foveoschisis. Jpn J Ophthalmol. 2008;52:269-76.
22. Ikuno Y, Tano Y. Vitrectomy for macular holes associated with myopic foveoschisis. Am J Ophthalmol. 2006;141:774-6.
23. Ikuno Y, Tano Y. Early macular holes with retinoschisis in highly myopic eyes. Am J Ophthalmol. 2003;136:741-4.
24. Sakaguchi H, Ikuno Y, Choi JS, et al. Multiple components of epiretinal tissues detected by triamcinolone and indocyanine green in macular hole and retinal detachment as a result of high myopia. Am J Ophthalmol. 2004;138:1079-81.
25. Sayanagi K, Morimoto Y, Ikuno Y, et al. Spectral-domain optical coherence tomographic findings in myopic foveoschisis. Retina. 2010;30:623-8.

27

Submacular Hemorrhage Removal and Pneumatic Displacement of Submacular Hemorrhage

Osamu Sawada, Masahito Ohji

Introduction

Submacular hemorrhage is defined as hemorrhage located in the space between the retinal pigment epithelium and the neurosensory retina involving macula. Submacular hemorrhage is a complication of a range of ocular pathologies like age-related macular degeneration (AMD),[1] polypoidal choroidal vasculopathy (PCV),[2] retinal artery macroaneurysm,[1] pathogenic myopia[3] and traumatic choroidal rupture.[4] Increasing size, thickness and duration of the submacular hemorrhage result in a poor prognosis in visual acuity.[4,5] The natural history of untreated submacular hemorrhage is especially poor in patients with submacular hemorrhage resulting from AMD.[1,4,5]

Choroidal neovascularization (CNV) is common cause of subretinal hemorrhage. Ibanez et al.[1] reported a series of 47 consecutive cases of submacular hemorrhage. In this report, 41 of 47 cases were secondary to AMD and others were secondary to retinal arterial macroaneurysm, presumed ocular histoplasmosis syndrome, angioid streaks and idiopathic condition. Myopic choroidal neovascularization and PCV have been reported to cause submacular hemorrhage.[2,3] Trauma caused the choroidal rupture in some cases and the development of CNV at the rupture site. When the CNV due to choroidal rupture occurred in the macular area, submacular hemorrhage might be complicated.[4] The visual outcome, in the natural course of submacular hemorrhage with AMD, was very poor.[1,4,5] In a natural course series of 60 cases of submacular hemorrhage secondary to AMD reported by Scupola et al.[5] visual acuity ranged from 20/70 to light perception (mean 20/240) at the initial examination and had worsened in 80% in the eyes with a mean final visual acuity of 20/1250 (range from 20/100 to light perception). Size and thickness of the hemorrhage were important prognosis factors and influenced negatively the natural prognosis.

Poor prognosis due to submacular hemorrhage is contributed to several factors. At first, visual dysfunction is induced by clot formation with diffusion disturbance between photoreceptor and retinal pigment epithelium. In the second phase, photoreceptors are damaged directly by toxic iron ions from erythrocyte degradation,[6-8] ripped by fibrin construction.[9] Irreversible change in the outer retinal layers was observed within 24 hours after subretinal injection of blood in the rabbit model,[10] 3 days with retraction of fibrin strands in cat model.[9] Experimental reports with animal models showed that subretinal blood started to cause significant damage within 24 hours and experimental reports in a rabbit model with subretinal hemorrhage demonstrated irreversible damage to the photoreceptors within 7 days.[10] Existence of blood in subretinal space prevent the exchange of nutrients, oxygen and metabolites between the retina and choriocapillaris, iron released from the hemorrhage induces toxic effect to the retinal circulation and fibrin contraction derived from subretinal clot results in the irreversible damage of photoreceptor.

Therefore, to prevent irreversible permanent damage of retina, rapid removal or displacement of submacular hemorrhage from macula is recommended within 7 days after the bleeding onset. To prevent the irreversible vision loss caused by the submacular hemorrhage, effective options of surgical or pharmacological treatments have been attempted.[11-26] Author described some common treatments to be effective.

Surgical Steps

Initial surgical attempts involved standard three port vitrectomy, followed by making a retinotomy and removal of subretinal clot by subretinal forceps. The results in this attempt were disappointing, with few cases showing improvement in visual acuity.[11,12] Since the results in direct surgical approach were disappointing, available adjuvants were studied to assist removal surgery of subretinal clots. After the safety in subretinal injection of tissue plasminogen activator (tPA) was demonstrated in experimental models of subretinal hemorrhage in animals,[6,7,27] Peyman et al.[13] for the first time reported the experience of patients with submacular hemorrhage using tPA as surgical adjuvant. They performed a standard pars plana vitrectomy, injected tPA into the subretinal space. After the dissolution of clot, they removed the retinal hemorrhage from retinal hole via irrigation of balanced salt solution. In this report, visual outcome was a disappointing in cases with AMD. The following reports by Lewis and Lim et al.[14,15] presented the visual outcome favorably compared to surgical treatment without tPA. Lewis[14] reported the improvement in visual acuity in 20 eyes out of 24 eyes with AMD and the worsening in one eye. Lim et al.[15] reported that visual acuity improved or remained unchanged in 11 eyes of 16 eyes with AMD and decreased in 5 eyes.

To evaluate the benefit of vitrectomy for removal of submacular hemorrhage, the Submacular Surgery Trials (SST) Group B was started in 1997. This study was multicenter, prospective, randomized clinical trial and the purpose was to determine whether vitrectomy to remove submacular hemorrhage secondary to AMD improved visual outcome versus observation over 2 years or more. Major inclusion criteria in SST Group B included evidence of AMD, blood more than equal to 50% of lesion, blood or choroidal neovascularization extends through center of fovea, size of lesion more than equal to 3.5 macular photocoagulation study (MPS) disc areas and less than equal to 9 MPS disc areas, more than equal to 75% of lesion posterior to equator and visual acuity range 20/100 to light perception. The defined surgical method was a standard three port pars plana vitrectomy, the making of a retinotomy, manual extraction of the blood clot so the fovea was free of thick subretinal hemorrhage and manual extraction of CNV when possible. The use of tPA and the choice of long acting postoperative tamponade were left to the surgeon's own choice. Three hundred thirty six patients were enrolled in the SST Group B Trial, 168 were assigned to each treatment arm. Loss of 2 lines or more of visual acuity occurred in 56% of surgery eyes, versus 59% of observation eyes examined at 24 months. The study group concluded that submacular surgery did not increase the chance of stable or improved visual acuity. Additionally, of initially phakic eyes, 44% in the surgery arm compared with 6% in the observation arm had undergone cataract surgery in 24 months. Sixteen percent in the surgery arm compared with 2% in the observation arm had a rhegmatogenous retinal detachment. Otherwise, although severe loss of visual acuity was not the primary outcome of interest in the study, surgery prevented such loss with occurring 36% in the observation arm versus 21% in the surgery arm at the 24 month examination. SST research group concluded that submacular surgery as performed in the SST Group B Trial did not increase the chance of stable or improved visual acuity and was associated with a high risk of rhegmatogenous retinal detachment, but reduced the risk of severe visual acuity loss in comparison with observation[16]

In 1996 Heriot[17] presented the results from a small clinical series of a novel, minimally invasive, outpatient procedure of intravitreal tPA and perfluoropropane (C_3F_8) gas injection for the treatment of submacular hemorrhage. Submacular hemorrhage would be liquefied enzymatically and then be pneumatically displaced inferiorly in the subretinal space without vitrectomy. Indeed, it had been presented that clinical evidence of clot lysis in subretinal hemorrhage after intravitreal injection of tPA in several experimental models.[28,29] Hesse et al.[18] reported their experience with intravitreal tPA and perfluoropropane gas injection of massive subretinal hemorrhage in 11 patients presenting with AMD. The described method involved intravitreal injection of tPA in a dose of 50 or 100 mg and injection of C_3F_8 or sulfur hexafluoride (SF_6) gas, either immediately or the following day after tPA injection following by 24 hours of face-down positioning. In this series, visual acuity improved by two or more lines in 5 of the 11 eyes (45%). Recently Chen et al.[19] reported a retrospective clinical case series examining 104 eyes of intravitreal tPA and expansile gas injection for submacular hemorrhage. In this study, 2 Snellen lines or more improvement were achieved postoperatively in 51% at 1 week, 63% at 3 months and 64% at 12 months and the complications included breakthrough vitreous hemorrhage in 8% and retinal detachment in 3%.

The details of retinal toxicity of intravitreal tPA in human beings are uncertain. Dose-dependent retinal toxicity of intravitreal tPA has been reported in rabbit and cat eyes with intravitreal injection of tPA greater or equal to 50 µg.[30-32] In human there was presented a case report of retinal toxicity in a patient with submacular hemorrhage complicating idiopathic polypoidal choroidal vasculopathy treated with two intravitreal injections (50 µg each) of tPA 3 days apart and by pneumatic displacement. The clinical condition in this case included diffuse retinal pigment epithelium (RPE) perturbations, poor recovery of visual acuity and decreased photopic and scotopic A-waves and B-waves in electroretinogram.[33]

Ohji et al.[20] presented an alternative in-office method, pneumatic displacement without intravitreal injection of tPA. They described a small case series of five patients treated with pure C_3F_8 gas (0.3–0.4 mL) and face down positioning. Submacular hemorrhage was displaced completely or partially in all five patients. This treatment was simple and safe and lead to improvement in visual acuity. Ron et al.[21] reported a 24 case series with submacular hemorrhage secondary to AMD treated by injection of C_3F_8 (11 patients) or SF_6 gas (13 patients). This case series showed a statistically significant improvement in mean visual acuity.[21] In a 20 case series with submacular hemorrhage secondary to various etiologies presented by Gopalakrishan et al.[22] mean visual acuity improved from 1.6–0.72 logarithm of the minimum angle of resolution, which was statistically significant.

Several modified surgical treatments have been proposed for management of submacular hemorrhage. Haupert et al.[23] reported an alternative technique to achieve maximal clot lysis and displacement of subretinal hemorrhage from fovea while minimizing the risk of trauma to retina and RPE. They performed pars plana vitrectomy, subretinal tPA injection without clot manipulation and fluid-gas exchange with postoperative prone positioning for management of thick submacular hemorrhage in 11 patients with AMD. In their case series, subretinal hemorrhage was displaced from the fovea in all 11 cases with improvement of visual acuity in eight (73%) cases, no change in one case and worsening in two cases. Olivier et al.[24] described a minor modified procedure. They injected tPA used by 39-gauge flexible translocation cannula to create a bullous retinal detachment encompassing the entire blood clot. In this series of 29 eyes in 28 patients with thick submacular hemorrhage secondary to AMD, total subfoveal blood displacement was achieved in 25 eyes, with subtotal displacement in the others. 17 eyes improved more than 2 lines of visual acuity, whereas 3 had lost more than 2 lines and difference in between preoperative and 3 months postoperative mean visual acuity was statistically significant.

When a subretinal hemorrhage develops massively and extends peripherally to form large hemorrhagic retinal detachments, it is hard to display or remove the subretinal clots using the conventional techniques. Oshima et al.[25] performed a newly modified surgical procedure consisting of intravitreal injection of tPA 12–24 hours preoperatively and subsequent vitrectomy to force the subretinal hemorrhage through the peripheral small retinotomy using perfluorocarbon liquid (PFCL) and long-acting gas for management of eight eyes in eight patients with a massive subretinal hemorrhage. Most of subretinal hemorrhage was evacuated to the vitreous cavity via the peripheral retinotomy using PFCL. Residual subretinal hemorrhage if existed was drained from anterior chamber at the bedside after prone positioning overnight. The final visual acuity improved in seven eyes of eight eyes.[25]

Neovascular AMD is one of the most common causes of submacular hemorrhage. With the widespread use of intravitreal bevacizumab in treatment of neovascular AMD, Chawla et al.[26] reported the efficacy of treating of submacular hemorrhage secondary to choroidal neovascular membrane with pneumatic displacement using SF_6 gas and intravitreal injection of bevacizumab. In this series in four patients with submacular hemorrhage, postoperative best corrected visual acuity improved in all cases with complete or partial displacement of submacular hemorrhage out of the foveal area.

To avoid the permanent irreversible damage to retina in macular area, removal or displacement of the blood from subretinal space is required. The pneumatic displacement with/without intravitreal injection of tPA might been recommended for the treatment of submacular hemorrhage because this technique is simple, safe, effective to displace the subretinal hemorrhage and improve the visual acuity. However when the duration of submacular hemorrhage was long and it is difficult to display the subretinal clots using pneumatic technique, surgical treatment with tPA is selected. Otherwise when a subretinal hemorrhage is extremely massive and extends peripherally to form large hemorrhagic retinal detachments, it might been recommended to perform

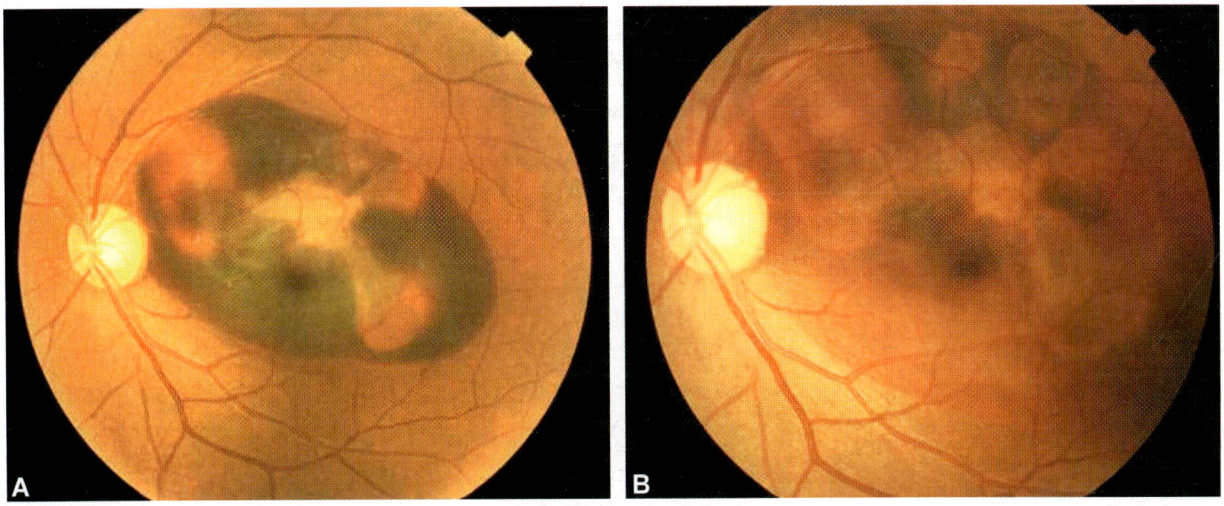

▲ **Figures 27.1A and B**

(A) A 56-year-old man experienced sudden painless loss of vision in the left eye. LogMAR VA was 1.00. Submacular hemorrhage secondary to polypoidal choroidal vasculopathy was detected; (B) This eye underwent injection of 0.4 mL 100% C_3F_8 gas with face-down positioning. LogMAR VA improved to 0.82 one month later

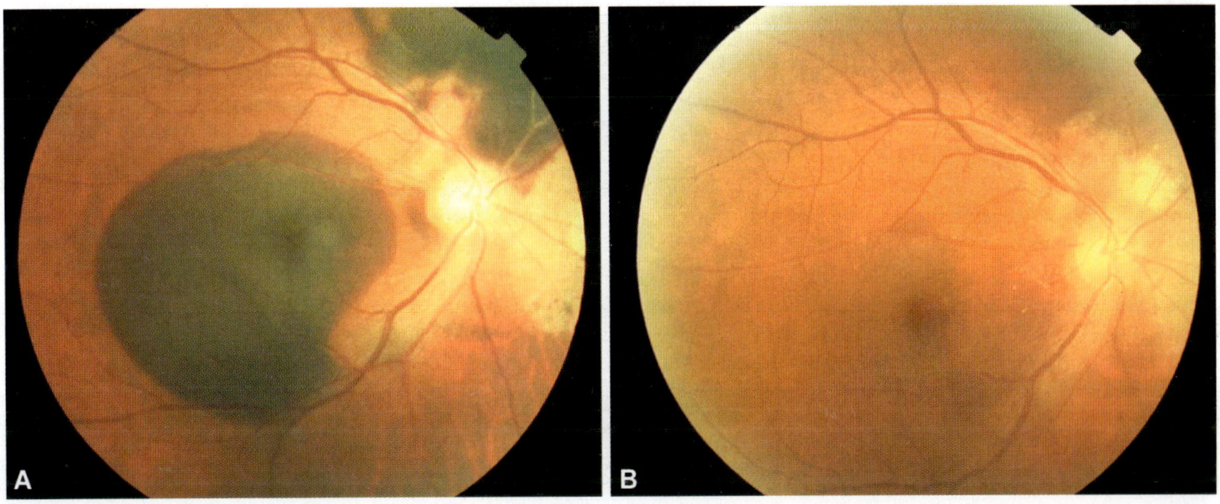

▲ **Figures 27.2A and B**

(A) A 67-year-old man experienced sudden painless loss of vision in the right eye. LogMAR VA was 1.70. Submacular hemorrhage secondary to polypoidal choroidal vasculopathy was detected; (B) This eye underwent injection of 0.3 mL 100% C_3F_8 gas and 25 mg of tPA with face-down positioning. LogMAR VA improved to 0.82 one month later

a modified surgical procedure consisting of intravitreal injection of tPA preoperatively and subsequent vitrectomy to force the subretinal hemorrhage through the peripheral small retinotomy using PFCL and long-acting gas (Figs 27.1 and 27.2).

References

1. Ibanez HE, Williams DF, Thomas MA, et al. Surgical management of submacular hemorrhage: a series of consecutive cases. Arch Ophthalmol. 1995;113:62-9.

2. Shiraga F, Matsuo T, Yokoe S, et al. Surgical treatment of submacular hemorrhage associated with idiopathic polypoidal choroidal vasculopathy. Am J Ophthalmol. 1999;128:147-54.
3. Hayasaka S, Uchida M, Setogawa T. Subretinal hemorrhage with or without choroidal neovascularization in the maculas of patients with pathologic myopia. Graefes Arch Exp Ophthalmol. 1990;228:277-80.
4. Bennett SR, Folk JC, Blodi CF, et al. Factors prognostic of visual outcome in patients with subretinal hemorrhage. Am J Ophthalmol. 1990;109:33-7.
5. Scupola A, Coscas G, Soubrane G, et al. Natural history of macular subretinal hemorrhage in age-related macular degeneration. Ophthalmologica. 1999;213:97-102.
6. Lewis H, Resnick SC, Flannery JG, et al. Tissue plasminogen activator treatment of experimental subretinal hemorrhage. Am J Ophthalmol. 1991;111:197-204.
7. Johnson MW, Olsen KR, Hernandez E. Tissue plasminogen activator treatment of experimental subretinal hemorrhage. Retina. 1991;11:250-8.
8. Cibis PA, Yamashita T. Experimental aspects of ocular siderosis and hemosiderosis. Am J Ophthalmol. 1959;48:465-80.
9. Toth CA, Morse LS, Hjielmeland LM, et al. Fibrin directs early retinal damage after experimental subretinal hemorrhage. Arch Ophthalmol. 1991;109:723-9.
10. Glatt H, Machemer R. Experimental subretinal hemorrhage in rabbits. Am J Ophthalmol. 1982;94:762-73.
11. Wade EC, Flynn HW, Olsen KR, et al. Subretinal hemorrhage management by pars plana vitrectomy and internal drainage. Arch Ophthalmol. 1990;108:973-8.
12. Vander JF, Federman JL, Greven C, et al. Surgical removal of massive subretinal hemorrhage associated with age-related macular degeneration. Ophthalmology. 1991;98:23-7.
13. Peyman GA, Nelson NC, Alturki W, et al. Tissue plasminogen activating factor assisted removal of subretinal hemorrhage. Ophthalmic Surg. 1991;22:575-82.
14. Lewis H. Intraoperative fibrinolysis of submacular hemorrhage with tissue plasminogen activator and surgical drainage. Am J Ophthalmol. 1994;118:559-68.
15. Lim JI, Drews-Botsch C, Sternberg P, et al. Submacular hemorrhage removal. Ophthalmology. 1995;102:1393-9.
16. Submacular Surgery Trials (SST) Group. Surgery for hemorrhagic choroidal neovascular lesions of age-related macular degeneration: ophthalmic findings: SST report no. 13. Ophthalmology. 2004;111:1993-2006.
17. Heriot WJ. Intravitreal gas and tPA: an outpatient procedure injection for subretinal haemorrhage. In: Vail Vitrectomy Meeting;1996; Vail, CO.
18. Hesse L, Schmidt J, Kroll P. Management of acute submacular hemorrhage using recombinant tissue plasminogen activator and gas. Graefe's Arch Clin Exp Ophthalmol. 1999;237:273-7.
19. Chen CY, Hooper C, Chiu D, et al. Management of submacular hemorrhage with plasminogen activator and expansile gas. Retina. 2007;27:321-8.
20. Ohji M, Saito Y, Hayashi A, et al. Pneumatic displacement of subretinal hemorrhage without tissue plasminogen activator. Arch Ophthalmol. 1998;116:1326-32.
21. Ron Y, Ehrlich R, Axer-Siegel R, et al. Pneumatic displacement of submacular hemorrhage due to age-related macular degeneration. Ophthalmologica. 2007;221:57-61.
22. Gopalakrishan M, Giridhar A, Bhat S, et al. Pneumatic displacement of submacular hemorrhage. Retina. 2007;27:329-334.
23. Haupert CL, McCuen BW, Jaffe GJ, et al. Pars plana vitrectomy, subretinal injection of tissue plasminogen activator, and fluid-gas exchange for displacement of thick submacular hemorrhage in age-related macular degeneration. Am J Ophthalmol. 2001;131:208-15.
24. Oliver S, Chow DR, Packo KH, et al. Subretinal recombinant tissue plasminogen activator injection and pneumatic displacement of thick submacular hemorrhage in age-related macular degeneration. Ophthalmology. 2004;111:1201-8.
25. Oshima Y, Ohji M, Tano Y. Pars plana vitrectoy with peripheral retinotomy after injection of preoperative intravitreal tissue plasminogen activator: a modified procedure to drain massive subretinal haemorrhage. Br J Ophthalmol. 2007;91:193-8.
26. Chawla S, Misra V, Khemchandani M. Pneumatic displacement and intravitreal bevacizumab: a new approach for management of submacular hemorrhage in choroidal neovascular membrane. Indian J Ophthalmol. 2009;57:155-7.
27. Benner JD, Hay A, Landers MB, et al. Fibrinolytic-assisted removal of experimental subretinal hemorrhage within seven days reduces outer retinal degeneration. Ophthalmology. 1994;101:672-81.
28. Coll GE, Sparrow JR, Marinovic A, Chang S. Effect of intravitreal tissue plasminogen activator on experimental subretinal hemorrhage. Retina. 1995;15:319-26.
29. Boone DE, Boldt HC, Ross RD, et al. The use of intravitreal tissue plasminogen activator in the treatment of experimental subretinal hemorrhage in the pig model. Retina. 1996;16:518-24.
30. Johnson MW, Olsen KR, Hernandez E, et al. Retinal toxicity of recombinant tissue plasminogen activator in rabbit. Arch Ophthalmol. 1990;108:259-63.
31. Irvine WD, Johnson MW, Hernandez E, et al. Retinal toxicity of human tissue plasminogen activator in vitrectomized rabbit eyes. Arch Ophthalmol. 1991;109:718-22.
32. Hrach CJ, Johnson MW, Hassan AS, et al. Retinal toxicity of commercial intravitreal tissue plasminogen activator solution in cat eyes. Arch Ophthalmol. 2000;118:659-63.
33. Chen SN, Yang TC, Ho CL, et al. Retinal toxicity of intravitreal tissue plasminogen activator : case report and literature review. Ophthalmology. 2003;110:704-8.

Anti-VEGF Therapy for Neovascular Age-related Macular Degeneration

28

Pearse A Keane, Srinivas R Sadda

Introduction

Neovascular age-related macular degeneration (AMD) is a disorder characterized by choroidal neovascularization (CNV), a process where abnormal blood vessels develop from the choroidal circulation and result in structural damage to the overlying retina.[1] Neovascular (or "wet") AMD is a leading cause of visual loss in people aged 50 years or older and, until recently, there existed no effective treatment for the majority of patients with this disorder.[2,3]

In the 1980s, results of the macular photocoagulation study demonstrated that thermal ablation of CNV using laser was effective in halting disease progression.[4] However, this approach resulted in destruction of both retinal pigment epithelium (RPE) and photoreceptors in the treated area, and was thus suitable only for the minority of cases with exclusively extrafoveal involvement. Furthermore, despite initially successful treatment, in many cases subsequent CNV recurrence was associated with irreversible visual loss.[5] In the late 1990s, a significant advance was made, when the treatment of age-related macular degeneration with photodynamic therapy (TAP study) and verteporfin in photodynamic therapy studies demonstrated that photodynamic therapy (PDT) with verteporfin (Visudyne; Novartis AG, Basel, Switzerland) could be effective for the treatment of subfoveal CNV.[6,7] Unfortunately, however, while PDT was successful in reducing the risk of moderate to severe visual acuity (VA) loss in selected patients with subfoveal CNV, only a small percentage of patients achieved an improvement in VA.

More recent advances in the management of neovascular AMD have been achieved by adopting pharmacological methods aimed at inhibition of the vascular growth process underlying CNV, in particular, blockade of the glycoprotein vascular endothelial growth factor (VEGF).[8] In 2004, the first evidence of the efficacy of this approach was provided by the VEGF inhibition in ocular neovascularization study (VISION). In this study, pegaptanib (Macugen, OSI Pharmaceuticals, Inc., Melville, NY, USA) was shown to be effective in preventing moderate visual loss in patients with neovascular AMD.[9] The more clinically significant breakthrough, however, occurred in 2006 with the publication of minimally classic/occult trial of the anti-VEGF antibody ranibizumab in the treatment of neovascular AMD (MARINA) and anti-VEGF antibody for the treatment of predominantly classic CNV in AMD (ANCHOR). These studies demonstrated that inhibition of VEGF by regular treatment with ranibizumab (Lucentis, Genentech, Inc., South San Francisco, CA, USA) could lead to significant visual improvement in a substantial number of patients.[10,11] Coincident with this, a number of small retrospective studies demonstrated that intravitreal injection of bevacizumab (Avastin, Genentech, USA), an anti-VEGF drug approved for the treatment of colorectal cancer, could lead to potentially similar visual gain, but at a lower cost.[12,13] As a result, bevacizumab was rapidly adopted worldwide as an additional agent for the treatment of neovascular AMD despite the absence of evidence from clinical trials.[14]

In this review, author begins by providing an overview of the events involved in new blood vessel formation and then highlights the role of VEGF in this process; they then described the manner in which these events are critical to CNV pathophysiology. Author continues by describing the pharmacology of VEGF inhibition and by summarizing the principal findings from clinical trials for the use of anti-VEGF pharmacotherapy. Perhaps most importantly, author then provides recommendations on how the results from these trials may be best applied in everyday clinical practice. Author concludes with a description of clinical trials for anti-VEGF therapies that are still underway and provide an overview of future directions in the field.

Angiogenesis and Vascular Endothelial Growth Factor

In the past 20 years, significant progress has been made in our understanding of the process by which new blood vessel formation occurs in adults, termed angiogenesis.[15] This has been driven by realization that the control of this process might allow new treatment of many, previously intractable conditions, both in ophthalmology and in other medical specialties.

Angiogenesis is the process by which new blood vessels form from existing vessel networks in adults (as opposed to vasculogenesis, a form of de novo blood vessel formation that is typically seen in the embryo).[16] Angiogenic processes are initiated by an angiogenic stimulus, most commonly hypoxia, which leads to the upregulation of growth factor expression. Growth factor production, in turn, leads to vasodilatation and increases vascular permeability as well as the activation, and proliferation of endothelial cells. These changes are accompanied by degradation of the surrounding extracellular matrix, facilitating endothelial cell migration. The migrating endothelial cells assemble, form cords, and ultimately acquire lumens; further differentiation to accommodate local requirements then occurs, supported by a surrounding network of similarly differentiated periendothelial cells and matrix. After further remodeling, a complex vascular network is ultimately formed.

Each step of the angiogenic sequence is controlled by a delicate balance between pro- and anti-angiogenic growth factors, the most important of which is VEGF-A.[16] VEGF-A, first isolated in 1989 by Ferrara et al,[17] is a glycoprotein produced by cells in response to hypoxia (cells deficient in oxygen produce a transcription factor, hypoxia inducible factor, which stimulates its production and release). Circulating extracellular VEGF-A then binds to receptors on endothelial cells leading to increased vascular permeability and proliferation of the endothelial cells.

VEGF-A is the prototype member of a gene family (i.e. a group of genes with shared sequences and with similar biochemical functions) that also includes placenta growth factor, VEGF-B, VEGF-C, VEGF-D, and VEGF-E (prior to the discovery of others, VEGF-A was known simply as VEGF and the terms are used interchangeably in this review).[18] VEGF-A has four major isoforms; different forms produced by alternative gene splicing. Isoforms 165 and 121 are freely diffusible outside the cell, whereas isoforms 189 and 206 are almost completely sequestered in the extracellular matrix. $VEGF_{165}$ is the predominant isoform and binds to heparin with high affinity. Although multiple growth factors other than VEGF-A have been implicated in the angiogenic process (e.g. basic fibroblast growth factor, angiopoietin-2, pigment-epithelium derived factor, and platelet-derived growth factor), VEGF-A appears critical for a number of reasons: its production is driven by hypoxia; it is highly selective for endothelial cells and possesses diffusion characteristics that allow it to reach its target, and it affects multiple aspects of the angiogenic process. VEGF also causes vascular dilatation and promotes vasopermeability, both of which facilitate a rich environment for the growth of new vessels. Thus, despite the complexity of the angiogenic process and the potential redundancy of the growth factors involved, blockade of VEGF-A was quickly recognized as a promising approach for the restriction of blood vessel formation in a variety of pathologic scenarios.[15,19]

Pathogenesis of Choroidal Neovascularization

A large number of clinical and epidemiological studies have investigated potential risk factors for AMD;[20] it is clear from these studies that AMD is a multifactorial disorder that involves a complex interaction between environmental (e.g. smoking), genetic (e.g. positive family history), and metabolic (e.g. the high nutritional demands and turnover of cells in the macular region) factors that result in characteristic degenerative changes in the macula.[21,22] The clinical hallmark of these alterations is the deposition of acellular, polymorphous material, termed drusen, between the RPE and Bruch's membrane.[20] In early AMD, drusen are often accompanied by focal retinal pigmentary abnormalities; as the disease progresses, such abnormalities often accumulate resulting in the loss of large areas of RPE and outer retina, a phenomenon termed geographic atrophy (GA). In a subset of patients with AMD, these abnormalities in the outer retina, Bruch's membrane and choroid may also be accompanied by the development of CNV, the characteristic feature of neovascular AMD.[23]

In neovascular AMD, abnormal blood vessels develop from the choroidal circulation, pass anteriorly through breaks in Bruch's membrane, and then proliferate in the sub-RPE and/or subretinal space; such vessels are structurally immature and their growth is often accompanied by hemorrhage and/or fluid exudation.[24,25] In addition, the angiogenic process may also involve significant degradation and remodeling of the extracellular space as well as the incursion of cellular components, such as fibroblasts, which ultimately results in disciform scar formation. Thus, CNV commonly results in loss of the RPE and overlying photoreceptors as well as significant disorganization of the overlying retinal architecture leading to irreversible visual loss.

The processes that instigate development of the CNV lesion remain poorly understood. It appears that an elaborate interaction of pathologic states, such as oxidative stress, ischemia and chronic inflammation result in cellular damage, accumulation of extracellular debris, and modification of the extracellular matrix.[21,22] In patients who develop neovascular AMD, the interplay of such changes leads to overexpression of pro-angiogenic growth factors, such as VEGF and the formation of CNV. In recent years, much evidence has emerged implicating the changes associated with chronic inflammation in this process, for example recent studies have shown that drusen contain bioactive fragments of complement components (C3a and C5a) that lead to increased expression of VEGF.[26] These complement components also issue a chemotactic signal for inflammatory cells, such as macrophages; macrophage activation may, in turn, lead to attenuation of and breaks in Bruch's membrane through the release of proteolytic enzymes.

From the results of clinical trials,[9-11] and from earlier animal studies,[27,28] it is clear that VEGF plays a key role in CNV formation; blockade of VEGF thus offers an attractive pathway to target in the treatment of neovascular AMD.

Pegaptanib

Pegaptanib is an oligonucleotide (aptamer) that binds to a specific target molecule, in this case, the heparin-binding domain of VEGF-A.[29,30] In this way, pegaptanib is capable of preventing the predominant $VEGF_{165}$ isoform from binding to VEGF receptors; unlike other agents, pegaptanib is thus a selective inhibitor of VEGF. Selective inhibition of a single isoform offers the theoretical advantage that "normal" vessels may be maintained by $VEGF_{121}$ and other isoforms, while pathologic neovascularization may be suppressed. Indeed, prior to clinical trials in humans, basic research demonstrated that intravitreal administration of pegaptanib could lead to both reduced vascular permeability and inhibition of retinal neovascularization.[29] It has subsequently been shown, however, that various proteases activated during angiogenesis may cleave $VEGF_{165}$ (and longer isoforms) to generate non-heparin binding fragments; such fragments may be sufficient to drive angiogenesis while evading pegaptanib blockade.[31,32]

Efficacy

In 2004, following publication of the VISION study results, pegaptanib (Macugen, OSI Pharmaceuticals Inc., Melville, NY, USA) was licensed for use in USA by the Food and Drug Administration. The VISION trials, two large-scale, multi-center, randomized, controlled, clinical trials, demonstrated that intravitreal administration of 0.3 mg of pegaptanib at 6 weekly intervals for a period of 48 weeks was effective in reducing moderate vision loss in patients with neovascular AMD.[9,33] In these studies, 70% of pegaptanib-treated patients avoided further moderate visual loss (defined in most AMD studies as a loss of fewer than 15 letters of VA) compared with 55% of sham-treated patients. This effect was seen regardless of angiographic CNV classification, lesion size, or level of VA at baseline. However, treated eyes still lost, on average, 1.5 lines of VA over the course of a year of treatment. Other studies have replicated many of the visual outcomes seen in the VISION trials and evaluated other endpoints, such as vision-related quality of life, with similarly underwhelming results.[34-37]

Anatomic Outcomes

Anatomic endpoints were also evaluated in the VISION studies. On fluorescein angiography (FA), administration of pegaptanib led to "a slowing of the growth" of the CNV lesion and reduction in the severity of CNV leakage as compared with the control group.[9] In other words, despite the use of pegaptanib, the CNV lesion continued to grow and remain active, albeit at a lesser rate. More recently, the effects of pegaptanib on CNV leakage have also been evaluated using optical coherence tomography (OCT), which has demonstrated modest reductions in central foveal thickness following treatment.[38]

Safety

Prior to the testing of first anti-VEGF agents in humans, the possibility of significant systemic toxicity was a major concern; use of the non-selective VEGF antagonist, bevacizumab, in the treatment of colorectal cancer had been associated with increased incidence of hypertension, bleeding, and thromboembolic events.[39] While the doses employed with intravitreal administration are many times less than when used systemically, pegaptanib also offers the potential safety advantage of selective VEGF inhibition. Indeed, the VISION trials failed to highlight any serious safety concerns, both from an intraocular and systemic perspective.[40,41] Furthermore, doses ten times greater than that recommended by the VISION study have been employed clinically without evidence of increased systemic adverse effects.[42] The requirement for long-term VEGF inhibition in the treatment of neovascular AMD and the positive safety profile of pegaptanib has led to proposals that an initial inductive treatment with non-selective VEGF inhibitors could be followed by maintenance therapy with pegaptanib.[43,44] The results of the phase IV, evaluation of efficacy and safety in maintaining visual acuity with sequential treatment of neovascular AMD (LEVEL study), provide some justification for this approach, although patients still lost VA in the maintenance phase.[45] Furthermore, only patients who initially responded to treatment with ranibizumab were included in the study. Despite these caveats, the use of pegaptanib maintenance therapy may be a useful option for patients with significant cardiovascular risk factors, particularly when the long-term systemic adverse effects of non-selective intravitreal VEGF inhibition remain unclear.

Ranibizumab

Ranibizumab (formerly known as rhuFAb V2) is an antibody fragment that binds and inhibits all isoforms of VEGF-A.[18,46] It is a chimeric molecule, consisting of an antigen-binding murine component and a non-binding human component that serves to make it less antigenic (in Greek mythology, the chimera was a monster with a lion's head, a goat's body, and a serpent's tail). Ranibizumab was developed by alteration of bevacizumab, a humanized version of a murine monoclonal antibody first derived in 1996.[18] This requirement for the alteration of bevacizumab was driven by preclinical studies suggesting that a full-size antibody would be unable to penetrate the retina.[47] Substitution of targeted amino acids was also performed in a bid to maximize the binding affinity of ranibizumab for VEGF, in the hope that this change would lead to improved outcomes [the VEGF binding affinity of ranibizumab is approximately 100 times that of bevacizumab (Figs 28.1A to D to 28.3A to D)].[18]

Efficacy

In 2006, ranibizumab was licensed for use in United States by the Food and Drug Administration following publication of the MARINA and ANCHOR studies.[10,11] The MARINA trial was a multi-center, 2-year, double-blind, sham-controlled study, where patients with either minimally classic or occult with no classic CNV were randomized to receive either 24 monthly intravitreal injections of ranibizumab (either 0.3 mg or 0.5 mg) or sham injections.[11] At 12 months in this study, 94.5% of the group given 0.3 mg of ranibizumab and 94.6% of those given 0.5 mg avoided further moderate visual loss (i.e. lost fewer than 15 letters of VA), as compared with 62.2% of patients receiving sham injections. VA improved by 15 or more letters in 24.8% of the 0.3 mg group and 33.8% of the 0.5 mg group, as compared with 5.0% of the sham-injection group. The mean increase in VA was 6.5 letters in the 0.3 mg group and 7.2 letters in the 0.5 mg group (as compared with a decrease of 10.4 letters in the sham-injection group). These VA benefits were maintained at 24 months.

The ANCHOR trial was also a multi-center, 2-year, double-blind, sham-controlled study, where patients with predominantly classic CNV were randomized to receive either 24 monthly intravitreal injections of ranibizumab (either 0.3 mg or 0.5 mg) or PDT with verteporfin.[10] 94.3% of those given 0.3 mg of ranibizumab and 96.4% of those given 0.5 mg lost fewer than 15 letters, as compared with 64.3% of those in the verteporfin group. VA improved by 15 letters or more in 35.7% of the 0.3 mg group and 40.3% of the 0.5 mg group (as compared with 5.6% of the verteporfin group). Mean VA increased by 8.5 letters in the 0.3 mg group and 11.3 letters in the 0.5 mg group (as compared with a decrease of 9.5 letters in the verteporfin group).

Subgroup analysis were performed in both the MARINA and ANCHOR studies with the aim of evaluating the relationship between selected baseline characteristics and final VA outcomes.[48,49] In both studies, use of ranibizumab was associated with an average increase from baseline VA in all subgroups evaluated, and was also superior to the control

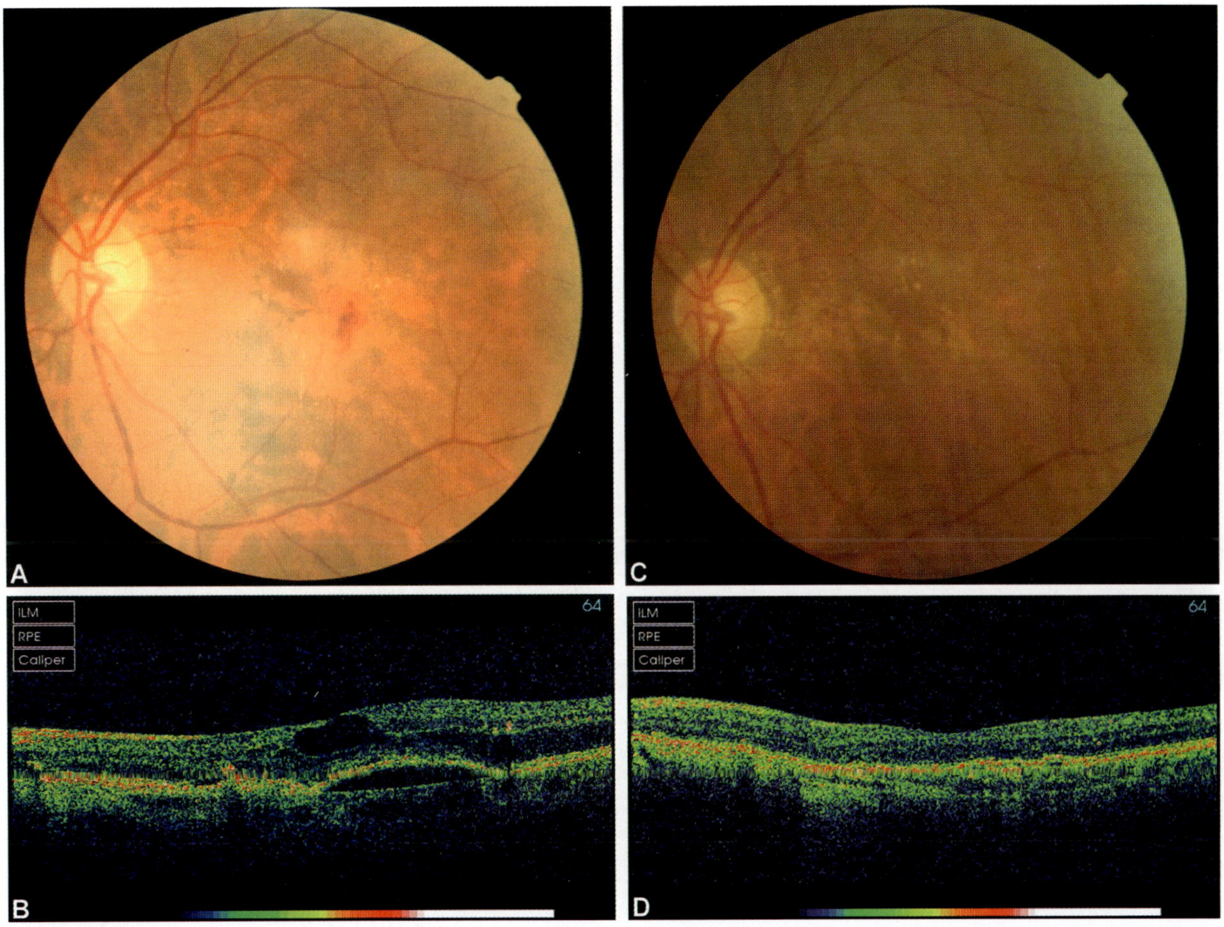

▲ **Figures 28.1A to D**

(A and B) Color fundus photographs and OCT images (3D-OCT 1000, Topcon Medical Systems, Japan) from an 84-year-old woman diagnosed with retinal angiomatous proliferation in her left eye; (C and D) Following treatment with four intravitreal injections of ranibizumab her VA had improved from 20/60 to 20/40 and there was resolution of cystoid macular edema, pigment epithelium detachment, and subretinal fluid

groups in each case. The most important predictors of final VA outcomes were, in decreasing order of importance, baseline VA score, CNV lesion size, and patient age – i.e. younger patients with smaller lesions and relatively preserved VA tended to have superior outcomes. The findings of the subgroup analyses thus highlight the importance of prompt diagnosis and treatment in patients with neovascular AMD, a conclusion that has subsequently been confirmed in other studies. The MARINA and ANCHOR study groups have also analyzed the characteristics of the small percentage of patients who suffered moderate visual loss despite monthly treatment with ranibizumab for 2 years.[50] In these cases, vision loss was associated with lesion characteristics commonly associated with CNV suppression, such as pigmentary abnormalities and atrophic scar formation; the authors speculate that further VA improvements in such patients may require strategies aimed at preservation of photoreceptor and RPE function rather than CNV targeting.

In addition to objectively measured visual outcomes, patients treated with ranibizumab in the MARINA and ANCHOR studies also reported clinically relevant improvements in vision-related quality of life measures as determined using the National Eye Institute Visual Function Questionnaire 25.[51]

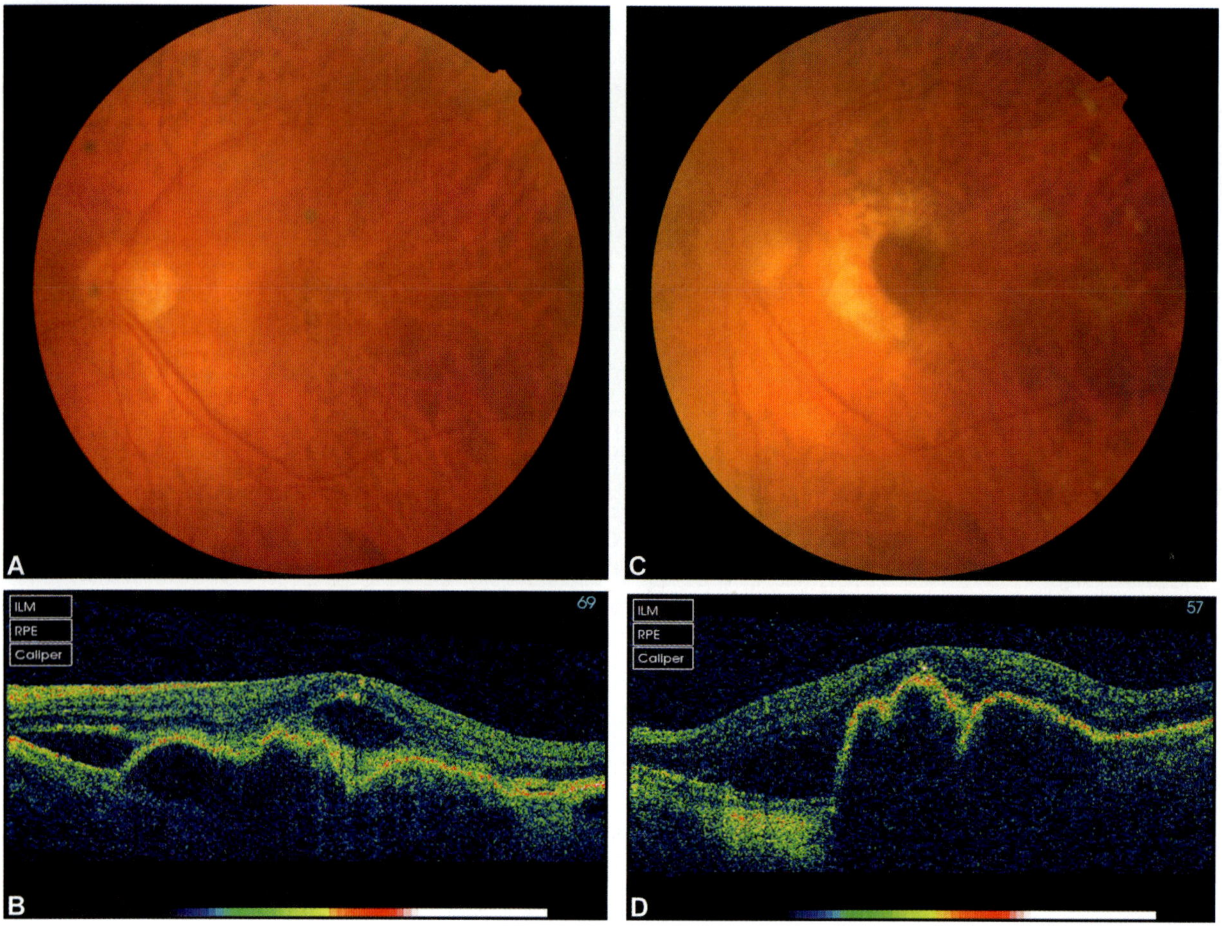

▲ Figures 28.2A to D

(A and B) Color fundus photographs and OCT images (3D-OCT 1000, Topcon Medical Systems, Japan) from an 85-year-old woman diagnosed with neovascular AMD in her left eye; (C and D) Following treatment with intravitreal ranibizumab she developed a tear of the RPE despite her left VA was maintained at 20/80

Anatomic Outcomes

Anatomic endpoints based on FA and OCT were also evaluated in the MARINA and ANCHOR studies.[52,53] In patients treated with ranibizumab, the CNV lesion did not recede or disappear, but did demonstrate less fibrosis and less exudation as evidenced by CNV leakage area on FA and decreased central retinal thickness on OCT. Furthermore, in contrast to the prior treatments for neovascular AMD, the size of the CNV lesion was stabilized with ranibizumab treatment, as determined by planimetric measurements on FA.

Safety

Results of the MARINA and ANCHOR studies, and the safety assessment of intravitreal Lucentis for AMD (SAILOR) study, indicate a high benefit-to-risk ratio for the treatment of neovascular AMD with ranibizumab.[10,11,54] A low rate of serious ocular adverse events has been demonstrated for the use of 0.5 mg of ranibizumab in the MARINA and ANCHOR studies, the most common of these were presumed endophthalmitis (1.3% in MARINA; 1.4% in ANCHOR) and uveitis (1.3% in MARINA; 0.7% in ANCHOR). Other less serious, but potentially more common, adverse events reported include vitreous floaters (from the medication itself or from vitreous hemorrhage), subconjunctival hemorrhage, discomfort from the antiseptic used to prepare the eye prior to the injection. In the MARINA and ANCHOR trials, the incidence of serious adverse effects was similar between treatment and control groups—for arterial thromboembolic events (e.g. nonfatal

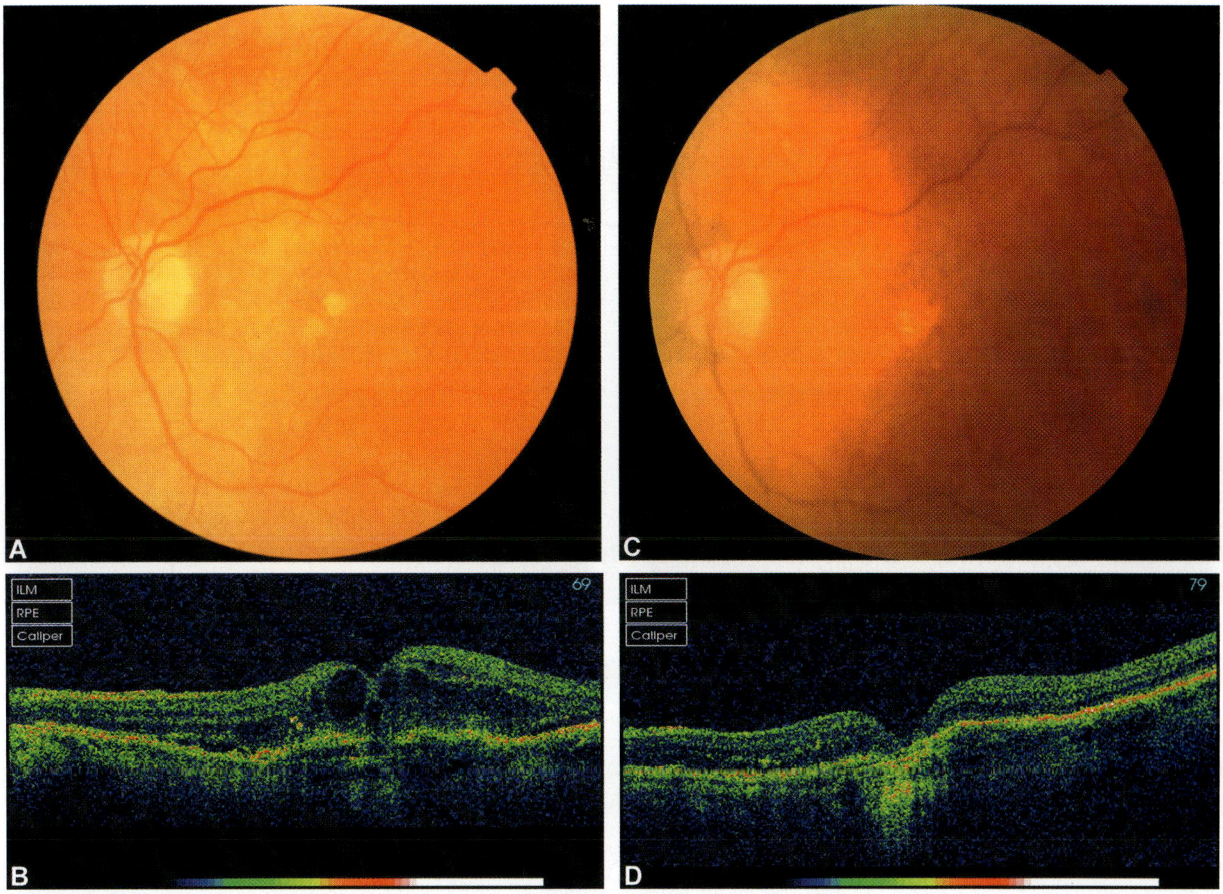

▲ **Figures 28.3A to D**

(A and B) Color fundus photographs and OCT images (3D-OCT 1000, Topcon Medical Systems, Japan) from an 85-year-old man diagnosed with neovascular AMD in his left eye; (C and D) To date, he has received 17 injections of intravitreal ranibizumab and has maintained a VA of 20/60 despite the presence of foveal atrophy

myocardial infarctions, nonfatal stroke and death from a vascular or unknown cause) incidence was 3.8% (sham) versus 4.6% (0.3 mg ranibizumab) and 4.6% (0.5 mg ranibizumab) in MARINA; and 4.2% (PDT) versus 4.4% (0.3 mg ranibizumab) and 5.0% (0.5 mg ranibizumab) in ANCHOR. An interim analysis from the SAILOR study showed a trend for an increase in the incidence of stroke in the group treated with 0.5 mg of ranibizumab. Moreover, the incidence of stroke was higher with pre-existing risk factors, in particular, a previous history of stroke or arrhythmia. These findings, and recent studies reporting an association between AMD itself and higher risk of stroke, suggest that extra discussion of risk-to-benefit ratios may be warranted prior to ranibizumab treatment in patients with a history of stroke.

Bevacizumab

Bevacizumab is a full-length monoclonal antibody, first derived from a murine source and prepared for intravenous administration that binds to and inhibits the biologic activity of all isoforms of VEGF-A.[18] Bevacizumab was originally developed and approved for the treatment of metastatic colorectal cancer, but it is now also used in the treatment of non-small cell lung cancer and in patients with metastatic breast cancer.[39] The results of preliminary studies suggested that bevacizumab, due to its large size, would not be fully distributed within the retinal layers; hence, the development of an antibody fragment, ranibizumab, for the treatment of neovascular AMD.[18] Furthermore, the longer half-life of a complete antibody, versus an antibody fragment raised

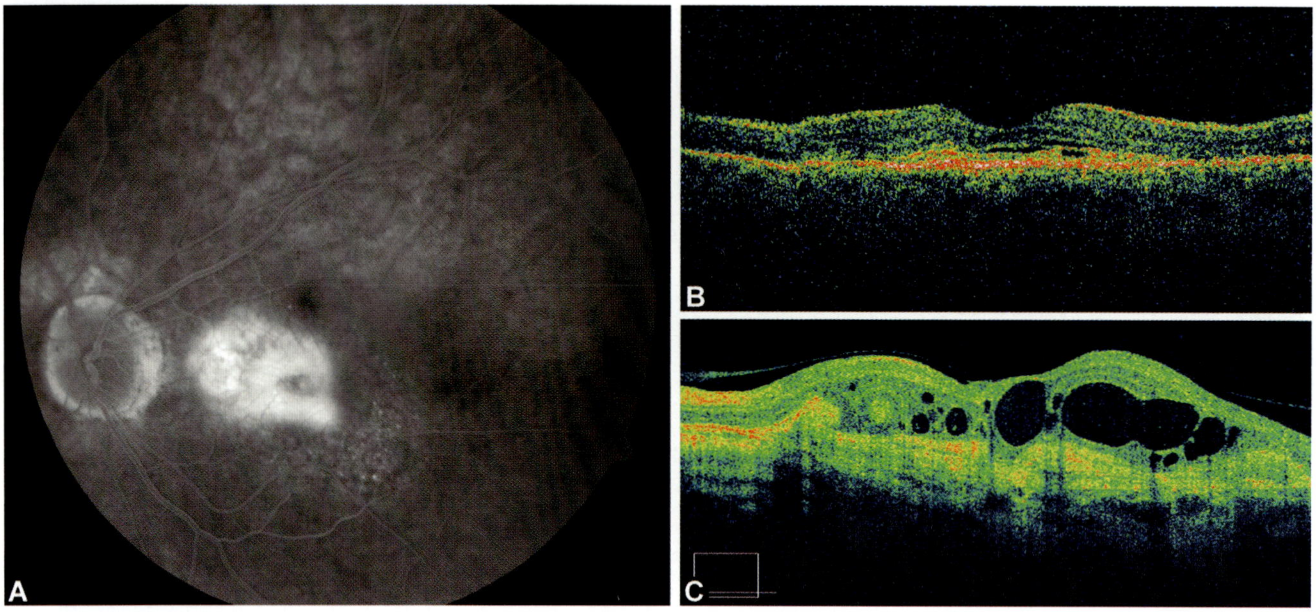

▲ **Figures 28.4A to C**

(A to B) Fluorescein angiographic and OCT images (Stratus OCT and Cirrus HD-OCT, Carl Zeiss Meditec, Dublin, CA) from a 77-year-old man diagnosed with predominantly classic choroidal neovascularization; (C) This failed to respond to treatment with intravitreal bevacizumab

concerns regarding systemic toxicity in patients requiring long-term anti-VEGF blockade (Figs 28.4A to C and 28.5A to C).[18]

▶ Efficacy

In 2005, Rosenfeld et al.[55] reported that intravitreal administration of bevacizumab led to rapid resolution of abnormalities on OCT in a patient with neovascular AMD; other studies subsequently confirmed the apparent beneficial effects of bevacizumab administration in this context.[12,13] On the basis of these reports and on the anecdotal experiences of ophthalmologists worldwide, intravitreal bevacizumab was quickly adopted as a treatment for neovascular AMD, driven in large part by its low-cost relative to ranibizumab. A large number of off-label, short-term, uncontrolled, retrospective case series have evaluated the efficacy of intravitreal bevacizumab in neovascular AMD.[56-78] Until recently, however, no evidence from randomized controlled clinical trials existed for its use. In 2010, the results of the Avastin (bevacizumab) for treatment of CNV (ABC) trial provided the first level I evidence for the efficacy of intravitreal bevacizumab in neovascular AMD.[79,80] In this prospective, double-masked, multi-center, randomized, controlled trial, 32% of patients treated with bevacizumab gained 15 or more letters from baseline VA. More than 45% of patients treated with bevacizumab improved 10 or more letters, a threshold that exceed the variability of the measurement of VA and represents the proportion of patients recovering vision. In addition, 91% of patients receiving bevacizumab lost fewer than 15 letters of VA from baseline. Mean VA increased by 7 letters in the bevacizumab group with a median of seven injections over a 54-week period. Among the 65 patients treated with bevacizumab in the trial, there were no cases of endophthalmitis or serious uveitis related to the intervention. Three serious systemic adverse events occurred in the bevacizumab group (two myocardial infarctions and one atrial fibrillation) and seven in the control group (five unexpected admissions to hospital, one atrial fibrillation, and one episode of prolonged bleeding after excision of a benign neck tumor). The results of the ABC trial thus support immediate implementation of bevacizumab in healthcare systems where budgetary limitations prevent access to ranibizumab. What remains unresolved, however, is how the efficacy and safety of bevacizumab compare to that of ranibizumab. A number

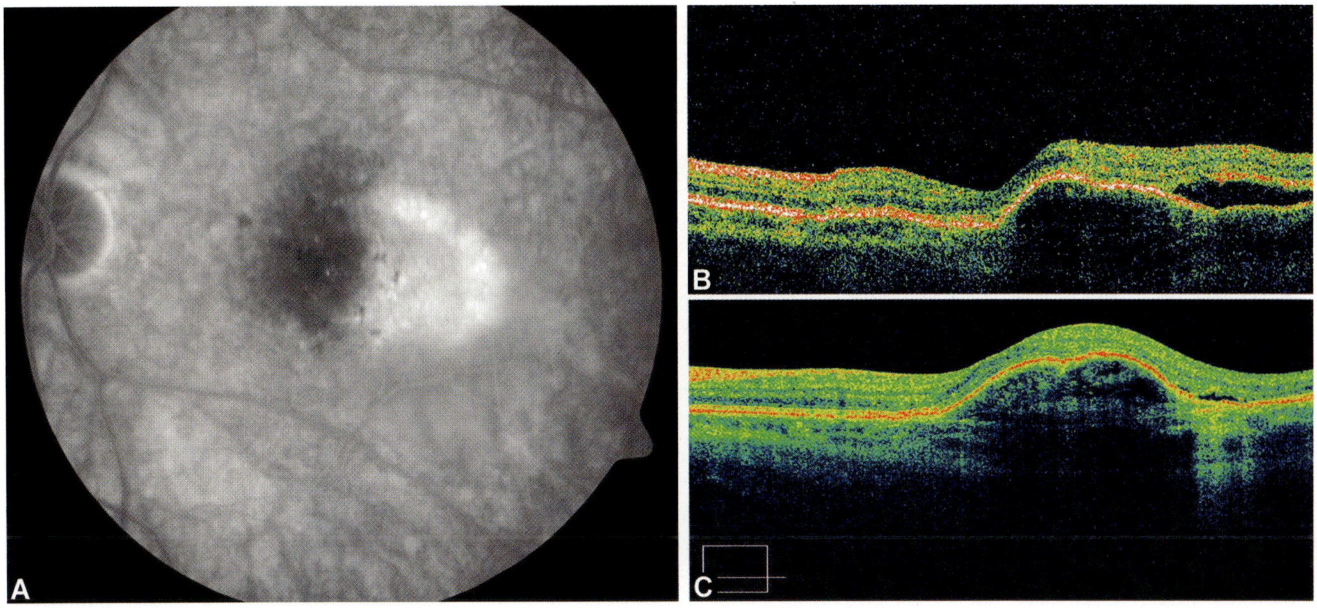

▲ **Figures 28.5A to C**

(A and B) Fluorescein angiographic and optical coherence tomography images (Stratus OCT and Cirrus HD-OCT, Carl Zeiss Meditec, Dublin, CA) from a 73-year-old woman diagnosed with occult choroidal neovascularization; (C) Over a 5-year period she received nine treatments with intravitreal bevacizumab, followed by 13 treatments with intravitreal ranibizumab, allowing her to maintain a VA of 20/40

of small retrospective comparison studies have evaluated the ranibizumab versus bevacizumab for the treatment of neovascular AMD,[81-83] but the results of large, randomized controlled trials, such as the comparison of AMD treatments trials (CATT) and inhibit VEGF in age-related CNV (IVAN) studies will be required to settle this issue.

Use of Anti-VEGF Therapies in Clinical Practice

▶ Initiation

Assessment of patients at risk of neovascular AMD requires careful history taking (especially the nature and duration of symptoms) and slit-lamp biomicroscopy, followed by FA and OCT. In selected cases, indocyanine green angiography may also provide useful diagnostic information. VA should also be assessed—logMAR VAs obtained using ETDRS charts with protocol refraction are preferable to Snellen VAs in this context. A recent study by Falkenstein et al.[84] has reported that Snellen VA was consistently lower (worse) than the ETDRS VA in patients with AMD, and that this discrepancy was more marked in patients with VA worse than 20/100. Accurate assessment of VA is an important consideration in healthcare systems where anti-VEGF therapy can only be provided for VA within a certain prespecified range [e.g. the National Institute for Health and Clinical Excellence (NICE) guidelines in the United Kingdom].[85]

Traditionally, FA has been required for the diagnosis of neovascular AMD, however, with the advent of OCT, some have questioned this dogma. Despite this, it is clear that FA provides unique information that is useful in the management of neovascular AMD. In particular, FA can provide information about lesion size, location and classification. Determination of CNV location is critical; for well-demarcated lesions located in an extrafoveal location, consideration may be given to the use of laser photocoagulation as per the MPS guidelines. Such an approach may allow the patient to avoid the need for monthly intravitreal injections over an extended follow-up period.[4] Consideration of angiographic lesion classification is also important when considering whether to initiate treatment. In lesions classified as "occult" on FA, the decision to treat may be influenced by whether there is evidence of recent disease progression (in the MARINA study of minimally classic and occult lesions, despite requiring evidence of recent disease progression, only 35% of sham-treated patients lost fewer than 15 letters).[11] Therefore, careful monitoring would appear prudent in patients with occult CNV, but without evidence of disease progression. Finally, evaluation of lesion size prior to treatment may provide a useful baseline parameter against which future lesion growth can be assessed, particularly in difficult cases where repeat FA is required.

Fluorescein angiography may also be useful for the exclusion of other macular diseases that can mimic the features of neovascular AMD. Diseases that can lead to diagnostic confusion in this respect include retinal macro-aneurysms resulting in submacular hemorrhage, central serous chorioretinopathy resulting in subretinal and sub-RPE fluid, pattern dystrophies where there is progressive staining of vitelliform-like material.[86] FA can also highlight those cases where CNV is present, but due to other etiologies than neovascular AMD, e.g. pathologic myopia, inflammatory disorders, trauma etc. CNV related to non-AMD sources may respond differently to treatment with ranibizumab and may also benefit from alternative or supplementary treatment regimens. Finally, indocyanine green angiography may be useful in the assessment of selected cases at baseline, for example in the context of substantial submacular hemorrhage where the presence or extent of underlying CNV is unclear.[87] Many authors have also suggested that indocyanine green angiography is helpful for the assessment of disease variants, such as polypoidal choroidal vasculopathy, or retinal angiomatous proliferation.[88,89]

If clinical examination and imaging studies confirm the presence of subfoveal CNV secondary to AMD, and the disease appears active, treatment with intravitreal ranibizumab or bevacizumab should be initiated without delay (treatment delay has been shown to have detrimental effects on final visual outcomes).[90,91] In neovascular AMD, signs of disease activity include deterioration in VA; abnormal retinal thickness with the presence of intraretinal, subretinal, or sub-RPE fluid on OCT; presence (or recurrence) of intraretinal or subretinal hemorrhage, and evidence of CNV leakage on FA.[92]

In routine practice, physicians will often encounter clinical scenarios not evaluated in the MARINA and ANCHOR studies (or, in some cases, scenarios that were specifically excluded from consideration); thus, the results of these studies must often be extrapolated to other contexts. For example, ranibizumab or bevacizumab therapy may be of benefit in patients with predominantly hemorrhagic lesions, although such lesions were excluded from MARINA and ANCHOR.[93-95] Caution is still required, the hemorrhage may be present as a result of an underlying RPE tear; furthermore, the toxic effect of blood on the RPE may also limit the final visual outcome. In addition, consideration should also be given to other management options, such as pneumatic displacement of the hemorrhage, with or without the use of tissue plasminogen activator.[96] Caution is also required in treating CNV lesions where greater than 50% of the lesion is made up of serous pigment epithelium detachment; such lesions were excluded from the MARINA and ANCHOR trials and may be at greater risk of RPE tear development.[97] Other lesions falling outside the MARINA and ANCHOR treatment criteria include those with advanced subretinal fibrosis or GA involving the foveal center; a trial of anti-VEGF therapy may be indicated but, in general, such cases are unlikely to benefit from continued treatment. Similarly, patients with initial VAs worse than 20/320 were excluded from the MARINA and ANCHOR studies and are less likely to benefit from treatment (in some countries, treatment of such patients may be restricted: in the United Kingdom, the NICE recommends that patients with logMAR VAs worse than 1.2 do not receive treatment).[98,99] Conversely, patients with initial VAs better than 20/40 were not evaluated in the MARINA and ANCHOR studies. Treatment of such patients should, however, always be considered in the case of active subfoveal or juxtafoveal disease.

Maintenance

In the MARINA and ANCHOR studies, monthly treatments were provided over a 2-year period, each patient thus received a total of 24 injections. Other large clinical trials have since evaluated the benefits of ranibizumab in less-frequent retreatment regimens, e.g. the PIER, efficacy and safety of ranibizumab in patients with subfoveal CNV secondary to AMD (EXCITE), and SAILOR studies. In these studies, patients were initially treated with three injections of ranibizumab on a monthly basis, often termed the loading phase. Subsequently, patients received retreatments on a quarterly basis. The results of the PIER study suggested that intravitreal ranibizumab on a fixed quarterly retreatment regimen led to visual improvement in many patients with neovascular AMD and prevented visual loss in the majority of patients.[100,101] However, the mean improvement in VA and the percentage of patients experiencing greater than 15 letters of visual gain was less than that of the MARINA and ANCHOR studies. Furthermore, the initial visual gain attained during the loading phase was not maintained during the remainder of the study. The EXCITE study compared monthly maintenance therapy with 0.3 mg of intravitreal ranibizumab to the PIER study quarterly regimen (0.3 mg and 0.5 mg) reduced frequency fixed dose schedule and found better mean VA gains in patients receiving monthly retreatment.[92] Similarly, the SAILOR study evaluated a loading phase of three consecutive monthly injections followed by quarterly monitoring with retreatment determined by physician's discretion (Cohort 2) or by VA and OCT criteria (Cohort 1). The results of this study provided further confirmation that quarterly visits are insufficient for optimal monitoring of disease progression.[54]

Despite the compelling evidence from the MARINA and ANCHOR studies, fixed, monthly ranibizumab retreatment regimens have not been widely adopted. While a variety of retreatment protocols are in use, the dosing schedule described in the [Prospective optical coherence tomography imaging of patients with neovascular AMD treated with intraocular ranibizumab (Lucentis) PrONTO study is perhaps the most widely known.[102,103] In the PrONTO study, an OCT-guided variable dosing regimen was assessed for the treatment of neovascular AMD with ranibizumab. In this small single-center study, subjects with subfoveal CNV secondary to AMD and a central retinal thickness of at least 300 µm as measured by OCT were enrolled to receive three consecutive monthly injections of intravitreal ranibizumab (the results of the fixed monthly ranibizumab treatment regimens have consistently shown that the majority of VA gain occurs during this initial treatment period). Thereafter, ranibizumab retreatment was performed, in part, based on OCT criteria: a loss of five letters of VA in conjunction with intraretinal fluid on OCT, or an increase on OCT of central retinal thickness of at least 100 µm, being indications for retreatment. FA was only required when there was significant or unexplained VA loss. The results of this study suggested that results similar to the MARINA and ANCHOR trials could be obtained but requiring fewer injections, however, the small, open-label, nature of this study, and significant differences in the trial design, limit the comparisons that can be made or conclusions that can be drawn. Major issues with this study include the small sample size (n = 40) with resulting large confidence intervals, and the lack of comparison group receiving fixed monthly retreatment. In addition, a number of single center studies with similar designs have failed to replicate the PrONTO study findings.

The results of the Study of Ranibizumab in Patients With Subfoveal CNV Secondary to AMD (SUSTAIN) and HORIZON studies also suggest that the chance of substantial VA gain seems less likely with retreatments that occur less than monthly, whether they be determined on a reduced frequency, fixed dosing schedule, or when retreatment decisions are influenced by imaging parameters, such as OCT or FA.[86,92] For example, the HORIZON extension study demonstrated that one year after entry into the study, when monthly treatments were replaced by physician-determined retreatment decisions, median VA decreased by five letters after one year and by a further three letters after 2 years.

Although there is an absence of evidence from clinical trials, a wide variety of other retreatment regimens, often tailored to healthcare system-specific logistical factors, have been adopted worldwide. In an attempt to minimize both the number of intravitreal injections required and the number of office visits, a "treat and extend" approach has recently been described.[104] In this method, monthly injections with ranibizumab are provided until all signs of exudation have resolved as seen with OCT. The treatment interval is then sequentially lengthened by 1–2 weeks as long as there are no signs of recurrent exudation. When recurrent exudation is detected on a follow-up visit, the treatment interval is reduced to the prior interval. Thus, treatment is rendered at every visit, but the time between visits is individualized based on a given patient's response to treatment. To date, this approach has only been evaluated in the context of single-center retrospective studies.[104-108]

In conclusion, the current evidence suggests that monthly retreatment with ranibizumab results in the best VA outcomes. However, when a monthly retreatment regimen is not possible, a flexible strategy with monthly monitoring may be feasible, although the visual benefits may be reduced. When pursuing a strategy of flexible retreatment, frequent monitoring of patients is required to determine signs of disease activity. Disease monitoring should include history, VA assessment, clinical examination and OCT imaging; if active disease is present or recurs, further treatment should be provided urgently; if the disease remains quiescent over long time periods, extending the follow-up intervals may be justified.

Termination

Although there is a considerable body of work documenting the natural history of untreated neovascular AMD, the duration of disease activity in patients receiving anti-VEGF therapy is less clear. Similarly, the frequency and likelihood of disease recurrence remains unknown. Evidence from the HORIZON extension study suggests that neovascular AMD may remain active for a number of years. In this study, 61% of patients treated with monthly ranibizumab for 2 years, required further ranibizumab treatment in the 3rd year.[86] Thus, careful monitoring of patients with neovascular AMD is required for extended time periods, although reduction in the frequency of follow-up may be justified when the disease has been quiescent for a protracted period. On occasion, termination of treatment for situations other than lack of disease activity may also be required. For example, treatment may be deferred or terminated in situations where further visual improvement appears unlikely, e.g. severe RPE tears involving the foveal center, or in the context of significant co-existing GA or subfoveal scar formation.[109] Limited evidence exists evaluating the benefits of continued treatment with ranibizumab in the case of RPE tears (although no data suggest that such an approach should be contraindicated).

CNV Activity "Refractory" to Treatment

The findings of the PrONTO study suggest that 70% of patients treated with intravitreal ranibizumab will have resolution of macular edema within 1 month of their first injection (as demonstrated using OCT); similarly, more than 90% of patients will have resolution of all fluid following three consecutive monthly injections.[102] In a small minority of patients, however, the anatomical signs of fluid exudation (and hence disease activity) appear refractory to anti-VEGF therapy, Such patients may have polypoidal choroidal vasculopathy, a disease variant best detected using indocyanine green angiography.[110,111] Polypoidal choroidal vasculopathy, characterized by the presence of "polyps" found just below the RPE, and seen most commonly in Asians and African Americans, is increasingly believed to be a structural variant of neovascular AMD.[112] Freund et al.[113] have recently suggested that the polyps in polypoidal choroidal vasculopathy originate from long-standing type 1 (sub-RPE) neovascular tissue rather than from the choroidal circulation. They hypothesize that differences in the structure of the RPE monolayer in Asians and African Americans relative to Caucasians, render the RPE somewhat resistant to penetration by underlying neovascular tissue. As a result, CNV lesions in these populations often demonstrate slow lateral growth with eventual development of saccular dilatations, polyps, and finally to fluid exudation and hemorrhage. According to this theory, CNV lesions with features of polypoidal choroidal vasculopathy would be less responsive to anti-VEGF therapy due to the relative maturity of the neovascular tissue present (evidence from preclinical studies suggests that coverage by pericytes is one of the key events resulting in the loss of VEGF dependence in the angiogenic process).[114] The treatment of polypoidal choroidal vasculopathy has not yet been adequately addressed in clinical trials to date, although many authorities recommend the use of anti-VEGF therapy in combination with verteporfin PDT. The results of the EVEREST study, a phase IV clinical trial investigating the use of ranibizumab in PCV, should provide further clarification regarding this.[92]

Anti-VEGF Tachyphylaxis

Recent evidence suggests that treatment with ranibizumab leads to rapid early reductions in retinal thickness, that this effect may be attenuated over time, suggesting the presence of tachyphylaxis.[115,116] Other studies have produced similar findings with regard to bevacizumab.[117,118] In patients who show initial anatomic improvement on treatment with ranibizumab, subsequent regression of these improvements is strongly correlated with decrease in VA.[115] Hence, the presence of a putative tachyphylaxis is of clinical importance. A number of strategies may prove useful in dealing with such phenomenon. Anecdotal evidence suggests that patients exhibiting signs of ranibizumab tachyphylaxis may benefit from being switched to bevacizumab (and vice versa). Similarly, patients with anatomical evidence of tachyphylaxis may benefit from the use of "treatment holidays", or the use of ranibizumab at higher doses. In the ongoing HARBOR trial, OCT-guided therapy is being used to compare the typical dose of ranibizumab (0.5 mg) with an increased dose (2 mg).[86]

Future Directions and Conclusions

Role of Combination Therapy

A number of authors have recently suggested that, in neovascular AMD, combining treatments with different mechanisms of action may result in synergistic benefits including better visual outcome, reduced frequency of treatments, lower risk of adverse events, decreased likelihood of "escape" (i.e. the development of alternative pathways by which cells allow themselves to overcome iatrogenic inhibition).[22,119,120]

To date, much of the work on combination therapies has focused on the use of verteporfin PDT in combination with VEGF blockade.[119] Preliminary results suggest that this approach may reduce the number of treatments required to render the CNV lesion quiescent, but at the expense of achieving maximum visual gain. The 12-month results of the DENALI study were recently reported.[22] In this phase IIIb study, patients receiving PDT in combination with ranibizumab gained an average of 5.3 letters in VA from baseline for the standard fluence group and 4.4 letters for the reduced fluence group, compared with 8.1 letters for the patients receiving ranibizumab monotherapy. On average, patients in the combination group received 2.2 (standard fluence) or 2.8 (reduced fluence) additional ranibizumab injections after the loading phase compared with 7.6 additional injections in the ranibizumab monotherapy cohort.

VEGF blockade is also being combined with macular radiation therapy, either from an internal approach via pars plana vitrectomy and the introduction of a radioactive probe, or from an external approach which is delivered from the inferior sclera.[121] Evidence from early studies suggests that epiretinal intraocular radiation, in combination with ranibizumab, may result in a reduced need for intravitreal injections.[122] Caution is still required, particularly with regard to potential ocular adverse effects, and phase III clinical trials are currently underway.

Other Anti-VEGF Therapies – VEGF Trap

VEGF Trap (Regeneron Pharmaceuticals, Tarrytown, NY, USA) is a fusion protein comprising segments of the extracellular domains of human VEGF receptor-1 and VEGF receptor-2, fused to the constant region of human immunoglobulin G1.[123] VEGF Trap binds to all isoforms of VEGF-A with a higher affinity than either bevacizumab or ranibizumab (VEGF Trap also binds placental growth factors 1 and 2), thereby offering a theoretically longer interval between doses. The use of intravitreal "VEGF Trap-Eye" (a formulation of VEGF Trap for intraocular delivery) has been evaluated in Phase I/II studies, and has demonstrated a mean increase in VA of 13.5 letters as well as a mean time to retreatment of 150 days.[124] No serious ocular or systemic adverse effects were noted. A phase III clinical trial evaluating VEGF Trap-Eye in the treatment of neovascular AMD is currently underway.

Other Therapies

Since the revolutionary introduction of ranibizumab, much of the focus in neovascular AMD management has been on the development of optimal treatment regimens and use of combination therapies. With this focus, it is becoming increasingly clear that the development and progression of CNV lesions occurs in the context of a more slowly-evolving underlying disorder, atrophic or "dry" AMD.[50] It appears likely that, even with early diagnosis and optimal treatment, the visual benefits achievable with anti-VEGF therapies will reach a plateau and, in some patients, inexorable visual loss may occur. Thus, further visual gains among patients undergoing anti-VEGF therapy may require novel treatment strategies that promote RPE and photoreceptor survival rather than targeting CNV. In this regard, a number of therapies now in development for dry AMD, using neuroprotective, anti-inflammatory and visual-cycle targeted strategies, may be of benefit.[22]

Conclusion

The introduction of anti-VEGF therapy was a massive first step in the successful management of neovascular AMD, it is likely that this advance will be the first of many exciting developments in the field. Numerous population-based epidemiological studies have described AMD as the leading cause of blindness in elderly populations in the developed world, while it is too soon to evaluate the effects of anti-VEGF therapy in this context; it appears likely that, with further breakthroughs in pathway-based therapies for neovascular AMD, neovascular AMD will lose its "standing" in such studies of "irreversible" visual loss.

References

1. de Jong PT. Age-related macular degeneration. N Engl J Med. 2006;355:1474-85.
2. Jager RD, Mieler WF, Miller JW. Age-related macular degeneration. N Engl J Med. 2008;358:2606-17.
3. Fine SL. Age-related macular degeneration 1969-2004: a 35-year personal perspective. Am J Ophthalmol. 2005;139:405-20.
4. Argon laser photocoagulation for neovascular maculopathy. Five-year results from randomized clinical trials. Macular Photocoagulation Study Group. Arch Ophthalmol. 1991;109:1109-14.
5. Persistent and recurrent neovascularization after laser photocoagulation for subfoveal choroidal neovascularization of age-related macular degeneration. Macular Photocoagulation Study Group. Arch Ophthalmol. 1994;112:489-99.
6. Photodynamic therapy of subfoveal choroidal neovascularization in age-related macular degeneration with verteporfin: one-year results of 2 randomized clinical trials—TAP report. Treatment of age-related macular degeneration

with photodynamic therapy (TAP) Study Group. Arch Ophthalmol. 1999;117:1329-45.
7. Verteporfin therapy of subfoveal choroidal neovascularization in age-related macular degeneration: two-year results of a randomized clinical trial including lesions with occult with no classic choroidal neovascularization—verteporfin in photodynamic therapy report 2. Am J Ophthalmol. 2001;131:541-60.
8. Schmidt-Erfurth UM, Pruente C. Management of neovascular age-related macular degeneration. Prog Retin Eye Res. 2007;26:437-51.
9. Gragoudas ES, Adamis AP, Cunningham ET, et al. Pegaptanib for neovascular age-related macular degeneration. N Engl J Med. 2004;351:2805-16.
10. Brown DM, Kaiser PK, Michels M, et al. Ranibizumab versus verteporfin for neovascular age-related macular degeneration. N Engl J Med. 2006;355:1432-44.
11. Rosenfeld PJ, Brown DM, Heier JS, et al. Ranibizumab for neovascular age-related macular degeneration. N Engl J Med. 2006;355:1419-31.
12. Avery RL, Pieramici DJ, Rabena MD, et al. Intravitreal bevacizumab (Avastin) for neovascular age-related macular degeneration. Ophthalmology. 2006;113:363-72. e5.
13. Spaide RF, Laud K, Fine HF, et al. Intravitreal bevacizumab treatment of choroidal neovascularization secondary to age-related macular degeneration. Retina. 2006;26:383-90.
14. Canning C, Lotery A. Bevacizumab: a new way of doing business? Eye. 2006;20:985-7.
15. Ferrara N, Kerbel RS. Angiogenesis as a therapeutic target. Nature. 2005;438:967-74.
16. Carmeliet P. Mechanisms of angiogenesis and arteriogenesis. Nat Med. 2000;6:389-95.
17. Ferrara N, Henzel WJ. Pituitary follicular cells secrete a novel heparin-binding growth factor specific for vascular endothelial cells. Biochem Biophys Res Commun. 1989;161:851-8.
18. Ferrara N, Damico L, Shams N, et al. Development of ranibizumab, an anti-vascular endothelial growth factor antigen binding fragment, as therapy for neovascular age-related macular degeneration. Retina. 2006;26:859-70.
19. Miller JW. Vascular endothelial growth factor and ocular neovascularization. Am J Pathol. 1997;151:13-23.
20. Connell PP, Keane PA, O'Neill EC, et al. Risk factors for age-related maculopathy. J Ophthalmol. 2009;2009:360764.
21. Zarbin MA. Current concepts in the pathogenesis of age-related macular degeneration. Arch Ophthalmol. 2004;122: 598-614.
22. Zarbin MA, Rosenfeld PJ. Pathway-based therapies for age-related macular degeneration: an integrated survey of emerging treatment alternatives. Retina. 2010;30:1350-67.
23. Holz FG, Pauleikhoff D, Klein R, et al. Pathogenesis of lesions in late age-related macular disease. Am J Ophthalmol. 2004;137:504-10.
24. Green WR, Wilson DJ. Choroidal neovascularization. Ophthalmology. 1986;93:1169-76.
25. Grossniklaus HE, Green WR. Choroidal neovascularization. Am J Ophthalmol. 2004;137:496-503.
26. Nozaki M, Raisler BJ, Sakurai E, et al. Drusen complement components C3a and C5a promote choroidal neovascularization. Proc Natl Acad Sci U S A. 2006;103:2328-33.
27. Lopez PF, Sippy BD, Lambert HM, et al. Transdifferentiated retinal pigment epithelial cells are immunoreactive for vascular endothelial growth factor in surgically excised age-related macular degeneration-related choroidal neovascular membranes. Invest Ophthalmol Vis Sci. 1996;37:855-68.
28. Kvanta A, Algvere PV, Berglin L, et al. Subfoveal fibrovascular membranes in age-related macular degeneration express vascular endothelial growth factor. Invest Ophthalmol Vis Sci. 1996;37:1929-34.
29. Group ES. Preclinical and phase 1A clinical evaluation of an anti-VEGF pegylated aptamer (EYE001) for the treatment of exudative age-related macular degeneration. Retina. 2002;22:143-52.
30. Group ES. Anti-vascular endothelial growth factor therapy for subfoveal choroidal neovascularization secondary to age-related macular degeneration: phase II study results. Ophthalmology. 2003;110:979-86.
31. Lee S, Jilani SM, Nikolova GV, et al. Processing of VEGF-A by matrix metalloproteinases regulates bioavailability and vascular patterning in tumors. J Cell Biol. 2005;169:681-91.
32. Park JE, Keller GA, Ferrara N. The vascular endothelial growth factor (VEGF) isoforms: differential deposition into the subepithelial extracellular matrix and bioactivity of extracellular matrix-bound VEGF. Mol Biol Cell. 1993;4:1317-26.
33. Group VISION CT, Chakravarthy U, Adamis AP, et al. Year 2 efficacy results of 2 randomized controlled clinical trials of pegaptanib for neovascular age-related macular degeneration. Ophthalmology. 2006;113:1508. e1-25.
34. Ehlers JP, Fintak DR, Gupta OP, et al. Pegaptanib for choroidal neovascularization in treatment-naïve exudative age-related macular degeneration. Ophthal Surg Lasers Imaging. 2007;38:371-7.
35. Leys, Zlateva, Shah, et al. Quality of life in patients with age-related macular degeneration: results from the VISION study. Eye. 2008;22:792-8.
36. Quiram PA, Hassan TS, Williams GA. Treatment of naïve lesions in neovascular age-related macular degeneration with pegaptanib. Retina. 2007;27:851-6.
37. Sivaprasad S, Hykin P, Saeed A, et al. Intravitreal pegaptanib sodium for choroidal neovascularisation secondary to age-related macular degeneration: Pan-European experience. Eye. 2010;24:793-8.
38. Emerson GG, Flaxel CJ, Lauer AK, et al. Optical coherence tomography findings during pegaptanib therapy for neovascular age-related macular degeneration. Retina. 2007;27:724-9.
39. Gordon MS, Cunningham D. Managing patients treated with bevacizumab combination therapy. Oncology. 2005;69(Suppl 3):25-33.
40. D'Amico DJ, Masonson HN, Patel M, et al. Pegaptanib sodium for neovascular age-related macular degeneration: two-year safety results of the two prospective, multicenter,

controlled clinical trials. Ophthalmology. 2006;113:992-1001.

41. Singerman LJ, Masonson H, Patel, et al. Pegaptanib sodium for neovascular age-related macular degeneration: third-year safety results of the VEGF Inhibition Study in Ocular Neovascularisation (VISION) trial. Br J Ophthalmol. 2008;92:1606-11.
42. Apte RS, Modi M, Masonson H, et al. Pegaptanib 1-year systemic safety results from a safety-pharmacokinetic trial in patients with neovascular age-related macular degeneration. Ophthalmology. 2007;114:1702-12.
43. Farah SE. Treatment of neovascular age-related macular degeneration with pegaptanib and boosting with bevacizumab or ranibizumab as needed. Ophthal Surg Lasers Imaging. 2008;39:294-8.
44. Hughes MS, Sang DN. Safety and efficacy of intravitreal bevacizumab followed by pegaptanib maintenance as a treatment regimen for age-related macular degeneration. Ophthal Surg Lasers Imaging. 2006;37:446-54.
45. Friberg TR, Tolentino M, Group LS. Pegaptanib sodium as maintenance therapy in neovascular age-related macular degeneration: the LEVEL study. Br J Ophthalmol. 2010; 94:1611-7.
46. Gaudreault J, Fei D, Rusit J, et al. Preclinical pharmacokinetics of Ranibizumab (rhuFabV2) after a single intravitreal administration. Invest Ophthalmol Vis Sci. 2005;46:726-33.
47. Mordenti J, Cuthbertson RA, Ferrara N, et al. Comparisons of the intraocular tissue distribution, pharmacokinetics, and safety of 125I-labeled full-length and Fab antibodies in rhesus monkeys following intravitreal administration. Toxicol Pathol. 1999;27:536-44.
48. Boyer DS, Antoszyk AN, Awh CC, et al. Subgroup analysis of the MARINA study of ranibizumab in neovascular age-related macular degeneration. Ophthalmology. 2007;114:246-52.
49. Kaiser PK, Brown DM, Zhang K, et al. Ranibizumab for predominantly classic neovascular age-related macular degeneration: subgroup analysis of first-year ANCHOR results. Am J Ophthalmol. 2007;144:850-7.
50. Rosenfeld PJ, Shapiro H, Tuomi L, et al. Characteristics of patients losing vision after 2 years of monthly dosing in the phase iii ranibizumab clinical trials. Ophthalmology. 2011; 118:523-30.
51. Bressler NM, Chang TS, Fine JT, et al. Improved vision-related function after ranibizumab vs photodynamic therapy: a randomized clinical trial. Arch Ophthalmol. 2009;127:13-21.
52. Kaiser PK, Blodi BA, Shapiro H, et al. Angiographic and optical coherence tomographic results of the MARINA study of ranibizumab in neovascular age-related macular degeneration. Ophthalmology. 2007;114:1868-75.
53. Sadda SR, Stoller G, Boyer DS, et al. Anatomical benefit from ranibizumab treatment of predominantly classic neovascular age-related macular degeneration in the 2-year anchor study. Retina. 2010;30:1390-9.
54. Boyer DS, Heier J, Brown D, et al. A phase iiib study to evaluate the safety of ranibizumab in subjects with neovascular age-related macular degeneration. Ophthalmology. 2009;116:1731-9.
55. Rosenfeld PJ, Moshfeghi AA, Puliafito CA. Optical coherence tomography findings after an intravitreal injection of bevacizumab (avastin) for neovascular age-related macular degeneration. Ophthal Surg Lasers Imaging. 2005;36:331-5.
56. Arevalo JF, Fromow-Guerra J, Sanchez JG, et al. Primary intravitreal bevacizumab for subfoveal choroidal neovascularization in age-related macular degeneration: results of the Pan-American Collaborative Retina Study Group at 12 months follow-up. Retina. 2008;28:1387-94.
57. Arevalo JF, Sánchez JG, Wu L, et al. Intravitreal bevacizumab for subfoveal choroidal neovascularization in age-related macular degeneration at twenty-four months: the Pan-American Collaborative Retina Study Group. Ophthalmology. 2010;117:1974-81. e1.
58. Arias L, Caminal JM, Casas L, et al. A study comparing two protocols of treatment with intravitreal bevacizumab (Avastin) for neovascular age-related macular degeneration. Br J Ophthalmol. 2008;92:1636-41.
59. Costagliola C, Romano M, Corte MD, et al. Intravitreal bevacizumab for treatment-naive patients with subfoveal occult choroidal neovascularization secondary to age-related macular degeneration: a 12-month follow-up study. Retina. 2009;29:1227-34.
60. Emerson MV, Lauer AK, Flaxel CJ, et al. Intravitreal bevacizumab (Avastin) treatment of neovascular age-related macular degeneration. Retina. 2007;27:439-44.
61. Goff MJ, Johnson RN, McDonald HR, et al. Intravitreal bevacizumab for previously treated choroidal neovascularization from age-related macular degeneration. Retina. 2007;27:432-8.
62. Lai TYY, Liu DTL, Chan KP, et al. Visual outcomes and growth factor changes of two dosages of intravitreal bevacizumab for neovascular age-related macular degeneration: a randomized, controlled trial. Retina. 2009;29:1218-26.
63. Lux, Llacer, Joussen H. "Non-responders" to Bevacizumab (AvastinTM) therapy of choroidal neovascular lesions. Br J Ophthalmol. 2007;91:1318-22.
64. Madhusudhana KC, Hannan SR, Williams CPR, et al. Intravitreal bevacizumab (Avastin) for the treatment of choroidal neovascularization in age-related macular degeneration: results from 118 cases. Br J Ophthalmol. 2007;91:1716-7.
65. Modarres M, Naseripour M, Falavarjani KG, et al. Intravitreal injection of 2.5 mg versus 1.25 mg bevacizumab (Avastin) for treatment of CNV associated with AMD. Retina. 2009;29:319-24.
66. Tao Y, Jonas JB. Intravitreal bevacizumab for exudative age-related macular degeneration: effect on different subfoveal membranes. Retina. 2010;30:1426-31.
67. Yoganathan P, Deramo VA, Lai JC, et al. Visual improvement following intravitreal bevacizumab (Avastin) in exudative age-related macular degeneration. Retina. 2006;26:994-8.

68. Rich RM, Rosenfeld PJ, Puliafito CA, et al. Short-term safety and efficacy of intravitreal bevacizumab (Avastin) for neovascular age-related macular degeneration. Retina. 2006;26:495-511.
69. Abrahám-Marin ML, Cortés-Luna CF, Alvarez-Rivera G, et al. Intravitreal bevacizumab therapy for neovascular age-related macular degeneration: a pilot study. Graefes Arch Clin Exp Ophthalmol. 2007;245:651-5.
70. Aggio F, Melo S. Intravitreal bevacizumab for exudative age-related macular degeneration after multiple treatments. Graefes Arch Clin Exp Ophthalmol. 2006;245:215-20.
71. Aisenbrey S, Ziemssen F, Völker M, et al. Intravitreal bevacizumab (Avastin) for occult choroidal neovascularization in age-related macular degeneration. Graefes Arch Clin Exp Ophthalmol. 2007;245:941-8.
72. Lazic R, Gabric N. Intravitreally administered bevacizumab (Avastin) in minimally classic and occult choroidal neovascularization secondary to age-related macular degeneration. Graefes Arch Clin Exp Ophthalmol. 2007;245:68-73.
73. Cleary CA, Jung K, Kumar R. Intravitreal bevacizumab in the treatment of neovascular age-related macular degeneration, 6- and 9-month results. Eye. 2007;22:82-6.
74. Bashshur Z, Haddad Z, Schakal AJ. Intravitreal bevacizumab for treatment of neovascular age-related macular degeneration: the second year of a prospective study. Am J Ophthalmol. 2009;148:59-65. e1.
75. Bashshur ZF, Bazarbachi A, Schakal A, et al. Intravitreal bevacizumab for the management of choroidal neovascularization in age-related macular degeneration. Am J Ophthalmol. 2006;142:1-9.
76. Bashshur ZF, Haddad ZA, Schakal A, et al. Intravitreal bevacizumab for treatment of neovascular age-related macular degeneration: a one-year prospective study. Am J Ophthalmol. 2008;145:249-56.
77. Melamud A, Stinnett S, Fekrat S. Treatment of neovascular age-related macular degeneration with intravitreal bevacizumab: efficacy of three consecutive monthly injections. Am J Ophthalmol. 2008;146:91-5.
78. Pedersen K, Sjølie A, Møller F. Intravitreal bevacizumab (Avastin) for neovascular age-related macular degeneration in treatment-naive patients. Acta Ophthalmol. 2008;87:714-9.
79. Patel P, Bunce C, Tufail A, et al. A randomised, double-masked phase III/IV study of the efficacy and safety of Avastin(R) (Bevacizumab) intravitreal injections compared to standard therapy in subjects with choroidal neovascularisation secondary to age-related macular degeneration: clinical trial design. Trials. 2008;9:56.
80. Tufail A, Patel PJ, Egan C, et al. Bevacizumab for neovascular age related macular degeneration (ABC Trial): multicentre randomised double masked study. BMJ. 2010;340:c2459.
81. Fong DS, Custis P, Howes J, et al. Intravitreal bevacizumab and ranibizumab for age-related macular degeneration a multicenter, retrospective study. Ophthalmology. 2010;117: 298-302.
82. Subramanian M, Ness S, Abedi G, et al. Bevacizumab vs ranibizumab for age-related macular degeneration: early results of a prospective double-masked, randomized clinical trial. Am J Ophthalmol. 2009;148:875-82. e1.
83. Subramanian ML, Abedi G, Ness S, et al. Bevacizumab vs ranibizumab for age-related macular degeneration: 1-year outcomes of a prospective, double-masked randomised clinical trial. Eye. 2010;24:1-8.
84. Falkenstein IA, Cheng L, Morrison VL, et al. Standardized visual acuity results associated with primary versus secondary bevacizumab (avastin) treatment for choroidal neovascularization in age-related macular degeneration. Retina. 2007;27:701-6.
85. Amoaku W. The Royal College of Ophthalmologists interim recommendations for the management of patients with age-related macular degeneration. Eye. 2008;22:864-68.
86. Bressler NM. Antiangiogenic approaches to age-related macular degeneration today. Ophthalmology. 2009;116:S15-23.
87. Reichel E, Duker JS, Puliafito CA. Indocyanine green angiography and choroidal neovascularization obscured by hemorrhage. Ophthalmology. 1995;102:1871-6.
88. Harding SP. Neovascular age-related macular degeneration: decision making and optimal management. Eye. 2010;24:497-505.
89. Stanga PE, Lim JI, Hamilton P. Indocyanine green angiography in chorioretinal diseases: indications and interpretation: an evidence-based update. Ophthalmology. 2003;110:15-21.
90. Muether PS, Hermann MM, Koch K, et al. Delay between medical indication to anti-VEGF treatment in age-related macular degeneration can result in a loss of VA. Graefes Arch Clin Exp Ophthalmol. 2011;249:633-7.
91. Arias L, Armada F, Donate J, et al. Delay in treating age-related macular degeneration in Spain is associated with progressive vision loss. Eye. 2009;23:326-33.
92. Mitchell P, Korobelnik JF, Lanzetta P, et al. Ranibizumab (Lucentis) in neovascular age-related macular degeneration: evidence from clinical trials. Br J Ophthalmol. 2009;94:2-13.
93. Chang MA, Do DV, Bressler SB, et al. Prospective one-year study of ranibizumab for predominantly hemorrhagic choroidal neovascular lesions in age-related macular degeneration. Retina. 2010;30:1171-6.
94. McKibbin M, Papastefanou V, Matthews B, et al. Ranibizumab monotherapy for sub-foveal haemorrhage secondary to choroidal neovascularisation in age-related macular degeneration. Eye. 2010;24:994-8.
95. Sacu S, Stifter E, Vecsei-Marlovits PV, et al. Management of extensive subfoveal haemorrhage secondary to neovascular age-related macular degeneration. Eye. 2009;23:1404-10.
96. Tennant MT, Borrillo JL, Regillo CD. Management of submacular hemorrhage. Ophthalmol Clin North Am. 2002;15:445-52.
97. Chang LK, Sarraf D. Tears of the retinal pigment epithelium: an old problem in a new era. Retina. 2007;27:523-34.

98. Galbinur T, Averbukh E, Banin E, et al. Intravitreal bevacizumab therapy for neovascular age-related macular degeneration associated with poor initial visual acuity. Br J Ophthalmol. 2009;93:1351-2.
99. Ehrlich R, Weinberger D, Priel E, et al. Outcome of Bevacizumab (Avastin) injection in patients with age-related macular degeneration and low visual acuity. Retina. 2008;28:1302-7.
100. Abraham P, Yue H, Wilson L. Randomized, double-masked, sham-controlled trial of ranibizumab for neovascular age-related macular degeneration: PIER study year 2. Am J Ophthalmol. 2010;150:315-24.
101. Regillo CD, Brown DM, Abraham P, et al. Randomized, double-masked, sham-controlled trial of ranibizumab for neovascular age-related macular degeneration: PIER Study year 1. Am J Ophthalmol. 2008;145:239-48.
102. Fung AE, Lalwani GA, Rosenfeld PJ, et al. An optical coherence tomography-guided, variable dosing regimen with intravitreal ranibizumab (Lucentis) for neovascular age-related macular degeneration. Am J Ophthalmol. 2007;143:566-83.
103. Lalwani G, Rosenfeld P, Fung AD, et al. A Variable-dosing Regimen with Intravitreal Ranibizumab for Neovascular Age-related Macular Degeneration: Year 2 of the PrONTO Study. Am J Ophthalmol. 2009;148:43-58.
104. Brown DM, Regillo CD. Anti-VEGF agents in the treatment of neovascular age-related macular degeneration: applying clinical trial results to the treatment of everyday patients. Am J Ophthalmol. 2007;144:627-37.
105. Engelbert M, Zweifel SA, Freund KB. "Treat and extend" dosing of intravitreal antivascular endothelial growth factor therapy for type 3 neovascularization/retinal angiomatous proliferation. Retina. 2009;29:1424-31.
106. Engelbert M, Zweifel SA, Freund KB. Long-term follow-up for type 1 (subretinal pigment epithelium) neovascularization using a modified "treat and extend" dosing regimen of intravitreal antivascular endothelial growth factor therapy. Retina. 2010;30:1368-75.
107. Gupta OP, Shienbaum G, Patel AH, et al. A treat and extend regimen using ranibizumab for neovascular age-related macular degeneration clinical and economic impact. Ophthalmology. 2010;117: 2134-40
108. Oubraham H, Cohen SY, Samimi S, et al. Inject and extend dosing versus dosing as needed: a comparative retrospective study of ranibizumab in exudative age-related macular degeneration. Retina. 2011;31:26-30.
109. Gaudric A, Cohen SY. When should anti-vascular endothelial growth factor treatment be stopped in age-related macular degeneration? Am J Ophthalmol. 2010;149:4-6.
110. Cho M, Barbazetto IA, Freund KB. Refractory neovascular age-related macular degeneration secondary to polypoidal choroidal vasculopathy. Am J Ophthalmol. 2009;148:70-8.
111. Stangos AN, Gandhi JS, Nair-Sahni J, et al. Polypoidal choroidal vasculopathy masquerading as neovascular age-related macular degeneration refractory to ranibizumab. Am J Ophthalmol. 2010;150:666-73.
112. Gomi F, Tano Y. Polypoidal choroidal vasculopathy and treatments. Curr Opin Ophthalmol. 2008;19:208-12.
113. Freund KB, Zweifel SA, Engelbert M. Do we need a new classification for choroidal neovascularization in age-related macular degeneration? Retina. 2010;30:1333-49.
114. Benjamin LE, Golijanin D, Itin A, et al. Selective ablation of immature blood vessels in established human tumors follows vascular endothelial growth factor withdrawal. J Clin Invest. 1999;103:159-65.
115. Keane PA, Chang KT, Liakopoulos S, et al. Effect of ranibizumab retreatment frequency on neurosensory retinal volume in neovascular AMD. Retina. 2009;29:592-600.
116. Keane PA, Liakopoulos S, Ongchin SC, et al. Quantitative subanalysis of optical coherence tomography after treatment with ranibizumab for neovascular age-related macular degeneration. Invest Ophthalmol Vis Sci. 2008;49:3115-20.
117. Forooghian F, Cukras C, Meyerle CB, et al. Tachyphylaxis after intravitreal bevacizumab for exudative age-related macular degeneration. Retina. 2009,29.723-31.
118. Schaal S, Kaplan HJ, Tezel TH. Is there tachyphylaxis to intravitreal anti-vascular endothelial growth factor pharmacotherapy in age-related macular degeneration? Ophthalmology. 2008;115:2199-205.
119. Kaiser PK. Combination therapy with verteporfin and anti-VEGF agents in neovascular age-related macular degeneration: where do we stand? Br J Ophthalmol. 2010;94:143-5.
120. Spaide RF. Rationale for combination therapies for choroidal neovascularization. Am J Ophthalmol. 2006;141:149-56.
121. Do DV. Antiangiogenic approaches to age-related macular degeneration in the future. Ophthalmology. 2009;116:S24-6.
122. Avila MP, Farah ME, Santos A, et al. Twelve-month short-term safety and visual-acuity results from a multicentre prospective study of epiretinal strontium-90 brachytherapy with bevacizumab for the treatment of subfoveal choroidal neovascularisation secondary to age-related macular degeneration. Br J Ophthalmol. 2009;93:305-9.
123. Dixon JA, Oliver SC, Olson JL, et al. VEGF trap-eye for the treatment of neovascular age-related macular degeneration. Expert Opin Investig Drugs. 2009;18:1573-80.
124. Nguyen QD, Shah SM, Browning DJ, et al. A phase I study of intravitreal vascular endothelial growth factor trap-eye in patients with neovascular age-related macular degeneration. Ophthalmology. 2009;116:2141-8.

SECTION 6

Trauma

Vitrectomy in the Management of the Injured Eye

29

Ferenc Kuhn, Nicholas Marchase

Introduction

Mechanical vitrectomy (i.e. one performed using a machine-driven handpiece rather than that utilizing a sponge and scissors) has been around for some four decades.[1] It has increasingly been employed in the treatment of patients with severe injuries; in 1999, an entire book dedicated to the subject was published.[2]

Vitrectomy represented a revolution in ophthalmology, a 180° change in our understanding of, and treatment for, conditions involving primarily the vitreous and the retina. Trauma has been an especially fertile ground for this new management modality since injuries require innovation, creative thinking and an unbiased, non-dogmatic approach to solving problems for which no prescribed recipe may have been reported. Vitrectomy opened the door to the treatment for many pathologies that previously resulted in the loss of vision or even the eyeball.

This chapter provides a broad overview of selected conditions for which vitrectomy techniques can and should be used. Since a lone book chapter cannot do justice for such a broad topic, the reader is referred to the literature for more details.

Instrumentation

Until a few years ago, this issue could have been addressed by stating that "standard (i.e. 20-gauge) three-port vitrectomy" is to be employed. Today, however, there is a variety of gauges (23,[3] and 25,[4] with 27[5] in the pipelines) and monomanual techniques have also resurfaced (injector,[6] slit-lamp illumination). There is a huge variety of hand tools, in addition to intraoperative liquids (e.g. triamcinolone acetonide, perfluorocarbons) and dyes (e.g. indocyanine green, brilliant peel), postoperative tamponades (silicone oil, heavy silicone oil, various gases). The visualization technology has also evolved (wide-angle viewing, illuminated instruments, chandelier systems); finally, endoscopy has reached a point where it can offer complete surgery in many cases.[7] Intraoperative replacement of the cornea with the temporary keratoprosthesis[8,9] has also become routine.

Of all these, let us address in a little more detail only one issue here: transconjunctival ("small-gauge") surgery.

There are several advantages to perform transconjunctival vitreoretinal surgery for many indications.[3,4] Some of the advantages such as reduced trauma to the eye and faster healing do not manifest themselves as prominently as they do in elected cases. Conversely, these instruments also have certain disadvantages, among others:

- Reduced shaft stiffness (i.e. flexibility and consequent difficulty manipulating the eyeball)
- Presence of cannula for instrument entry with two important consequences:
  1. The inability of using certain hand instruments such as scissors with long angled blades
  2. The inability of performing complete vitrectomy underneath the scleral incision in the phakic eye
- The availability of a less full armamentarium than with 20-gauge
- Increased risk of postoperative hypotony.

These difficulties do not render smaller-gauge vitrectomy unusable for trauma cases as the surgeon can typically work around some of them. However, it is an error to use a 23- or 25-gauge system just because the ophthalmologist also employs them for other indications. A conscious, individual decision regarding the choice of the instrument system must be made in every case. In other words: as always, the technique must be adapted to the specific eye or situation and not vice versa.[10]

As the instrumentation evolves, it is likely that transconjunctival surgery will be a more commonly accepted option offering comprehensive solutions to all issues facing the surgeon who performs vitrectomy on the severely injured eye.

A final note concerns the type of vitrectomy machine. As a general rule, using a flow-control system (peristaltic pump) gives the surgeon much more precise control over what occurs inside the eye when the vitrectomy probe is activated. A machine with a Venturi pump (aspiration-based system) limits the control the surgeon possesses over tissue removal and while this may be compensated by high-frequency cutting (reducing, for instance, the "flickering" of the detached retina when vitreous is removed in its proximity), the high speed sacrifices the completeness of vitreous removal (shaving, rather than removal, is achieved).

Vitrectomy for Ocular Trauma: Conditions and Techniques

The pathologies for which vitrectomy is indicated are listed in an anterior-posterior order based on tissue location or the appearance of signs. In addition to the brief description of the surgical technique, we also cover issues such as basic concepts and timing.

▶ Vitreous Prolapse Through the Wound

Basic Concepts

The traditional sponge-scissors method (Fig. 29.1), while able to remove vitreous form the ocular surface, has two main disadvantages:

1. Traction transmitted to the vitreous base and thus the retinal periphery as the vitreous is lifted (i.e. there is a risk of creating an iatrogenic retinal break and detachment);
2. Inability to do a complete job underneath the wound (i.e. vitreous is left adhering to the inside of the wound: the risk of traction is not eliminated).

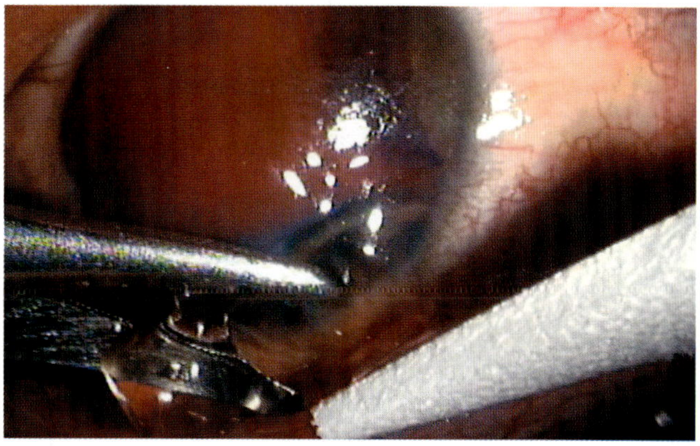

▲ **Figure 29.1**

Sponge-scissors removal of the prolapse vitreous. The sponge is immersed (dipped) in the prolapsed vitreous; the scissors is being ready to cut the vitreous that is about to be elevated with the sponge

The vitrectomy probe, on the other hand, is able to accomplish both goals without inflicting additional damage on the eye.

Technique

The vitrectomy probe is immersed in the prolapsed vitreous (Fig. 29.2), which is cut and removed; this is followed by dealing with the vitreous caught between the wound lips and, finally, underneath them.

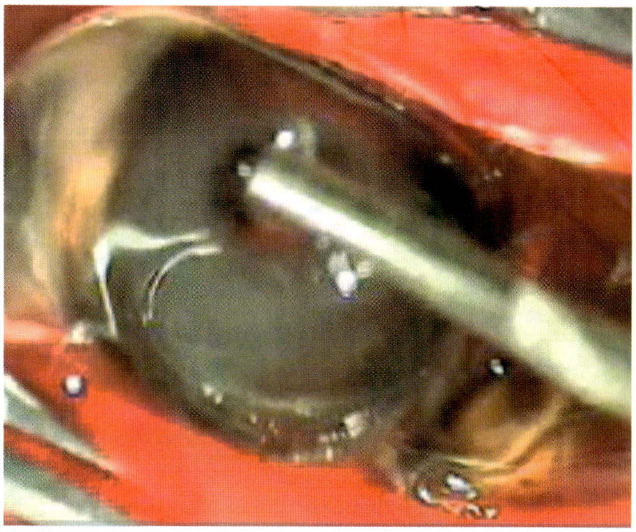

▲ **Figure 29.2**

Vitrectomy-probe removal of the prolapse vitreous. The vitrectomy probe is able to remove vitreous from the ocular surface, in-between the wound lips and from the anterior chamber

If the wound is corneal, the surgeon should consider removing the vitreous from the entire anterior chamber; in this case, it is usually preferable to close the wound at this point and complete the procedure through a strategically placed paracentesis.

If the wound is scleral, no vitreous removal from deep inside the eye is recommended.

Timing

Immediate; this is the first step of restoring the integrity of the injured eye. The only exception to this rule is the occurrence of an expulsive choroidal hemorrhage, in which case the eye must instantly be closed, regardless of whether any tissue prolapse is present.

Hyphema

Basic Concepts

In most cases, there is no need for surgery, the blood resolves spontaneously. In cases requiring surgery, the blood may be liquid and a simple washout is sufficient. In eyes with an anterior chamber filled mostly or completely and with clotted blood, however, vitrectomy offers the best option to remove it.

As a general rule, this surgery should be performed by an experienced vitreoretinal, rather than an anterior segment, specialist. While the surgery appears quite easy, it is not unless one is comfortable with posterior segment (vitreoretinal) surgical techniques.

Technique

The first thing is to introduce an infusion line into the anterior chamber, usually an anterior chamber maintainer. Any (especially sudden) drop of the intraocular pressure is to be avoided (see above: flow-, rather than aspiration control).

In a phakic eye, it is advisable to have the position of the tip of the irrigation cannula be continually monitored by the assistant or nurse so as to avoid iatrogenic injury—the surgeon's attention is focused on the movements of the vitrectomy probe. This is especially true if a sharp needle is used in lieu of an anterior chamber maintainer.

The clot should be engaged in the periphery, over the iris, keeping the port of the probe horizontally (i.e. do not turn it downwards; Fig. 29.3). Initially, the clot should be gently moved to break its adherence to the iris and/or angle. Aspiration should be activated only when the clot is engaged and the cutting frequency should be low. Direct contact with the iris is to be avoided as much as possible, to reduce the risk of rebleeding and prevent causing miosis.

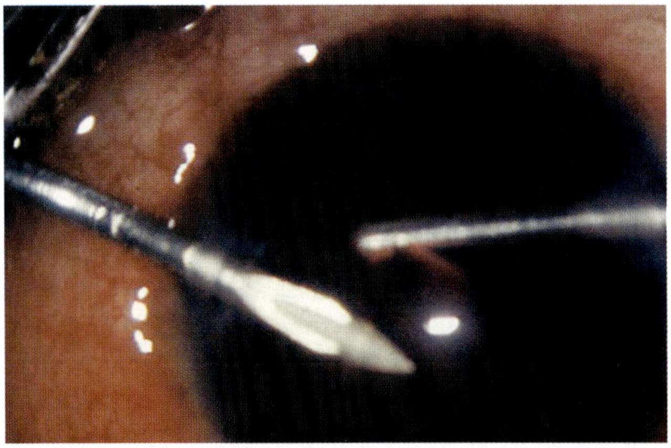

▲ **Figure 29.3**

Vitrectomy-probe removal of a clotted hyphema. A sharp needle is used for infusion; it is turned toward the cornea and its tip's position is continually monitored by the assistant. The vitrectomy probe is turned sideways and its flow is not activated unless the port engages the blood clot

In the pseudo or aphakic eye the surgeon's job is easier; the crucial tissue to avoid touching is the cornea.

Timing

Ideally, surgery is performed before the cornea becomes blood-stained ("imbibition", Fig. 29.4). In this context, surgery is rarely urgent; however, should the intraocular

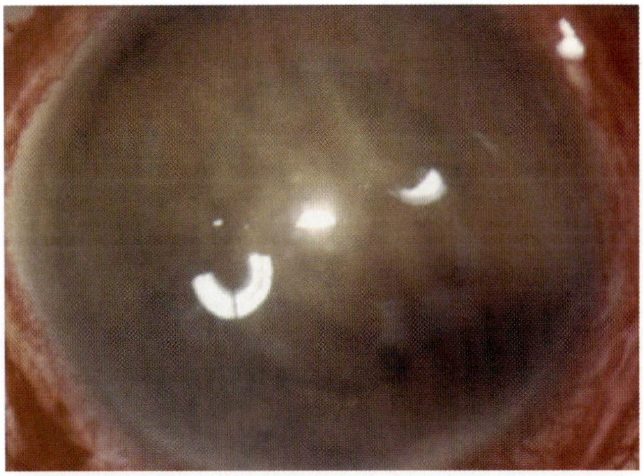

▲ **Figure 29.4**

Corneal blood-staining. Due a few days' delay in surgery for hyphema removal, even mild elevation of the intraocular pressure in this eye with total hyphema was enough to make it impossible to view details of the inside of the globe. The temporary keratoprosthesis was necessary to perform vitrectomy for a coexisting retinal detachment pressure become elevated and impossible to reduce with conservative methods, vitrectomy-hyphema removal becomes an emergency. It is best to prevent this by early surgery.

Lens Trauma

Basic Concepts

It is crucial for the surgeon to understand and accept that a traumatic cataract is very different from an elective one. Techniques perfected for the latter may cause serious iatrogenic complications if indiscriminately employed in the trauma setting.[11] In eyes with a substantial posterior capsule lesion the vitreous can prolapse into the lens, which may be unknown to the surgeon not only preoperatively but its intraoperative recognition is also very difficult.

A study on a large series of eyes operated on for traumatic cataract found that a careful preoperative examination was able to identify 23% of eyes with such a posterior capsule lesion; intraoperatively, this rate almost doubled (45%).[12] This should give pause to the surgeon: it is preferable to "unnecessarily" use the vitrectomy probe for lens removal rather than to be "brave" and perform phacoemulsification and thus aspirate vitreous and cause traction (see above).

If the lens is subluxed, it need not be removed unless the patient has visual complains. In the latter a case, again, caution is in order. While a capsular tension ring may be a good option in nontraumatic cases, its use in trauma is questionable at least: how would the surgeon know the condition of the remaining zonules?[13] Should the entire capsular bag, including capsular tension ring and intraocular lens become dislocated later (Figs 29.5A to D), the anterior segment surgeon will not see the patient and thus remain convinced that he chose the correct technique by using the capsular tension ring. Again, removal using the vitrectomy probe is safe and the alternative techniques (iris-clip, scleral-fixated, anterior chamber) of intraocular lens implantation to the otherwise desired "in-the-bag option" offer safe and excellent outcomes.

Whether vitreous prolapse alone justifies vitrectomy depends on its size: if it does not cause corneal touch, observation is usually thought to suffice. However, since the vitreous is stuck to the iris, the presence of traction must always be considered and vitrectomy may be indicated.

Before surgery, it must be decided whether a limbal or pars plana approach is to be used. As a general rule, the latter requires more experience but has more advantages:

- Instant access to the vitreal cavity if posterior segment pathologies require it
- Preservation of the corneal endothelium
- Preservation of the anterior capsule without exerting traction on the zonules.

The technique described below is for a pars plana entry.

If the lens is luxated into the vitreous, its removal must be preceded by a complete vitrectomy.

Technique

First, an infusion line must be introduced. If the surgeon is unable to verify the position of the pars plana cannula, an anterior chamber maintainer should be used. Alternatively, a bimanual approach can be used: a needle is connected to the infusion line and the needle is inserted into the lens. It is kept inside the capsular bag until the all lens material has been removed.

Traumatic cataract with a definite or suspected posterior capsular lesion: the following are the steps:

- The vitrectomy probe is advanced into the lens after the creation of an opening in the capsular bag with a microvitrectomy blade.
- The cortex or nucleus is removed using a "nibbling" technique: The probe is slowly advanced while continually engaging lens material. The port is not turned toward the surgeon, neither is it turned toward the vitreous to avoid opening of the capsule too soon; this helps prevent loss of lens material posteriorly.
- Injection of triamcinolone into the capsular bag (Fig. 29.6) helps identify any prolapsed vitreous. If the nucleus is too hard for the vitrectomy probe to handle—again, this is an advantage for a 20-gauge probe—and ultrasound is necessary (phacofragmentation), this is especially important. Vitreous removal must be complete before aspiration-without-cutting can be used.
- Once the nucleus and most of the cortex are removed, a large opening in the posterior capsule is made. Especially in children, an anterior vitrectomy is also performed.
- Depending on the situation and the surgeon's intentions, either an anterior capsulectomy is made or the anterior capsule is cleaned with the vitrectomy port, using the following technique:
  - Reduce the flow (~3 ml/min) or the aspiration (~30 mm Hg)
  - Turn the port toward the capsule (the probe is behind the capsule);

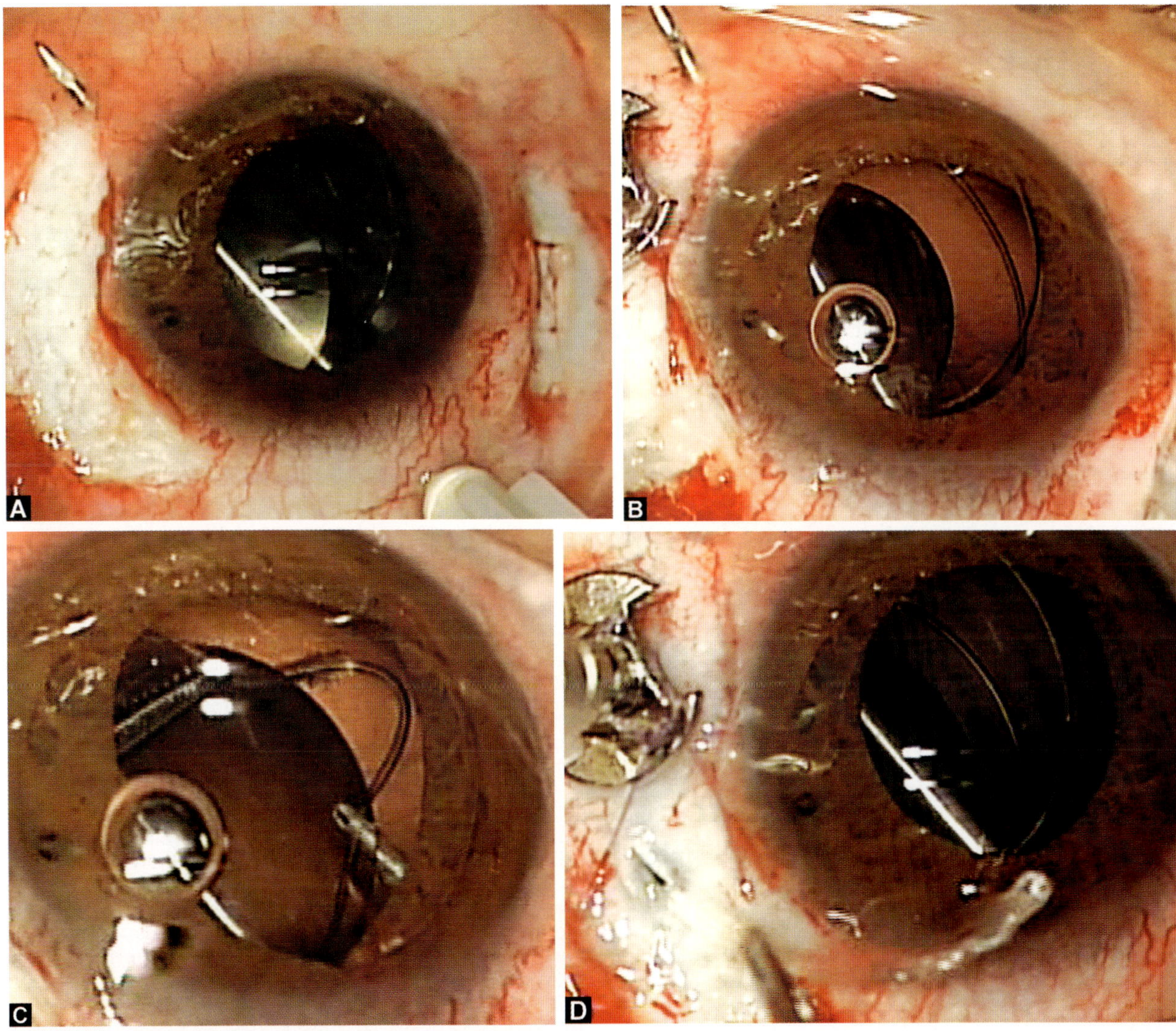

▲ **Figures 29.5A to D**

Subluxation of the capsule-intraocular lens-capsular tension ring complex. This patient with traumatic cataract underwent phacoemulsification and in-the-bag implantation of an intraocular lens by a well-known anterior segment specialist. During surgery, lens material was lost into the vitreous; the patient was referred for vitreoretinal surgery weeks later as the inflammation would not subside. (A) A 25-gauge needle is holding the intraocular lens and the capsular bag in place. The edge of the intraocular lens and the inferior haptic are well visible; (B) Surgical surprise: The discharge summary did not mention that the lens was also dislocated and a capsular tension ring had been implanted; (C) Two intraocular forceps are used to locate the tip of the capsular tension ring; (D) The capsular tension ring is being removed through the pars plana; part of it is visible outside the eye superiorly, still connected to capsular and cortex material

- Advance the probe slowly as the flow or aspiration is activated; this will clean the capsule and reduce the risk of opacification.

Subluxed lens with or without cataract: the technique is very similar to the description above, but complete removal of the anterior capsule should also be considered.

Lens luxated into the vitreous: perform a complete vitrectomy, including removal of the posterior hyaloid face and the peripheral vitreous:

- Remove the lens either using the vitrectomy probe or the phacofragmentor
- Examine the retinal periphery by scleral indentation for iatrogenic breaks.

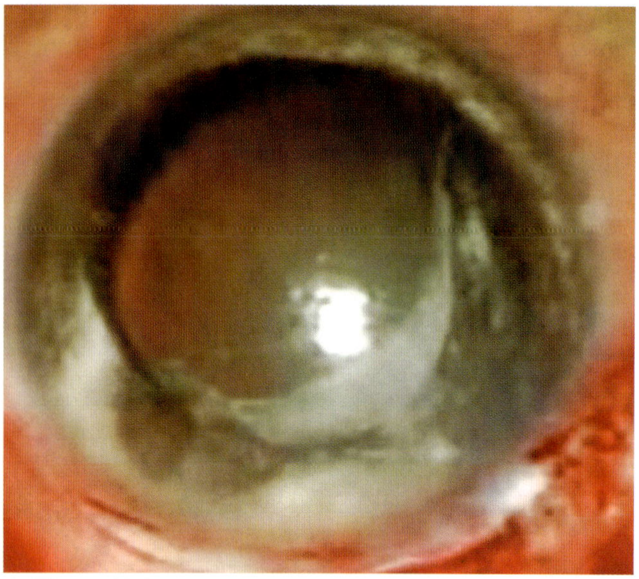

▲ Figure 29.6

Triamcinolone acetonide to delineate vitreous prolapsed into the lens. The otherwise invisible vitreous prolapse is clearly seen when marked by the white crystals of triamcinolone; this determines the method of lens removal (vitrectomy probe)

Timing

The intervention is rarely acute, except if the lens is swelling and causes a significant rise in the intraocular pressure. It can occur rapidly in children. Less commonly, such a pressure elevation can occur because of a severe inflammation or, occasionally, due to a pupillary block. Vitrectomy is urgent in the latter but less so in the former.

Endophthalmitis

Basic Concepts

The diagnosis may be much more difficult than in a post-operative setting, due to corneal opacity and/or intracameral blood or inflammatory debris. Consequently, the surgeon's bar for vitrectomy should be set very low.

The goal is to systematically clear the inside of the eye, advancing from anterior to posterior. As a general rule, it is more dangerous to leave pus behind than to cause a peripheral retinal break, although every effort should be made to avoid this complication. Surgery is not a substitute for the proper antibiotic therapy; the latter is not discussed here.

Technique

- Scrape the corneal epithelium.
- Dry the corneal stroma if necessary (40% glucose).
- Introduce an anterior chamber maintainer.
- Remove any blood and inflammatory debris from the anterior chamber (see above).
- Remove any fibrinous membrane, both from the surface of the (intraocular) lens and iris as well as from the angle.
- Dilate the pupil; use iris retractors if necessary.
- Introduce a pars plana infusion; as soon as its tip can be visualized, turn it on and remove the anterior chamber maintainer.
- If the eye is pseudophakic, make a large posterior capsulectomy and irrigate the bag copiously.
- Perform careful anterior-posterior vitrectomy. Always be "on the lookout" for detached retina, even if the pre-operative ultrasonography was negative.
- Try to detach the posterior hyaloid, especially in the macular area. This is a sensitive, difficult maneuver and must be done with great caution. Pus always accumulates here (macular hypopyon; Fig. 29.7) since it is heavy; leaving vitreous here significantly interferes with the eye achieving its full visual potential.
- Carefully trim the vitreous in the periphery, but remain on the conservative side here.
- If a retinal break or detachment is present, irrigate the vitreous cavity with antibiotics or corticosteroids and

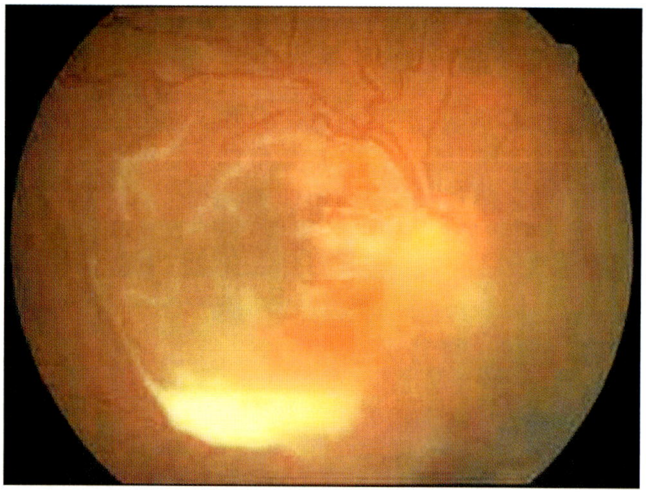

▲ Figure 29.7

Macular hypopyon in an eye with traumatic endophthalmitis. Pus has accumulated on the macular surface; this picture was taken at the slit lamp and thus clearly imitates the image of a hypopyon. However, when the patient is in bed, the heavy material covers the fovea, explaining the poor outcome even if the organism is relatively benign implant silicone oil;[14] inject antibiotics or corticosteroids (1/3 of the normal dose) into the oil.

Timing

Vitrectomy for traumatic endophthalmitis is an absolute emergency.

▶ Glaucoma

Basic Concepts

The rise in intraocular pressure may be related to blood or inflammatory debris in the anterior chamber or caused by the lens (swelling, subluxation); these are discussed above.

In addition, the cause of the glaucoma may be degenerated (ghost) red blood cells in the vitreous that enter the anterior chamber and block the aqueous outflow in the trabecular meshwork. Aqueous misdirection (malignant glaucoma) is another cause: the aqueous then pushes the vitreous/lens/iris forward.

Technique

Obviously, the cause must be addressed (material accumulating in the anterior chamber, lens-related). In the other cases described in the previous paragraph, a complete vitrectomy must be performed.

Timing

Unless the pressure is very high, the vitrectomy is rarely acute.

▶ Vitreous Hemorrhage

Basic Concepts

Vitreous bleeding has several negative consequences; it:

- Reduces vision;
- Blocks the view of the retina;
- Causes amblyopia in young children;
- Increases the risk of cataract, siderosis and glaucoma;[15]
- Increases the risk of epimacular proliferation, proliferative vitreoretinopathy and retinal detachment.[16-19]

Removal of the blood helps treating or, preferably, preventing these complications. In a traumatic setting, this otherwise straightforward surgery can be a lot more difficult.

Technique

The standard technique does not differ from complete vitreous removal for other indications. However, in young individuals whose vitreous has been healthy prior to the injury, it is not easy to distinguish between layers of vitreous and a detached retina; the preoperative ultrasound is notoriously unreliable in these cases.

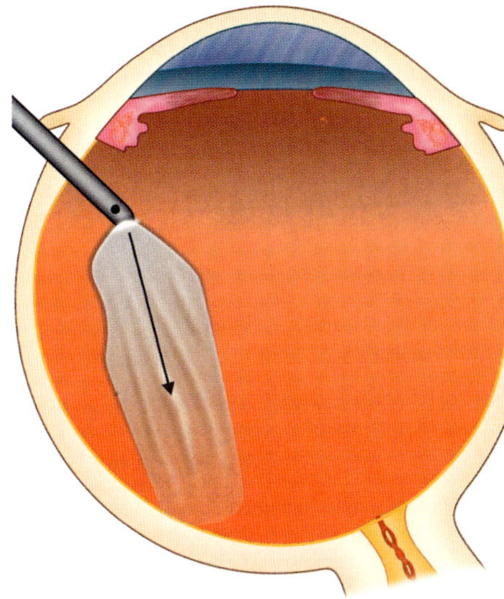

▲ **Figure 29.8**
The "vertical digging" technique for eyes with severe vitreous hemorrhage

The intraoperative difficulty distinguishing the two tissues is caused by several factors:

- The vitreous looks like layers of onion and an individual layer appears similar to a detached retina;
- The layers have blood streaks on them, similar to the appearance of blood vessels in the retina;
- There is unclotted blood trapped between the vitreous layers; when released, this can imitate retinal bleeding;
- The retina may be partially necrotic with consequent lack of bleeding when bitten into.

For these reasons, the surgeon should overcome his instinct to progress in a "careful horizontal" fashion and dig instead a vertical "well" on the nasal side (Fig. 29.8). Holding the wall of this well open with the two instruments, the surgeon can hopefully identify the attached or detached retina before actually causing a retinectomy. In the latter case the surgeon at least knows immediately the location of the retina and the iatrogenic damage is restricted to a small and relatively insignificant area.

The posterior hyaloid face has been reportedly described as detaching within a week or so; in reality, it rarely does, even weeks after the injury (see below).

Timing

There is no disagreement in the literature: eyes with open globe injury require early removal of the vitreous hemorrhage. The traditional interpretation of "early", however, is debated; usually it is understood as waiting 7–10 days. The authors of this chapter tend to agree with Coleman[20] and prefer performing vitrectomy within 4 days, often performing comprehensive primary vitrectomy (i.e. during the initial, wound-closure surgery).

For eyes with closed globe (contusion) injury, the traditional recommendation is to wait a few months to allow for spontaneous clearing and to allow spontaneous detachment of the posterior hyaloid. The latter maneuver is deemed dangerous by many surgeons in young individuals.

A recent study, however, showed that even weeks after (open globe) injury, less than a quarter of eyes developed spontaneous detachment of the posterior hyaloid.[21] The argument of postponing vitrectomy for the sake of spontaneous posterior vitreous detachment therefore does not seem to hold water; furthermore, early surgery allows rapid functional recovery for the injured person and a detailed examination of the retina for the ophthalmologist. Contusion is a well-known risk factor for retinal break and subsequent detachment development, which can be prevented by early recognition and proper laser treatment.

For all these reasons, early surgery should be considered for contusion-related vitreous hemorrhage as well as for eyes with open-globe trauma and be best discussed with the patient (counseling).

Intraocular Foreign Body

Basic Concepts

The presence of an object left in the eye after trauma always brings extra excitement for both patient and ophthalmologist. In reality, in most cases it is not the presence of a foreign object inside the eye that determines the outcome but the concurrent damage to intraocular tissues. The only reasons why special consideration should be given to the eye with an intraocular foreign body (IOFB) are:

- An increased risk of endophthalmitis;
- The potential for toxicosis;
- The need or demand to remove the foreign object.

The increased endophthalmitis risk is real; presence of the IOFB roughly doubles the risk compared to similar penetrating injuries. However, proper postinjury antibiotic therapy allows the surgeon to carefully weigh other factors (equipment availability, patient's systemic condition, etc.) without increasing the risk.[21]

Toxicosis a long-term issue; with the exception of the IOFB being copper and threatening acute retinal necrosis, a delay of a few days or even weeks does not increase the risk.

As a general rule, all fresh IOFBs should be removed. Exceptions can be made, though: an intralenticular IOFB need not lead to cataract formation,[22] although the risk of siderosis is still an issue to deal with if the IOFB is ferrous. Similarly, an inert intravitreal IOFB in an eye that has no major pathology may be left behind—but all these issues are best discussed with the patient.

Technique

An intracameral IOFB is usually removed through a paracentesis created at some distance away to allow for greater manipulation; use of viscoelastics should always be considered to protect the corneal endothelium.

An IOFB in the posterior segment represents a more complex situation. Unless a free-floating intravitreal IOFB is encountered with no retinal injury present, a complete vitrectomy is recommended, during which the IOFB is removed once all traction has been eliminated. This is achieved by performing some vitrectomy, grabbing the IOFB with an intraocular magnet of forceps, bringing it anteriorly and performing complete vitrectomy around it before extraction. Use of a third hand (chandelier) greatly simplifies the procedure.

An epiretinal IOFB is removed after all vitreous around it has been removed. To avoid retinal injury by an IOFB falling back on the retina, the IOFB must securely be grabbed; for ferrous IOFBs, a strong intraocular magnet with a short working distance and directional magnetic force is recommended.[23] Non-ferrous IOFBs must be removed using a forceps; several designs should be available for the surgeon so that the most ideal one can be selected. Significant dexterity is needed to lift a sharp IOFB from the retinal surface; perfluorocarbon liquid use is generally not recommended since they may submerge the IOFB or push it sideways.

An intraretinal IOFB requires its careful freeing and separating the object from the surrounding tissue (retina, capsule) before actual removal. As with a deep-impact IOFB (Fig. 29.9), which causes choroidal or even scleral pathology, prophylactic chorioretinectomy should be considered (see below).

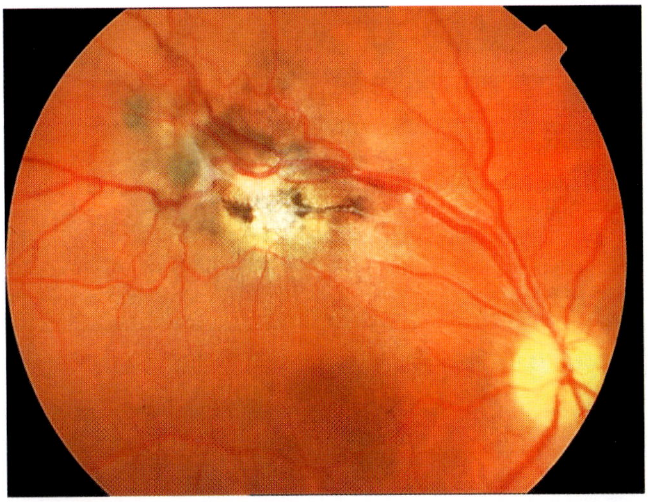

▲ Figure 29.9

A deep-impact intraocular foreign body's aftermath. The object has been extracted (it bounced back and was found lying on the retinal surface). The primary impact site shows naked sclera centrally, reactive pigmentation around it, and epimacular proliferation, which causes retinal fold formation reaching into the macula and dragging of the retinal vessels. The patient is fortunate that proliferative vitreoretinopathy did not develop

Timing

As mentioned above, an IOFB usually does not constitute an emergency if proper antibiotic treatment has been initiated. Nevertheless, early surgery has definite advantages and is indicated for all cases with a high-risk for endophthalmitis: soil contamination or rural injury,[24] organic IOFB, or lens injury in a patient over 50 years with a traumatic cataract.[25]

Retinal Break/Macular Hole

Basic Concepts

The retina may suffer a break due to impact or, more commonly, due to subsequently developing traction. The former is obviously a possibility to consider in eyes with open globe trauma; the latter can occur both in eyes with open- or closed globe injury. In contusions, the retina may also become necrotic; in this case vitrectomy is usually contraindicated to avoid creating a retinal detachment during surgery.

Vitrectomy for a retinal break is not indicated unless a detachment ensues; proper laser treatment suffices. However, vitrectomy may be necessary for eyes with a macular hole, even if there are other macular pathologies present (hemorrhage, contusion maculopathy, choroidal rupture).

Technique

Complete vitrectomy, combined with removal of the internal limiting membrane (ILM) around the hole. Staining of the ILM makes the procedure not only easier, it allows for a more complete removal. Gas tamponade and proper positioning are part of the procedure.

Timing

There is no agreement whether a traumatic macular hole can be observed for months due to a presumed tendency of spontaneous hole closure or very early vitrectomy to prevent deterioration of the macular function. Again, counseling the patient and common decision-making are the ideal path to arrive at the decision.

Retinal Detachment

Basic Concepts

It is best to prevent the retinal detachment by early surgery. Should it have occurred by the time of vitrectomy, the surgeon must understand that the tractional element in the pathogenesis is key to the success of surgery.

Technique

The vitrectomy should be as complete as possible, including removal of the vitreous:

- Posteriorly (cortical vitreous facing the retina)
- In the periphery (using scleral indentation)
- Behind the lens in the pseudo or phakic eye to prevent the postoperative development of circumferential traction

It is highly recommended to use triamcinolone to visualize the posterior hyaloid (Fig. 29.10) so that it can be detached and removed in its entirety. A traumatic retinal detachment has a higher-than-normal risk of recurrence so the choice of tamponade should be considered accordingly: the bar for silicone oil implantation should be low.

Timing

If prevention was unsuccessful, surgery is urgent, although it does not represent an absolute emergency.

Proliferative Vitreoretinopathy

Basic Concepts

Not considering pathologies occurring directly at the time of the injury, proliferative vitreoretinopathy (PVR) represents

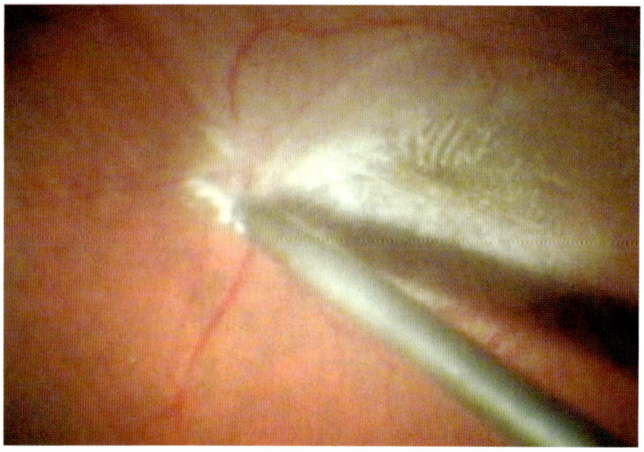

▲ **Figure 29.10**

Attached posterior vitreous in an eye with retinal detachment. Contrary to commonly held dogma, the posterior vitreous is attached in most eyes with retinal detachment; the image clearly shows the triamcinolone-marked vitreous to adhere to the detached retina posteriorly

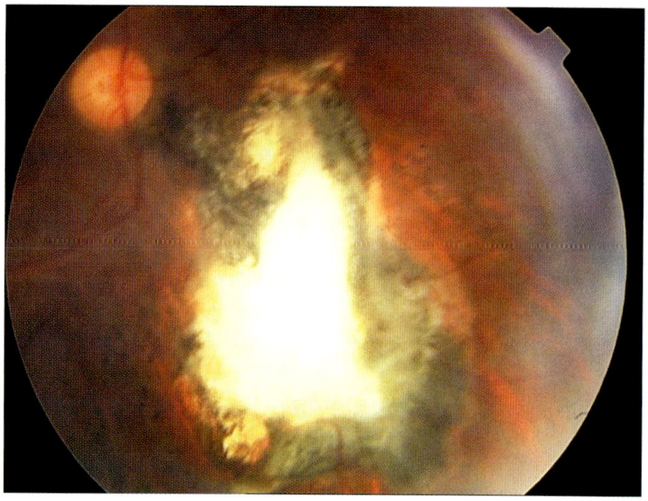

▲ **Figure 29.11**

Long-term follow-up after prophylactic chorioretinectomy. The central area shows bare sclera, surrounded by reactive pigmentation, but there is neither proliferative vitreoretinopathy nor retinal fold formation (compare to Fig. 29.9)

the most important reason for failure in ocular traumatology. It should be prevented if possible (see below); once it occurs, surgery usually involves retinectomy and a high risk of recurrence. Prevention is achieved via prophylactic chorioretinectomy. The goal is to prevent retinal incarceration in the wound and to prevent the retinal pigment epithelial cells as well as the sclera-originated fibroblasts to reach the retina and grow on it (apparently, the fibroblasts do not cross the barrier of the bare sclera to invade the retina away from the scleral scar).

Technique

Prevention: Although ideally this should be achieved pharmacologically, so far this has not proved successful. Surgical prevention using prophylactic chorioretinectomy has shown to be remarkably effective.[26] The procedure is to be employed in all eyes with high PVR risk:

- A rupture or laceration with postequatorial extension;
- An IOFB injury with deep impact (see above);
- A perforating injury with a posterior exit wound.

The surgical steps are as follows:

- Complete the vitrectomy (see above).
- Use the highest setting of the endodiathermy probe to create a continual, one-burn wide barrier around the scleral wound (rupture/laceration), exit wound (perforation), or deep-impact IOFB lesion (Fig. 29.11).

Treatment: Once PVR is present, complex vitreoretinal surgery is necessary. Its description is beyond the scope of this chapter.

Timing

Prophylactic chorioretinectomy should be performed within 4 days of the injury to effectively prevent scar formation related to the wound or impact site. Once PVR occurs, there is no consensus regarding the optimal time to intervene. If there is no macular detachment, it may be advisable to wait with surgery until the PVR cycle is over (this is typically a 3-month period). This is generally the case if the eye is already filled with silicone oil; if the macula is involved or quickly threatened, surgery should be performed urgently.

References

1. Machemer R, Buettner H, Norton E, et al. Vitrectomy: a pars plana approach. Ophthalmology. 1971;75:813-5.
2. Alfaro D, Liggett P. Vitreoretinal surgery of the injured eye. Philadelphia: Lippincott-Raven; 1999.
3. Eckardt C. Transconjunctival sutureless 23-gauge vitrectomy. Retina. 2005;25:208-11.
4. Fujii GY, De Juan E, Humayun M, et al. Initial experience using the transconjunctival sutureless vitrectomy system for vitreoretinal surgery. Ophthalmology. 2002;109:1814-20.

5. Oshima Y, Wakabayashi T, Sato T, et al. A 27-gauge instrument system for transconjunctival sutureless microincision vitrectomy surgery. Ophthalmology. 2010;117:93-102.
6. Koch F, Scholtz S, Singh P, et al. Combined intravitreal therapy for age-related macular disease. Klin Monbl Augenheilkd. 2008;1003-8.
7. Boscher C, Kuhn F. Endoscopy. In: Kuhn F (Ed). Ocular traumatology. Berlin: Springer; 2008. pp. 473-86.
8. Eckardt C. A new temporary keratoprosthesis for pars plana vitrectomy. Retina. 1987;7:34-7.
9. Landers M, Foulks G, Landers D, et al. Temporary keratoprosthesis for use during pars plana vitrectomy. Am J Ophthalmol. 1981;91:615-9.
10. Kuhn F. Strategic thinking in ocular traumatology. In: Kuhn F (Ed). Ocular Traumatology. Berlin: Springer; 2008. pp. 79-104.
11. Kuhn F. Traumatic cataract: what, when, how. Graefe's Arch Clin Exp Ophthalmol. 2010;248:1221-3.
12. Kuhn F. Lens. In: Kuhn F (Ed). Ocular Traumatology. Berlin: Springer; 2008. pp. 245-8.
13. Kuhn F. The proper time for capsular tension rings. EyeNet; 2008.p.12.
14. Yan H, Lu Y, Yu J, et al. Silicone oil in the surgical treatment of traumatic endophthalmitis. Eur J Ophthalmol. 2009;19:496-7.
15. Cibis P, Yamashita T, Rodriguez F. Clinical aspects of ocular siderosis and hemosiderosis. Arch Ophthalmol. 1959;62:46-53.
16. Clarkson JG, Flynn HW, Daily MJ. Vitrectomy in Terson's syndrome. Am J Ophthalmol. 1980;90:540-52.
17. Ehrenberg M, Tresher RJ, Machemer R. Vitreous hemorrhage nontoxic to retina as a stimulator of glial and fibrous proliferation. Am J Ophthalmol 1984;97:611-26.
18. Isernhagen RD, Smiddy WE, Michels RG. Vitrectomy for nondiabetic vitreous hemorrhage. Not associated with vascular disease. Retina 1988;8:81-7.
19. Spraul CW, Grossniklaus HE. Vitreous Hemorrhage. Surv Ophthalmol. 1997;42:3-39.
20. Coleman D. Early vitrectomy in the management of the severely traumatized eye. Am J Ophthalmol. 1982;93:543-51.
21. Colyer M, Weber E, Weichel, et al. Delayed intraocular foreign body removal without endophthalmitis during Operations Iraqi Freedom and Enduring Freedom. Ophthalmology. 2007;114:1439-47.
22. Pieramici D, Capone AJ, Rubsamen P, et al. Lens preservation after intraocular foreign body injuries. Ophthalmology. 1996;103:1563-7.
23. Kuhn F, Heimann K. Ein neuer Dauermagnet zur Entfernung intraokularer ferromagnetischer Fremdkoerper. Klin Mbl Augenheilk. 1991;198:301-3.
24. Boldt H, Pulido J, Blodi C, et al. Rural endophthalmitis. Ophthalmology. 1989;101:332-41.
25. Thompson W, Rubsamen P, Flynn H, et al. Endophthalmitis after penetrating trauma. Risk factors and visual acuity outcomes. Ophthalmology. 1995;102:1696-701.
26. Kuhn F, Mester V, Morris R. A proactive treatment approach for eyes with perforating injury. Klin Monatsbl Augenheilk. 2004;221:622-8.

SECTION

7

Endophthalmitis

Vitreoretinal Surgery in Endophthalmitis

30

Dimple Modi, Benjamin J Ernst, Stephen S Feman

Introduction

Endophthalmitis is an intraocular inflammation and can be infectious or noninfectious. The noninfectious variety can occur from sources such as retained lens particles after cataract extraction, or from other materials that may be toxic to the intraocular cavity. Endophthalmitis is a response to an infectious agent originating from a source that is either exogenous or endogenous to the patient. Exogenous endophthalmitis results from the direct inoculation of an infectious agent into the intraocular contents, such as when the eye is physically penetrated from trauma or surgery. Endogenous causes are less common; they occur when microorganisms located originally elsewhere in the patient, travel to the eye, usually through the blood stream.

Clinical Presentation

Most often the symptoms of acute endophthalmitis include eye pain, conjunctival injection, decreased vision, eyelid and conjunctival swelling and ocular discharge. Patients with this presentation should undergo a thorough eye exam to search for a potential etiologic agent. Signs on examination may include decreased visual acuity, conjunctival and corneal edema, anterior chamber inflammation, afferent pupillary defect, vitritis, retinitis, retinal edema and decreased red reflex. In some cases endophthalmitis can result in permanent ocular tissue damage within 24–48 hours and as a result acute emergent intervention is often needed; however, other forms may be more indolent and difficult to diagnose.

Infectious Endophthalmitis

Infectious endophthalmitis is a severe inflammation of the internal structures of the eye caused by infectious agents that propagate intraocular damage. Bacteria, fungi, viruses and parasites can all invade and replicate in the eye, leading to an inflammatory response. When an intraocular infection spreads to involve the cornea, sclera and extraocular structures, it is termed a panophthalmitis.

Exogenous Endophthalmitis

These are the following factors causing exogenous endophthalmitis

Postoperative

The majority of endophthalmitis cases occur after a previous surgical procedure has been performed on the eye; that is, approximately 67% of all patients with this infection have a history of a previous operation.[1] Although any ocular surgery can be related to this problem, cataract extraction is the most common immediate cause.[1] Acute postoperative endophthalmitis is defined as a case that occurs within 6 weeks of surgery; while chronic cases occur after 6 weeks. Studies suggest that the incidence of postoperative endophthalmitis have decreased over the past half century because of the increased attention given to sterile techniques, such as the preparation of the surgical field and the use of povidone-iodine application prior to operating.

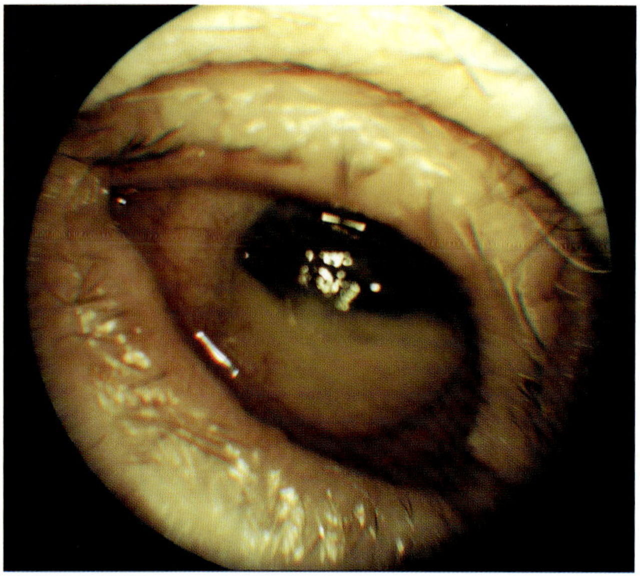

▲ **Figure 30.1**
Hypopyon as presenting sign of endophthalmitis

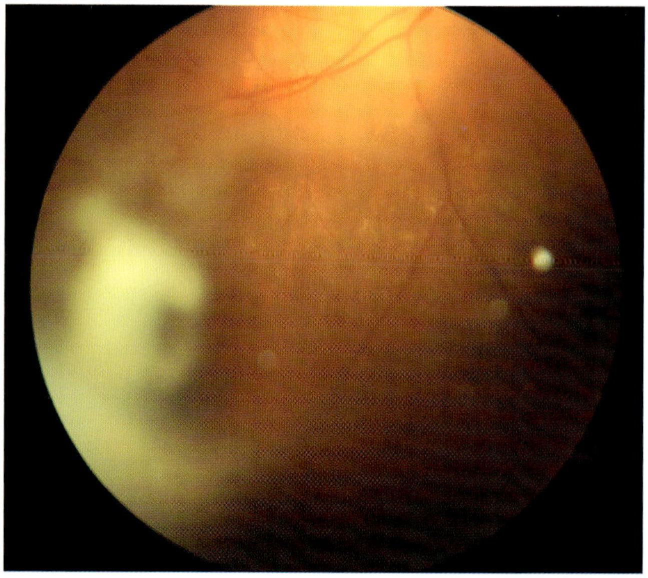

▲ **Figure 30.2**
Endophthalmitis in vitreous

Cataract Extraction

Acute endophthalmitis post cataract surgery typically presents with pain, eyelid edema, yellow conjunctival discharge, increased conjunctival injection and chemosis; usually appearing between 24 hours to 1 week after surgery. Corneal edema and keratic precipitates may be evident. There is anterior chamber inflammation usually, with white blood cells, red blood cells and fibrin, which can layer to form a hypopyon (Fig. 30.1). Exudates may leak from a dehiscence of the surgical wound. Vitritis with debris and vitreous opacification may obstruct a view of the retina and lead to a decreased red reflex. Inflammation around retinal vessels and cotton-wool spots in the retina may be masked because of this increased vitreous inflammation (Fig. 30.2).

It is important to distinguish infectious endophthalmitis after cataract extraction from toxic anterior segment syndrome (TASS), a sterile anterior segment inflammation after cataract surgery. Patients with TASS will develop symptoms within 12–24 hours after surgery, also; but this disorder is thought to be associated with toxic solutions entering the intraocular cavity during the operation, rather than from an infectious etiology.[2]

Chronic endophthalmitis, occurring 6 weeks postoperatively may be secondary to the presence of a vitreous wick in the anterior chamber, a wound leak, an infection around the suture at the surgical wound, or from the formation of a filtering bleb.

The Endophthalmitis Vitrectomy Study (EVS) assessed the benefits of pars plana vitrectomy (PPV) surgery versus tap (vitreous biopsy) with the injection of intravitreal antibiotics in patients with bacterial endophthalmitis within 6 weeks of surgery.[3] The study concluded that for those patients with light perception visual acuity, or worse, on presentation, PPV should be the preferred treatment mode whereas those with hand motion vision, or better, should undergo tap with injection[3] (Table 30.1).

Filtering Surgery

Endophthalmitis after filtering surgery typically presents months to years after the operation and can present with symptoms of eye pain, redness, headache and brow ache. The filtering bleb may be filled with exudates and thus will appear white against the injected red eye. Although grossly the bleb may appear to be intact, a microscopic leak may be present when stained with fluorescein. Increased risk factors for this problem include blebs that are avascular, thin, located inferiorly, leaking and associated with the use of antifibrotic agents, such as mitomycin, during the surgery.[4]

Corneal Transplant

Endophthalmitis following penetrating keratoplasty (PK) can be acute or chronic and the hallmark finding is a severe anterior chamber reaction, usually with the presence of a hypopyon. Pain is less prominent but the dense inflammation

TABLE 30.1: Results of endophthalmitis vitrectomy study (EVS)

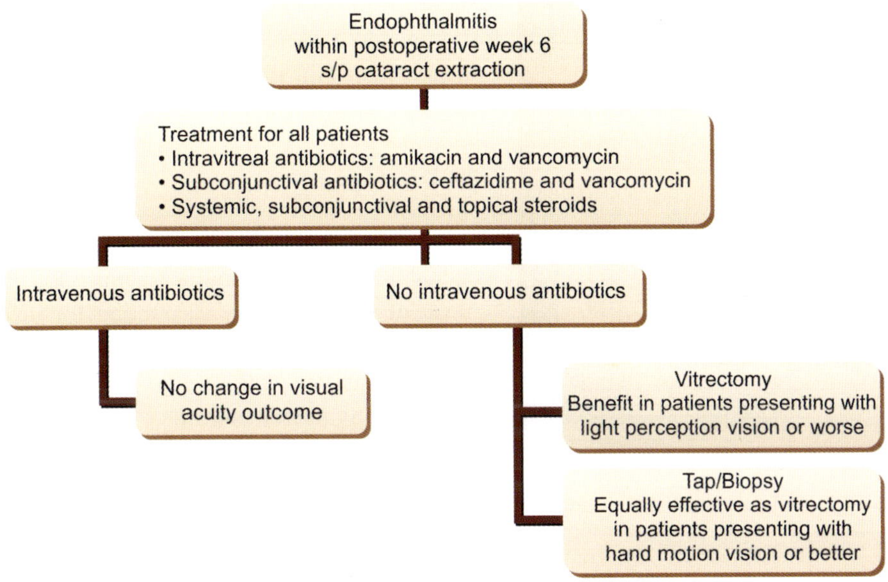

in the anterior chamber may cause a decreased red reflex. The acute onset may be the result of organisms introduced into the eye during surgery while chronic cases tend to result from a wound dehiscence, suture abscess, presence of a vitreous wick, or a corneal ulcer. Reports have demonstrated that pseudophakic or aphakic patients that undergo PK are at a higher risk of endophthalmitis than those that are phakic.[5]

Pterygium Surgery

Endophthalmitis following pterygium removal is caused, more often, by fungal micro-organisms. Infection can spread through necrosis of the sclera where the pterygium was removed and treatment typically requires a combination of surgical debridement and antifungal medication.[6]

Pars Plana Vitrectomy

Endophthalmitis after vitrectomy is rare, but when it occurs, may be difficult to diagnose. Normal postoperative symptoms of a pars plana vitrectomy (PPV) procedure can include pain and poor visual acuity, which may mask symptoms of endophthalmitis. One should be suspicious if the inflammation is more prominent, in the presence of exudates in the vitreous cavity and when there is increased fibrin formation in the anterior chamber. Studies found that risk factors for endophthalmitis post-PPV include diabetes, previous intraocular surgery and increased complexity and duration of the surgery.[7] Outcomes tend to be poor because, in addition to endophthalmitis, patients typically have existing advanced vitreoretinal disease.

Retinal Detachment Repair

There are reports of endophthalmitis after scleral buckling and pneumatic retinopexy procedures used to repair retinal detachments.[8,9] The associated clinical findings are similar to those in post-PPV endophthalmitis; pain and severe inflammation out of proportion to the usual postoperative retinal detachment repair symptoms. Endophthalmitis secondary to scleral buckling tends to occur on the extra-scleral implant.[9] Inadvertent perforation of the sclera during the procedure may also allow for direct inoculation of organisms (Fig. 30.3). Gas contamination or a defect in the filter used to pass the gas into the eye may lead to endophthalmitis after pneumatic retinopexy.[8]

Intraocular Injections

Intraocular injections may create a tract for organisms to pass into the globe and cause endophthalmitis, also. Hypopyon formation as a sign of endophthalmitis must be distinguished

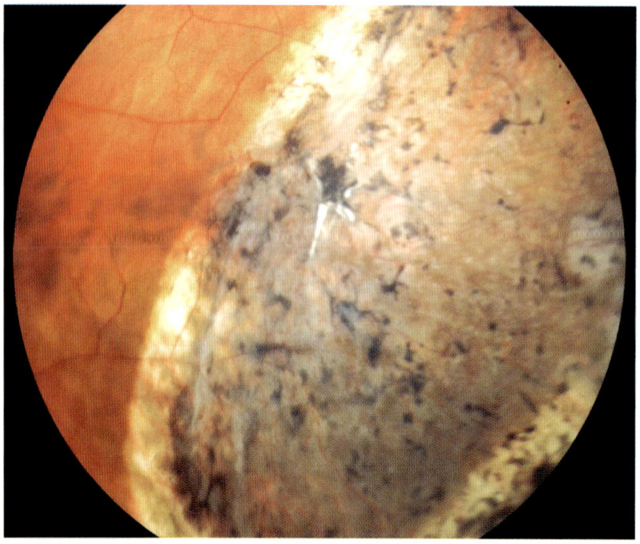

▲ **Figure 30.3**

Retinal detachment secondary to endophthalmitis, treated with laser therapy

from pseudohypopyon, which may form from inadvertent injection or deposition of the material from the syringe into the anterior chamber.[10]

Strabismus Surgery

Endophthalmitis following strabismus surgery is rare but can have a poor prognosis because of nonspecific symptoms,[11] such as lethargy, asymmetric eye redness, fever and lid swelling, with delayed diagnosis. Globe perforation by scleral sutures is most likely the underlying mechanism for inoculation of micro-organisms inside the globe.[11] Scleral abscess in an area of thin sclera where the suture is passed may also lead to endophthalmitis.[11]

▶ Post-traumatic

Nonsurgical trauma is the second most frequent cause of endophthalmitis.[1] Penetrating trauma is the primary causative mode of this infection, accounting for up to a quarter of cases.[12] Eyes with traumatic endophthalmitis tend to have poorer visual prognosis than those with postoperative infections. Symptoms may vary in severity depending on the virulence of the organism but symptoms typically include increased pain, hypopyon, anterior chamber inflammation and vitritis. Also there may be evidence of a retained intraocular foreign body (IOFB) material with any penetrating injury.[12] Gram-positive organisms can account for up to 75% of the micro-organisms cultured from these eyes.[12] Bacillus cereus infection tends to be associated with IOFB retention and can cause an even more serious sight-threatening complication. Factors leading to an increased risk of intraocular infection following penetrating trauma include retained IOFB, delayed primary repair of wound and lens disruption[12] (Figs 30.4A and B).

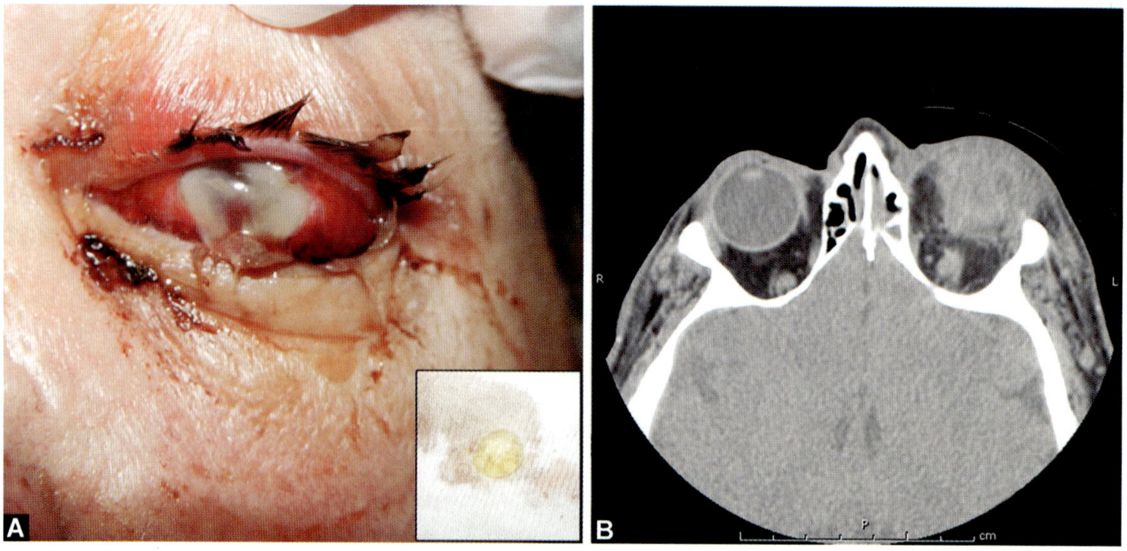

▲ **Figures 30.4A and B**

(A) Fifty-year-old male with endophthalmitis secondary to Clostridium species after trauma to left eye. Subset—Patient's lens prolapsed out of globe and found on shirt upon presentation to clinic; (B) CT scan of orbits axial view 1 mm cut. Left globe is disorganized, unformed with haze in vitreous, representation endophthalmitis

Causes of Endogenous Endophthalmitis

Endogenous endophthalmitis is caused by the spread of infection from elsewhere in the body to the intraocular tissue; hence it is also known as metastatic endophthalmitis. Infection occurs when micro-organisms seed into the vasculature of the retina and choroid, as opposed to exogenous endophthalmitis where infection is directly introduced into the vitreous. The organisms can then produce a breakdown of the blood-ocular barrier and penetrate into the intraocular cavity.

Patients who develop endogenous endophthalmitis tend to have systemic diseases associated with immunosuppression, although cases can occur in healthy individuals too. Fungal organisms are the most frequent causes of this problem and occur through hematogenous dissemination.[13] *Candida albicans* is the most common fungus followed by *Aspergillus* species.[13] Bacterial infections are less common than fungal.[13]

There are several identified risk factors that predispose patients to develop fungal endophthalmitis. The use of intravenous therapy produces a route for the spread of an infection throughout the patient.[13] A majority of patients with this disorder have undergone some form of surgical intervention, allowing for this hematogenous seeding. The use of intravenous catheters also allows a source for infection. Steroid use stimulates the growth of micro-organisms and many patients who developed endophthalmitis have a history of being treated with steroids. In a similar manner, immunosuppressive medications depress the immune system, decreasing the normal response to defend against infection.

▶ Sterile Endophthalmitis

Inflammation occurring in the absence of infection may be acute or chronic and mild to moderately severe. This disorder has been reported to occur postoperatively or after intravitreal injection and most often is detected within 3–4 days after a procedure.[14,15] It can present with hypopyon and cloudy vitreous, but usually there is no corneal edema, chemosis, or lid swelling. Unlike infectious endophthalmitis, aseptic endophthalmitis is not severely and progressively painful. Secondary aseptic endophthalmitis is related, most often, to toxic foreign materials inoculated or implanted into the eye, either as a retained lens particle after cataract extraction or as an inflammatory response to preservatives from an injected intravitreal substance.[14,15] Sterile endophthalmitis may occur, also, weeks or months after intraocular surgery and has been associated with late rupture of the anterior hyaloid membrane and vitreous adhesion to the wound in aphakic patients, degradation of implant materials, the withdrawal of topical steroid therapy, or the dislocation of an intraocular lens (IOL).

▶ Organisms

Bacteria

Bacteria are the most common micro-organisms causing endophthalmitis and account for over 90% of all cases.[16] Gram-positive organisms are grouped together based on their characteristic gram stain reaction, presence of a thick cell wall made of proteoglycan and shape, appearing as either pairs, clusters, or chains. Gram-negative organisms lack the proteoglycan cell wall and thus stain differently with gram stain.

Gram-positive cocci

Staphylococci are gram-positive cocci in grape-like clusters that are classified based on the coagulase test. There are 23 recognized species members of the family *Micrococcaceae*. *S. aureus* are coagulase positive non-spore-forming facultative anaerobic organisms whereas the other members of the staphylococci family are coagulase negative. *S. aureus* is part of the natural skin flora and can be found on mucous membranes including the conjunctiva. It is a virulent pyogenic organism releasing toxins that cause scalded skin syndrome and food poisoning. It is the second most common micro-organism causing postoperative bacterial endophthalmitis. *S. epidermidis* endophthalmitis is the most common cause of postoperative endophthalmitis[16] and more often occurs in the presence of foreign bodies, such as catheters, prosthetic valves, or IOFB. *S. saprophyticus* adhere to urothelial cells and are involved in urinary tract infections.

Streptococci are gram-positive cocci in pairs or chains. One classification system is based on the hemolytic activity of these agents. Alpha hemolysis results in incomplete lysis, beta hemolysis causes complete lysis and gamma hemolysis is nonhemolytic. Another classification system groups streptococci on the antigenic characteristics of the carbohydrate content of their cell wall. Group A streptococci, also known as *S. pyogenes*, are extremely virulent beta hemolytic organisms that cause diseases such as impetigo, rheumatic fever and necrotizing fasciitis. Group B streptococci are *S. agalactiae* and found in the oral cavity, gastrointestinal tract and vaginal tract. Rare cases of endophthalmitis are caused by this group which more commonly causes meningitis, endocarditis and pneumonia. Group C beta-hemolytic streptococci are often the cause of endophthalmitis in the elderly and immunocompromised patients. Group D streptococci are divided into enterococcal and non-enterococcal species. Enterococcal organisms include *S. faecalis, S. faecium* and *S. durans*. Increasingly they are becoming multidrug resistant because of the nosocomial infections they cause. Non-enterococcal species are *S. bovis* and *S. equinus*. The viridans streptococci are alpha hemolytic and are not classified into the above scheme. They produce toxins to increase virulence and are found in the respiratory tract.

Gram-positive bacilli

The ***bacillus* species** are one of two different varieties of spore-forming bacteria. They are found in soil, water, vegetable matter and human intestines. Risk factors for infection with this species include immunosuppression, intravenous drug use, chronic catheter placement and corticosteroid use. Commonly identified bacilli are *B. anthracis*, *B. cereus* and *B. subtilis*, the latter two are known to be associated with endophthalmitis. *B. anthracis*, the organism known to cause anthrax, has recently been discussed as a biohazardous weapon and can cause cutaneous, respiratory and gastrointestinal infection. Whereas *B. anthrax* is non-motile, *B. cereus* is a motile organism that causes food poisoning through toxin release. It is the second most common cause of post-traumatic endophthalmitis, following *S. epidermidis,* and runs a rapidly destructive course within the eye. Patients may develop corneal abscess and destruction within 48 hours and typically have an extremely poor visual prognosis. *B. subtilis* has also been identified in culture of endophthalmitis cases.

Clostridium, the other spore-forming gram-positive organism, is found in water, soil, vegetative material and the gastrointestinal tract. It causes ocular tissue destruction through release of exotoxin. *C. perfringens* is known to cause gas gangrene panophthalmitis and associated with post-traumatic infection following penetrating injury. Signs and symptoms include severe pain, coffee-colored discharge, intraocular gas production causing increased intraocular pressure, significant eyelid swelling and severely decreased visual acuity within 24–48 hours after trauma (Figs 30.5A to D).

Corynebacterium produces exotoxins and is known to cause subacute postoperative endophthalmitis. Humans are the only known natural host and this micro-organism resides in the upper respiratory tract and skin.

Listeria endophthalmitis is known to occur, mostly, in immunocompromised hosts. *L. monocytogenes* is the only subspecies that is pathogenic to humans. It is found in soil, water and sewage and is also known to cause listeriosis, occurring in newborns, the elderly and in immunocompromised patients.

Proprionibacterium organisms are found on skin and mucosal surfaces and are known to cause acne, osteomyelitis and endocarditis. *P. acnes* is the most common subspecies and causes chronic granulomatous postoperative endophthalmitis.[17] It can present as a granulomatous reaction on the endothelial surface of the cornea and/or as a hypopyon with plaque-formation on the posterior lens capsule and thickening of the capsule around the lens implant and beading of fibrin strands in the anterior chamber. Nd:YAG capsulotomy may propagate the infection by introducing the organism further into the eye when it may have adhered, originally, to the posterior capsule during surgery.

Gram-negative cocci

Neisseria are diplococci that grow best in moist warm environments on chocolate agar. *N. gonorrhoeae* and *N. meningitidis* are the two subspecies most commonly seen clinically. *N. meningitis* is a natural inhabitant of the nasopharynx and is transmitted through respiratory droplets. It is the second leading cause of septic meningitis. *N.* gonorrhoeae is found in the oropharynx, nasopharynx, urethral tract and rectum. Both have been reported to be a rare cause of endogenous endophthalmitis.

Moraxella species are found in the respiratory tract and can be found on the skin and urogenital tract. More commonly they cause angular blepharitis and they rarely penetrate the intraocular contents.

Gram-negative bacilli

Actinobacter are non-motile bacteria and are known to cause hospital-acquired infections in immunocompromised patients. There are only a few case reports of exogenous endophthalmitis secondary to actinobacter infection[16] and they tend to present similar to *P. acnes* endophthalmitis.

Enterobacteriaceae are natural inhabitants of the human gastrointestinal tract yet are the most common cause of nosocomial infections. Species include *Escherichia coli, Klebsiella, Morganella, Proteus* and *Serratia*. Most cases of

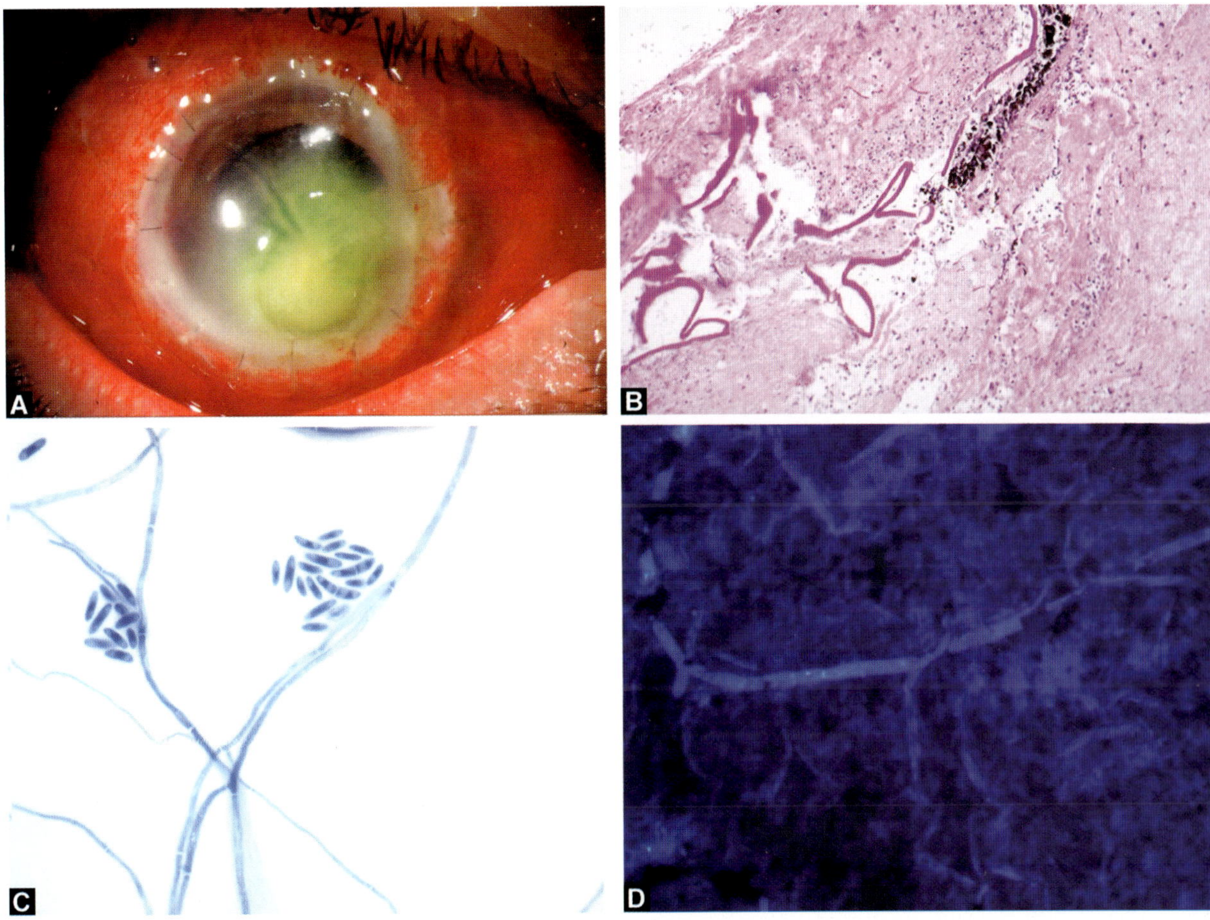

▲ **Figures 30.5A to D**

(A) Photomicrograph of the right eye showing large diameter limbus-to-limbus tectonic corneal transplant and recurrent, deep central corneal ulcer in the corneal graft; (B) Histopathology of right corneal button from penetrating keratoplasty. Note fibrinopurulent exudate and iris adherent to the cornea. Also note disruption of Descemet's membrane with PAS positive fungal hyphae present on both sides of the disrupted membrane. (Magnification x 200); (C) Lactophenol cotton blue stain. Note the septate hyphae and canoe-shaped conidia, or spores; (D) Calcofluor white stain. Note the filamentous hyphae with septation

reported endophthalmitis from this group are secondary to Klebsiella or Serratia.

Haemophilus species are characterized by their capsular properties and are parasites of the human respiratory tract. *H. influenzae* has best been known to cause bleb-associated endophthalmitis but has also caused cases of post-strabismus and post-traumatic endophthalmitis. *Haemophilus* can also cause meningitis, epiglottitis and cellulitis. Since the advent of the *H. influenzae* vaccination, the number of systemic infections secondary to this species has dramatically declined.

Pseudomonas species are gram-negative motile rods that are found in soil, water, plant and animal surroundings. Their virulence is determined by the presence of adhesions, invasions, ability to be motile and toxin production. This micro-organism tends to cause infection in immunocompromised patients, those with cystic fibrosis, burn victims and people with chronic indwelling catheters or on respirators. *Pseudomonas* is the most common cause of gram-negative endophthalmitis and *P. aeruginosa* is the most common subspecies, although others have been reported.[18]

Actinobacteria

The actinobacteria are all gram-positive non-spore-forming rod-shaped bacteria that undergo filamentous branching, similar to fungi. Three major families of this genus include *Actinomyces,* Mycobacteria, and *Nocardia.*

Actinomyces can be found in the soil and play a role in degradation of plant material. They populate the oral cavity of humans and can lead to formation of oral abscesses, mostly secondary to *A. israelii.*

Mycobacteria species have a thick hydrophobic cell wall which allows them to survive through harsh conditions. They are known to cause leprosy and tuberculosis and both typical and atypical strains can be associated with endophthalmitis. An immunocompromised state is a risk factor for atypical mycobacterium endophthalmitis.

Nocardia is a weakly staining acid-fast bacterium and most cases occur as an opportunistic infection in immunocompromised patients. *N. asteroides* is the species most frequently found in humans and leads to a slowly progressive pneumonia, but can also cause encephalitis celluitis, skin abscess, or brain abscess.

▶ Fungi

Fungal micro-organisms are the most common cause of endogenous endophthalmitis. In this situation the disease course may be acute or indolent and should be suspected in immunocompromised patients or those with traumatic injury with plant or soil-contaminated material. Fungi may grow as molds, yeast, or be dimorphic. Molds are filamentous branching hyphae whereas yeasts are round or oval buds. They have the ability to reproduce asexually or sexually.

Candida are dimorphic organisms that have the capability of forming yeast, hyphae and pseudohyphae. They can live symbiotically in humans but can also cause nosocomial infections or be found in soil and food. *Candida* is the most common cause of fungal endophthalmitis and tends to cause endophthalmitis following a systemic infection, spreading to the eye via the hematogenous route. The typical clinical finding of *Candida* endophthalmitis includes chorioretinitis with deep white fluffy infiltrative lesions and vitreous haze.

Aspergillus is the second most common source of fungal endophthalmitis. It is a mold found in soil, vegetable material, fecal material and air-condition filters. Aspergillus may be cultured from traumatic fungal corneal ulcers as well. Endogenous aspergillosis endophthalmitis may present with discrete pale yellow fluffy elevated lesions and may eventually lead to exudative retinal detachment or vitreous abscess formation.

Cryptococcus is a yeast found in bird droppings, contaminated soil and vegetative material. *C. neoformans* is the most common species with dissemination occurring to the central nervous system and is known to cause cryptococcosis and meningitis in patients with AIDS. Cases of exogenous endophthalmitis post-penetrating keratoplasty have been reported.[5]

Histoplasma are dimorphic fungi found particularly in the Ohio and Mississippi river valley from bat and pigeon excretions. The clinical triad of ocular histoplasmosis includes punched-out mid-peripheral retinal lesions, macular scarring and peripapillary scarring. Endogenous endophthalmitis has been reported via hematogenous spread.

Blastomyces are dimorphic fungi that are found in soil, most prominent in the woods. The infection spreads through respiratory droplets to the lungs and can disseminate hematogenously to involve the skin, bone, genital tract and rarely cause endophthalmitis.

Fusarium are filamentous fungi found in plants. They cause aggressive infection that may be difficult to treat, especially in immunocompromised patients.

Helminths and Protozoa

Helminths are worms that live inside the host. There are three groups of worms: cestodes (tapeworms), nematodes (roundworms) and trematodes (flukes). The human host responds to these worms through an inflammatory cascade. *Toxocara*, predominantly found in cats and dogs, can produce a chronic granulomatous intraocular inflammatory reaction and is most prevalent in children. *Onchocerca,* transmitted through larvae from blackfly bites, can lodge in the skin and travel to the eye to cause "river blindness." Cystercercosis, caused by *taenia solium*, a trematode, can be ingested by humans through undercooked pork and larvae can migrate to the vitreous to cause retinal edema and inflammation.

Protozoa are single-cell micro-organisms that can infect plants and animals. *Toxoplasmosis gondii* is the most common protozoa affecting the eye. Cats are the host of this species and it can be transmitted to humans through contact with cat feces or ingestion of undercooked meats. The cysts of *Toxoplasma* can then spread through the blood-stream through the gastrointestinal tract. The classical clinical triad includes chorioretinitis, cerebral calcifications and seizures.

Management of Infectious Endophthalmitis

Once the clinical diagnosis of infectious endophthalmitis is made, management is tailored to the etiology, severity and course of the infection. Obtaining specimens can identify the causative organism to guide therapy. Appropriate, safe and efficacious antimicrobial therapy is initiated urgently. The goals of treatment are to eradicate the infectious microbes and to limit damage both from microbial toxins and host inflammatory mediators.

A vitreous specimen provides material to identify the causative micro-organism. An aqueous specimen may also be obtained and in some cases is the only specimen to result in a positive culture.[19] The vitreous specimen is obtained via either a needle tap biopsy through the pars plana, vitreous biopsy with an automated vitrector, or during a pars plana vitrectomy (PPV). In the Endophthalmitis Vitrectomy Study (EVS),[20] the rate of positive cultures was similar with each method.[21] Slides for gram stain and culture media are inoculated with the specimen as soon as it is obtained. Microbiologic evaluation to identify the organism and antibiotic sensitivities can guide the antibiotic regimen. Polymerase chain reaction (PCR) testing, which has the potential to increase yield and provide rapid results, may be performed if capable facilities are available. PCR has been shown to have greater yield than culture with both undiluted and dilute vitreous samples, even after prior intravitreal antibiotic administration.[22]

▶ Pars Plana Vitrectomy

In addition to obtaining specimens for culture, PPV can be therapeutic in selected cases. The rationale for vitrectomy includes reducing the load of infectious organisms, lessening toxic infectious and inflammatory products and removing opacities.[1] The disadvantages of PPV for endophthalmitis include the need for expensive equipment and an operating room, surgical complications and a theoretical risk of decreased antibiotic half-life in vitrectomized eyes, as shown in rabbits treated with intravitreal vancomycin and ceftazidime.[23,24] The EVS guides the decision to proceed with PPV for acute, post-cataract surgery or secondary intraocular lens placement. Since the EVS did not include endophthalmitis due to other causes, such as following other surgeries and chronic infections, the optimal role of vitrectomy in these cases is yet to be defined.

The EVS showed that PPV was beneficial in patients presenting with light perception only vision. The chance of 20/40 or better visual acuity was three times greater with PPV than vitreous tap or biopsy (33% vs 11%, respectively).[20] Obtaining at least moderate visual acuity of 20/100 or better improved to 56% for vitrectomy compared to 30% for vitreous tap. The risk of poor visual outcome (< 5/200) was decreased from 47% in the vitreous tap group to 20% in the PPV group. For patients with hand motions visual acuity [defined as correctly identifying hand motions at ≥ 2 feet (≥60 cm) four out of five times] or better vision at presentation, there was no significant difference in final visual acuity in the vitrectomy group compared to the vitreous tap group.[20] The results of the EVS do not directly apply to cases such as bleb-related endophthalmitis, chronic postoperative endophthalmitis and traumatic endophthalmitis. Therefore, clinical judgment is critical in determining the optimal management for each particular patient.

▶ Antibiotics

Once a vitreous specimen has been obtained, treatment with antimicrobial agents is initiated. Until the causative organism is identified, broad-spectrum antibiotics covering both gram-positive and gram-negative organisms should be selected. The common pathogens and antibiotic resistance rates may vary by region and this should be taken into account when choosing empiric agents.[25,26] If fungal endophthalmitis is suspected, antifungal medications should be given instead of, or concurrently with antibiotics, depending on the clinical situation.

Intravitreal antibiotics are the mainstay of treatment for exogenous endophthalmitis. Typical antibiotics for empiric therapy are vancomycin 1 mg/0.1 mL for gram-positive coverage and ceftazidime 2.25 mg/0.1 mL for gram-negative coverage. Aminoglycosides provide effective gram-negative coverage, but are associated with greater retinal toxicity than ceftazidime.[27] In particular, macular infarction, which appears as whitening of the retina, can occur even at low concentrations of gentamicin, amikacin and tobramycin.[27] Nonetheless, in patients with cephalosporin allergy, amikacin 400 μg/0.1 mL is an effective alternative for gram-negative coverage.[1]

Newer antibiotics, such as the fourth-generation fluoroquinolones are under investigation for intravitreal use in endophthalmitis. Gatifloxacin and moxifloxacin have been demonstrated to be safe in rabbit studies and have broad-spectrum coverage of gram-positive and gram-negative organisms. However, resistance among gram-positive organisms is common.[28] Linezolid, a synthetic antibiotic with gram-positive coverage, may be beneficial in rare cases of vancomycin resistance. Linezolid has been shown to be safe in rabbit eyes.[29] Further work is required to determine the appropriate intraocular use of this agent in human patients.

The administration of antibiotics through other routes may be beneficial, depending on the clinical situation. However, in the EVS, systemic amikacin and either ceftazidime or ciprofloxacin provided no significant improvement in final visual acuity.[20] It is possible that other antibiotics with better vitreal penetration, such as oral moxifloxacin, could be useful adjuncts. Oral gatifloxacin and oral moxifloxacin were shown to achieve therapeutic levels for a wide variety of pathogens in uninflamed eyes.[30,31] However, statistically valid controlled studies showing a benefit for visual acuity are lacking.

Subconjunctival antibiotics were used in all patients in the EVS. Since that time, two case series have suggested that their use, in addition to intravitreal antibiotics, did not result in an improved final visual acuity.[32,33] Similarly, topical antibiotics, while routinely used, have not been rigorously evaluated in endophthalmitis. In fact, topical administration of the fourth-generation fluoroquinolones did not result in therapeutic vitreous levels in one study.[34] However, it is reasonable to think that subconjunctival or topical antibiotics may be efficacious in treating cases with anterior segment infections, such as blebitis and keratitis.

Corticosteroids

Since endophthalmitis results in intense inflammation, corticosteroids may modulate the host response and limit damage from toxic inflammatory mediators. Systemic, intravitreal, periocular and topical steroids have been used with varying reports of efficacy. In the EVS, all patients were treated with oral prednisone. One nonrandomized case series suggested better outcomes in patients receiving systemic steroids.[35] Intravitreal dexamethasone 400 µg/0.1 mL has been evaluated in multiple small studies with some showing a benefit, some no difference and some harm.[36-38] Topical corticosteroids are used more often, although data regarding efficacy are limited.

Other Causes

For exogenous endophthalmitis following other surgeries or trauma, clinical judgment is required since there is a lack of information from controlled clinical trials. For example, since bleb-related endophthalmitis often has more virulent pathogens, some authors feel vitrectomy may have a larger role.[1] Frequent topical antibiotics may be important to treat the infected bleb, as well. In the case of chronic postoperative endophthalmitis, evaluation for anaerobic and fungal organisms is important, since they are present more commonly than in acute postoperative endophthalmitis.[39] *Proprionibacterium acnes* sequestered in the lens capsule after cataract surgery can present months to years postoperatively. Since most antibiotics may not penetrate the capsular remnants well, PPV with capsulectomy along with intravitreal vancomycin injection is often the preferred treatment. The presence of fluffy, white infiltrates should raise suspicion for fungal infection. In the past, amphotericin B 5 µg/0.1 mL has been the only available intravitreal agent. Unfortunately, retinal toxicity is common with this agent, especially with repeated injections.[40] Newer antifungals, such as voriconazole 100 µg/0.1 mL have been shown, recently, to be safe in animal models and have been used intravitreally with success in some case reports.[41,42] Traumatic endophthalmitis has a poor outcome, largely due to the initial injury. Intraocular foreign bodies may bring infectious material directly into the vitreous. In addition, Bacillus species are more common in such injuries and they are more virulent, often resulting in poor vision or loss of the eye despite prompt, aggressive treatment.[43] Some authors recommend vitrectomy for many of these cases in light of the poor prognosis.[44]

Endogenous Endophthalmitis

While intravitreal antibiotics and vitrectomy play crucial roles in managing exogenous endophthalmitis, in endogenous endophthalmitis, identifying and treating the systemic source of infection is critical. Fungal endogenous endophthalmitis is more common, but pathogens vary by region.[45] Systemic cultures (blood, urine and cerebrospinal fluid) and specific tests to identify the source of infection should be performed. In some cases, a vitreous specimen may provide the only identification of the causative organism. Often, prolonged systemic treatment is required.[46] For endogenous fungal endophthalmitis, systemic voriconazole 400 mg/day has been successfully used in recent reports, even without vitrectomy and intravitreal therapy.[47] When there is significant vitreal involvement or progression on systemic therapy, PPV with intravitreal antifungal injection may be needed. As mentioned above, while amphotericin B frequently damages the retina, intravitreal voriconazole has been well-tolerated and efficacious in recent case reports.[48] Endogenous bacterial endophthalmitis is uncommon and has a poor prognosis. Systemic antibiotics are required; however a large, prospective case series showed that vitrectomy allowed more eyes to retain useful vision and was able to avoid a need for evisceration or enucleation when compared to treatment with antibiotics alone.[49]

Outcomes

Visual outcomes depend on the causative organism, source of infection, and prompt, effective therapy. Additional therapy is required in some patients. Initial therapy may take more than 24 hours to show a significant response. If no improvement or progression occurs, repeated intravitreal antibiotics should be considered, guided by culture results. Vitrectomy may be performed or repeated as well. In the EVS, 10% of all patients required an additional procedure in the first week, and approximately one-third required additional surgery overall. Loss of the eye does occur, with 1% of patients undergoing evisceration or enucleation in the EVS.[20] These risks may be higher in other situations, particularly following trauma.

Prompt diagnosis and treatment are critical for managing infectious endophthalmitis. The EVS provides a very useful guide for treating acute postcataract and secondary IOL placement endophthalmitis. Vitrectomy has an important therapeutic role in the care of such patients, but its true role continues to be defined. In every particular case, clinical judgment must be applied to best treat each patient.

References

1. Lemley CA, Han DP. Endophthalmitis: a review of current evaluation and management. Retina. 2007;27:662-80.
2. Mamalis N, Edelhauser HF, Dawson DG, et al. Toxic Anterior Segment Syndrome. J Cataract Refract Surg. 2006;32:324-33.
3. Haimann MH, Weiss H, Miller JA. Endophthalmitis Vitrectomy Study. Arch Ophthalmol. 1991;109:1060-1.
4. Prasad N, Latina MA. Blebitis and endophthalmitis after glaucoma filtering surgery. Int Ophthalmol Clin. 2007;47:85-97.
5. Taban M, Behrens A, Newcomb RL, et al. Incidence of acute endophthalmitis following penetrating keratoplasty: a systematic review. Arch Ophthalmol. 2005;123:605-9.
6. Tarr KH, Constable IJ. Late complications of pterygium treatment. Br J Ophthalmol. 1980; 64:496-505.
7. Cohen SM, Flynn HW, Murray TG, et al. Endophthalmitis after pars plana vitrectomy. The Postvitrectomy Endophthalmitis Study Group. Ophthalmology. 1995;102:705-12.
8. Eckardt C. Staphylococcus epidermidis endophthalmitis after pneumatic retinopexy. Am J Ophthalmol. 1987;103:720-1.
9. Kearney JJ, Lahey JM, Borirakchanyavat S, et al. Complications of hydrogel explants used in scleral buckling surgery. Am J Ophthalmol. 2004;137:96-100.
10. Lad EM, Moshfeghi DM. Minimizing the risk of endophthalmitis following intravitreal injections. Compr Ophthalmol Update. 2006;7:277-84.
11. Ing MR. Infection following strabismus surgery. J Ophthalmic Nurs Technol. 1991;10:211-4.
12. Waheed NK, Young LH. Intraocular foreign body related endophthalmitis. Int Ophthalmol Clin. 2007;47:165-71.
13. Smith SR, Kroll AJ, Lou PL, et al. Endogenous bacterial and fungal endophthalmitis. Int Ophthalmol Clin. 2007;47:173-83.
14. Bilge AH, Aykan U, Akin T, et al. Review of sterile, postoperative, anterior segment inflammation following cataract extraction and intraocular lens implantation. Eur J Ophthalmol. 2005;15:224-7.
15. Wang LC, Yang CM. Sterile endophthalmitis following intravitreal injection of triamcinolone acetonide. Ocul Immunol Inflamm. 2005;13:295-300.
16. Callegan MC, Engelbert M, Parke DW d, et al. Bacterial endophthalmitis: epidemiology, therapeutics, and bacterium-host interactions. Clin Microbiol Rev. 2002;15:111-24.
17. Deramo VA, Ting TD. Treatment of Propionibacterium acnes endophthalmitis. Curr Opin Ophthalmol. 2001;12:225-9.
18. Eifrig CW, Scott IU, Flynn HW, et al. Endophthalmitis caused by Pseudomonas aeruginosa. Ophthalmology. 2003;110:1714-7.
19. Barza M, Pavan PR, Doft BH, et al. Evaluation of microbiological diagnostic techniques in postoperative endophthalmitis in the Endophthalmitis Vitrectomy Study. Arch Ophthalmol. 1997;115:1142-50.
20. Endophthalmitis Vitrectomy Study Group. Results of the Endophthalmitis Vitrectomy Study. A randomized trial of immediate vitrectomy and of intravenous antibiotics for the treatment of postoperative bacterial endophthalmitis. Arch Ophthalmol. 1995;113:1479-96.
21. Han DP, Wisniewski SR, Kelsey SF, et al. Microbiologic yields and complication rates of vitreous needle aspiration versus mechanized vitreous biopsy in the Endophthalmitis Vitrectomy Study. Retina. 1999;19:98-102.
22. Chiquet C, Maurin M, Thuret G, et al. French Institutional Endophthalmitis Study (FRIENDS) group. Analysis of diluted vitreous samples from vitrectomy is useful in eyes with severe acute postoperative endophthalmitis. Ophthalmology. 2009;116:2437-41.
23. Shaarawy A, Meredith TA, Kincaid M, et al. Intraocular injection of ceftazidime. Effects of inflammation and surgery. Retina. 1995;15:433-8.
24. Aguilar HE, Meredith TA, el-Massry A, et al. Vancomycin levels after intravitreal injection. Effects of inflammation and surgery. Retina. 1995;15:428-32.
25. Recchia FM, Busbee BG, Pearlman RB, et al. Changing trends in the microbiologic aspects of postcataract endophthalmitis. Arch Ophthalmol. 2005;123:341-6.
26. Anand AR, Therese KL, Madhavan HN. Spectrum of aetiological agents of postoperative endophthalmitis and antibiotic susceptibility of bacterial isolates. Ind J Ophthalmol. 2000;48:123-8.

27. Campochiaro PA, Lim JI. Aminoglycoside toxicity in the treatment of endophthalmitis. The Aminoglycoside Toxicity Study Group. Arch Ophthalmol. 1994;112:48-53.
28. Miller D, Flynn PM, Scott IU, et al. In vitro fluoroquinolones resistance in staphylococcal endophthalmitis isolates. Arch Ophthalmol. 2006;124:479-83.
29. Duke S, Kump L, Yuan Y, et al. The Safety of Intraocular Linezolid in Rabbits. Invest Ophthalmol Vis Sci; 2009.
30. Hariprasad SM, Mieler WF, Holz ER. Vitreous and aqueous penetration of orally administered gatifloxacin in humans. Arch Ophthalmol. 2003;121:345-50.
31. Hariprasad SM, Shah GK, Mieler WF, et al. Vitreous and aqueous penetration of orally administered moxifloxacin in humans. Arch Ophthalmol. 2006;124:178-82.
32. Iyer MN, Han DP, Yun HJ, et al. Subconjunctival antibiotics for acute postcataract extraction endophthalmitis: is it necessary? Am J Ophthalmol. 2004;137:1120-1.
33. Smiddy WE, Smiddy RJ, Ba'Arath B, et al. Subconjunctival antibiotics in the treatment of endophthalmitis managed without vitrectomy. Retina. 2005;25:751-8.
34. Costello P, Bakri SJ, Beer PM, et al. Vitreous penetration of topical moxifloxacin and gatifloxacin in humans. Retina. 2006;26:191-5.
35. Koul S, Philipson BT, Philipson A. Visual outcome of endophthalmitis in Sweden. Acta Ophthalmol. 1989;67:504-9.
36. Irvine WD, Flynn HW, Miller D, et al. Endophthalmitis caused by gram-negative organisms. Arch Ophthalmol. 1992;110: 1450-4.
37. Das T, Jalali S, Gothwal VK, et al. Intravitreal dexamethasone in exogenous bacterial endophthalmitis: Results of a prospective randomised study. Br J Ophthalmol. 1999;83: 1050-5.
38. Shah GK, Stein JD, Sharma S, et al. Visual outcomes following the use of intravitreal steroids in the treatment of postoperative endophthalmitis. Ophthalmology. 2000;107: 486-9.
39. Fox GM, Joondeph BC, Flynn HW, et al. Delayed onset pseudophakic endophthalmitis. Am J Ophthalmol. 1991;111: 163.
40. Souri EN, Green WR. Intravitreal amphotericin B toxicity. Am J Ophthalmol. 1974;78:77-81.
41. Gao H, Pennesi ME, Shah K, et al. Intravitreal voriconazole: an electroretinographic and histopathologic study. Arch Ophthalmol. 2004;122:1687-92.
42. Hariprasad SM, Mieler WF, Lin TK, et al. Voriconazole in the treatment of fungal eye infections: a review of current literature. Br J Ophthalmol. 2008;92:871-8.
43. Thompson JT, Parver LM, Enger CL, et al. Infectious endophthalmitis after penetrating injuries with retained intraocular foreign bodies. National Eye Trauma System. Ophthalmology. 1993;100:1468-74.
44. Reynolds DS, Flynn HW. Endophthalmitis after penetrating ocular trauma. Curr Opin Ophthalmol. 1997;8:32-8.
45. Wong JS, Chan TK, Lee HM, et al. Endogenous bacterial endophthalmitis: an east Asian experience and a reappraisal of a severe ocular affliction. Ophthalmology. 2000;107:1483-91.
46. Chee SP, Jap A. Endogenous endophthalmitis. Curr Opin Ophthalmol. 2001;12:464-70.
47. Hariprasad SM, Mieler WF, Holz ER, et al. Determination of vitreous, aqueous, and plasma concentration of orally administered voriconazole in humans. Arch Ophthalmol. 2004;122:42-7.
48. Scott IU, Cruz-Villegas V, Flynn HW, et al. Delayed-onset, bleb-associated endophthalmitis caused by Lecythophora mutabilis. Am J Ophthalmol. 2004;137:583-5.
49. Jackson TL, Eykyn SJ, Graham EM, Stanford MR. Endogenous bacterial endophthalmitis: a 17-year prospective series and review of 267 reported cases. Surv Ophthalmol. 2003;48:403-23.

SECTION

8

Pediatric Vitreoretinal Surgery

Vitreoretinal Surgery for Retinopathy of Prematurity

31

Michael T Trese

Introduction

Management of retinopathy of prematurity in great part depends on identification of children who are at risk of developing retinal detachment that can result in blindness. The current techniques involve examination in the neonatal intensive care unit (NICU) by an individual physician and indirect ophthalmoscopy or a combination of retinal photography by an NICU nurse and indirect ophthalmoscopy. In the future, it may be that genetic testing and following the rate of weight gain may also play a role to identify children at higher risk of developing retinopathy of prematurity, particularly severe retinopathy of prematurity, due to the accident of premature birth.

When children are identified according to the criteria of the Early Treatment Retinopathy of Prematurity (ETROP) Study, peripheral retinal ablation is currently recommended.[1] This can be done with any indirect laser, although author favors using a red diode laser to avoid lenticular damage due to persistent tunica vasculosa lentis absorption of green laser light. The laser pattern is a near confluent pattern, which minimizes problems of varying degrees of anterior segment ischemia resulting in flocculent cataract and hypotony, although a very rare complication, it can be quite severe. The technique involves placing laser spots approximately one-half laser spot apart and treating the horizontal meridians with a somewhat less intense pattern as we feel that this may contribute to the gradation of anterior segment ischemia.

Once eyes have been lasered, the child is followed very closely with weekly examination as this population represents children who may go on to retinal detachment. The success rate of early laser treatment based on the ETROP Study suggests that about 10% of treated eyes will go on to retinal detachment.[1] These eyes then would be candidates for early vitrectomy. The clinical manifestations of children who are developing retinal detachment generally show vitreous organization at the juncture of the vascularized and avascular retina as well as vitreous organization over the area of the optic nerve and extending up into the vitreous cavity. It should be remembered that the vitreous of premature children is not the homogeneous solid vitreous of a term infant, but rather sheets of solid and liquid vitreous that can be organized into tractional planes, which can cause retinal elevation in a tractional fashion. In addition however the vascular shunt contained within the ridge tissue can also be quite permeable allowing blood and blood products to leak into the subretinal space causing an effusive retinal detachment. In addition, typical stage 3 neovascularization that is elevated from the retinal surface posterior to the ridge tissue can also be intertwined in this vitreous organization again leading to traction exerted along the retinal surface.

With more posterior disease, stage 3 neovascularization lies flat along the retinal surface, often without ridge tissue being present. This is most likely seen in zone 1 and very posterior zone 2 retinopathy of prematurity. These neovascular fronds can also organize and exert traction posteriorly on the retina.

Surgical Technique

The techniques of early vitrectomy can be accomplished with both two-port vitreous surgery as well as three-port

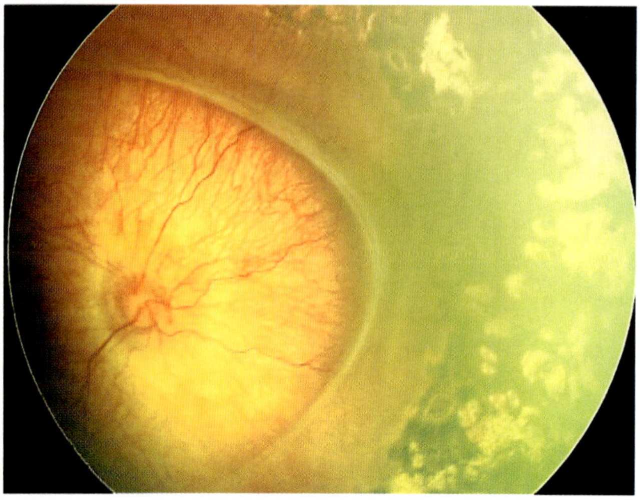

▲ **Figure 31.1**

Shows an extensive 4A retinal detachment with old laser treatment

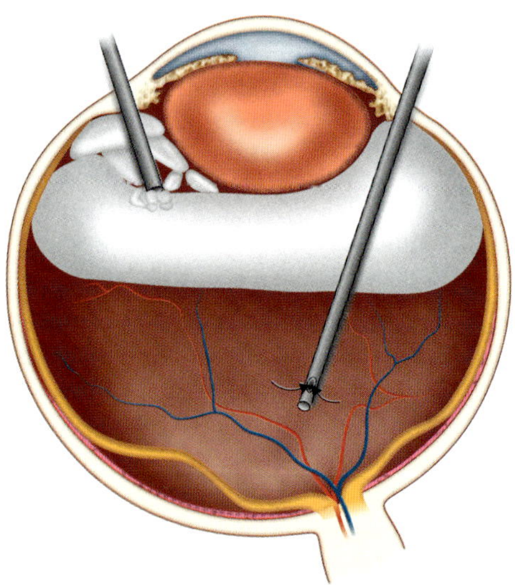

▲ **Figure 31.2**

Shows an artist drawing of 2-port vitreous surgery entry through the pars plicata, using an infusion light pipe and vitrector

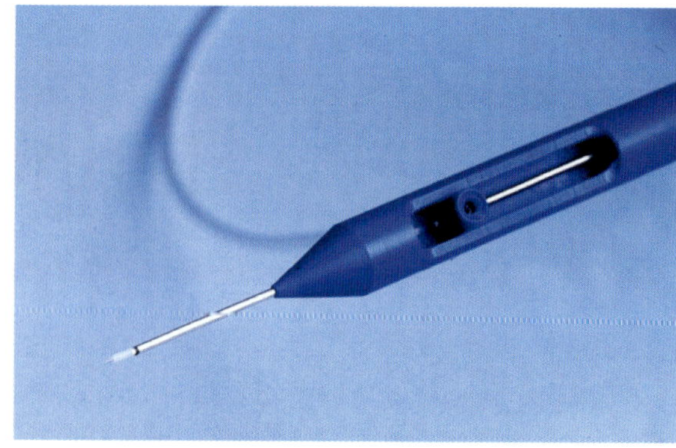

▲ **Figure 31.3**

Shows a wide-angle infusion light pipe that is 19-gauge, but gives good wide angle illumination

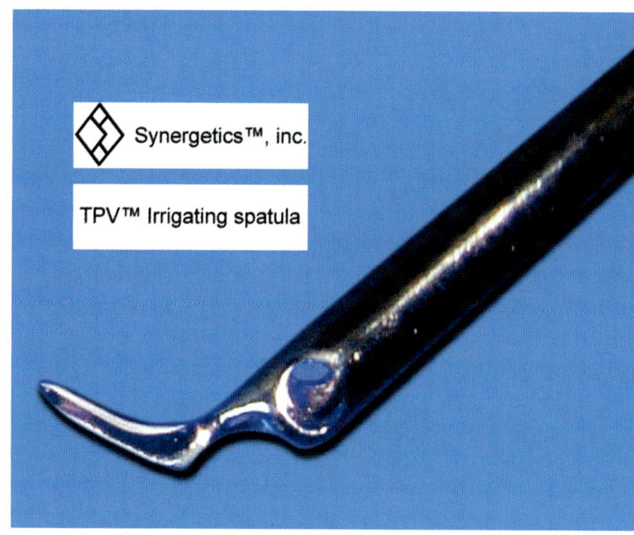

▲ **Figure 31.4**

Shows the infusion spatula that allows lamellar dissection

vitreous surgery as other authors have pointed out (Figs 31.1 to 31.6). The two-port vitreous surgery allows the surgeon to manipulate the eye in the vitreous in the orbit without being concerned with damage from a third port.[2] The approach of vitrectomy is to relieve traction most likely without using enzymatic adjunct (plasmin or microplasmin) without removal of the posterior hyaloid, which in authors opinion generally remains attached at the end of vitreous surgery unless enzyme is used. Upon entry into the eye through the pars plicata, as these children are usually operated on such a young age that they do not have a developed para plana, the entry is achieved when the lens is spared by an incision approximately one-half to one mm posterior to the surgical limbus. This incision is extended directly posteriorly and then angled to the mid vitreous cavity. Following entry, author uses a wide-angle high flow light pipe, which is 19-gauge, the incisions themselves that author makes are

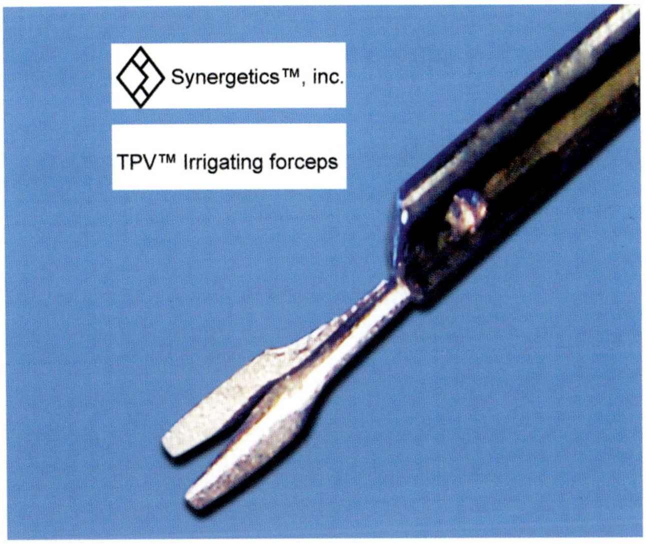

▲ Figure 31.5

Shows the infusion forceps used for 2-hand dissection with a light or lighted pick

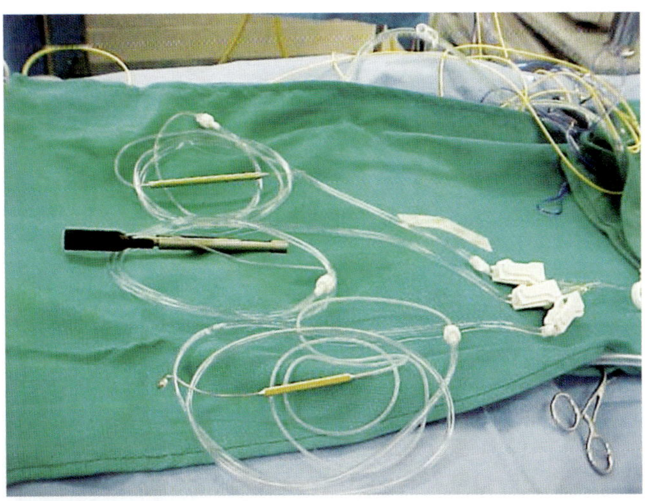

▲ Figure 31.6

Shows the 3 line manifold that allows hanging one fluid bottle to supply three infusion instruments

19-gauge and a 20-gauge vitrector as in many eyes the proliferative tissue is very dense and unable to deform into a smaller port, although 23-gauge instruments may be able to handle much of the vitreous organization.

The approach to the vitreous is first to remove some of the central vitreous while observing the width of the trough between the ora serrata and the elevated peak of the retinal detachment customarily in the area of ridge tissue. If the gap between the ridge tissue, the ora serrata and the lens is quite small, then initially the tissue in the trough is dissected. This can be done with the vitrector usually or may require using MPC scissors or other scissors to open the trough initially. When that traction is relieved, the trough generally falls posteriorly and then more peripheral vitreous can be removed. It is important to isolate stalk tissue centrally, which often can be subtle to identify and this can be done by elevating layers of vitreous collagen around the area of the optic nerve. These layers of the solid vitreous are often thought to be the posterior hyaloid; however, frequently multiple layers of this tissue can be peeled before traction is relieved. It is extremely important to divide the tissue between the disc and the ridge, which if not divided can result in the retinal detachment rolling in a posterior fashion as time goes on. When this dissection is completed, fluid-gas exchange is performed to allow ease of closing these two-port treated eyes. The ridge of detachment following vitrectomy if traction is well relieved will stand straight up at approximately 90° from the tangent at its base. This can be appreciated nicely using the BIOM system, which we find to be the best system for peripheral dissection.[3] Author often uses a contact lens, infusion type to treat the posterior areas and to do dissection around the areas of the optic nerve. When dissection is complete and fluid-air exchange is performed, we then close both the scleral and conjunctival wounds using a fine vicryl suture.

These children are then placed in either a face down, sitting-up, or lateral position, depending on how author likes the air bubble to be used to displace subretinal fluid from the macular area. Drainage of subretinal fluid is very rarely performed and then only on eyes that have extensive stage 5 retinal detachment or very severe stage 4B. If drainage is attempted, it is attempted externally and care must be taken to avoid perforation of an attached lasered or cryoed peripheral retina. Drainage is performed very infrequently, but when performed, a 21 needle with syringe is used through the sclera. This wound is not sutured following drainage and a 21 needle is used due to the very viscous nature of the subretinal fluid, which is blood of varying degrees of viscosity. This blood is potentially toxic to the retinal pigment epithelium (RPE) and outer retina. Following surgery, the child is protected from ocular trauma by using a metal shield and elbow restraints. The child would then be followed for several months to determine reabsorption of subretinal fluid and resolution of vitreous organization and vitreous traction.

This subretinal fluid is the rate limiting feature of final visual acuity as the iron in the blood of the subretinal fluid is toxic to the rods and cones and RPE making the importance of operating at the 4A stage even more appropriate.

Author has published the success rates for stage 4A eyes at 90% anatomic attachment or more importantly, a lack of foveal detachment. This procedure results in an average visual acuity of approximately 20/50.[4,5] Others have confirmed these excellent results for 4A vitreous surgery.[1,2]

Discussion

The management of retinopathy of prematurity in 2011 is basically a combination of peripheral ablative treatment for the early stages of retinopathy of prematurity and vitreous surgery for the later stages of retinopathy of prematurity. This combination can yield a very good success rate and visual outcome for this previously devastating disease. Currently peripheral ablation results in a 90% success rate and of the 10% failures, 90% can achieve lack of foveal detachment or resolution of 4A retinal detachment, leaving fortunately a very small percentage of eyes totally blind from retinopathy of prematurity.

Although the current surgical results are quite good, the posterior hyaloid is rarely removed from the retinal surface, which may contribute to retinal dragging and distortion of the foveal area. Plasmin and microplasmin enzymes have been shown to be effective in cleaving the vitreoretinal interface. In adult vitreoretinal surgery, it has been shown that cleavage of the vitreoretinal junction can be important in terms of resolution of many retinal diseases. It is not know what the long-term (40–50 years) issues of leaving the posterior hyaloid attached in these children may be. Author has seen a few eyes that have detached posterior hyaloid following vitrectomy for retinopathy of prematurity leaving a large amount of debris in the vitreous cavity. The use of an enzyme atraumatically cleaving the vitreoretinal juncture may be a potential benefit of enzyme-assisted vitreous surgery in the future. Currently there is a microplasmin (ocriplasmin) study in the United States to assess the use of microplasmin in children less than 16 years of age for any indication for vitreous surgery.

To date however, early laser and early vitrectomy for 4A retinopathy of prematurity can yield good anatomic and visual results.[6] The use of anti-VEGF is still being evaluated, although the mechanism of disease makes great sense. Whether there are other issues relative to other organ effects or delayed or aggravated tractional component to detachment is yet to be resolved.

References

1. Early Treatment for Retinopathy of Prematurity Cooperative Group. Revised indications for the treatment of retinopathy of prematurity: results of the Early Treatment for Retinopathy of Prematurity Randomized Trial. Arch Ophthalmol. 2003;121:1684-94.
2. Lakhanpal RR, Sun R, Albini T, et al. Anatomic success rate after 3-port lens-sparing vitrectomy in stage 4A or 4B ROP. Ophthalmology. 2005;112:1569-73.
3. BIOM System, Insight Instruments, Stuart, Florida, 800-255-8354.
4. Capone A, Trese MT. Lens-sparing vitreous surgery for tractional stage 4A retinopathy of prematurity retinal detachments. Ophthalmology. 2001;108:2068-70.
5. Prenner JL, Capone, Trese MT. Visual outcomes after lens-sparing vitrectomy for stage 4A retinopathy of prematurity. Ophthalmology. 2004;111:2271-3.
6. Hubbard GB, Cherweck DH, Burion G. Lens-sparing vitrectomy for stage 4A ROP. Ophthalmology. 2004;111:2274-7.

SECTION

9 Surgical Techniques in Viral Retinitis

32

Surgical Management of Cytomegalovirus Related Retinal Detachment in Patients with AIDS

Humeyra Karacal, Eylem Yaman Pinarci, Levent Akduman

Introduction

Thirty three million people were estimated to be living with HIV/AIDS as of December 2008 and about 35 million people had died since the beginning of the epidemic, in 1981.[1] Globally, more than 6800 people are infected with HIV everyday and more than 5700 people die from complications of AIDS.[1] Highly Active Antiretroviral Therapy (HAART) which combines a protease inhibitor with nucleoside analog agents has decreased the mortality and AIDS associated opportunistic infections and improved the quality of life of HIV patients.[2]

Eye is a target organ in AIDS; the most common ocular finding is HIV retinopathy, but the most devastating complications are ocular opportunistic infections, especially Cytomegalovirus (CMV) retinitis (Figs 32.1A and B).[3,4] Other infectious agents account for less than 1% of HIV-related retinal infections.

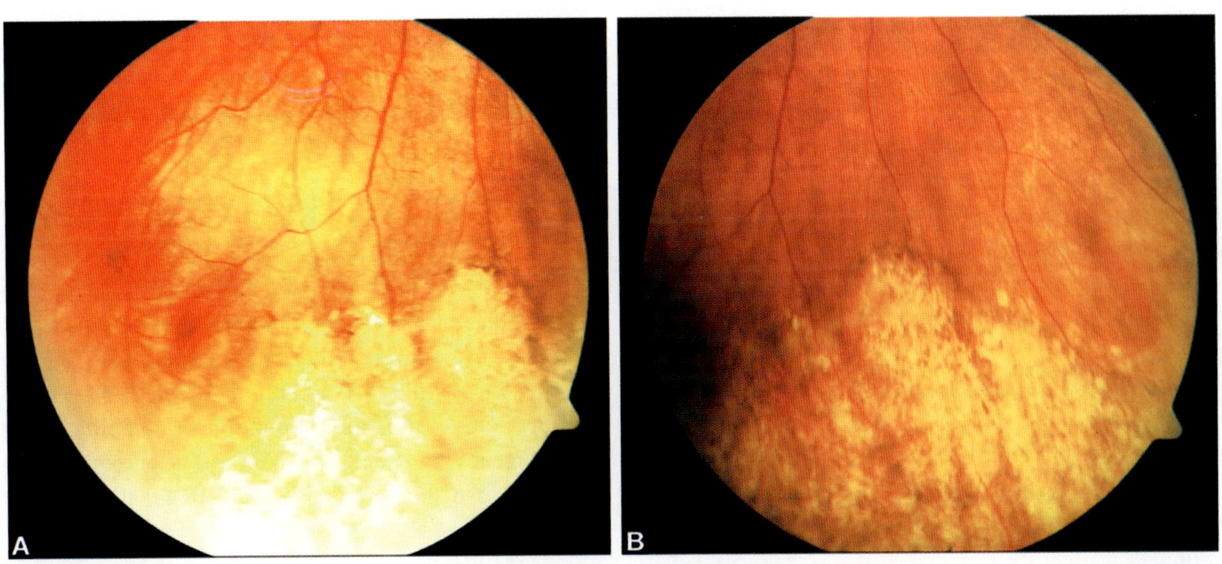

▲ **Figures 32.1A and B**

(A) Active CMV retinitis with involvement of inferior peripheral retina. The lesion appears as granular, confluent, yellow-white retinitis; (B) Same lesion in Fig. 32.1A is seen after anti-CMV treatment (with oral Valganciclovir). The lesion appears as well demarcated atrophic RPE and necrotic retina

In the pre-HAART era, CMV retinitis (Figs 32.1A and B) would develop in about 30% of patients with AIDS.[5] There has been a 75–80% decline in CMV retinitis with HAART and ensuing immune recovery.[6,7] The Longitudinal Studies of the Ocular Complications of AIDS (LSOCA) has reported the incidence of CMV retinitis as 5.6 cases/100 person years (PY) in the HAART era.[8] CMV retinitis usually occurs in HIV-infected people with CD4+ T-lymphocyte counts of less than 50 cells/μl.[9] In the HAART era, CMV retinitis occurs in patients who are HAART intolerant or unresponsive/resistant to HAART.[10,11] With HAART, the rates of retinitis progression and retinal detachment have declined and we have been able to even discontinue anti-CMV maintenance therapy in some patients with immune recovery.[12-14] Patients who achieved a sustained response to HAART, defined as a CD4+ cell count greater than 100–150 cells/mm^3 for at least 6 months, can be considered to discontinue secondary prophylaxis of CMV therapy if they remain disease free for 5–16 months.[15] However, factors like the location of retinitis, vision in the fellow eye, the duration and magnitude of the CD4+ cell count should still be considered before a decision for discontinuation is made. The anti-CMV treatment should be resumed if the CD4+ cell count decreases to below 100–150 cells/mm or CMV retinitis recurs.[16] This highlights the importance of continued surveillance, as there have been reports of recurrent CMV retinitis despite CD4+ counts higher than 100 cells/mm^3 and undetectable HIV RNA level. These cases are probably due to loss of CMV-specific immunity.[17]

There are newer antiretroviral medications like fusion inhibitors, integrase inhibitors (raltegravir) and CCR5 receptor antagonists (maraviroc and vicriviroc). There are ongoing clinical trials with these agents in treatment—naïve as well as treatment-experienced patients.[18,19]

CMV retinitis accounts for 40% of vision loss to 20/200 or worse among LSOCA subjects.[20] The main reasons of vision loss in patients with CMV retinitis are involvement of fovea, optic nerve (zone 1 disease) and retinal detachment (Fig. 32.2).[21]

Despite these advances, AIDS is still a growing problem in other areas of the world, including Eastern Europe, Southeast Asia and India and the bulk of new disease is occurring in the developing world.[9] Access to medical care in these areas of the world is limited; drugs are expensive with limited availability.

It is possible, incidence of CMV retinitis will rise again, as HIV resistance to antiretroviral drugs increases and HIV infects vulnerable patients with limited access to screening, medical care; minorities and teenagers.[9]

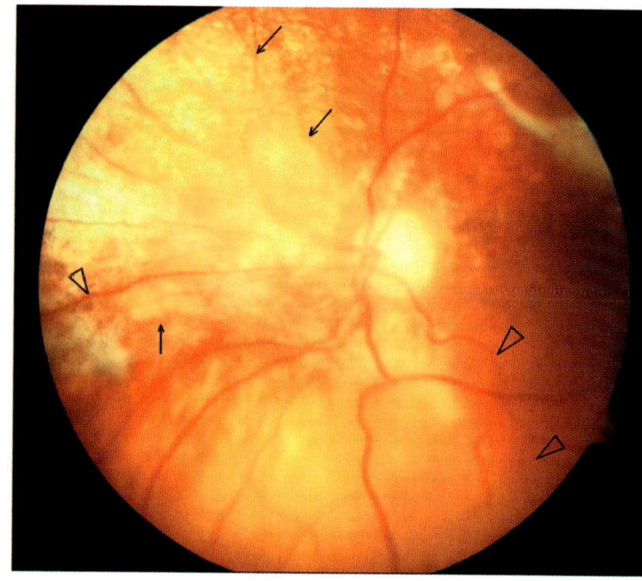

▲ **Figure 32.2**

Retinal detachment along with active CMV retinitis. Arrows show area of retinitis. There is also retinitis in part of the detached retina. Arrowheads show area of retinal detachment

The World Health Organization (WHO) and the Joint United Nations Program on HIV/AIDS (UNAIDS) have announced the largest ever HIV vaccine clinical trial results, in September of 2009. The RV144 HIV vaccine study results revealed a 31.2% vaccine efficacy in preventing HIV infections, which is modestly protective.[22] However, this should not deter health care professionals and people at risk from seeking and implementing prevention measures.

Incidence of Retinal Detachment in Cytomegalovirus Retinitis

The Studies of the Ocular Complications of AIDS (SOCA) was the first clinical trial which enrolled and followed-up 234 patients with CMV retinitis between 1990 and 1992.[23] In the SOCA trial, the cumulative probability of retinal detachment (Fig. 32.2) was 57–66% at one year.[24] Labs et al.[25] reported the cumulative risk of retinal detachment as 50%, one year after the diagnosis.

There has been a modest decrease in the rate of retinal detachment in CMV retinitis after the introduction of HAART. The rate of retinal detachment in pre-HAART was 0.50 per person-year (0.50/PY) compared to 0.06/PY in the HAART era.[4,26] This is due to better control of infection, resulting in smaller, inactive lesions.[27] In a relatively larger study of 147 patients, 41 patients (28%) developed retinal detachment; with a median time of 25 weeks and a rate of 40% one year after diagnosis.[28] Jabs et al.[29] reported an overall retinal detachment rate of 0.06/PY in a multicenter, prospective, observational study of 271 patients with AIDS. The retinal detachment rate was 0.30/PY among patients with CD4+ T-cell counts of less than equal to 50/μl as compared to 0.02/PY among those with CD4+ T-cell counts of more than or equal to 200/μl; indicating lower rates of retinal detachment with immune reconstitution. For patients with CD+T-cell counts of 50–200/μl, the rate was 0.12/PY.

The incidence of bilateral detachments is variable; between 17% and 67%, making retinal detachments major cause of visual disability in patients with CMV retinitis.[25,30]

Risk Factors for Retinal Detachment in CMV Retinitis

Involvement of more than half of the retina increased the risk of retinal detachment by sixfold.[23]

Freeman et al.[31] reported the degree of peripheral retina involvement and the presence of active retinitis on the most recent examination, as the best predictors of retinal detachment. In another study, active retinitis seemed to increase the risk of retinal detachment by 2.9 times; involvement of zone 2 (retina extending from 2,000 μ from optic nerve to the equator) increased the risk to more than 25%; and involvement of 25% of retina increased the risk of detachment by 8.3 times.[31]

Other risk factors for retinal detachment were older age, lower CD4+ T-lymphocyte count.[32] Irvine et al.[33] had suggested myopia as a risk factor; however this was not verified in larger studies. Higher hemoglobin levels were also suggested.[34] Treatment of CMV retinitis with either foscarnet or ganciclovir did not influence the rate of detachment.[23] The overall risk of retinal detachment was not higher in patients with ganciclovir implant than in patients treated with only intravenous ganciclovir.[9]

Clinical Features of Retinal Detachment in CMV Retinitis

CMV related retinal detachments are relatively atypical rhegmatogenous detachments by their distinctive features.

Retinal surgeons have reported multiple retinal breaks which are difficult to visualize even during the surgery and thus may be missed. They are mostly located within or at the junction between normal and necrotic, gliotic retina. As the border of the retinal detachment is sharply demarcated and retinal breaks are hard to find, there may be a false impression of exudative detachment. CMV infects and destroys full thickness retina and spares the choroid. The vitreous may be seeping through the necrotic or gliotic retina which has been infected with CMV. These retinal detachments progress slowly because of the adherence of posterior hyaloid to retina in these young patients. Inferior retina shows mild fibrosis and foreshortening.[35-39]

Severe proliferative vitreoretinopathy (PVR) has infrequently been reported; some degree of PVR has been found in less than 20% of CMV retinitis associated retinal detachments.[25,40,41] This might be related to decreased number and function of lymphocytes in AIDS,[42] as most eyes are "not inflamed".

It is important for the surgeon to be aware of these features and plan the approach in CMV related retinal detachments.

Pathophysiology of CMV Related Retinal Detachments

Freeman et al.[43] published the results of endoretinal biopsies which were obtained in seven eyes undergoing vitrectomy for CMV related retinal detachment. The vitreous was found to be strongly attached to the retina; there were active areas of retinitis at the junction of normal and atrophic retina, small breaks were located in the area of thinning at border between healing and normal retina. These help explain the mechanical factors related to CMV retinitis associated retinal detachments. Vitreous traction is responsible for most CMV-related detachments. When this traction overcomes the chorioretinal adhesion in areas of scarring, retinal breaks and detachment will occur.

Occasionally, multiple small holes form in active or atrophic retinitis areas; coalesce and then cause entry of vitreous into the subretinal space even without traction.[34]

Another mechanism may be vitreous inflammation in eyes with immune recovery. This inflammation may cause vitreous detachment and traction and lead to horseshoe tears.[34] As more patients go into remission and develop immune recovery uveitis or vitritis with HAART, we are yet to find out how this will change the rates of retinal detachment, in such patients.

Management of Retinal Detachments in CMV Retinitis

The difficulty of management of retinal detachment stems from many factors in patients with AIDS. These factors are mainly difficulty in identifying the breaks, posterior location of the breaks, vitreous adherence to the necrotic or gliotic retina, lack of posterior vitreous detachment and poor health of the patient.

In the pre-HAART era, the goal in such retinal detachment was to stabilize the extent of detachment and preserve vision till the patient expired which was as short as 6 weeks after the diagnosis of CMV retinitis.[44] In the HAART era, with longer life expectancies in these patients, procedures that guarantee the maximum amount of vision in both eyes for an indefinite time are needed. This will require collaboration of the infectious disease specialist, primary physician and the ophthalmologist.

The options for repair of retinal detachment in CMV retinitis include pneumatic retinopexy, laser photocoagulation, scleral buckle, vitrectomy with intraocular tamponade or combination of these procedures.

Pneumatic Retinopexy and Laser Photocoagulation

As the retinal detachments in CMV retinitis are distinct from typical rhegmatogenous retinal detachments, pneumatic retinopexy has limited application in AIDS patients. However, in few patients with limited visual potential and survival, it should be reserved as a viable option.

McAuliffe et al.[45] reported pneumatic retinopexy to delay surgical repair of a retinal detachment associated with the ganciclovir intraocular device. They proposed pneumoretinopexy may benefit patients when the break was located superiorly and in the retina not involved with CMV.

There are some patients who may benefit from laser photocoagulation due to their medical conditions, especially if they cannot undergo prolonged surgery. Laser photocoagulation may be employed to barricade a peripheral retinal detachment if the macula is attached. Thermal laser burns should be applied to surround the retinal detachment as well as areas of retinitis and atrophic retina. This should extend as anterior as the ora serrata. However, this may not be feasible if there is no healthy retina left.

Orellana et al.[46] applied laser photocoagulation to demarcate the retinal detachment in 22 eyes with CMV retinitis. They were not able to visualize holes, preoperatively. The outcome was limited with a short median survival time; 17 eyes (77%) had no further advancement of detachment. They recommended laser to treat non-bullous CMV-related detachments.

Irvine treated five eyes with peripheral retinal detachments with barrier laser photocoagulation. In three patients (60%), the detachment progressed through the laser 2–4 weeks after the treatment despite absence of active retinitis.[31]

McCluskey[47] used laser photocoagulation only if less than one quadrant of retina was involved and if less than 50% of the retinitis area was detached. He reported five such patients; all patients retained a visual acuity of 6/18 or better, with a median survival of 7 months.

There are two comparative studies for laser photocoagulation versus pars plana vitrectomy (PPV) and silicone oil. Davis et al.[48] reviewed 63 eyes with macula sparing CMV-related retinal detachment. Twenty-three eyes had barrier laser photocoagulation, 24 had PPV with silicone oil and 16 had no treatment. Initial and final visual acuity were better in laser treated eyes, although half of these retinal detachments progressed and a third (30%) went on to have PPV. Median time to progressive detachment was 175 days.

In another series by Vrabec,[49] seven eyes treated with laser photocoagulation were spared from visual loss. Only one patient (14%) showed progression of retinal detachment during the mean follow-up of 9 months. Two patients (28%) had decreased vision due to retinal detachment and progressive CMV retinitis, compared to 5 of 7 eyes (71%) experiencing decreased vision after PPV with silicone oil due to above mentioned complications. The author addressed the importance of proper laser technique with three rows of confluent 200 μ grey-white laser burns in healthy retina posterior and peripheral to the entire detached area and all contiguous areas of active and inactive retinitis.

There have been reports on prophylactic laser photocoagulation in CMV retinitis to prevent retinal detachment. Althaus et al.[50] performed prophylactic laser photocoagulation in twenty AIDS patients (22 eyes) with medically treated CMV retinitis. In half of the eyes, smoldering CMV retinitis crossed the laser scars. The laser scar did not prevent smoldering disease from progressing. Retinal hole formation with retinal detachment occurred in 4 of 22 eyes (18%). In three of these cases, the laser scar prevented further progression of detachment for about 6.5 months. However, it is not clear if such laser in these patients could initiate new retinal holes or breaks, as they observed a schisis-like splitting central to the laser scar. Mefferet and Ai reported 24 patients with nonmacular-threatening CMV retinitis and no retinal detachment. They assigned half of the patients to control group. Four retinal detachments (33%) occurred in the control group as opposed to one (8%) in the treated group; this was not statistically different.[51] There is no evidence that laser photocoagulation increases the retina-choroidal adhesion in eyes with CMV retinitis, so prophylactic laser treatment to prevent retinal detachment is currently not recommended in CMV retinitis.

Scleral Buckle

The rationale for an encircling scleral buckle is to offset traction and support necrotic retina. Scleral buckling alone may be employed in cases with small peripheral retinal detachment and with inactive CMV retinitis; which are those with less complicated pathophysiology. This, unfortunately, represents a very small group of patients.

Scleral buckle alone has not been shown to be effective in CMV-related retinal detachments.[52] In a small series, Irvine was able to reattach retina after scleral buckling and sponge in one eye with a small area of CMV retinitis; however this approach failed in 2 eyes.[53] Orellena et al.[46] performed scleral buckling in 9 patients with extramacular retinal detachment with CMV retinitis and reattached retina in 7 cases (77%); two patients had recurrent retinal detachments.

In a report by Ross et al.[54] three of the four patients (75%) who underwent scleral buckling remain attached at the end of follow-up, which was reported as 6 months to until death. The breaks in this group were well defined and were consistent with the configuration of the detachment.

It has been proposed that scleral buckle in eyes of patients with AIDS may cause ocular ischemia is in patients with sickle cell disease.[55] Patients who are anemic, who have intra-operative hypotension and those who undergo general anesthesia are especially vulnerable. Segmental buckles can also be considered an alternative to avoid such ischemia.

As there are multiple, invisible breaks in patients with CMV-related retinal detachments, these patients are not the best candidates for scleral buckling alone. Some retinal breaks are recognized only at the time of vitrectomy because of their location in the necrotic retina.[42] The reattachment rate with scleral buckling is lower than with PPV and silicone oil.

Pars Plana Vitrectomy with Silicone Oil Injection

Pars plana vitrectomy with silicone oil tamponade has been the standard of care in many patients with CMV-related retinal detachments. This involves three-port vitrectomy with removal of posterior hyaloid. As most of those patients are young, the vitreous gel is adherent to the necrotic retina. This may create more retinal breaks. If the retina is taut due to necrosis and gliosis, retinotomy may be required. Creation of retinotomy would allow internal drainage of subretinal fluid, otherwise a pre-existing retinal break may also be used. Laser photocoagulation should be performed in uninvolved, healthy retina adjacent to areas of CMV retinitis and to barricade the retinotomy sites.

This should be coupled with fluid-air or fluid-silicone oil exchange. Either 1,000- or 5,000-centistoke silicone oil can be infused for retinal tamponade. Although a randomized comparison has not been performed, there has been no difference in surgical outcome based on the type of silicone oil.[56] It is important to achieve a complete fill, as these patients may have invisible breaks and the posterior hyaloid may still be attached. Infusion of oil till it is visualized in the infusion cannula may assure complete fill. Lensectomy should be avoided when complete fill of vitreous cavity is important. Presence of the lens and the zonules will prevent anterior segment complications of silicone oil.[36] If lensectomy is required, the posterior capsule should be preserved. If this is not possible, then an inferior iridectomy should be performed.[36]

Advantages of silicone oil are numerous. In atypical retinitis cases, retinal biopsy may be required and silicone oil would adequately tamponade the biopsy site. Postoperative positioning requirements are not as stringent with silicone oil as with intraocular gases, this is a major benefit in debilitated patients. Permanent tamponade may be achieved as long as the silicone oil stays in the eye; this may avoid future retinal breaks due to ongoing retinal traction by active retinitis or proliferative retinopathy. Despite the fact that inferior breaks may not be fully tamponaded with silicone oil, further entry of fluid into the macular subretinal space may be blocked with silicone oil, thus macula may stay attached despite the residual inferior retinal detachment.[56] Intravitreal injections can be performed and ganciclovir sustained drug delivery device can be implanted in eyes with silicone.[57]

A prospective multicenter trial of 407 eyes (350 patients) reported the safety and efficacy of PPV with either 1,000- or 5,000-centistokes silicone oil, in HIV patients with CMV-related retinal detachment.[56] Follow-up was variable; three hundred ninety-three eyes (97%) had at least one follow-up examination; fifty-four eyes (13%) had their last eye exam at 1 week, 129 (32%) at 1 month, 113 (28%) at 3 months, 65 (16%) at 6 months, 28 (7%) at 1 year and four (1%) at 2 years. Seventy-three percent of eyes had completely attached retina at the last follow-up examination and 94% of eyes had attached maculae. Ambulatory vision was achieved in 68% of eyes; visual acuity was preserved or improved in 56% of eyes.[56]

There are other smaller series reporting on rates of retinal reattachment, ambulatory vision and preservation of vision. Jabs et al.[15] reported a rate of 70% of retinal attachment with PPV with silicone oil, Dugel et al.[58] reported an 89% reattachment rate, however 95% of eyes had optic atrophy with poor vision. Freeman et al.[36] reported their results on 29 eyes of 24 patients; they used silicone oil as tamponade in most, except two eyes with in which sulfur hexafluoride (SF_6) was used. They achieved a macular attachment rate of 90%, total retinal reattachment of 76%. After a mean follow-up of 29 weeks, 62% of eyes had final visual acuity of 20/100 or better.

Kuppermann et al.[59] reported their experience on 65 eyes; 50% had half of the retina involved with CMV retinitis. A macula reattachment rate of 92% was achieved. Interestingly, preoperative macular detachment did not seen to affect postoperative visual acuity. They attributed this to the relatively shallow nature of the detachment associated with formed vitreous and also to the short duration of detachment. Similar results were reported by Lim et al.[60] they found the visual outcomes were better unless the optic nerve was involved.

Potential postoperative complications related to silicone oil include cataract formation, corneal decompensation, silicone oil emulsification, ocular hypertension or glaucoma, hypotony, refractive shifts. The most common complication is cataract formation which is reported in 30% of eyes at a median interval of 7 months.[56] Cataract surgery is possible in eyes with permanently implanted silicone oil if certain precautions are taken.

There are some authors who perform primary cataract surgery during initial repair of retinal detachment with vitrectomy, silicone oil injection.[61] This may improve long-term visual rehabilitation, allows better visualization of the posterior pole and avoids an additional cataract procedure in the future. Axial length measurements should be modified and silicone IOLs should be avoided due to potential emulsification of silicone oil, on silicone lenses.

Silicone oil was considered toxic to the retina by the electroretinographic (ERG) data, however this was probably due to the insulative effects of the oil.[56] Other studies showed that ERG results recovered upon removal of silicone oil.[62,63] Davis et al.[56] reported retention of vision for 2 years with silicone oil.

Garcia et al.[35] compared the results of retinal detachment repair with (56 eyes) and without scleral buckle (22 eyes) in addition to PPV in CMV related retinal detachments. The results in respect to retinal reattachment, mean and median best postoperative visual acuity were not statistically different. This was a retrospective, nonrandomized study, the preoperative differences between the two groups were not reported; the authors applied additional endolaser to the inferior retina in eyes which did not receive scleral buckle. Those patients without scleral buckle had a larger percentage of macula on retinal detachments. Nevertheless, elimination of scleral buckle theoretically decreases operative time, patient discomfort and accidental needle stick on the surgeon. However, encircling scleral buckle should be considered in eyes with residual traction especially in the inferior retina where silicone oil may not provide adequate tamponade due to its buoyancy.

Planned Removal of Silicone Oil

The longevity of patients with HIV/AIDS has significantly increased; oil removal will eventually be required to restore vision secondary to hyperopic shift or the development of complications such as corneal decompensation, glaucoma, cataract formation.

Silicone oil can be removed in patients who attained complete retinal attachment with initial surgery. Oil removal is more likely to succeed if the original breaks were located superiorly, as these are well tamponaded with the silicone oil.[34] The immune status of these patients should be improved prior to the removal of oil; this will assure long-term stability without recurrence or progression of retinitis and retinal redetachment. Laser photocoagulation should be performed in the normal retina surrounding the areas of retinitis.[34] These patients may also undergo peripheral laser photocoagulation in the clinic before oil removal.[34]

Morrison et al.[64] studied the risk factors for retinal redetachment after silicone oil removal in eyes with CMV-related retinal detachment. They reviewed 15 eyes of 14 patients with HIV and CMV retinitis. About half of the eyes (53%) redetached after a median of 4 months following silicone oil removal. They performed cataract surgery, scleral buckling, endolaser, membrane peeling, intraocular gas (C_3F_8, SF_6) or air injection, in some patients during oil removal. They found cataract surgery as a significant risk factor for redetachment. They also recorded a trend for lower CD4+ T lymphocyte counts to be associated with a higher risk of retinal detachment. The use of scleral buckle did not prevent future retinal detachment. The presence of proliferative vitreoretinopathy (PVR) or duration of oil tamponade was unrelated to the risk of redetachment.

Pars Plana Vitrectomy with Intraocular Gas Tamponade

Pars plana vitrectomy with intraocular gas is another option for CMV-related retinal detachments. PPV with intraocular gas may be considered if the breaks are adequately visualized; they are superiorly located and are consistent with the configuration of the detachment. Laser photocoagulation should be used and scleral buckling should be considered especially if there is retinal traction. These patients will need to position for sometime after the surgery, so this may not be the best option for debilitated patients. Patients may need to be away from work for longer time, due to positioning requirements. Some patients may choose this type of surgery to avoid a second surgery to remove silicone oil. Many phakic patients develop cataract after intraocular gas installation, even sooner than silicone oil.

There are few reports on surgical repair of CMV-related retinal detachments in patients with AIDS, without silicone oil but with perfluoropropane (C_3F_8) or sulfur hexafluoride (SF_6). Canzano et al.[65] analyzed visual and anatomic results of 5 such cases (6 eyes). All patients had low CD4+ T lymphocyte counts and were receiving HAART. They were on systemic ganciclovir, foscarnet; 2 patients had ganciclovir implants. They were able to reattach retina in five of six eyes (83%), without using silicone oil. Mean postoperative visual acuity was 20/40 (range 20/30–20/60) during a mean follow-up of 12 months. Orellana et al.[46] reported one out of three cases failed after vitrectomy and gas surgery. On the other hand, Parke[66] showed an 80% success rate with vitrectomy, scleral buckle and gas tamponade.

Retinal Detachment After Ganciclovir Implant

The ganciclovir implant (Vitrasert®; Bausch and Lomb, Inc., San Dimas, California, USA) for local drug delivery was approved by Food and Drug Administration, in 1996. The ganciclovir implant has shown higher intravitreal drug concentration than can be achieved with standard intravenous ganciclovir therapy in CMV retinitis.[67] Randomized trials have shown efficacy and safety of the intraocular device. The risk of progression was approximately three times higher in patients treated with intravenous ganciclovir as among those treated with an implant. A randomized clinical trial by NEI has shown that the median time to progression was 15 days in the deferred treatment group versus 226 days in the immediate treatment with ganciclovir implant.[67] A phase 3 multicenter controlled randomized clinical trial confirmed the lower rate of retinitis progression with ganciclovir impant; that there was neither increased ocular morbidity nor decreased patient survival. However, 50% of patients developed CMV retinitis in the fellow eye in 6 months and 31% of patients developed systemic CMV disease without concomitant systemic anti-CMV therapy.[67]

Potential complications of ganciclovir implant surgery are retinal detachment, endophthalmitis, vitreous hemorrhage and cataract, erosion of the implant strut or sutures, hypotony, macular edema, temporary astigmatism.[68] The rates of retinal detachment after ganciclovir implant vary between 5% and 11%.[67-69] In a retrospective review of outcomes associated with ganciclovir implants revealed the overall (7 year) incidence of retinal detachment as 0.079 per patient year. This incidence was lower in patients who were on HAART and those who had immune-reconstitution.[70] There was no association between implant exchange, multiple implants and retinal detachment.[70] The overall risk of retinal detachment was no higher in patients with ganciclovir implant than in patients treated with intravenous ganciclovir alone.[9]

Anand[71] recommended the retinal detachment repair procedure be modified in eyes that had undergone implantation of the device. He proposed a traditional PPV followed by insertion of the infusion cannula in the inferior nasal quadrant or at 12 o'clock position. Silicone oil is injected to a 90% fill to avoid contact between the oil and the device; inferior 180° of the retina is demarcated with endolaser as silicone oil would partially support this area. As the device will be in contact with the aqueous in upright position, there should be adequate diffusion of ganciclovir.

Martidis et al.[72] reported 10 patients who underwent PPV with silicone oil tamponade and simultaneous placement of ganciclovir implant. They performed a standard PPV, detachment of posterior hyaloid, endodrainage through a nasal retinotomy, endolaser, followed by infusion of silicone oil. The implant was implanted in the inferior temporal quadrant prior to PPV or after air or fluid exchange. They were able to achieve anatomic reattachment in all cases; best post-operative visual acuity was better than 20/100 in 70% of patients. Seven patients (70%) had active retinitis preoperatively; all showed diminished retinitis or were inactive after the surgery although most patients were treated before the HAART era. They proposed ganciclovir diffuses into the peripheral vitreous and is redistributed along the retinal surface at the oil-retina interface. The kinetics of implants and injections in eyes filled with silicone oil is uncertain, so these patients should be followed closely and timely intervention with systemic therapy should be employed if progressive disease is encountered.

Visual Outcome After Retinal Detachment in CMV Retinitis

There has been a decline in visual impairment in patients with CMV retinitis; it is estimated at a rate of 0.10 case/eye-year (EY) and blindness at 0.06 case/EY.[73,74] This is associated with improved control of retinitis and decline in complications. A SOCA trial has reported involvement of the posterior pole with CMV retinitis (zone 1 retinitis) accounted for approximately half of visual acuity loss of 20/50 or worse, 20/200 or worse and of doubling of the visual angle. Cataract and retinitis-related retinal detachment were the second and third most common causes of vision loss.[75] Retinal detachment appears to be a definite risk factor for reduced vision in CMV retinitis.[76] Goldberg et al.[77] prospectively studied the long-term visual outcome of 63 AIDS patients with CMV retinitis who received HAART. Severe vision loss (loss of 6 or more ETDRS lines) occurred in 69% of eyes with retinal detachment compared to 8% of eyes without retinal detachment. In another study by Thorne et al.[75] eyes that developed retinal detachment had the highest risk of vision loss, with 100% of eyes developing visual impairment (20/50 or worse vision) and 42% of eyes developing legal blindness (20/200 or worse vision) in 12 months after the diagnosis of the retinal detachment. In a pre-HAART study by Davis et al.[56] 407 eyes of 350 AIDS patients with retinal detachment associated with CMV retinitis (96%) were prospectively reviewed. These patients underwent repair with PPV (98%) and injection of silicone oil, as well as laser photocoagulation in 80%, scleral buckle in 11%. At final evaluation, which varied between 1 week to 2 years, the retina was completely reattached in 73%; the macula was reattached in 94%, and 68% had ambulatory vision (defined as $\geq$ 4/200). Only 12% of patients had visual acuity of 20/50 or better. This study did not specifically address factors related to poor vision other than macular detachment and media opacities. The median survival after retinal detachment was about 7 months. This might be related to the poor control of systemic CMV disease due to lack of HAART, which may also account for limited visual improvement after surgical intervention.

In another study by Kuppermann et al.[59] macula was reattached in 92% of 65 eyes after PPV and silicone oil injection. The mean final postoperative visual acuity was 20/100 (range 20/25–no light perception-NLP). Mean post-operative follow-up was 20 weeks (1–138 weeks) and mean survival time was 30 weeks (5–146 weeks) after surgery. The final visual acuity was equal to or worse than "count fingers" in 20/65 eyes (31%). The high rate of visual loss was attributed to the extent of retinitis and involvement of the optic nerve. Thirty percent had vision of count fingers or worse. They stated visual outcomes are better unless macula or macula-papillary bundle is affected. Interestingly, post-operative vision was not affected by the presence of preoperative macular detachment.

Anatomic reattachment rates do not correlate well with visual results. Dugel et al.[78] reported the anatomic success rate as 89.5% (17 of 19 patients). Fifteen of 19 patients (79%) had lost at least two lines of Snellen visual acuity at time of death. The mean survival time after surgery was 4 months. The visual acuity was worse than 5/200 in 58% of eyes at the time of death. Jabs et al.[25] reported only 20% of eyes with vision better than 5/200. Freeman et al.[39] noted better outcomes with visual acuity of 20/100 or better in 62% of eyes.

There are few studies looking into visual outcomes after retinal detachment repair, in the HAART era. In one study, almost all eyes developed visual impairment (20/50 or worse vision) and 42% of eyes develop legal blindness (20/200 or worse vision) at 12 months.[75]

As the control of HIV infection has much improved, patients with AIDS have improved quality of life and increased longevity. The mean survival after diagnosis of

CMV retinitis was 265 days in patients who were not on HAART as opposed to 914 days in those who took a protease inhibitor.[79] Patients with HIV are now estimated to live for at least 15 years.[80]

Significant success has been achieved with the reconstitution of immune status and thus life expectancy in patients with AIDS. Visual preservation or restoration is not the ultimate goal, we should be seeking ways to improve vision in both eyes, for an indefinite time in these patients.

The management of retinal detachment in patients with CMV retinitis[81] and AIDS should be tailored to each patient based on the number and location of retinal breaks; extent of detachment and of the necrotic retina; and overall health of the patient. Prevention, early intervention and close follow-up, as well as education of the patients on the importance of these issues are paramount.

Despite the increased success of therapy in AIDS and AIDS associated complications in the US, it is still a major problem in the developing world. We should share our experience and means with our colleagues in other areas of the world.

References

1. AIDS epidemic update, Joint United Nations Programme on HIV/AIDS (UNAIDS) and World Health Organization (WHO) December, 2009.
2. Belfort R. The ophthalmologist and the global impact of the AIDS epidemic LV Edward Jackson Memorial Lecture. Am J Ophthalmol. 2000;129:1-8.
3. Holland GN, Gottlieb MS, Yee RD, et al. Ocular disorders associated with a new severe acquired cellular immunodeficiency syndrome. Am J Ophthalmol. 1982;93:393-402.
4. Jabs DA. Ocular manifestations of HIV infection. Trans Am Ophthalmol Soc. 1995;93:623-83.
5. McCannel CA, Holland GN, Helm CJ, et al. Causes of uveitis in the general practice of ophthalmology. UCLA Community-Based Uveitis Study Group. Am J Ophthalmol. 1996;121:35-46.
6. Holtzer CD, Jacobson MA, Hadley WK, et al. Decline in the rate of specific opportunistic infections at San Francisco General Hospital, 1994-1997. AIDS. 1998;12:1931-3.
7. Jabs DA. AIDS and ophthalmology in 2004. Arch Ophthalmol. 2004;122:1040-2.
8. Jabs DA, Van Natta ML, Holbrook JT, et al. Studies of the Ocular Complications of AIDS Research Group. Longitudinal study of the ocular complications of AIDS: 1. Ocular diagnoses at enrollment. Ophthalmology. 2007;114:780-6.
9. Holland GN. AIDS and ophthalmology: the first quarter century. Am J Ophthalmol. 2008;145:397-408.
10. Jabs DA, Van Natta ML, Kempen JH, et al. Characteristics of patients with cytomegalovirus retinitis in the era of highly active antiretroviral therapy. Am J Ophthalmol. 2002;133:48-61.
11. Holland GN, Vaudaux JD, Jeng SM, et al. UCLA CMV Retinitis Study Group. Characteristics of untreated AIDS-related cytomegalovirus retinitis. I. Findings before the era of highly active antiretroviral therapy (1988 to 1994). Am J Ophthalmol. 2008;145:5-11.
12. Jabs DA, Van Natta ML, Thorne JE, et al. Studies of Ocular Complications of AIDS Research Group. Course of cytomegalovirus retinitis in the era of highly active antiretroviral therapy: 1. Retinitis progression. Ophthalmology. 2004;111:2224-31.
13. Jabs DA, Bolton SG, Dunn JP, et al. Discontinuing anti-cytomegalovirus therapy in patients with immune reconstitution after combination antiretroviral therapy. Am J Ophthalmol. 1998;126:817-22.
14. Torriani FJ, Freeman WR, Macdonald JC, et al. CMV retinitis recurs after stopping treatment in virological and immunological failures of potent antiretroviral therapy. AIDS; 2000.pp.173-80.
15. 2001 US Public Health Service Infectious Diseases Society of America guidelines for the prevention of opportunistic infections in persons infected with human immunedeficiency virus. www.hivats.org/guidelines (accessed 2001 Nov 30).
16. Palella FJ, Chmiel JS, Moorman AC, et al. HIV Outpatient Study Investigators. Durability and predictors of success of highly active antiretroviral therapy for ambulatory HIV-infected patients. AIDS. 2002;16:1617-26.
17. Jouan M, Savès M, Tubiana R, et al. RESTIMOP study team. Discontinuation of maintenance therapy for cytomegalovirus retinitis in HIV-infected patients receiving highly active antiretroviral therapy. AIDS. 2001;15:23-31.
18. Hicks C, Gulick RM. Raltegravir: the first HIV type 1 integrase inhibitor. Clin Infect Dis. 2009;48:931-9.
19. Dolin R. A new class of anti-HIV therapy and new challenges. N Engl J Med. 2008;359:1509-11.
20. Thorne JE, Holbrook JT, Jabs DA. Studies of Ocular Complications of AIDS Research Group. Effect of cytomegalovirus retinitis on the risk of visual acuity loss among patients with AIDS. Ophthalmology. 2007;114:591-8.
21. Thorne JE, Jabs DA, Kempen JH. Studies of Ocular Complications of AIDS Research Group. Causes of visual acuity loss among patients with AIDS and cytomegalovirus retinitis in the era of highly active antiretroviral therapy. Ophthalmology. 2006;113:1441-5.
22. Press statement by UNAIDS/WHO: "Largest ever HIV vaccine trial results very encouraging", September 24, 2009.
23. The Studies of Ocular Complications of AIDS (SOCA) Research Group in Collaboration with the AIDS Clinical Trials Group (ACTG). Rhegmatogenous retinal detachment in patients with cytomegalovirus retinitis: the Foscarnet-Ganciclovir Cytomegalovirus Retinitis Trial. Am J Ophthalmol. 1997;124:61-70.

24. Foscarnet-Ganciclovir Cytomegalovirus Retinitis Trial. 4. Visual outcomes. Studies of Ocular Complications of AIDS Research Group in collaboration with the AIDS Clinical Trials Group. Ophthalmology. 1994;101:1250-61.
25. Jabs DA, Enger C, Haller J, et al. Retinal detachments in patients with cytomegalovirus retinitis. Arch Ophthalmol. 1991;109(6):794-9.
26. Jabs DA, Van Natta ML, Thorne JE, et al. Studies of Ocular Complications of AIDS Research Group. Course of cytomegalovirus retinitis in the era of highly active antiretroviral therapy: 2. Second eye involvement and retinal detachment. Ophthalmology. 2004;111:2232-9.
27. Martin DF, Parks DJ, Mellow SD, et al. Treatment of cytomegalovirus retinitis with an intraocular sustained-release ganciclovir implant. A randomized controlled clinical trial. Arch Ophthalmol. 1994;112:1531-9.
28. Sandy CJ, Bloom PA, Graham EM, et al. Retinal detachment in AIDS-related cytomegalovirus retinitis. Eye. 1995;9 (Pt 3):277-81.
29. Jabs DA, Van Natta ML, Thorne JE, et al. Studies of Ocular Complications of AIDS Research Group. Course of cytomegalovirus retinitis in the era of highly active antiretroviral therapy: 2. Second eye involvement and retinal detachment. Ophthalmology. 2004;111:2232-9.
30. Sidikaro Y, Silver L, Holland GN, et al. Rhegmatogenous retinal detachments in patients with AIDS and necrotizing retinal infections. Ophthalmology. 1991;98:129-35.
31. Freeman WR, Friedberg DN, Berry C, et al. Risk factors for development of rhegmatogenous retinal detachment in patients with cytomegalovirus retinitis. Am J Ophthalmol. 1993;116: 713-20.
32. Díaz-Llopis M, Chipont E, Sanchez S, et al. Intravitreal foscarnet for cytomegalovirus retinitis in a patient with acquired immunodeficiency syndrome. Am J Ophthalmol. 1992;114:742-7.
33. Irvine AR. Treatment of retinal detachment due to cytomegalovirus retinitis in patients with AIDS. Trans Am Ophthalmol Soc. 1991;89:349-63.
34. Davis JL. Management of CMV retinal detachments in the new era of antiretroviral therapy. Ocul Immunol Inflamm. 1999;7:205-13.
35. García RF, Flores-Aguilar M, Quiceno JI, et al. Results of rhegmatogenous retinal detachment repair in cytomegalovirus retinitis with and without scleral buckling. Ophthalmology. 1995;102:236-45.
36. Freeman WR, Quiceno JI, Crapotta JA, et al. Surgical repair of rhegmatogenous retinal detachment in immunosuppressed patients with cytomegalovirus retinitis. Ophthalmology. 1992;99:466-74.
37. Baumal CR, Reichel E. Management of cytomegalovirus-related rhegmatogenous retinal detachments. Ophthalmic Surg Lasers. 1998;29:916-25.
38. Freeman WR. Retinal detachment in cytomegalovirus retinitis: should our approach be changed? Retina. 1999;19:271-3.
39. Freeman WR, Henderly DE, Wan WL, et al. Prevalence, pathophysiology and treatment of rhegmatogenous retinal detachment in treated cytomegalovirus retinitis. Am J Ophthalmol. 1987;103:527-36.
40. Regillo CD, Vander JF, Duker JS, et al. Repair of retinitis-related retinal detachments with silicone oil in patients with acquired immunodeficiency syndrome. Am J Ophthalmol. 1992;113:21-7.
41. Geier SA, Klauss V, Goebel FD. Risk factors for development of rhegmatogenous retinal detachment in patients with cytomegalovirus retinitis. Am J Ophthalmol. 1994;117:820-1.
42. Shah GK, Vander J. Rhegmatogenous retinal detachments with cytomegalovirus retinitis. Curr Opin Ophthalmol. 1998;9:6-10.
43. Freeman WR, Henderly DE, Wan WL, et al. Prevalence, pathophysiology, and treatment of rhegmatogenous retinal detachment in treated cytomegalovirus retinitis. Am J Ophthalmol. 1987;103:527-36.
44. Holland GN, Pepose JS, Pettit TH, et al. Acquired immune deficiency syndrome. Ocular manifestations. Ophthalmology. 1983;90:859-73.
45. McAuliffe PF, Heinemann MH. Ophthalmic Surg Lasers. The use of pneumatic retinopexy to delay surgical repair of a retinal detachment associated with the ganciclovir intraocular device. 1998;29:244-6.
46. Orellana J, Teich SA, Lieberman RM, et al. Treatment of retinal detachments in patients with the acquired immune deficiency syndrome. Ophthalmology. 1991;98:939-43.
47. McCluskey P, Grigg J, Playfair TJ. Retinal detachments in patients with AIDS and CMV retinopathy: a role for laser photocoagulation. Br J Ophthalmol. 1995;79:153-6.
48. Davis JL, Hummer J, Feuer WJ. Laser photocoagulation for retinal detachments and retinal tears in cytomegalovirus retinitis. Ophthalmology. 1997;104:2053-60.
49. Vrabec TR. Laser photocoagulation repair of macula-sparing cytomegalovirus-related retinal detachment. Ophthalmology. 1997;104:2062-7.
50. Althaus C, Loeffler KU, Schimkat M, et al. Prophylactic argon laser coagulation for rhegmatogenous retinal detachment in AIDS patients with cytomegalovirus retinitis. Graefes Arch Clin Exp Ophthalmol. 1998;236:359-64.
51. Meffert SA, Ai E. Laser photocoagulation prophylaxis for CMV retinal detachments. Ophthalmology. 1998;105:1353-5.
52. Meredith TA, Aaberg TM, Reeser FH. Rhegmatogenous retinal detachment complicating cytomegalovirus retinitis. Am J Ophthalmol. 1979;87:793-6.
53. Irvine AR. Treatment of retinal detachment due to cytomegalovirus retinitis in patients with AIDS. Trans Am Ophthalmol Soc. 1991;89:349-63.
54. Ross WH, Bryan JS, Barloon AS. Management of retinal detachments secondary to cytomegalovirus retinitis. Can J Ophthalmol. 1994;29:129-33.
55. Davis J, Chuang E. Repair of retinal detachment caused by cytomegalovirus retinitis in patients with the acquired immunodeficiency syndrome. Am J Ophthalmol. 1992;113: 468-70.

56. Davis JL, Serfass MS, Lai MY, et al. Silicone oil in repair of retinal detachments caused by necrotizing retinitis in HIV infection. Arch Ophthalmol. 1995;113:1401-9.
57. Duker JS, Robinson M, Anand R, et al. Initial experience with an eight-month sustained-release intravitreal ganciclovir implant for the treatment of CMV retinitis associated with AIDS. Ophthalmic Surg Lasers. 1995;26:442-8.
58. Dugel PU, Liggett PE, Lee MB, et al. Repair of retinal detachment caused by cytomegalovirus retinitis in patients with the acquired immunodeficiency syndrome. Am J Ophthalmol. 1991;112:235-42.
59. Kuppermann BD, Flores-Aguilar M, Quiceno JI, et al. A masked prospective evaluation of outcome parameters for cytomegalovirus-related retinal detachment surgery in patients with acquired immune deficiency syndrome. Ophthalmology. 1994;101:46-55.
60. Lim JI, Enger C, Haller JA, et al. Improved visual results after surgical repair of cytomegalovirus-related retinal detachments. Ophthalmology. 1994;101:264-9.
61. Engstrom RE, Goldenberg DT, Parnell JR, et al. Clear lens extraction with intraocular lens implantation during retinal detachment repair in patients with Acquired Immune Deficiency Syndrome (AIDS) [correction of autoimmune deficiency syndrome] and cytomegalovirus retinitis. Ophthalmology. 2002;109(4):666-73.
62. Foerster MH, Esser J, Laqua H. Silicone oil and its influence on electrophysiologic findings. Am J Ophthalmol. 1985;99:201-6.
63. Frumar KD, Gregor ZJ, Carter RM, et al. Electroretinographic changes after vitrectomy and intraocular tamponade. Retina. 1985;5:16-21.
64. Morrison VL, Labree LD, Azen SP, et al. Results of silicone oil removal in patients with cytomegalovirus retinitis related retinal detachments. Am J Ophthalmol. 2005;140:786-93.
65. Canzano JC, Morse LS, Wendel RT. Surgical repair of cytomegalovirus-related retinal detachment without silicone oil in patients with AIDS. Retina. 1999;19:274-80.
66. Parke DW. Management of retinal detachments in patients with AIDS. Presented at the 10th annual Meeting of the Vitreous Society, 21 October 1992, Laguna Nigel, CA, USA.
67. Martin DF, Parks DJ, Mellow SD, et al. Treatment of cytomegalovirus retinitis with an intraocular sustained-release ganciclovir implant. A randomized controlled clinical trial. Arch Ophthalmol. 1994;112:1531-9.
68. Dunn JP, Van Natta M, Foster G, et al. Studies of Ocular Complications of AIDS Research Group. Complications of ganciclovir implant surgery in patients with cytomegalovirus retinitis: the Ganciclovir Cidofovir Cytomegalovirus Retinitis Trial. Retina. 2004;24:41-50.
69. Lim JI, Wolitz RA, Dowling AH, et al. Visual and anatomic outcomes associated with posterior segment complications after ganciclovir implant procedures in patients with AIDS and cytomegalovirus retinitis. Am J Ophthalmol. 1999;127:288-93.
70. Kappel PJ, Charonis AC, Holland GN, et al. Southern California HIV/Eye Consortium. Outcomes associated with ganciclovir implants in patients with AIDS-related cytomegalovirus retinitis. Ophthalmology. 2006;113:683.e1-8.
71. Anand R. Treatment of cytomegalovirus retinitis with the intraocular ganciclovir implant. Curr Opin Ophthalmol. 1997;8:8-14.
72. Martidis A, Danis RP, Ciulla TA. Treating cytomegalovirus retinitis-related retinal detachment by combining silicone oil tamponade and ganciclovir implant. Ophthalmic Surg Lasers. 2002;33:135-9.
73. Srivastava SK, Martin DF, Mellow SD, et al. Pathological findings in eyes with the ganciclovir implant. Ophthalmology. 2005;112:780-6.
74. Kempen JH, Jabs DA, Wilson LA, et al. Mortality risk for patients with cytomegalovirus retinitis and acquired immune deficiency syndrome. Clin Infect Dis. 2003;37:1365-73.
75. Thorne JE, Jabs DA, Kempen JH, et al. Studies of Ocular Complications of AIDS Research Group: incidence of and risk factors for visual acuity loss among patients with AIDS and cytomegalovirus retinitis in the era of highly active antiretroviral therapy. Ophthalmology. 2006;113:1432-40.
76. Matsuo T, Morimoto K, Matsuo N. Factors associated with poor visual outcome in acute retinal necrosis. Br J Ophthalmol. 1991;75:450-4.
77. Goldberg DE, Wang H, Azen SP, et al. Long term visual outcome of patients with cytomegalovirus retinitis treated with highly active antiretroviral therapy. Br J Ophthalmol. 2003;87:853-5.
78. Dugel PU, Liggett PE, Lee MB, et al. Repair of retinal detachment caused by cytomegalovirus retinitis in patients with the acquired immunodeficiency syndrome. Am J Ophthalmol. 1991;112:235-42.
79. Walsh JC, Jones CD, Barnes EA, et al. Increasing survival in AIDS patients with cytomegalovirus retinitis treated with combination antiretroviral therapy including HIV protease inhibitors. AIDS. 1998;12:613-8.
80. Braithwaite RS, Roberts MS, Chang CC, et al. Influence of alternative thresholds for initiating HIV treatment on quality-adjusted life expectancy: a decision model. Ann Intern Med. 2008;148:178-85.
81. Musch DC, Martin DF, Gordon JF, et al. Treatment of cytomegalovirus retinitis with a sustained-release ganciclovir implant. The Ganciclovir Implant Study Group. N Engl J Med. 1997;337:83-90.

SECTION 10

Miscellaneous

Management of Dislocated Lens, Lens Fragments and Intraocular Lens

33

Astha Jain, Sandeep Saxena

Introduction

The problems facing the dislocated lens, nucleus, lens fragments and intraocular lens is different and hence each needs to be managed by a different technique. The clinical presentation can be as follows:

A. Dislocated crystalline lens
   a. Spontaneous
   b. Post-traumatic
   c. Associated with certain hereditary conditions.
B. Dislocated lens fragments/ nucleus/ cortex
   a. As an intraoperative complications of cataract surgery
   b. Spontaneous absorption of lens matter and dislocated nucleus secondary to hypermaturity.
C. Dislocated intraocular lens
   a. Dislocated intraocular lens with vitreous disturbance
   b. Dislocation of intraocular lens along with capsule following zonular dehiscence due to capsular fibrosis
   c. Trauma-related dislocation.

Dislocated Crystalline Lens

The lens is considered dislocated or luxated when it lies completely outside the lens patellar fossa, in the anterior chamber, free-floating in the vitreous, or directly on the retina.

Disruption or dysfunction of the zonular fibers of the lens, regardless of the cause (trauma or heritable condition such as Marfan's syndrome, Marchesani syndrome, Homocystinuria etc.), is the underlying pathophysiology of ectopia lentis.

Dislocation of the lens following trauma can be associated with other complications such as retinal detachment, vitreous hemorrhage, macular damage, secondary glaucoma, etc. The dislocated lens may be clear or cataractous. The dislocated lens may be mobile or fixed to the retina in long standing cases.

Dislocated Nucleus, Lens Fragments and Cortex

In 0.1–1% of cases, cataract extraction is complicated by luxated lens fragments, also known as "dropped nucleus". Dropped nucleus can lead to severe complications such as glaucoma or retinal detachment.[1] This complication occurs most commonly during cataract surgery although trauma is also an important cause.[2] It has become fairly common with increased use of phacoemulsification with its relatively longer learning curve, especially in countries where it has just become a standard of care.[3] During phacoemulsification, the dislocation of a nucleus can occur in the peripheral sculpting stage or in central sculpting stage. A radial tear extending posteriorly from a discontinuous anterior capsulorhexis is the major risk factor predisposing to posterior dislocation of the nucleus or nuclear fragment.[4] The predisposing factors for dropped nucleus are hard cataracts (13.6%), polar cataracts (9.1%), previously vitrectomized eyes (4.5%) and high myopia (4.5%).[5]

Patients with retained lens fragments can present with complications such as glaucoma, uveitis, corneal edema, etc.

Margherio et al.[6] described an incidence of 52.4% of raised intraocular pressure beyond 25 mm Hg, 69.6% of uveitis, and 50.8% of corneal edema.

The cataract surgeon may be tempted to fish out the sinking lens without appropriate management of the vitreous. However this may create vitreoretinal traction and lead to retinal breaks and detachment. Anterior vitrectomy can be done to clear the anterior chamber and pupillary area of all vitreous. Care must be taken to remove the vitreous from the wound. Timely referral to vitreoretinal surgeon can result in good prognosis.[3]

Management of Dislocated Crystalline Lens, Dropped Nucleus and Lens Fragments

The basic technique for management of dislocated crystalline lens, dropped nucleus and lens fragments is the same and depends upon the hardness of the nucleus.

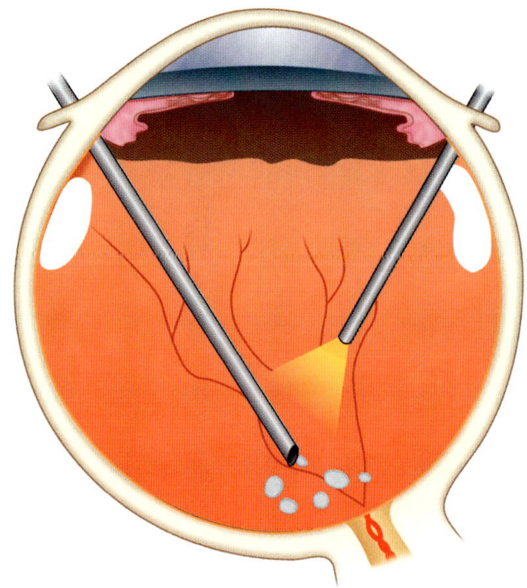

▲ **Figure 33.1**
Vitrectomy is done to access the dislocated lens fragments on retinal surface

▶ Observation

If the posterior dislocation of the crystalline lens or lens fragments is not associated with any complication it can just be visually rehabilitated by contact lenses or aphakic glasses. Cases of minimal cortex in the vitreous can be left untouched as the cortex itself gets absorbed without any sequel. However, presence of complications such as decreased visual acuity due to obstruction of visual axis, phacolytic uveitis, glaucoma, retinal detachment (RD) or cystoid macular edema (CME) is an indication for surgery. Studies have shown that removal of these before one week resulted in better visual results.[7]

▶ Surgery

Surgery to remove "dropped nucleus" must be performed as early as possible to prevent lens induced inflammation and glaucoma.[8] A higher incidence of glaucoma following vitrectomy for dropped nuclear fragments have been reported in cases where the vitrectomy was delayed for more than 3 weeks.[9]

Surgical Technique

A three port pars plana vitrectomy (PPV) is performed. Cortex and vitreous can be removed using the vitreous cutter. The nucleus is lifted into the mid-vitreous cavity and fragmented ultrasonically using 20-gauge fragmentor. However, this procedure might cause retinal damage from falling lens fragments. Perfluorocarbon liquid (PFCL) can be used instead to float the nucleus to anterior vitreous and then the fragmentation is done. PFCL flattens out associated detached retina and also prevents the retina from damage by flying lens particles (Figs 33.1 and 33.2). However, small fragments are not removed with perfluorocarbon since they may slip over the bubble towards the periphery. Any vitreous adherent to the capsule remnants is cleaned to prevent vitreous traction. Vitrectomy must be as complete as possible. However, if there is no posterior segment injury and no posterior vitreous detachment, an aggressive approach to create vitreous detachment to remove all vitreous is not required as it may cause retinal injury.

Retinal periphery is inspected with an indirect ophthalmoscope using a scleral indenter to look for any peripheral break and also for any residual peripheral lens material. Any retinal tears are managed with cryotherapy and fluid-air exchange. If intraocular lens (IOL) has not been implanted during the first surgery, one decides on the possibility of the same at the stage after the successful removal of the lens remnants. The extent and location of the tear in the anterior

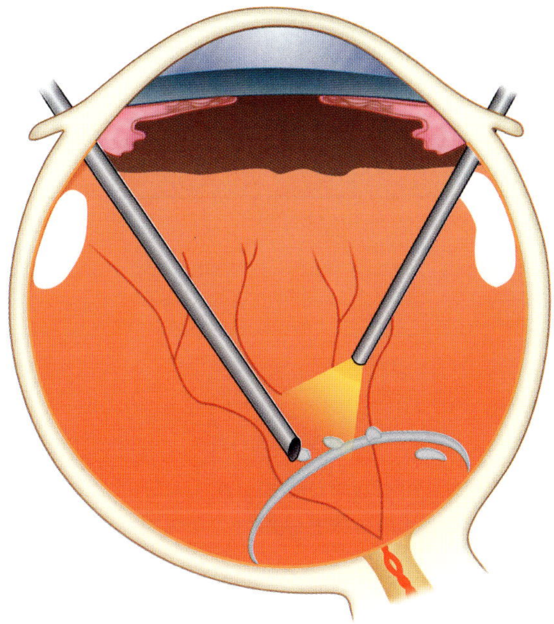

▲ **Figure 33.2**

Use of perfluorocarbon liquids helps to remove the lens fragments with ultrasonic fragmentor with relative safety

and posterior capsular should be inspected. One can place an anterior chamber intraocular lens (ACIOL) or a scleral fixated IOL if the capsular support is not enough.

The techniques of removing lens fragments by pars plana vitrectomy route are:[6,10]

- Ultrasonic fragmentation
- Crushing fragments between endoilluminator and cutter
- Vitrectomy cutter for cortex or soft nucleus
- Retrieval through limbal route.

The fragmentor is used only after performing core vitrectomy. The points to be kept in mind while performing fragmentation are:

- The nucleus should be lifted away from the retina with suction and then fragmented in the midvitreous cavity. Fragmentation should never be performed close to the retina.
- If lens milk appears, it indicates that the suction is blocked and continued use of the ultrasound energy can lead to scleral burns around the sclerotomy.
- The suction used to lift the lens from detached retina should be gentle to start with and increased to the desired level when the fragment is lifted up. PFCL must be used while fragmenting the lens with detached retina as there is risk of sucking and damaging the retina.
- Reducing fragmentation power to 5–10 %[11,12] minimizes chances of projectile fragments striking back the retina and causing further damage at the same time allowing nuclear extraction by continuous occlusion of the suction port.

Morris et al.[13] suggested prophylactic 360° laser retinopexy. The incidence of rhegmatogenous RD after PPV with 360° laser retinopexy prophylaxis was 1.3%, a significant reduction from the average 8.2% RD rate in the literature.

Dislocated Intraocular Lens

The incidence of dislocated intraocular lens (IOL) is between 0.2 to 1.8%.[14]

Posterior chamber IOLs can dislocate into the vitreous cavity if implanted in the setting of posterior capsular rupture or zonular dehiscence. This can occur during the surgery or in the early or late postoperative period. The cumulative incidence of dislocation over 10 years was found to be 1%. Although the risk is low, it may cause a relatively large public health problem because of the large number of cataract surgeries performed.[15]

During the surgery, dislocation may occur due to inadequate identification of capsular damage. Also the vitreous strands may pull the IOL posteriorly if it is not appropriately managed. Incorrect positioning of the IOL can also lead to posterior dislocation. The dislocated IOLs may lie in the vitreous gel or on the retinal surface if the vitreous is liquefied. Late, spontaneous dislocation of IOLs results from zonular insufficiency and zonulysis that has been associated with pseudoexfoliation, trauma and other risk factors.[16] Dislocation of IOL can also occur after Nd-YAG posterior capsulotomy.

Dislocated IOL is associated with complications such as a vitreous hemorrhage caused by mechanical contact with ciliary body vessels. The IOL may be related to RD or CME secondary to vitreous changes.

Management of Dislocated Intraocular Lens

There are several methods for the management of dislocated intraocular lens:

▶ Observation

The dislocated IOL might not be causing any posterior segment problem and the patient may be asymptomatic. Such patients may be observed and an ACIOL implanted for visual rehabilitation.

The most common indications for surgery include decreased visual acuity, persistent CME, increased IOP, inflammation coexisting RD, monocular diplopia, halo phenomenon and fluctuating vision caused by shifting IOL.[17] When surgery is planned for dislocated lens, vitreous loss is likely and the success of surgery most likely depends on how the vitreous loss is managed.

Retrieval of IOL

The technique of IOL retrieval depends upon the position of the dislocated IOL. If the IOL is in the anterior vitreous, it is first gripped with an intraocular forceps and vitrectomy is performed around it and then it is brought to the anterior segment. However, if the IOL is in the posterior vitreous or the retina, a different approach is required as trying to hold the IOL directly with the forceps may damage the retina. The vitreous is first removed in the center and a peripheral debulking is done. Then one edge of the optic is lifted and grasped by the forceps. This can be done by either using PFCL under the IOL to lift one edge or one can use the suction of a flute needle to gently lift the IOL (Figs 33.3 and 33.4). One may be able to easily grasp the haptic but this is not to be attempted as the haptic may break with disastrous results.

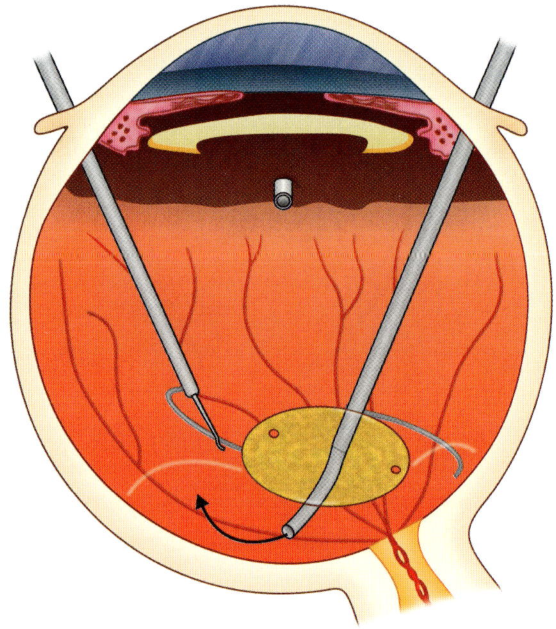

▲ **Figure 33.4**
Perfluorocarbon liquid injection can help float the intraocular lens making it easier to grip the same with forceps

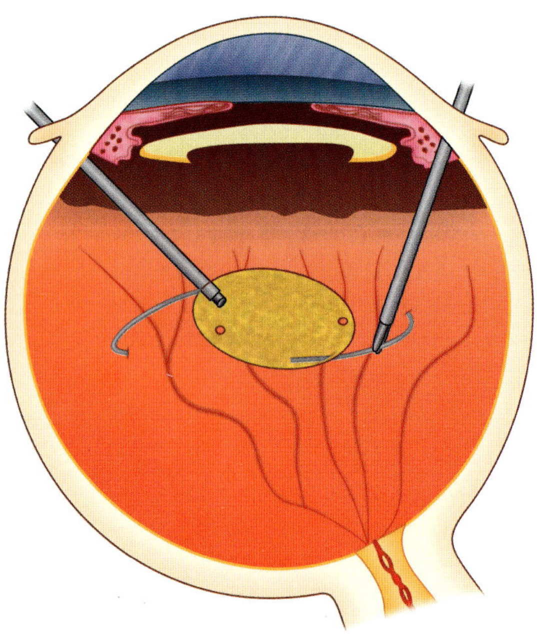

▲ **Figure 33.3**
A forceps can hold dislocated intraocular lens after vitrectomy

Explantation of IOL

The IOL is shifted from the grasp of an intraocular forceps to an external forceps and the lens is delivered by an ab externo incision. The cataract incision can also be reopened if the wound is not more than a week old. Once the dislocated IOL has been removed, aphakia can be corrected using an ACIOL or a sclera fixated IOL. However, if there is associated posterior segment problem, the eye may be left aphakic.

Repositioning of IOL

This technique minimizes ocular trauma and allows quicker recovery of vision. Presence of an intact rim of peripheral capsule allows the repositioning of the IOL. However, if the dislocation occurs several years after IOL implantation, even an intact capsule may not be able to support the IOL and there are chances of recurrent dislocation. If the capsular tear through which the IOL has dislocated has contracted due to fibrosis, the opening needs to be enlarged to bring forward the IOL.

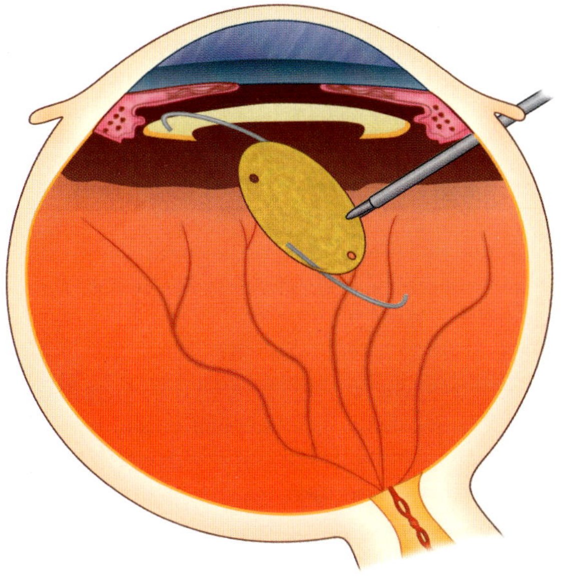

▲ Figure 33.5

The intraocular lens can be repositioned in the sulcus provided the capsular support is adequate

Repositioning of the IOL in the Sulcus

The IOL can be placed in front of the capsule in the sulcus. One haptic is brought anterior to the iris and the other haptic is placed in the sulcus over the capsular remnants. A sinskey hook is used to manipulate the other haptic into the sulcus. The orientation of the lens is confirmed to be in the axis of maximal capsular support. A bimanual technique can also be used for IOL repositioning where preset light is inserted in the inferonasal quadrant of the eye which leaves both hands free to grasp an IOL completely dislocated into the vitreous cavity. Both the haptics are directly placed in the sulcus (Fig. 33.5).

Sclera Fixation of the Dislocated Intraocular Lens

If the capsular support is inadequate, one has to consider sclera fixation of the same IOLs. One of the techniques described by Nikeghbal et al.[18] is haptic externalization by clear corneal incision. The haptic of the IOL is externalized temporarily through a clear corneal incision. A triangular limbal based sclera flap is made on both sides. 10-0 prolene suture is introduced in the eye through one sclera flap and exited from the opposite sclera flap. The suture is then withdrawn through the corneal incision and cut. The sutures are tied to the externalized haptics. The haptics are then repositioned into the anterior chamber followed by IOL reimplantation into the ciliary sulcus.

Another technique has been described by Lawrence and Hubbard called the lasso technique. It uses slipknots of 10-0 prolene that are made outside and taken inside through the sclerotomies and placed around the haptics of the IOL in the vitreous cavity.[19] The other end of the suture that is already passed through the ciliary sulcus is pulled to position the IOL.

Koh et al.[20] described the use of two corneal tunnels in which a double-armed 10-0 polypropylene suture loop is introduced through one corneal tunnel and placed around any accessible part of the haptic with the help of a bent 26-gauge needle. This technique is especially useful in cases of a dislocated capsular bag containing the IOL, a dislocated IOL with a large haptic, or a miotic pupil, where it is not easy to see the haptic ends to place the suture loop.

Tsukasa et al.[21] describe the use of cow hitch knot to engage the haptic of the IOLs that has been brought into the anterior chamber and then anchoring the IOLs to the scleral sulcus.

Implanting a New Intraocular Lens

This is done when either the IOL is damaged during retrieval or the IOL is of wrong power. An ACIOL or a sclera fixated IOL can be used.

Associated Retinal Detachment

Simple scleral buckling procedures should not be adopted in the presence of dislocated intraocular lens with retinal detachment. The IOLs should be removed and the RD managed internally. PFCL can be used to manage both the detachment and the dislocated IOLs.

Role of Perfluorocarbon Liquid in the Management of Dislocated Crystalline Lens, Nucleus and IOL

Perfluorocarbon liquid is injected into the vitreous cavity beneath the dislocated lens to float the lens on the anterior surface of PFCL bubble meniscus. The dislocated lens can now be removed by pars plana fragmentation. This technique of lens removal is particularly advantageous as:

- Perfluorocarbon liquid flattens the retina if the dislocated lens is associated with retinal detachment.

- The migration of lens fragment into subretinal space is prevented as PFCL seals off the breaks.
- Perfluorocarbon liquid prevents the macula from flying lens particle when it is being fragmented.
- The lens floats on the PFCL bubble meniscus allowing it to be grasped securely and then removed or repositioned.

Results

The timing of vitrectomy following nucleus drop has been controversial. While some advise immediate PPV, others show no difference in results.

Chen et al.[22] studied the outcome in patients with retained intravitreal lens fragments after phacoemulsification. He suggested that PPV performed immediately after cataract surgery for retained lens fragments showed better visual outcome and lesser complications compared to patients with PPV performed after 1 week who showed a higher complication rate (27% had CME, 36% developed RD).

Soliman et al.[23] stated that immediate intravitreal phacoemulsification with PPV in management of posteriorly dislocated nucleus or lens fragments is a surgical option in the management of posteriorly dislocated nucleus or lens fragments without much risk of retinal damage. The risk of postoperative complications including uveitis, secondary glaucoma and cystoid macular edema could be minimized.

However, Smiddy et al.[17] found that the timing of vitrectomy did not influence visual acuity outcomes. However vitrectomy done on the same day as cataract surgery yielded favorable visual outcomes. Also IOL inserted at the time of primary operation did not adversely affect the visual outcome.

Clinical presentation and treatment results of patients with dislocated IOL was also studied by Smiddy et al.[24] There were 18% "in the bag" IOL dislocations and it was associated with pseudoexfoliation, ocular trauma and time after implantation of IOL. The common complications were CME (10%) and RD (4%). However, the visual results were similar regardless of the surgical technique.

Chen et al.[23] showed that the timing of vitrectomy did not influence visual acuity outcomes. IOLs inserted at the primary operation did not adversely affect the visual outcome. However, vitrectomy on the same day as cataract surgery generally yielded favorable visual acuity outcomes and eliminated the need for a second operation at a later date. In most patients with retained lens fragments, management with vitrectomy allowed good visual acuity outcomes. However, another study by Seo et al.[25] showed visual rehabilitation earlier in late treated patients and except for very serious complication such as RD there is no need for immediate surgery following the occurrence.

Nikeghbali et al.[18] undertook a study to evaluate the results of trans-scleral fixation of dislocated posterior chamber IOLs by externalizing the haptics through a clear corneal incision. He found no statistically significant difference between mean visual acuity before IOL dislocation and after IOL refixation.

Gadre et al.[14] studied the clinical profile and visual outcome by different techniques in 60 dislocated IOL. They found that the incidence of intraoperative and postoperative IOL drop was more with IOL repositioning. However, the final visual outcome was more than >6/18 in 62% of patients with IOL repositioning as compared to IOL exchange (46%). The postoperative astigmatism was also less in cases of IOL repositioning (38%) as compared to IOL exchange (61.5%).

Modern vitreoretinal surgical techniques have improved removal of dislocated lens, dropped nucleus and lens fragments and retrieval of dislocated IOL. This has resulted in improved surgical and visual outcomes.

References

1. Hoeve M, Stilma J. Dropped nucleus on cataract extraction. Ned Tijdschr Geneeskd. 2010;154:1797.
2. Dada VK, Sharma N, Dada T. Retained nuclear fragments. J Cataract Refract Surg. 2000;26:1106-7.
3. Monshizadeh R, Samiy N, Haimovici R. Management of retained lens fragments after cataract surgery. Surv Ophthalmol. 1999;43:397-404.
4. Zhu X, Wei W, Shi Y, et al. Cause and management of dislocated nuclear fragments during phacoemulsification. Zhonghua Yan Ke Za Zhi. 2000;36:101-3.
5. Tajunisah I, Reddy SC. Dropped nucleus following phacoemulsification cataract surgery. Med J Malaysia. 2007;62:364-7.
6. Margherio RR, Margherio AR, Pendergast SD, et al. Vitrectomy for retained lens fragments after phacoemulsification. Ophthalmology. 1997;104:1426-32.
7. Monshizadeh R, Samiy N, Haimovici R. Management of retained lens fragments after cataract surgery. Surv Ophthalmol. 1999;43:397-404.
8. Vilar NF, Flynn HW, Smiddy WE, et al. Removal of retained lens fragments after phacoemulsification reverses secondary glaucoma and restores visual acuity. Ophthalmology. 1997;104:787-91.
9. Lim MC, Doe EA, Vroman DT, et al. Late onset lens particle glaucoma as a complication of spontaneous dislocation of

IOL in PXF Syndrome. Am J Ophthalmol. 2001;132:261-76.

10. Gillilan GD, Hulton WL, Fuller DG. Retained intravitreal lens fragments after cataract surgery. Ophthalmology. 1992;99: 1262-9.
11. Al-Khaier A, Wong D, Lois N, et al. Determinants of visual outcome after pars plana vitrectomy for posteriorly dislocated lens fragments in phacoemulsification. Cataract Refract Surg. 2001;27:1206-19.
12. Kapusta MA, Chen JC, Lam WC. Outcomes of dropped nucleus during phacoemulsification. Ophthalmology. 1996; 103:1184-7.
13. Morris RE, Shere JL, Witherspoon CD, et al. Intraoperative retinal detachment prophylaxis in vitrectomy for retained cataract fragments. J Cataract Refract Surg. 2009;35:491-5.
14. Gadre GA, Som V, Kulkarni A, et al. Clinical profile and visual outcome in different techniques of management of 60 dislocated intraocular implants. AIOC. 2010.pp.134-6.
15. Mönestam EI. Incidence of dislocation of intraocular lenses and pseudophakodonesis 10 years after cataract surgery. Ophthalmology. 2009;116:2315-20.
16. Davis D, Brubaker J, Espandar L, et al. Late in-the-bag spontaneous intraocular lens dislocation: evaluation of 86 consecutive cases. Ophthalmology. 2009;116:664-70.
17. Kim JE, Flynn HW, Smiddy WE, et al. Retained lens fragments after phacoemulsification. Ophthalmology. 1994; 101:1827-32.
18. Nikeghbali A, Falavarjani KG. Modified transscleral fixation technique for refixation of dislocated intraocular lenses. J Cataract Refract Surg. 2008;34:743-8.
19. Lawrence FC, Hubbaard WA. Lens Lasso repositioning of dislocated posterior chamber intraocular lenses. Retina. 1991;11:47-60.
20. Koh HJ, Kim CY, Lim SJ, et al. Scleral fixation technique using 2 corneal tunnels for a dislocated intraocular lens. J Cataract Refract Surg. 2000;26:1439-41.
21. Hanemoto T, Ideta H, Kawasaki T. Dislocated intraocular lens fixation using intra ocular cow hitch knot. Am J Ophthalmol. 2000;131:265-6.
22. Chen CL, Wang TY, Cheng JH, et al. Immediate pars plana vitrectomy improves outcome in retained intravitreal lens fragments after phacoemulsification. Ophthalmologica. 2008;222:277-83.
23. Soliman MM, Eid MZ, Shalaby KA, et al. Intravitreal phacoemulsification with pars plana vitrectomy for management of posteriorly dislocated nucleus or lens fragments. Eur J Ophthalmol. 2010;20:115-9.
24. Kim SS, Smiddy WE, Feuer W, et al. Management of dislocated intraocular lenses. Ophthalmology. 2008;115:1699-704.
25. Seo MS, Kim CR, Nah HJ, et al. Management of posteriorly dislocated intraocular lens using pars plana vitrectomy. Kor J Ophthalmol. 2000,14:80-4.

34

Surgery for Optic Disc Pit with Retinal Detachment

Edmund YM Wong, Claudine E Pang

Introduction

Optic disc pit is a rare congenital anomaly first described by Wiethe[1] in 1882. It has the distinctive feature of an excavation smaller than half a disc diameter in the optic disc and is often associated with juxtapapillary serous retinal detachments. It is usually included as part of a spectrum of congenital disc anomalies including the morning glory deformity, juxtapapillary staphyloma and optic disc coloboma[2] which are all associated with juxtapapillary and macular retinal detachments.

Etiology

Optic disc pits are congenital anomalies that likely occur in the first trimester of pregnancy. Two variants of abnormal embryological development have been postulated. Many believe, like Sugar, Apple and Rabb that they are due to incomplete closure of the superior end of the embryonic fissure as the normal fissure would normally have surrounded the developing disc.[3-5] They are felt to be similar to small colobomatous defects of the optic nerve head[6-8] and are also known as "atypical colobomas",[9] although optic disc pits and colobomas do differ in that optic pits are usually unilateral and are not associated with systemic anomalies. Gass, however, believed that optic pits were due to abnormal development of primordial optic nerve papillae and failure of complete resolution of peripapillary neuroectodermal folds, rather than being true coloboma from incomplete fissure closure.[10]

A genetic etiology has to be questioned, and although other optic disc anomalies such as morning glory disc have stronger genetic links, some evidence suggests a possible autosomal dominant hereditary pattern in optic disc pit. Slusher et al.[11] described a five-generation pedigree of 35 members who had optic disc pit, morning glory disc syndrome and optic nerve coloboma inherited in an autosomal dominant fashion. Jonas and Freisler[12] reported 2 monozygotic sibs aged 15 years with bilateral congenital optic nerve pits and phenotypically normal parents. The sibs had poorer visual acuity in the eye with the larger nerve and one twin had macular detachment.

Optic disc pit and other optic nerve abnormalities have been described in renal coloboma (papillorenal) syndrome, which is autosomal dominant in about half its patients.[13] Mutations in the gene encoding the paired box transcription factor, PAX2, located on chromosome 10q24-25, have been described. The PAX2 gene is involved in the embryonic development of the optic and otic vesicles, genital tracts, kidney and central nervous system.[14,15]

Renal assessment by a renal physician with creatinine clearance tests and cystograms to ascertain presence of vesicoureteric reflux should be considered in patients with optic disc pit or other cavitary optic nerve abnormalities especially in children. Genetic testing for PAX2 gene mutations should then be performed.

Clinical Features

Optic pits have been reported to occur in less than 1 in 10,000 patients seen in an ophthalmic setting[9] and occurred

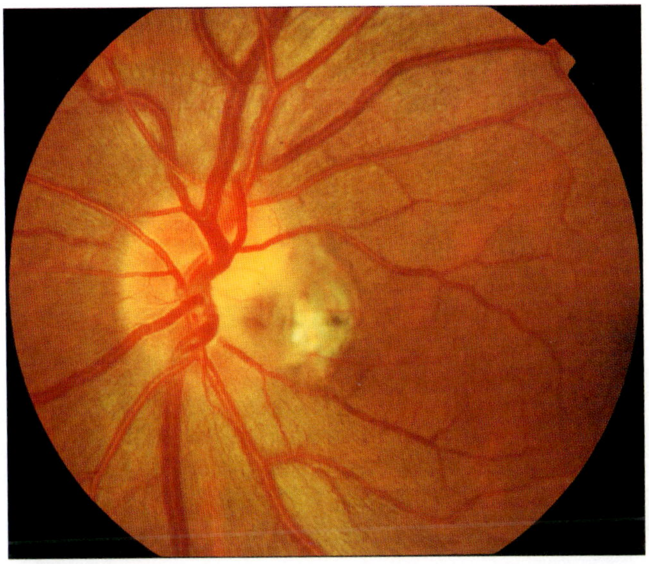

▲ **Figure 34.1**

An optic disc pit at the temporal margin of the optic nerve without macular detachment

unilaterally in 85–90% of cases.[6,16] Population based estimates ranged from 0.02% and 0.19% with similar distribution in males and females.[17-19]

Optic disc pits vary in size, occupying from one-quarter to one-half of the disc diameter. The depth of the optic pit can also vary. The pit can present as a slit or take the form of a round or oval depression.[20] The pit may appear olive-grey, yellow or white[9] (Fig. 34.1).

This depression is frequently situated in the temporal or infratemporal region of the optic disc. There is usually only one pit per optic disc, although two or three occasionally occur.[20] Circumpapillary chorioretinal atrophy with pigmentatory changes are seen in almost all cases where the pit is situated near the optic disc margin. In 60% of cases, a cilioretinal artery can be identified arising from the periphery of the pit.[9]

Visual acuity usually remains unaffected unless a serous retinal detachment of the macula develops. Approximately 25–75% of optic pits are associated with serous macular detachments.[7,8,10,19,21] These serous macular detachments are usually related to larger pits in the temporal region of the disc[22] and may occur during childhood or late in life[19,21,22] but are most common between the second and fourth decade.[9] Macular detachments have two components: an inner layer retinoschisis and an outer layer detachment.[23] Macular holes are usually in the outer layer, but can become full thickness if there is loss of inner retina and internal limiting membrane centrally. Successful hole closure and resolution of macular detachment can result in good visual acuity. Delayed closure and macula redetachment are associated with optic disc pit detachments.

Clinical Investigations

▶ Optical Coherence Tomography

Optical coherence tomography (OCT) of optic disc pit shows the depression of the pit into the substance of the nerve (Figs 34.2A to D and 34.3A and B). In cases with maculopathy, OCT has shown that macular elevation in the early stages of the disease seemed to be schisis-like with a splitting of the neurosensory retina emanating from the optic disc pit, with some patients demonstrating both a schisis cavity and outer-retinal detachment[9,24] (Figs 34.4A to D and 34.5A and B). This confirmed Lincoff's postulations[23] on inner schisis and outer layer detachment based on clinical examination.

Communication between a schisis cavity or subretinal space and the optic nerve pit was imaged in all eyes with serous macular detachment in the earliest reported OCT study, although no direct communication between the subretinal space and vitreous cavity was identified. Cystoid intraretinal spaces and bridging strands of presumed retinal tissue were identified in patients with macular detachment.[9] Subsequently, cyst formation alone or in association with lamellar holes could be found. A lamellar hole was shown to be a defect in the outer neurosensory retina. This study found that schisis cavities communicated with the optic disc pit but not the macular detachment.[25]

More recent OCT studies using higher resolution Fourier domain OCT have demonstrated a complete membrane traversing the optic disc cup in 3 of 5 eyes without maculopathy, in contrast to a deficient or absent membrane in eyes with no maculopathy.[26]

Spaide et al.[27] described high resolution OCT findings in 16 patients. Retinal detachment was noted in 11 eyes (69%), in whom only 3 of 11 (27%) had outer layer hole. Intraretinal fluid was demonstrated in 15 of 16 eyes (94%) in the outer nuclear layer, 13 eyes (81%) in the inner nuclear layer, 7 eyes (44%) in the ganglion cell layer, 2 eyes (13%) in the subinternal limiting membrane space. Eyes could retain 20/20 vision even in the presence of OCT demonstrated macular schisis and intraretinal cystic changes.[26,28]

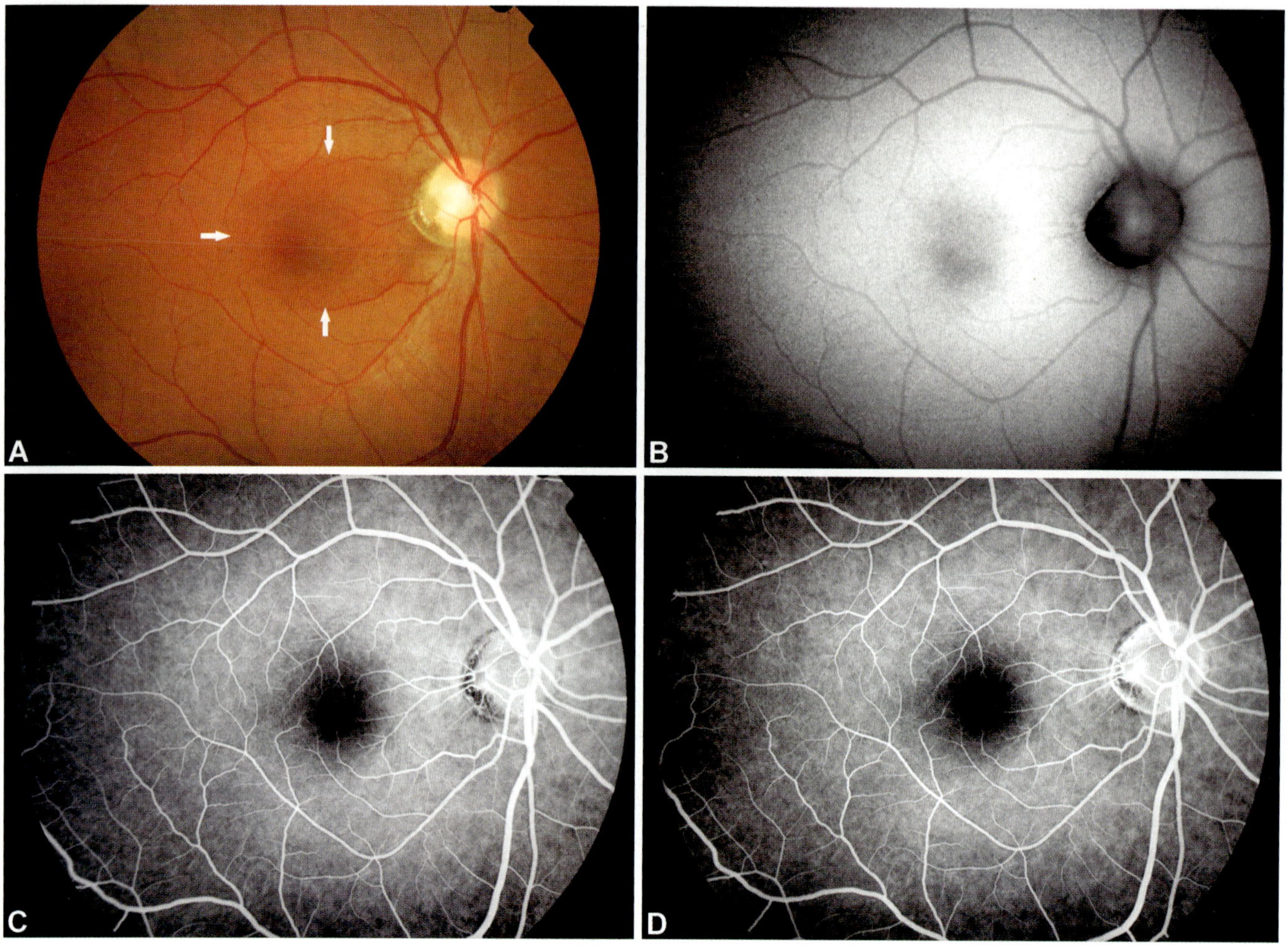

▲ **Figures 34.2A to D**

(A) Color photograph of optic disc pit. Oval reflex (arrows) noted extending from optic disc pit to macula. Clinically, no macular detachment on biomicroscopy; (B) Fundus autofluorescence. Fairly normal appearance, consistent with normal visual acuity in this patient; (C) Fluorescein angiography at 27 seconds. Hypofluorescence within optic disc pit. No leakage; (D) Fluorescein angiography at 5 minutes. Minimal staining around rim of optic disc pit (Dr Ranjana Mathur)

▶ Visual Field

Numerous visual field defects also exist. Reported changes included centrocecal defects, paracentral scotomas, arcuate defects, enlarged blind spots and nasal or temporal defects. Enlarged blind spots and arcuate scotomas were the most commonly reported defects.[10,13]

▶ Fluorescein and Indocyanine Green Angiography

Angiography of optic disc pits and maculopathies have been reported. Fluorescein angiography showed early hypofluorescence and late staining of the optic pit. Indocyanine green angiography showed absolute hypofluorescence of the optic disc. Both fluorescein and indocyanine green could demonstrate pooling of hyperfluorescence within the area of macular elevation. In other cases, the macular detachment area was silent[29] (Figs 34.2 and 34.4).

Pathogenesis

Histologically, optic pits[30] were demonstrated to consist of herniations of dysplastic retina into a collagen-lined pocket

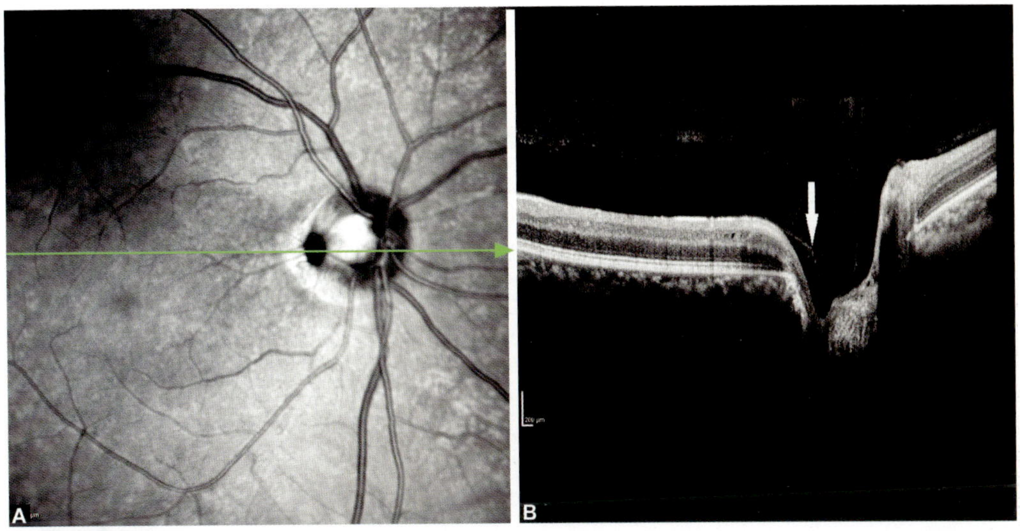

▲ **Figures 34.3A and B**

Optical coherence tomography of patient in **Figure 34.2**. Section through optic disc pit. No macular detachment. Thin membranous structure (arrow) arching over optic disc pit (Dr Ranjana Mathur)

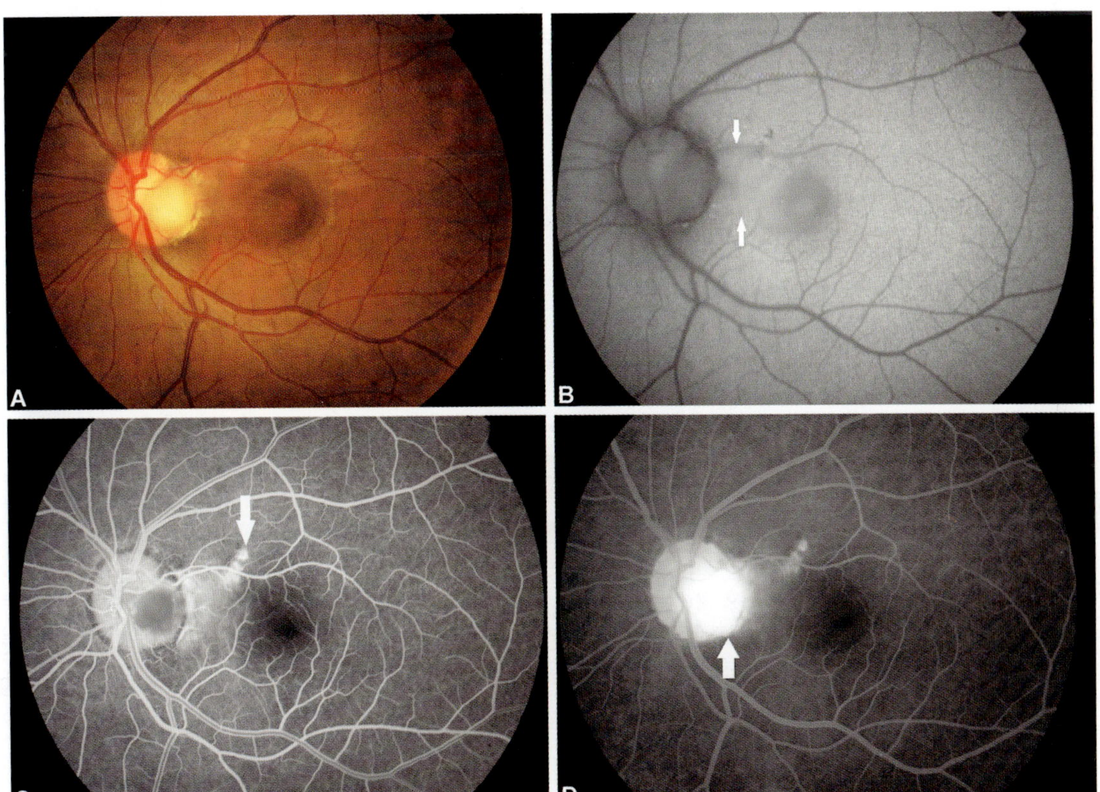

▲ **Figures 34.4A to D**

(A) Color photograph of optic disc pit with serous macular detachment; (B) Fundus autofluorescence. Slight masking of papillomacular area autofluorescence (arrows) due to serous detachment. Fairly normal appearance elsewhere over macula; (C) Fluorescein angiography at 27 seconds. Hypofluorescence over optic disc pit. Oblique hyperfluorescence under superotemporal macular vessel due to retinal pigment epithelium (RPE) transmission defect (arrow); (D) Fluorescein angiography at 8 minutes. Staining of optic disc pit (arrow). RPE transmission defect showing reduced hyperfluorescence with waning phase of angiograms (Dr Shu-Yen Lee)

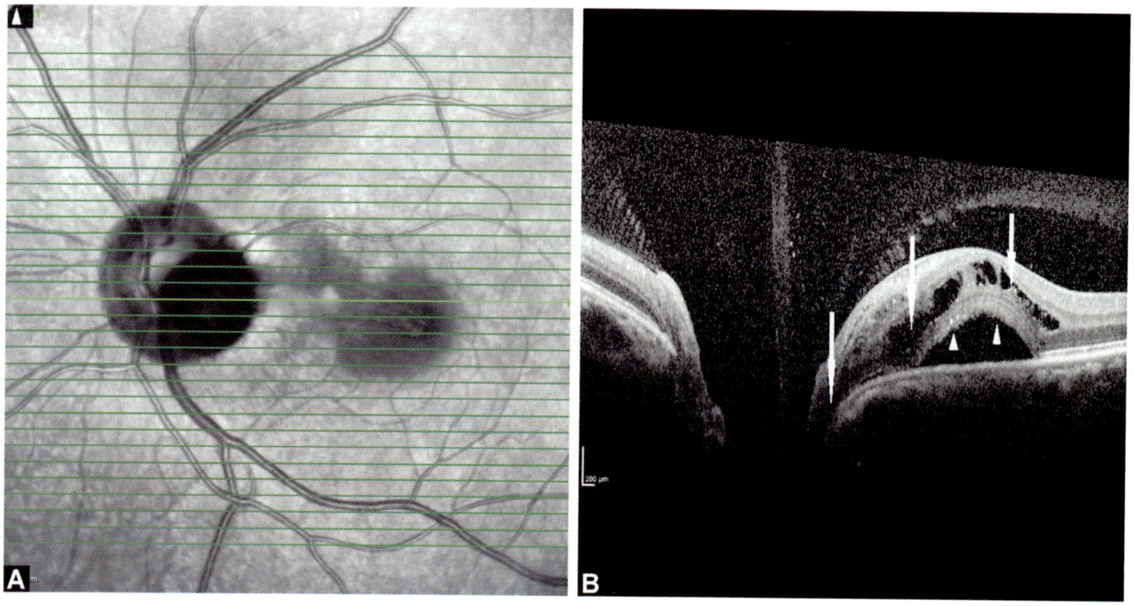

▲ Figures 34.5A and B

Optical coherence tomography of patient in **Figure 34.4**. Section through optic disc pit and macular detachment. Note inner layer cystic retinoschisis extending towards the optic disc pit (long arrows), outer layer detachment (arrowheads) (Dr Shu-Yen Lee)

extending posteriorly, often into the subarachnoid space, through a defect in the lamina cribosa.[10,31]

Close clinical examination and examination of magnified stereo images of the macular detachments in optic disc patients led Lincoff et al.[23] to postulate that these detachments actually had two components: a typically earlier, larger, oval shaped inner retina detachment connected to the optic disc pit, which they termed a retinoschisis, and a later, circle shaped outer, neurosensory retina detachment, which they termed outer layer detachment. Macular hole formation, when it occurred, occurred first in the outer layer detachment.

In contrast to the traditional view of retinoschisis, where there was an absolute scotoma in the area of retinoschisis, Lincoff and associates found that there was a relative scotoma in the retinoschisis area and an absolute scotoma only in the macular hole area on laser scotometry testing. They postulated that maintenance of visual sensitivity in the schisis area was possible due to vertical elongation, rather than total disconnection, of the Henle's fibers which were normally obliquely oriented. They proposed that at the macula hole area, the outer retina rim of the hole was turned inward towards the inner retina layer and that the photoreceptors in the base of the hole were destroyed, causing the absolute scotoma. OCT was able to demonstrate many of these clinical impressions later.

On the issue of the macula hole photoreceptors being destroyed, current thinking based on high resolution spectral domain OCT[32,33] in idiopathic macular hole is that the photoreceptor or outer segment layer is drawn up towards the inner retina rather than destroyed and it is likely similar in optic disc pit maculopathy. This postulate would explain the recovery of good visual acuity in cases with presumed centripetal repositioning of foveal photoreceptors that has been reported after successful reattachment.

▶ Source of Intraretinal Fluid

The source of the intraretinal fluid in optic disc pit detachments remains controversial. Commonly accepted possibilities include the vitreous fluid from the vitreous cavity, cerebrospinal fluid (CSF) from the perineural subarachnoid space and exudation from blood vessels at the base of the pit. Exudation from blood vessels is unlikely given that most reports of angiograms in these patients demonstrate little, if any, leakage and only occasional late staining.[19,29-31]

Cerebrospinal fluid as a source of fluid was postulated by Regenbogen and Gass, and supported in papers by Chang[34] and Irvine.[32] Normal intracranial pressure (ICP) varies between 5 mm Hg and 15 mm Hg. Ekstedt found that CSF pressure varied between 100 mm H_2O and 250 mm H_2O (7.4 to 18.4 mm Hg) in normal individuals at rest in the lateral recumbent position, with a mean of 141 mm H_2O (10.4 mm Hg).[35] With changes in body and head position from reclined to standing and the positive and negative intracranial changes that would induce, it is conceivable that CSF pressure can exceed intraocular pressure at certain peak times. This could lead to perineural subarachnoid CSF pressure exceeding intraocular pressure, creating the pressure gradient required for mean ingress of CSF into the intraocular intraretinal or subretinal compartment. In young children with optic disc pit maculopathy, it has been argued that since there was little vitreous degeneration and fluid, the CSF might reasonably be the source of intraretinal or subretinal fluid.

Some evidence from the related morning glory anomaly suggests the possibility of CSF in the pathogenesis of optic disc pit macular fluid. Two cases have been reported to prove communication between the subarachnoid space and vitreous cavity or subretinal space in morning glory disc anomaly. In one case, gas injected into the vitreous for treatment of retinal detachment by optic nerve fenestration was found in the subarachnoid space.[32] In another, metrizamide dye injected into the subarachnoid space migrated into the subretinal space, but not the vitreous.[34]

Similar direct evidence is lacking in optic disc pit, however, the close proximity of the herniated tissue of the optic pit extending into the perineural subarachnoid space separated only by variable multiloculated collagenous tissue makes it possible that CSF flows through the tissue into the dysplastic retina, causing retinoschisis and serous macular detachment.

The most accepted theory is that fluid from the vitreous leaks through the optic pit and fills the subretinal space.[3,19,21,22,36-38] The findings of a small tear in the diaphanous tissue over the pit has been substantiated in numerous reports and is consistent with findings in chorioretinal colobomas.[3,19,21,22,36-39] The transfer of the dye from the vitreous cavity to the subretinal space has been demonstrated in animal models.[34] However, these studies failed to identify, in the subretinal space, any glycosaminoglycan—an important component of the vitreous.[20]

Because optic nerve pits and related lesions are congenital, but macular detachment or schisis is usually a late phenomenon, a change must occur later in life that allows fluid movement beneath the retina or between layers of the retina. Sugar[3] was the first to suggest that the serous macular detachment associated with optic pits was a mechanical disorder, where fluid leaked through the pits into the subretinal space. Ferry postulated that traction resulted in macular detachment and demonstrated in one case Alcian blue staining of mucopolysaccharide material within the pit, suggesting fluid of vitreous origin.[40]

More recent studies supported this mechanical theory. A retinal rhegma (tear or hole) has been noted by multiple authors. Brockhurst[36] noted a small hole in the membrane overlying the pit in two cases and suggested that this might serve as a route of passage for fluid from the vitreous into the pit. Similarly, Brown et al.[19] detected holes in all cases with macular detachment in which a membrane was identified. A direct communication between the vitreous, the optic pit and the subretinal space was identified by Brown[41] after injection of India ink into the vitreous of collies and by Bonnet[21], who noted the passage of intravitreal gas through the optic pit and into the subretinal space. In addition, Bonnet[21] noted the presence of holes in the roofs of optic pits. Likewise, Postel et al.[39] reported small holes in the diaphanous tissue overlying the optic disc. Although these holes were extremely difficult to see because of their small size, lack of background pigmentation and location within the area of the optic nerve anomaly, they were nonetheless present in all cases. These findings support the rhegmatogenous theory of the pathogenesis of subretinal fluid associated with optic disc pits. Additional indirect support for this hypothesis comes from a study by Gopal et al.[42] who found that retinal detachments that occurred with choroidal colobomas were associated with breaks in the diaphanous retinal tissue overlying the coloboma. If juxtapapillary colobomas and various iterations of optic nerve colobomas did, indeed, fall within a spectrum of anomalies, it was likely that similar mechanisms would lead to retinal detachment in all of these conditions.[39]

Vitreous traction was also postulated as a cause of macular detachment in this condition. Joko and Kusaka reported a case of ophthalmoscopically observable tangential vitreous traction and cyst-like change at the macula without macula detachment treated with vitrectomy and posterior vitreous hyaloid separation. Although there had been a 10-year history of visual impairment, the cyst resolved after vitrectomy and visual acuity improved from 20/200 to 20/40.[43] Gordon[29] and Bonnet[21] found no posterior vitreous detachment in all cases studied, while Akiba[44] noted the vitreous to be completely attached in 15 of 17 eyes (88%). In the absence of a posterior vitreous detachment, a pocket of liquefied vitreous may overlie the optic disc anomaly. Theodossiadis et al.[45] reported OCT findings in patients with optic disc pit maculopathy treated with macular buckling. Preoperative OCT demonstrated vitreous traction between the optic disc and macula in 10 of 16 eyes (62%), which was relieved by surgery. Traction from the surrounding attached vitreous could open the tear in the diaphanous tissue overlying the excavation and allow fluid to percolate into the subretinal and/or intraretinal space.

A case of anomalous Cloquet's canal with a pulsating translucent membrane over the optic pit was reported.[44] An unusual posterior hyaloid strand tightly attached to the margin of the optic disc pit was documented in an 8-year old during triamcinolone acetonide-assisted pars plana vitrectomy (PPV), with the authors suggesting the posterior strand as a possible mechanism of macular traction and detachment.[46]

Further indirect support for this rhegmatogenous theory came from the observation of disappearance of the subretinal fluid with spontaneous or surgical detachment of the posterior vitreous.[21] This would explain the spontaneous resolution of macular detachment sometimes seen in this condition, as posterior vitreous detachment relieved traction on the torn roof of the optic pit, as well as the generally favorable results noted after vitrectomy.

Most recently, Johnson and Johnson[47] have postulated a unifying theory to account for the optic pit maculopathy variation in age of presentation, degree and physical features. They proposed that variations in CSF pressure in the perineural subarachnoid space acted on the herniated collagenous tissue of the optic disc pit, causing it to act like a bulb syringe pump to suck vitreous fluid into the optic pit and then pump it into the intraretinal space to create the retinoschisis. The intraoperative observation of Friberg and McLellan[48] that vitreous debris overlying the optic pit was intermittently sucked into the pit and later dislodged back into the posterior vitreous appear to support this theory. The anatomy, degree of differentiation and porosity of the herniated tissues were also suggested to relate to age of onset of macular detachment in these patients. Typical patients presenting in their third to fourth decades presumably had thicker, less permeable pit "capsules", requiring vitreous liquefaction before the pump action drew vitreous fluid through the pit and into the intraretinal schisis cavity. Children who presented at a younger age presumably had thinner capsules, and therefore behaved more like morning glory anomaly, with percolation of CSF through the permeable capsules into the pit and hence into the intraretinal schisis cavity from the pump action.

Natural History

Spontaneous resolution of macular detachments were estimated at approximately 25%. Reports of spontaneous visual improvement are uncommon,[4,9,10,49,50] but Patton et al.[49] reported a case of a 43-year-old male with visual acuity of 1/60, macular serous detachment with foveal cystic changes, who spontaneously improved to 6/18 over 2 years with resolution of subretinal fluid on OCT.

Most eyes with macular detachment associated with an optic nerve pit had a relatively poor visual prognosis.[9,10,19,37,43,51] The natural history of untreated optic disc pits is generally poor once there is macular detachment. Brown et al.[19] found that in 20 untreated eyes with optic pit associated macular detachment, 11 of 20 eyes (55%) had visual acuity less than or equal to 6/30 (20/100), 15 of 20 (75%) had subretinal fluid at the last visit. Sobol et al.[51] followed 15 eyes of 15 consecutive patients seen over 21 years with mean follow-up of 9 years. Twelve of 15 eyes (80%) lost 3 or more lines of vision within 6 months of serous macula detachment and had visual acuity of 20/200 or less at their last examination, compared to only 2 of 15 (5%) having initial visual acuity of 20/200 or less. Theodossiadis[37] reported 16 cases with persistent macular detachments followed over a mean of 9 years all of whom had eventual visual acuity of less than 6/60 (20/200). Seven of 16 (43.8%) had no significant change in visual acuity, while 9 of 16 (56.2%) had slight deterioration of vision.

In about 25% of eyes with a detachment, a lamellar or full thickness macular hole developed, further compromising vision.[19]

Management

An asymptomatic optic pit with no macular detachment can be monitored with routine ocular examinations. The patient should be counseled regarding the condition, and instructed on self-administered Amsler grid testing to detect the early development of metamorphopsia or central visual field changes which suggest macular detachment.

There is controversy regarding the treatment of retinal detachment associated with congenital pit of the optic disc. Due to its relative rarity, there are no randomized control trials to guide best management. The natural history of untreated optic disc pits is generally regarded as poor once there is macular detachment.

Treatment modalities such as external laser therapy alone[7], intravitreous gas injection alone,[9] laser therapy combined with gas,[28] vitrectomy associated with gas tamponade, with or without additional laser treatment[29-32] and scleral buckling[14] have been described in the literature and are discussed in detail in the paragraphs that follow. Systemic steroids have been tried and found to be ineffective.[52] Optic nerve fenestration was reported to relieve macular detachment in a child with morning glory disc anomaly and histological examination of the excised tissue revealed herniation of retinal tissue similar to that found in optic disc pit.[32] Its possible use in treating optic disc pit macular detachments is not well reported in the literature.

Laser Photocoagulation

Laser photocoagulation to treat serous macular detachments associated with optic disc pits was initially described in 1969 by Gass in 2 patients, but did not appear effective.[10] In 1972, Mustonen and Varonen reported 3 patients with optic disc pits treated with laser. One patient with macular detachment reaching the optic disc had macular reattachment and visual improvement after 2 years. The other 2 patients with macular detachments not reaching the optic disc had macular reattachment after 1–2 years but no visual improvement.[53] Brockhurst postulated the lack of visual improvement in the latter 2 cases could be due to nerve fiber layer damage from photocoagulation. In Brockhurst's own series, 5 of 6 patients treated with laser photocoagulation had macular reattachment after "strong" chorioretinal scarring and adhesion was achieved by repeated laser application where necessary in areas still detached. Interestingly, Brockhurst demonstrated that photocoagulation did not seem to produce significant corresponding visual field defects on Goldmann perimetry testing.[36]

Overall, laser photocoagulation alone has a success rate of about 33–37% in reattaching or improving a macular detachment.[39,54] Most authors described applying about 2–3 confluent rows of medium white laser burns with effective retinal spot sizes approximately 100–300 µm. The spots were applied at the temporal edge of the optic disc extending in a contiguous arc from the superotemporal to inferotemporal edge of the disc, with treatment extended to the superior and inferior borders of the macular detachment. Full 360° peripapillary laser has also been described as part of a vitrectomy procedure in this condition and could be considered if more limited laser were initially unsuccessful.[55]

Care has been recommended with regards to intensity of 360° peripapillary laser as one case which required repeated vitrectomies for recurrent retinal detachment and significant subretinal silicone oil, treated initially with segmental laser and finally 360° peripapillary laser, had eventual optic atrophy and no light perception.[47]

Eyes responding to laser treatment typically demonstrated reduction or resolution of macular detachment and visual acuity improvement in 6 weeks to 6 months, occasionally longer. Longer wavelength lasers, such as diode lasers, penetrate deeper with potentially less collateral damage to the nerve fiber layer.

Pneumatic Retinopexy

Pneumatic retinopexy has been described, often supplemented with peripapillary laser. Lincoff described his technique of using a temporary episcleral balloon explant device inflated till the central retinal artery was seen to pulsate, then removed after 1 hour. Up to 0.6 ml of expansile gas was then injected into the vitreous cavity, which would expand accordingly. For pure (100%) gas, expansion would be approximately 2 times for sulfur hexafluoride (SF_6), 3 times for perfluoroethane (C_2F_6) and 4 times for perfluoropropane (C_3F_8) over 24–48 hours. The eye position was alternated between gaze down and gaze forward to displace the submacular fluid beyond the inferior vascular arcade.

Overall, the procedure was successful in approximately 63–72% for attaching or improving macular detachments due to optic disc pits.[39,54] This was an improvement compared to laser alone, but less than the 81% reattachment rate for peripheral retinal breaks with detachments treated by pneumatic retinopexy and laser or cryopexy.[56] In addition, fairly frequent recurrence of macular serous detachments were also reported on long follow-up. The possible reasons for poorer success in optic pits include: chronicity and hence increased viscosity of subretinal fluid; more complex detachments combining both inner retinal schisis and outer neurosensory detachment; greater persistent anterior-posterior and tangential tractional forces over the macula and continuous ingress of fluid through the optic disc pit from the vitreous or subarachnoid space.

Ocular hypertension, postoperative infective endophthalmitis, vitreous hemorrhage, retinal breaks and detachments are potential complications but not widely reported in association with optic disc maculopathy treatment.

Macular Buckle

Macular buckle with a sponge episcleral explant has been described by Theodossiadis et al.[57] in optic pit maculopathy.

A 7.5 mm by 5.5 mm sponge was fixed temporal to the optic disc in the 6-12 o'clock meridian. Intraoperative buckle position was monitored intraoperatively by B-scan ultrasonography, and postoperatively by magnetic resonance imaging. Over a follow-up period of 9 months to 10 years, they reported complete macular reattachment in 20 of 23 eyes (87%), and visual improvement of 1–7 Snellen lines in 18 of 23 patients (78%). They postulated that the buckle acted mechanically to provide a barrier that prevented flow of fluid from the pit to the macula. Further consideration of the matter leads to another postulate: that the buckle relieved vitreoretinal traction causing the macular detachment, in a similar mechanism to its action in treatment of rhegmatogenous retinal detachments due to peripheral retinal breaks.

Potential complications include periocular hemorrhage, scleral perforation, optic nerve trauma and complications from extraocular muscle disinsertion. Again, complications are not widely reported.

Pars Plana Vitrectomy (PPV)

Pars plana vitrectomy to treat optic disc pit related macular detachment has been well-described by many groups over the years. Postel et al.[39] summarizing various studies, estimated vitrectomy success rate at 97%. More recent cases treated with vitrectomy and various adjunctive steps reported good success. An important point to keep in mind is that these reports represented anecdotal small case series at best. As anecdotal literature often under-reports treatment failures, over-estimation of vitrectomy success is likely. Slow resolution of subretinal fluid also made it difficult to be sure of its real efficacy. However, in the absence of better quality data, PPV at present seems to offer the highest likelihood of anatomical success and visual improvement in optic disc maculopathy.

The key step in all vitrectomy reports was complete removal of posterior cortical vitreous, thereby relieving posterior hyaloid traction on the macula area. Complete vitreous removal could be enhanced by intraoperative adjunctive intravitreal injection of triamcinolone acetonide to highlight vitreous.[46] In many cases, this was supplemented with internal gas tamponade and endolaser barricade of the temporal peripapillary area.[39,58-63] Successful therapy provided support for the rhegmatogenous and macular traction theories of optic disc pit maculopathy. Recurrences of submacular detachment were variable.

Variations of vitrectomy to reduce traction, seal the pit or drain subretinal fluid have been reported. Some groups have reported successful vitrectomy, posterior hyaloid separation and internal gas tamponade without peripapillary laser.[64-66] Peeling of the internal limiting membrane without laser over the detached macula has also been used to further relieve tangential macular traction, and the few cases reported appear to have recovered fairly well.[67-72]

Autologous blood[39] or platelets[73] have also been placed over the optic disc pit to close the pit. Fibrin glue[74] has recently been used for a similar purpose. The technique involved PPV, removal of posterior hyaloid, fluid-air exchange, drainage of subretinal fluid through optic disc pit, application of the fibrin sealant to the pit and air-perfluoropropane gas exchange with postoperative prone positioning.

Drainage of subretinal fluid with 39- and 42-gauge cannulas during vitrectomy has been described.[75-77] Inner retinal fenestration without intraoperative subretinal fluid drainage was reported to result in rapid resolution in 1 case,[77] but the fenestration was found to close within 3 weeks in another case without resolution of subretinal fluid.[78]

Overall, PPV has been reported to be successful in 87–97%,[39,54] however, recurrences similarly are reported in series with longer follow-up durations. Complications such as postoperative endophthalmitis, ocular hypertension, rhegmatogenous retinal detachment and vitreous hemorrhage are potential complications in any PPV procedure.

Various authors have described how intravitreal gas, silicone oil and perfluorocarbon liquids have been found in the subretinal space, presumably entering through the optic disc pit.[47,79,80] The presence of significant volumes of subretinal silicone oil and perfluorocarbon liquids has necessitated repeat procedures to drain these through the pit. It would be prudent to avoid use of silicone oil and perfluorocarbon liquids in these cases especially when the optic disc pit is large. Sealing the pit with autologous blood product or fibrin glue prior to injecting heavy liquids or silicone oil into these eyes may reduce these complications. One case of intracranial migration of silicone oil from an eye with optic pit was also reported.[81] Whether this is due to the optic disc pit or another mechanism is unknown, as migration of intraocular silicone oil into the brain in the absence of optic disc pit has been described.[82]

In summary, optic disc pit is a rare congenital anomaly associated with retinal schisis and serous detachment of the macula in 25–75%. OCT is very useful in defining the anatomical changes, typically a bilaminar macular detachment, preoperatively and postoperatively. Treatment with laser alone can be successful in about a third of patients, and is relatively noninvasive. PPV to completely relieve traction appears to give the best results at present. The optimal vitrectomy technique has not been conclusively established. Good visual recovery is possible even months after the onset of maculopathy and recurrence of serous macular detachment complicates any of the current treatment modalities.

References

1. Wiethe T. Ein Fall von angeborener Difformität der Sehnervenpapille. Arch Augenheilkd. 1882;11:14-9.
2. Gass JDM. Stereoscopic Atlas of Macular Diseases: Diagnosis and Treatment, 3rd edition. St Louis: Mosby; 1987. p. 732.
3. Sugar HS. Congenital pits in the optic disc with acquired macular pathology. Am J Ophthalmol. 1962;53:307-11.
4. Sugar HS. An explanation for the acquired macular pathology associated with congenital pits of the optic disc. Am J Ophthalmol. 1964;54:833-5.
5. Apple DJ, Rabb MF. Developmental anomalies. In: Ocular pathology: clinical applications and self-assessment. St Louis, MO: Mosby; 1998. pp. 24-6.
6. Greear JN. Pits, or crater-like holes, in the optic disk. Arch Ophthalmol. 1942;28:467-83.
7. Spencer WH. Ophthalmic Pathology: An Atlas and Textbook. Vol 3. 3rd edition. Philadelphia: Saunders; 1986. pp. 2355-7.
8. Kranenberg EW. Crater-like holes in the optic disc and central serous retinopathy. Arch Ophthalmol. 1960;64:132-44.
9. Krivoy D, Gentile R, Liebmann JM, et al. Imaging congenital optic disc pits and associated maculopathy using optical coherence tomography. Arch Ophthalmol. 1996;114: 165-70.
10. Gass JDM. Serous detachment of the macula secondary to congenital pit of the optic nerve head. Am J Ophthalmol. 1969;67:821-41.
11. Slusher MM, Weaver RG, Greven CM, et al. The spectrum of cavitary optic disc anomalies in a family. Ophthalmology. 1989; 96:342–7.
12. Jonas JB, Freisler KA. Bilateral congenital optic nerve head pits in monozygotic siblings. Am J Ophthalmol. 1997;124: 844-6.
13. Dureau P, Attie-Bitach T, Salomon R, et al. Renal coloboma syndrome. Ophthalmology. 2001;108:1912-6.
14. Eccles MR, Schimmenti LA. Renal-coloboma syndrome: a multi-system developmental disorder caused by PAX2 mutations. Clin Genet. 1999;56:1-9.
15. Samimi S, Antignac C, Combe C, et al. Bilateral macular detachment caused by bilateral optic nerve malformation in a papillorenal syndrome due to a new PAX2 mutation. Eur J Ophthalmol. 2008;18:656-8.
16. Lincoff H, Yanuzzi L, Singerman L, et al. Improvement in visual function after displacement of the retinal elevations emanating from optic pits. Arch Ophthalmol. 1993;111: 1071-9.
17. Wang Y, Xu L, Jonas JB. Prevalence of congenital optic disc pits in adult Chinese: The Beijing Eye Study. Eur J Ophthalmol. 2006;16:863-4.
18. Healey PR, Mitchell P. The prevalence of optic disc pits and their relationship to glaucoma. J Glaucoma. 2008;17:11-4.
19. Brown GC, Shields JA, Goldberg RE. Congenital pits of the optic nerve head.II. Clinical studies in humans. Ophthalmology. 1980;87:51-65.
20. Kritzinger EE, Beaumont HM. A Colour Atlas of Optic Disc Abnormalities. London: Wolfe Medical Publications; 1986.p. 332.
21. Bonnet M. Serous macular detachment associated with optic nerve pits. Graefes Arch Clin Exp Ophthalmol. 1991;229:526-32.
22. Theodossiadis GP. Treatment of maculopathy associated with optic disc pit by sponge explant. Am J Ophthalmol. 1996;121:630-7.
23. Lincoff H, Lopez R, Kreissig I, et al. Retinoschisis associated with optic nerve pits. Arch Ophthalmol. 1988;106:61-7.
24. Lincoff H, Kreissig I. Optical coherence tomography of pneumatic displacement of optic disc pit maculopathy. Br J Ophthalmol. 1998;82:367-72.
25. Rutledge BK, Puliafito CA, Duker JS, et al. Optical coherence tomography of macular lesions associated with optic nerve head pits. Ophthalmology. 1996;103:1047-53.
26. Doyle E, Trivedi D, Good P, et al. High-resolution optical coherence tomography demonstration of membranes spanning optic disc pits and colobomas. Br J Ophthalmol. 2009;93: 360-5.
27. Imamura Y, Zweifel SA, Fujiwara T, et al. High-resolution optical coherence tomography findings in optic pit maculopathy. Retina. 2010;30:1104-12.
28. Lalwani GA, Punjabi OS, Flynn HW, et al. Documentation of optic nerve pit with macular schisis-like cavity by spectral domain OCT. Ophthalmic Surg Lasers Imaging. 2007;38: 262-4.
29. Gordon R, Chatfield RK. Pits in the optic disc associated with macular degeneration. Br J Ophthalmol. 1969;53: 481-9.
30. Chen MS, Tsai WF. Congenital optic pits and central serous chorioretinopathy. Aust NZ J Ophthalmol. 1997;25:165-6.
31. Theodossiadis GP, Ladas ID, Panagiotidis DN, et al. Fluorescein and indocyanine green angiographic findings in congenital optic disk pit associated with macular detachment. Retina. 1999;19:6-11.
32. Irvine AR, Crawford JB, Sullivan JH. The pathogenesis of retinal detachment with morning glory disc and optic pit. Trans Am Ophthalmol Soc. 1986;84:280-92.
33. Ko TH, Fujimoto JG, Duker JS, et al. Comparison of ultrahigh and standard-resolution optical coherence tomography for imaging macular hole pathology. Ophthalmology. 2004;111: 2033-43.
34. Chang S, Haik BJ, Ellsworth RM, et al. Treatment of total retinal detachment with morning glory syndrome. Am J Ophthalmol. 1984;97:596-600.

35. Ekstedt J. CSF hydrodynamic studies in man, 2: normal hydrodynamic variables related to CSF pressure and flow. J Neurol Neurosurg Psychiatry. 1978;41:345-53.
36. Brockhurst RJ. Optic pits and posterior retinal detachment. Trans Am Ophthalmol Soc. 1975;73:264-91.
37. Theodossiadis G, Panopoulos M, Kollia A, et al. Long-term study of patients with congenital pit of the optic nerve and persistent macular detachment. Acta Ophthalmol. 1992;70: 495-505.
38. Hasegawa T, Akiba J, Ishiko S, et al. Abnormal vitreous structure in optic nerve pit. Jpn J Ophthalmol. 1997;41:324-7.
39. Postel EA, Pulido JS, McNamara JA, et al. The etiology and treatment of macular detachment associated with optic nerve pits and related anomalies. Tr Am Ophth Soc; 1998.pp.667-8.
40. Ferry AP. Macular detachment associated with congenital pit of the optic nerve head. Pathologic findings in two cases simulating malignant melanoma of the choroid. Arch Ophthalmol. 1963;70:346-57.
41. Brown GC, Shields JA, Patty BE, et al. Congenital pits of the optic nerve head. I: Experimental studies in collie dogs. Arch Ophthalmol. 1979;97:1341-4.
42. Gopal L, Badrinath SS, Sharma T, et al. Pattern of retinal breaks and retinal detachments in eyes with choroidal colobomas. Ophthalmology. 1995;102:1212-7.
43. Joko T, Kusaka S. Tangential vitreous traction observed in optic disc pit maculopathy without apparent serous detachment. Ophthalmic Surg Lasers. 1998;29:677-9.
44. Akiba J, Kakehashi A, Hikichi T, et al. Vitreous findings in cases of optic nerve pits and serous macular detachment. Am J Ophthalmol. 1993;116:38-41.
45. Theodossiadis PG, Grigoropoulos VG, Emfietzoglou J, et al. Vitreous findings in optic disc pit maculopathy based on optical coherence tomography. Graefes Arch Clin Exp Ophthalmol. 2007;245:1311-8.
46. Hirakata A, Hida T, Wakabayashi T, et al. Unusual posterior hyaloid strand in a young child with optic disc pit maculopathy: intraoperative and histopathological findings. Jpn J Ophthalmol. 2005;49:264-6.
47. Johnson TM, Johnson MW. Pathogenic implications of subretinal gas migration through pits and atypical colobomas of the optic nerve. Arch Ophthalmol. 2004;122:1793-800.
48. Friberg TR, McLellan TG. Vitreous pulsations, relative hypotony, and retrobulbar cyst associated with a congenital optic pit. Am J Ophthalmol. 1992;114:767-9.
49. Patton N, Aslam SA, Aylward GW. Visual improvement after long-standing central serous macular detachment associated with an optic disc pit. Graefes Arch Clin Exp Ophthalmol. 2008;246:1083-5.
50. Gass JDM. Optic nerve diseases that may masquerade as macular diseases. In: A stereoscopic atlas of macular disease. Diagnosis and Treatment. St Louis, MO: Mosby; 1997. pp. 976-83.
51. Sobol WM, Blodi CF, Folk JC, et al. Long-term visual outcome in patients with optic nerve pit and serous retinal detachment of the macula. Ophthalmology. 1990;97:1539-42.
52. Montenegro M, Bonnet M. Optic nerve pits: clinical and therapeutic review of 21 cases. J Fr Ophtalmol. 1989;12:411-9.
53. Mustonen E, Varonen T. Congenital pit of the optic nerve head associated with serous detachment of the macula. Acta Ophthalmol. 1972;50:689-98.
54. Sandali O, Barale PO, Bui Quoc E, et al. Long-term results of the treatment of optic disc pit associated with serous macular detachment: a review of 20 cases. J Fr Ophtalmol. 2011.
55. Bakri SJ, Beer PM. Vitreoretinal surgery for optic pit associated serous macular detachment: a discussion of two cases. Int Ophthalmol. 2004;25:143-6.
56. Tornambe PE, Hilton GF. Pneumatic retinopexy. A multicenter randomized controlled clinical trial comparing pneumatic retinopexy with scleral buckling. The retinal detachment study group. Ophthalmology. 1989;96:772-83.
57. Theodossiadis GP, Theodossiadis PG. The macular buckling technique in the treatment of optic disk pit maculopathy. Semin Ophthalmol. 2000;15:108-15.
58. Ghosh YK, Banerjee S, Konstantinidis A, et al. Surgical management of optic disc pit associated maculopathy. Eur J Ophthalmol. 2008;18:142-6.
59. Oshima Y, Emi K. Optical cross-sectional assessment of the macula by retinal thickness analyzer in optic disk pit maculopathy. Am J Ophthalmol. 1999;128:106-9.
60. García-Arumí J, Guraya BC, Espax AB, et al. Optical coherence tomography in optic pit maculopathy managed with vitrectomy-laser-gas. Graefes Arch Clin Exp Ophthalmol. 2004;242:819-26.
61. Lee KJ, Peyman GA. Surgical management of retinal detachment associated with optic nerve pit. Int Ophthalmol. 1993;17:105-7.
62. Schatz H, McDonald HR. Treatment of sensory retinal detachment associated with optic nerve pit or coloboma. Ophthalmology. 1988;95:178-86.
63. Snead MP, James N, Jacobs PM. Vitrectomy, argon laser, and gas tamponade for serous retinal detachment associated with an optic disc pit: a case report. Br J Ophthalmol. 1991;75:381-2.
64. Hirakata A, Okada AA, Hida T. Long-term results of vitrectomy without laser treatment for macular detachment associated with an optic disc pit. Ophthalmology. 2005;112: 1430-5.
65. Konno S, Akiba J, Sato E, et al. OCT in successful surgery of retinal detachment associated with optic nerve head pit. Ophthalmic Surg Lasers. 2000;31:236-9.
66. Bartz-Schmidt KU, Heimann K, Esser P. Vitrectomy for macular detachment associated with optic nerve pits. Int Ophthalmol. 1995-1996;19:323-9.
67. Gotzaridis EV. Perifoveal traction retinal detachment following successful optic disc pit surgery. Ophthalmic Surg Lasers. 2002;33:243-5.
68. Dai S, Polkinghorne P. Peeling the internal limiting membrane in serous macular detachment associated with congenital optic disc pit. Clin Experiment Ophthalmol. 2003;31:272-5.

69. Ishikawa K, Terasaki H, Mori M, et al. Optical coherence tomography before and after vitrectomy with internal limiting membrane removal in a child with optic disc pit maculopathy. Jpn J Ophthalmol. 2005;49:411-3.
70. Georgalas I, Petrou P, Koutsandrea C, et al. Optic disc pit maculopathy treated with vitrectomy, internal limiting membrane peeling, and gas tamponade: a report of two cases. Eur J Ophthalmol. 2009;19:324-6.
71. Kumar N, Al Sabti K. Optic disc pit maculopathy treated with vitrectomy, internal limiting membrane peeling, and gas tamponade: a report of two cases. Eur J Ophthalmol. 2009;19:897.
72. Georgalas I, Kouri A, Ladas I, et al. Optic disc pit maculopathy treated with vitrectomy, internal limiting membrane peeling, and air in a 5-year-old boy. Can J Ophthalmol. 2010;45:189-91.
73. Rosenthal G, Bartz-Schmidt KU, Walter P, et al. Autologous platelet treatment for optic disc pit associated with persistent macular detachment. Graefes Arch Clin Exp Ophthalmol. 1998;236:151-3.
74. Maia OO, Soriano DS, Takahashi WY, et al. Surgical treatment of macular detachment secondary to congenital pit of the optic disc: case report. Arq Bras Oftalmol. 2008;71:874-7.
75. Ziahosseini K, Sanghvi C, Muzaffar W, et al. Successful surgical treatment of optic disc pit maculopathy. Eye. 2009;23:1477-9.
76. Jalil A, Stavrakas P, Dhawahir-Scala FE, et al. Drainage of subretinal fluid in optic disc pit maculopathy using subretinal 42-gauge cannula: a new surgical approach. Graefes Arch Clin Exp Ophthalmol. 2010;248:751-3.
77. Spaide RF, Fisher Y, Ober M, et al. Surgical hypothesis: inner retinal fenestration as a treatment for optic disc pit maculopathy. Retina. 2006;26:89-91.
78. Slocumb RW, Johnson MW. Premature closure of inner retinal fenestration in the treatment of optic disk pit maculopathy. Retinal Cases and Brief Reports: Winter. 2010;4:37-9.
79. Dithmar S, Schuett F, Voelcker HE, et al. Delayed sequential occurrence of perfluorodecalin and silicone oil in the subretinal space following retinal detachment surgery in the presence of an optic disc pit. Arch Ophthalmol. 2004;122:409-11.
80. Becht C, Senn P, Lange AP. Delayed occurrence of subretinal silicone oil after retinal detachment surgery in an optic disc pit—a case report. Klin Monbl Augenheilkd. 2009;226:357-8.
81. Kuhn F, Kover F, Szabo I, et al. Intracranial migration of silicone oil from an eye with optic pit. Graefes Arch Clin Exp Ophthalmol. 2006;244:1360-2.
82. Eller AW, Friberg TR, Mah F. Migration of silicone oil into the brain: a complication of intraocular silicone oil for retinal tamponade. Am J Ophthalmol. 2000;129:685-8.

35

Vitreoretinal Surgery for Parasitic Diseases

Ajit Babu Majji

Introduction

Parasitic diseases as an indication for vitreoretinal surgery in rare usually constitute less than 1% of vitreoretinal surgeries in vitreoretinal surgical unit. The parasitic infections of the eye occur as zoonotic diseases with man as intermediate host or accidental host.[1-3] Most parasites get access to gastrointestinal tract by accidental ingestion through vegetables or uncooked meat. Parasites get access to bloodstream from gastrointestinal tract and reach liver and other organs which in most cases serve as end organs. Most parasites access to the eye through bloodstream either through choroidal blood flow into subretinal space then into vitreous cavity or through ophthalmic artery to retinal arteries and vitreous cavity or episcleral vessels into anterior chamber. Presence of the parasite can cause visual symptoms or the inflammation induced by the live or dead parasite, which can cause secondary effects which may require vitreoretinal interventions.[3] The vitreous retinal surgery may be needed to deal with the parasitic infections or inflammation secondary to presence of parasite or long-term effects of the secondary complications like development of vitreous membranes, traction retinal detachment or secondary rhegmatogenous retinal detachment. In this chapter author will provide the clinical aspects of intraocular parasite infections relevant to vitreoretinal surgery. Life cycle and pathology of individual parasitic infestations will not be touched upon in detail; however pathogenesis will be discussed as and when relevant.

Pathogenesis

Most frequent parasites encountered in Asia are Cysticercosis and Gnathostomiasis as regards to vitreoretinal surgery.[4-13] Toxoplasma infections both congenital and acquired form is more common but from vitreoretinal surgical point of view is less relevant.[1,3] Toxocara infections and hydatid cyst are less common in Asia.[14-19] *Thelazia*, *Baylisascaris* and malaria are very rare in occurrence.[17,18,20,21]

Cysticercosis is the most common platyhelminth infestation by cysticercus cellulosae larval form of pork tape worm *Taenia solium*, contracted by ingestion of uncooked pork, vegetables or water contaminated with eggs of *T. solium*.[2] Sites of predilection for the cysticerci to develop are central nervous system, subcutaneous tissue, skeletal muscles, heart muscle and eye.[2] Ocular manifestations can be devastating as the cysticercosis increases in size, leading to blindness in 3–5 years, if no intervention is contemplated. Location of intraocular cysticercosis may be in vitreous cavity (up to 60%) and subretinal space in 40%. Complications could be retinal detachment, proliferative vitreoretinopathy, vitreous inflammation (Figs 35.1A to C), macular scar (Figs 35.2A and B) and endophthalmitis-like picture.[11,13]

Gnathostoma is nematode causing ocular infection in addition to skin (migratory cutaneous nodules), brain (meningitis, meningoencephalitis and myeloencephalitis), gastrointestinal tract (abdominal mass) and respiratory system (bronchitis and pleurisy).[6,22] Ocular gnathostomiasis is rare but involves the eyelids, conjunctiva, cornea, anterior

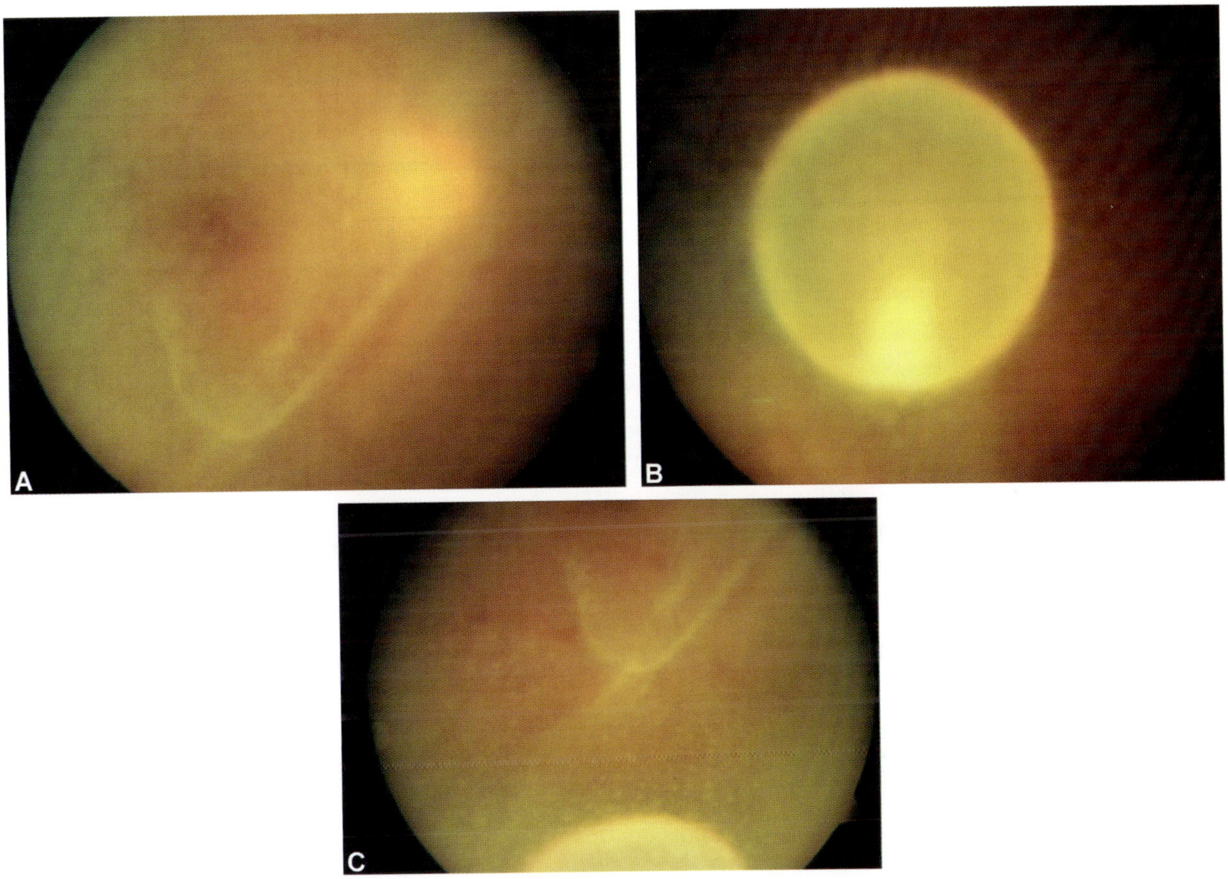

▲ **Figures 35.1A to C**

(A) Color fundus photograph showing vitreous inflammation with hazy view of the disc and partial posterior vitreous detachment; (B and C) Showing intravitreal cysticercosis inferiorly

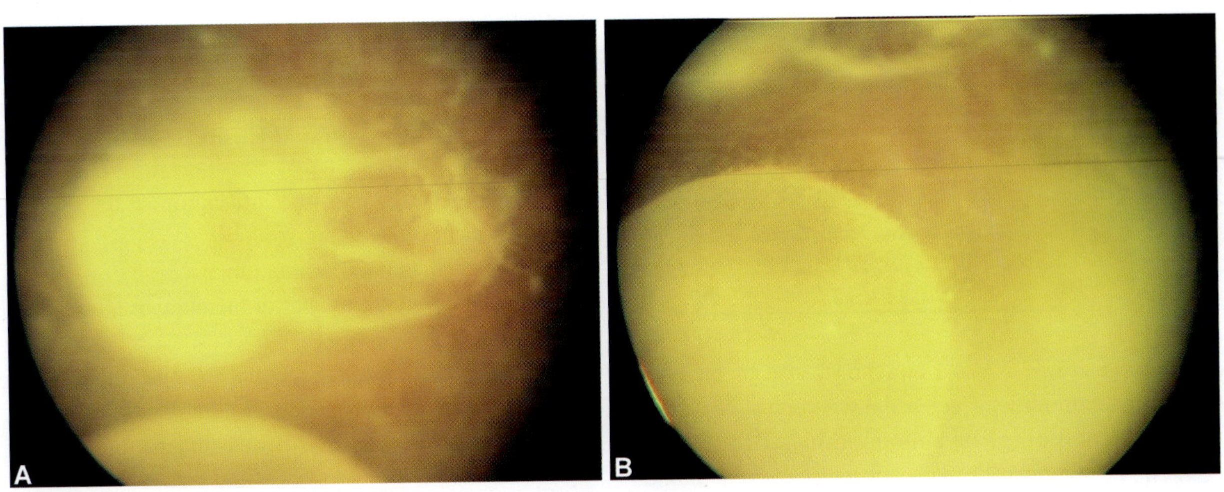

▲ **Figures 35.2A and B**

Color fundus photographs showing submacular scarring with vitreous inflammation and intravitreal cysticercosis chamber and vitreous cavity.[6] Most cases present as presence of parasite in the anterior chamber and few in vitreous cavity.[22] This parasitic infestation mostly observed in South-East Asian countries. Common definitive hosts are domestic cats, dogs and wild mammals. Man is an incidental host.[7] The infection in the eye is due to third stage larvae, which cannot mature in humans, but can remain viable for years.[6] The parasite is capable of migrating to various parts of the eye causing structural damage leading to severe intraocular inflammations, secondary glaucoma, formation of vitreous band leading to vitreoretinal traction and retinal detachment.[6,23]

Toxocara canis is a round worm forms an important cause of reduced visual acuity in young patients, involved in systemic visceral larva migrans causing infiltration of lungs and liver.[19] *T. canis* is a common ascarid of dogs having life cycle that cannot be completed in humans. The parasites are usually enclosed by an inflammatory granulomatous response that is primarily eosinophilic. The larva may remain viable for years within the granuloma.[19]

Toxocara can present as chronic endophthalmitis, posterior pole granuloma, peripheral inflammatory mass, optic nerve papillitis, presence of motile subretinal nematode and diffuse unilateral subacute neuroretinitis.[14,24-27] The inflammatory mass can resolve and may lead to fibrocellular membrane formation or traction retinal detachment or traction and rhegmatogenous retinal detachment, which may need vitreoretinal surgery.[15,28-30]

***T. canis* life cycle**

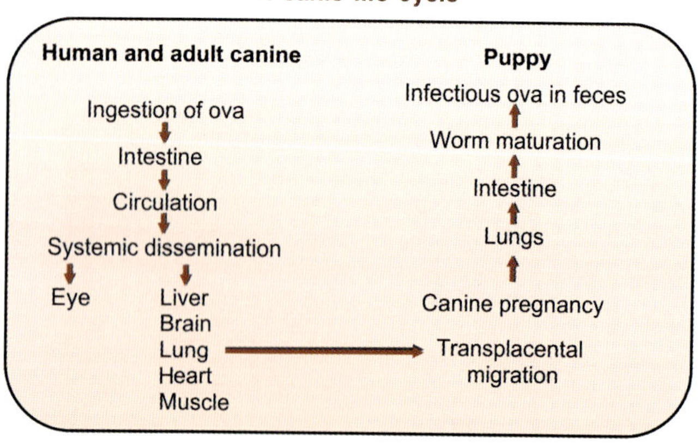

Toxoplasma gondii is most common cause of parasitic infective retinochoroiditis, which usually is controlled by oral medication including pyrimethamine/sulfadiazine/clindamycin in combination with corticosteroids or monotherapy.[1,3] Vitreous surgery in *T. gondii* infection is used for severe or persistent vitreous inflammation in patients with active lesions. More common indication for pars plana vitrectomy is however for removal of persistent vitreous opacities in otherwise quiet eye.[1]

Hydatid cyst is caused by *Echinococcus granulosus*. Liver lesions are most common (60–70%), followed by lungs, kidney, spleen, brain and other tissues.[16] Hydatid cysts occur rarely within the eye, although they are more common in the orbit. The cysts usually lies in the subretinal space but occasionally may develop in choroid or appear free in the vitreous cavity. Vitreous surgery may be needed to remove the cyst in vitreous cavity or subretinal or choroidal cyst.[16]

Alaria species are diplostomatid nematodes that as adults occur in the small intestine of carnivorous mammals. Alaria species have life cycles that involve succession of three hosts: snail first intermediate host, tadpole or frog second intermediate host and a carnivore is definitive host. Humans become infective by eating intermediate or paratenic host containing metacercariae. The most common means of infection of humans is by eating inadequately cooked frog's legs. Treatment may include oral anthelmintics like praziquantel and albendazole or laser photocoagulation to destroy the subretinal or intraretinal worms away from macula. Vitrectomy to remove intravitreal or subretinal worms has also been reported to be effective.[20]

Diffuse unilateral subacute neuroretinitis (DUSN) is characterized by progressive visual loss due to inflammatory changes in the retina, retinal vessels, retinal pigment epithelium and optic nerve.[18] DUSN is attributable to infestation by a solitary intraretinal or subretinal nematode. Several species of nematodes have been suggested as the etiological agent for DUSN including *Toxocara canis, Baylisascaris procyonis* and *Ancylostoma caninum*. Medical therapy, laser photocoagulation and cryotherapy may be indicated. Vitreous surgery is rarely indicated to remove the nematode.[17,18]

Indications for Vitreous Surgery

Vitreous surgery for parasitic infestation of the eye may be indicated for the following reasons:

- Persistent ocular inflammation
- Residual vitreous exudates or membranes after subsidence of inflammation.
- Removal of intra or subretinal or intravitreal parasites
- For management of secondary complications like traction or rhegmatogenous retinal detachment.

Persistent Ocular Inflammation

Initial phases of parasitic inflammation may be associated with severe intraocular inflammation mimicking endophthalmitis, which may be needing vitreous surgery apart from medical management. Such indication may arise in cases of *Toxocara* or *Toxoplasma* infections.[3,19] Cysticercosis cyst can present with severe intraocular inflammation if there is accidental rupture of the cyst.[2,12,13]

▶ Residual Vitreous Exudates or Vitreous Membranes

Residual vitreous exudates may persist in spite of resolution of active infection in cases of toxocara or toxoplasma retinochoroiditis.[3,19] Vitreous surgery is indicated to clear the vitreous exudates to improve the visual acuity. Vitreous membranes may form between the optic disc and peripheral granuloma in toxocariasis as well as epiretinal membrane formation in macular area.[15,19] Vitreous surgery is helpful in preventing secondary traction or rhegmatogenous retinal detachment in these cases.

▶ Removal of Intravitreal, Intraretinal or Subretinal Parasites

Most common indication for vitreous surgery among all indications. Common clinical condition requiring vitreous surgery is intravitreal (Figs 35.3A and B) or subretinal cysticercosis (Figs 35.4A and B).[8,10,11,13] DUSN due to varied

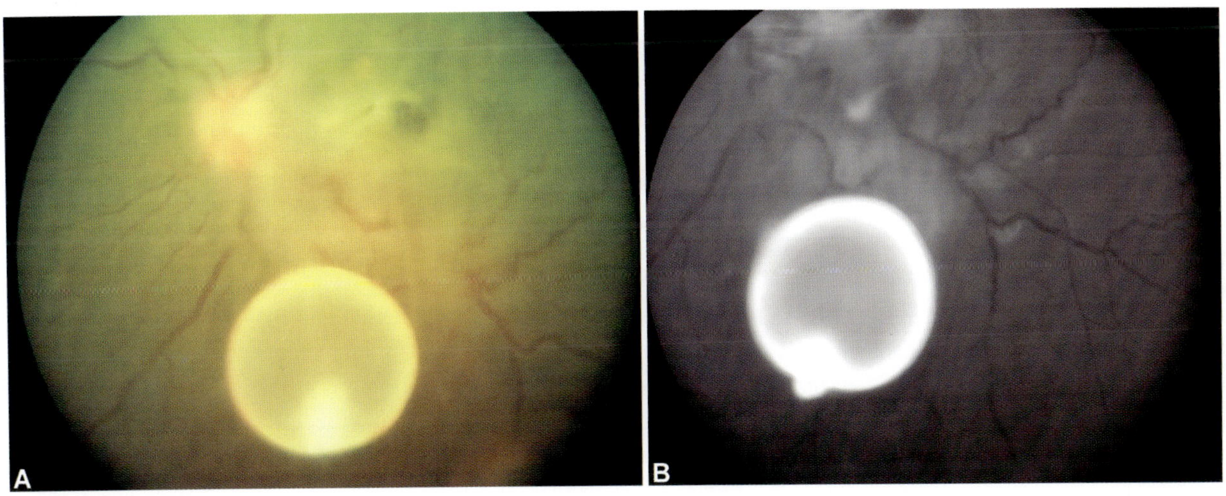

▲ **Figures 35.3A and B**
Color fundus photographs showing premacular scarring with partial posterior vitreous detachment and intravitreal cysticercosis

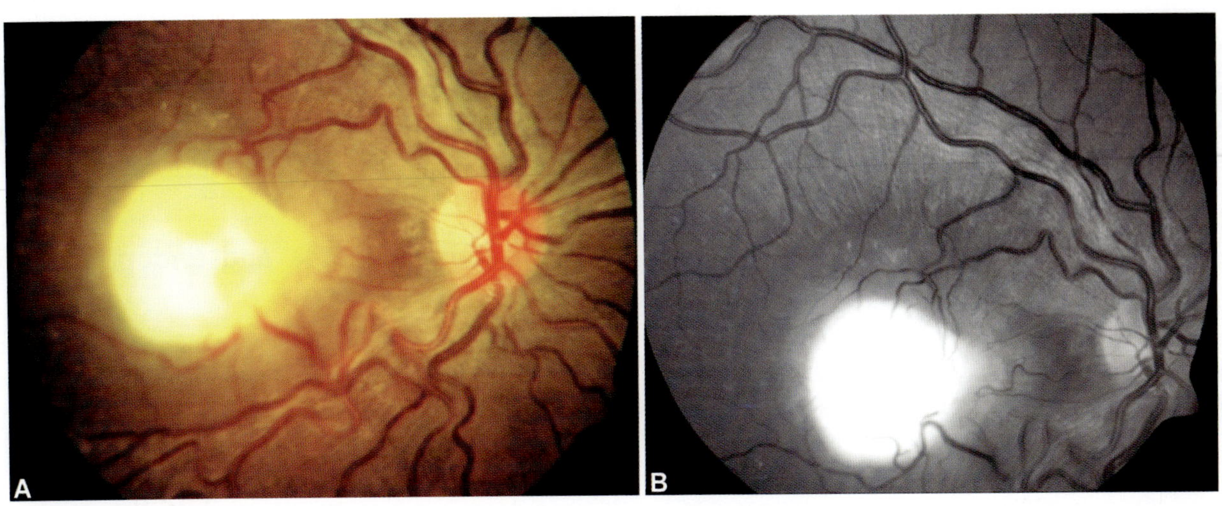

▲ **Figures 35.4A and B**
Color fundus photographs showing subretinal cysticercosis with retinal vessels coursing over the lesion. Note the vitreous cavity is free of inflammation

etiological organisms forms other major group requiring vitreous surgery.[18] Subretinal or intravitreal hydatid cyst is a rare clinical situation for vitreous surgery.[16] Intravitreal gnathostomiasis also forms an indication for vitreous surgery especially in Asian population.[5-7]

Secondary Complications

Secondary complications include tractional retinal detachment or rhegmatogenous retinal detachment. Retinal detachment found in 48.8% (22/45) eyes with intraocular cysticercosis.[13] In cases of toxocara infestation, retinal detachment is more often due to traction band development secondary to toxocara granuloma, with resultant retinal break formation leading to rhegmatogenous retinal detachment.[19,30]

Surgical Procedure

Intravitreal or Subretinal Cysticercosis

A standard 3 port pars plana vitrectomy (PPV) is recommended for intravitreal or subretinal cysticercosis. Vitreous need to be cleared in the anterior vitreous cavity and around the cysticercosis cyst in case of intravitreal cysticercosis. However, complete vitrectomy is advised before performing retinotomy for subretinal cysticercosis. The retinotomy should be adjacent to subretinal cyst and direct light of light pipe should be avoided over the area of retinotomy. Subretinal cysticercosis should be delivered into vitreous cavity with the help of extrusion cannula or active suction of the vitreous cutter. Once the cysticercosis cyst is delivered into vitreous cavity, the procedure of delivery is same as intravitreal cysticercosis. Delivery of intravitreal cysticercosis can follow two courses, after extending the sclerotomy, the cyst can be delivered with the help of flute needle or active suction of vitreous cutter or with the help of intravitreal cryoprobe. One can do a 23-gauge sutureless vitrectomy with cysticercosis contents sucked and cyst can be cut and removed with the help of 23-gauge cutter. In case one cuts and aspirates the cystcercosis cyst in vitreous cavity, a wash with steroids is recommended to reduce the postoperative inflammation. After removal of the cyst one should inspect the retina for retinal breaks and possible retinal scar due to presence of subretinal cysticercosis and they need to be managed properly with complete vitrectomy, intraocular tamponade with long acting gases or silicone oil injection and endolaser.

Vitreous Surgery for Live Nematodes

The most common live nematode infestation of the eye is by *Gnathostoma* and *Angiostrongylus*. The clinical condition is characterized by clinical features of multiple iris holes, uveitis, subretinal track lesions and rarely retinal detachment with multiple retinal holes. Vitreous surgery for removal of live worms involves standard 3 port pars plana vitrectomy and induction of posterior hyaloid detachment. The parasite can be aspirated into 19- or 20-gauge aspiration cannula or active suction by vitreous cutter. After removal of the worms one should carefully do a retina examination and identify all the retinal lesions and endophotocoagulation around the lesions and intraocular tamponade with long acting gases or silicone oil, depending on the intraocular condition. The worm obtained by surgery should be subjected to parasitology evaluation for species identification and patient should be subjected to systemic evaluation and appropriate systemic therapy.

Vitreous Traction Membranes and Epiretinal Membranes

Vitreous traction membranes may be extending from the disc to retinal periphery in patients with resolved toxocariasis warranting vitreous surgery. The vitreous surgery follow the general principles of vitrectomy for epiretinal and traction membranes except for in the area of healed granuloma. There will be full thickness retinochoroidal scar, where one needs to truncate and free the healed granulomatous area from rest of the retina and secure the area by 3–4 rows of contiguous laser photocoagulation burns. Depending on the amount of residual traction left around the healed granuloma, one should decide about whether to use or not to use any intraocular tamponading agents and whether to use long acting gases or silicone oil. The vitreous sample and the membranes removed during surgery should be subjected to histopathological and serological evaluation.

Vitreous Exudates and Endophthalmitis-Like Presentation

Parasitic infestations may present as endogenous endophthalmitis-like picture, however, may respond to initial therapy with antibiotics and steroids. As the clinical picture quietens the diagnosis becomes clear or certain times the persistent vitreous exudates may warrant PPV and the diagnosis may be made during surgery. The PPV in persistent vitreous exudates follow same principles as that of post-uveitis vitrectomy, however, one need to be careful while inducing posterior vitreous detachment. During vitrectomy or at the end of the surgical procedure one need to be observant about possible live parasites either in the vitreous cavity or intraretinal space, which need to be dealt with as required.

Traction or Rhegmatogenous Retinal Detachment

Traction and combined traction and rhegmatogenous retinal detachments are not an uncommon finding in parasitic infections of the eye. The scars resulting from toxocara granuloma or cysticercosis entry point into vitreous cavity from subretinal space are likely to be dense and involving all layers of retina and choroid. The residual scars cannot be removed in toto, so every attempt should be made to isolate the area and relieve all the traction bands extending into the healed granulomatous scar and photocoagulate around the scar so the rest of the retina will remain stable. Use of tamponading agents like long acting gas or silicone oil will depend on the status of the retina, location of the scar and relation of the scar to the surrounding retina. If there is any doubt about the complete clearance of traction, it would be better to inject silicone oil otherwise long acting gas would be the first option.

Results

Intraocular cysticercosis either intravitreal or subretinal location, the success rate for removal of cyst is nearly 100% and success of attachment of retina with modern day vitrectomy is about 85–90%.[13] Visual recovery depends on the location of the scar. If the scar is involving the macular center the visual acuity can be poor otherwise good visual recovery (better than 20/40) can be expected in 70% of the patients (Figs 35.5A and B and 35.6A and B).[13] Though literature is not concrete about the timing of the surgery, there is an indication towards early surgical intervention once diagnosed.

Reports on vitreous surgery for toxocariasis with vitreous traction membranes and traction detachment are rewarding with good anatomical outcome, with macular attachment in all eyes and relative good visual acuities (better than 20/70) in 50% of the eyes (5 out of 10 eyes).[17]

Literature available on vitrectomy for live nematodes or trematodes in the vitreous cavity constitutes either single case reports or small case series, showing successful removal of parasites with good anatomical and visual outcomes.[5-7,16,18,20,31]

Complications

In addition to complications related to vitreous surgery, vitrectomy in cysticercosis carries additional risk of cyst rupture and toxic reaction to cyst contents.[13] One should be thorough in irrigation and aspiration of vitreous cavity along with triamcinolone, to reduce possible postoperative inflammation. Recurrent epiretinal membrane formation is another risk factor frequently seen after removal of cysticercosis or after vitreous surgery for traction detachment in toxocriasis and following vitrectomy for live intraocular

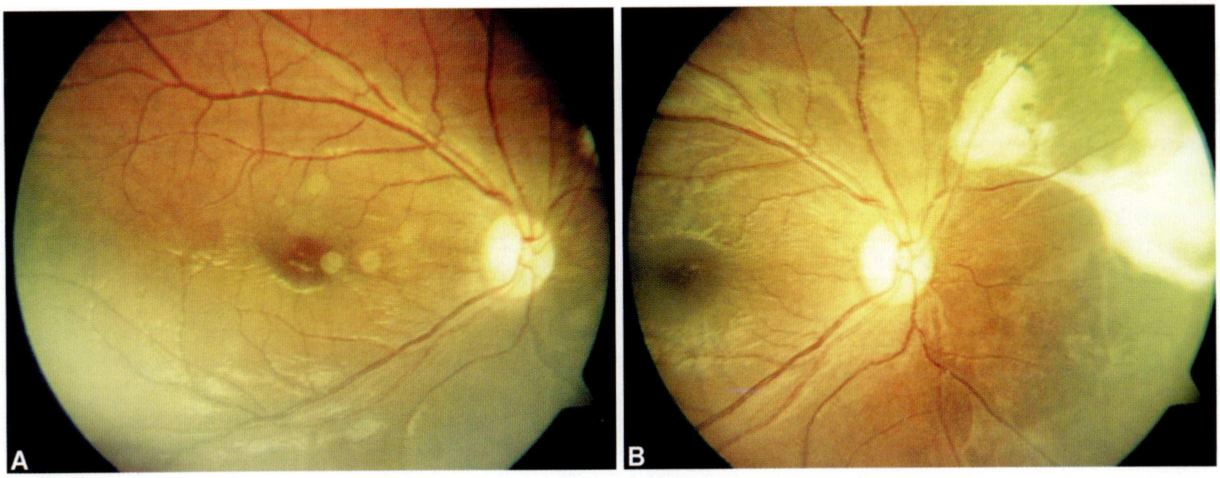

Figures 35.5A and B

Color fundus photographs showing residual subretinal scarring following vitreous surgery for subretinal cysticercosis. Note healthy condition of the macula. Postoperative visual acuity at 3 months follow-up was 20/20

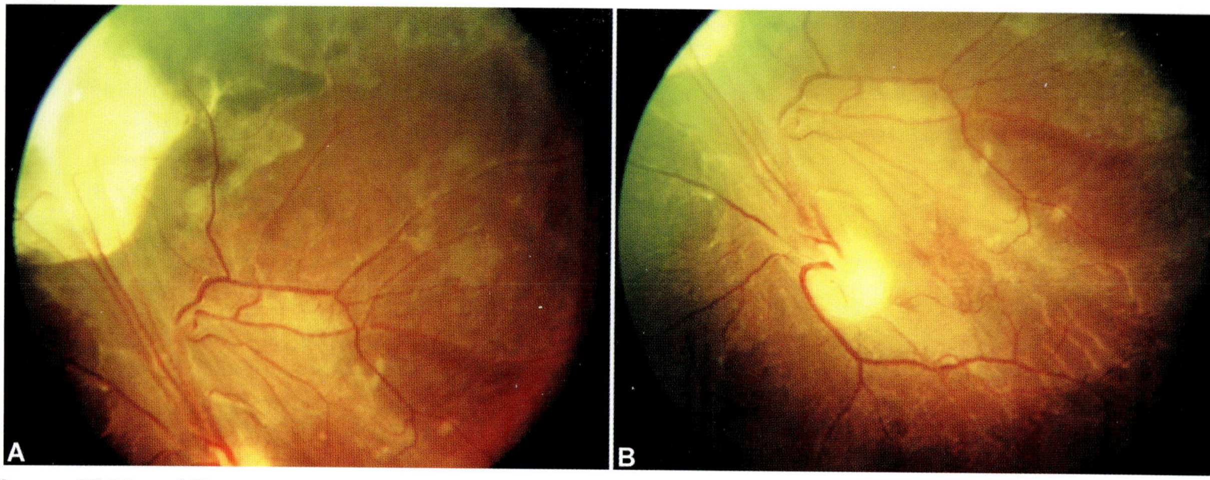

▲ **Figures 35.6A and B**

Color fundus photographs showing peripheral residual scarring following vitreous surgery for subretinal cysticercosis. Note macular heterotopia. Postoperative visual acuity at 3 months follow-up was 20/200

parasitic infestations.[13,17] Recurrent retinal detachment is another possible complication following vitrectomy for toxocara related traction retinal detachment and chorioretinal scars with traction retinal detachment associated with cysticercosis.[13,17] Subretinal cysticercosis with scarring is prone for more frequent occurrence of recurrent retinal detachment.[10]

Parasitic diseases as an indication for surgery constitute less than 1% of the surgeries in a vitreoretinal surgical unit. Intravitreal or subretinal cysticercosis and gnathostomiasis are frequent causes of indication for vitreous surgery in Asia. Indications for vitrectomy in parasitic diseases includes persistent ocular inflammation, residual vitreous exudates or membranes, intravitreal or subretinal parasites and for management of associated secondary complications like traction or rhegmatogenous retinal detachment. Anatomical outcomes are generally good after surgical intervention for parasitic diseases, but visual results are variable depending on the location of the residual scar.

References

1. Engstrom RE, Holland GN, Nussenblatt RB, et al. Current practices in the management of ocular toxoplasmosis. Am J Ophthalmol. 1991;111:601-10.
2. Cano MR. Ocular cysticercosis. In: Stephen J Ryan (Ed). Retina, 3rd edition. Mosby company; 2001. pp. 1553-7.
3. Jabs DA, Nguyen QD. Ocular toxoplasmosis. In: Stephen J Ryan (Ed). Retina, 3rd edition. Mosby; 2001. pp. 1531-44.
4. Ratra D, Phogat C, Singh M, et al. Intravitreal cysticercosis presenting as neovascular glaucoma. Indian J Ophthalmol. 2010;58:70-3.
5. Basak SK, Sinha TK, Bhattacharya D, et al. Intravitreal Live Gnathostoma Spinigerum. Indian J Ophthalmol. 2004;52:57-8.
6. Biswas J, Gopal L, Sharma T, et al. Intraocular Gnathostoma Spinigerum. Retina. 1994;14: 438-44.
7. Bhattacharjee H, Das D, Medhi J. Intravitreal gnathostomiasis and review of literature. Retina. 2007;27:67-73.
8. Nainiwal S, Chand M, Verma L, et al. Intraocular live cysticercus larva. Ophthalmic Surg Lasers Imaging. 2003;34:464-6.
9. George T, Mathai A, Challa JK, et al. Intravitreal cysticercosis: How did it get there? Aus and New Zealand J Ophthalmol. 1998;26:159-60.
10. Luger MHA, Stilma JS, Ringens PJ, et al. In-toto removal of a subretinal cysticercus cellulosae by pars plana vitrectomy. Br J Ophthalmol. 1991;75:561-3.
11. Natarajan S, Malpani A, Nirmalan PK, et al. Management of intraocular cysticercosis. Graefe's Arch Clin Exp Ophthalmol. 1999;237:812-4.
12. Messener KH, Kammerer WS. Intraocular cysticercosis. Arch Ophthalmol. 1979;97:1103-5.
13. Sharma T, Sinha S, Shah N, et al. Intraocular Cysticercosis: clinical charecteristics and visual outcome after vitreoretinal surgery. Ophthalmology. 2003;110:996-1004.
14. Maguire AM, Green WR, Michels RG, et al. Recovery of intraocular Toxocara canis by pars plana vitrectomy. Ophthalmology. 1990;97:675-80.
15. Werner JC, Ross RD, Green WR, et al. Pars plana vitrectomy and subretinal surgery for ocular toxocariasis. Arch Ophthalmol. 1999;117:532-4.
16. Muftuoglu G, Cicik E, Ozdamar A, et al. Vitreoretinal surgery for a subretinal hydatid cyst. Am J Ophthalmol. 2001;132: 435-7.

17. Amin HI, McDonald HR, Han DP, et al. Vitrectomy update for macular traction in ocular toxocariasis. Retina. 2000;20: 80-5.
18. de Souza EC, Nakashima Y. Diffuse unilateral subacute neuroretinitis. Ophthalmology. 1995;102:1183-6.
19. Wilkinson CP. Ocular toxocariasis. In: Stephen J Ryan (Ed). Retina, 3rd edition. Mosby company; 2001. pp. 1545-52.
20. McDonald HR, Kazacos KR, Schatz H, et al. Two cases of intraocular infection with alaria mesocercaria. Am J Ophthalmol. 1994;117: 447-55.
21. Lee J, Chung SH, Lee SC, et al. A technique for removal of a live nematode from the vitreous. Eye. 2006;20;1444-6.
22. Kean BH, Sun T, Ellsworth RM. Color Altas and Text Book of Ophthalmic Parasitology, New York: Igaku-Shoin; 1991. pp. 151-6.
23. Bathrick ME, Mango CA, Mueller JF. Intraocular gnathostomiasis, Ophthalmology 1981;8:1293-5.
24. Biglan AW, Glickman LT, Lobes LA. Serum and vitreous toxocara antibody in nematode endophthalmitis. Am J Ophthalmol. 1986;224:218-20.
25. Belmont JB, Irvine A, Benson W, et al. Vitrectomy in ocular toxocariasis. Arch Ophthalmol. 1982;100:1912-5.
26. Hagler WS, Pollard, ZF, Jarrett WH, et al. Results of surgery for ocular toxocara canis. Ophthalmology. 1981;88:1081-6.
27. Grand GM, Roper-Hall G. Pras plana vitrectomy for ocular toxocariasis. Retina. 1981;1:258-61.
28. Shields JA. Ocular toxocariasis: A review. Surv Ophthalmol. 1984;28:361-81.
29. Triester G, Machemer R. Results of vitrectomy for rare proliferative and hemorrhagic diseases. Am J Ophthalmol. 1977;84:394-412.
30. Small KW, McCuen BW, DE Juan E, et al. Surgical management of retinal traction caused by toxocariasis. Am J Ophthalmol. 1989;108:10-4.
31. Sallo F, Eberhard ML, Fok E, et al. Zoonotic intravitreal onchocerca in Hungary. Ophthalmology. 2005;112:502-4.

36 Surgery for Choroidal Coloboma and Retinal Detachment

Lingam Gopal

Introduction

Coloboma of the choroid is a congenital abnormality caused by defective closure of the embryonal fissure.[1] Retinal detachment has been reported in up to 40% of cases.[2] Retinal detachment can occur at any age. In order to understand the pathogenesis of retinal detachment associated with coloboma of the choroid, one should understand the pathology of the junction of the coloboma with the normal retina.

Anatomical Considerations

The area of the coloboma has no choroid and retinal pigment epithelium (RPE) and the retina in the area is replaced by variably fibrotic tissue called the intercalary membrane (ICM). The sclera in the area of the coloboma is ectatic to a variable degree. If one were to trace the normal retina on to the colobomatous area, the outer layer (towards the sclera) turns back and merges with the RPE, while the inner layer continues as the ICM. The point where the reversed outer retinal layer meets the RPE is called the "locus minoris resistentiae"[3] (Fig. 36.1).

The severity of the coloboma can vary. The optic disc can be within the coloboma of the choroid or outside the same and can also be colobomatous.[4] Presence or absence of the disc within the coloboma is an important feature that influences the treatment plan. Where in the disc is involved in the colobomatous area, the nerve fibers inserting into the disc will be occupying the upper border of the coloboma.

The macula may be totally within the coloboma, totally outside the coloboma or at the margin of the same. In eyes with large colobomata, the amount of functional retina is limited and the treatment should be tailored with minimal destruction of the functional retina.

The eyes affected by coloboma of the choroid very often are microphthalmic and have in addition coloboma of the

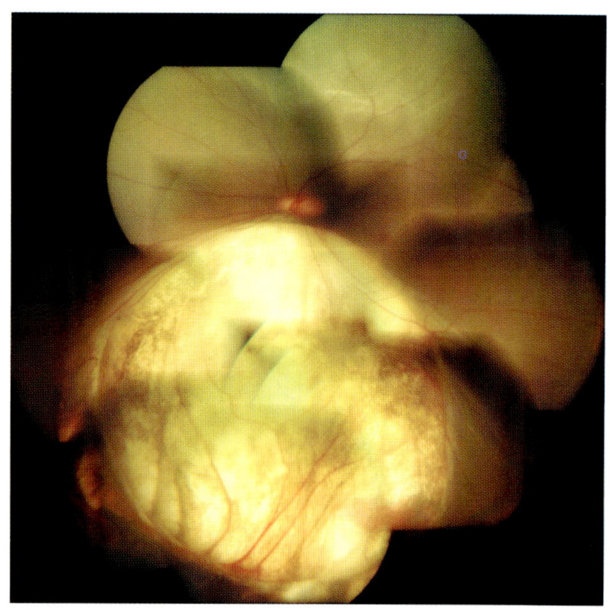

▲ **Figure 36.1**

Shows coloboma of the choroid sparing the optic disc and having partial retinal detachment. The intercalary membrane detachment is just about made out in the upper temporal part of the coloboma iris and zonules of the lens and ciliary body. Nystagmus can be coexistent when both eyes are affected by macular involvement.

Optical coherence tomography (OCT) in coloboma of choroid has helped to understand certain features of coloboma that are not obvious on clinical examination.

Studies have shown that the transition from normal retina to the intercalary membrane can be gradual or abrupt. The outer layers (towards the sclera) are lost early.

The communication between the subretinal space and subintercalary membrane space can be identified by careful examination with OCT.

Subclinical retinal detachment can sometimes be identified beyond the coloboma. These could be due to traction caused on the margin of coloboma by a taut ICM.

The eye wall near the margin of coloboma can sometimes overhang—seen as a hump on OCT. This can sometimes cause problems for photocoagulation.

Small colobomata can have ICM similar in thickness to retina but lacks the layering characteristic of normal retina.

Lesions similar to chorioretinal atrophic patches can be seen in the meridian of the coloboma and can be called "forme fruste" lesions. These lesions have normal looking retina on OCT with layering also noted.

Clinical Presentation of the Retinal Detachment

Retinal detachment can extend as ICM detachment into the colobomatous area or may stop at the coloboma margin. The presence of ICM detachment may not be obvious unless one carefully examines the margin. The extent of the ICM detachment can also vary. On occasions ICM detachment alone may be present without normal retina being detached. This would obviously be subclinical and be asymptomatic. The retinal detachment can be partial or total. Vitreous separation is usually absent. If the retinal detachment is restricted to the peri-colobomatous area, very often one sees signs of chronicity as evidenced by pigment demarcation lines and subretinal gliosis.

Retinal Breaks, Intercalary Membrane Breaks and Breaks at Locus Minoris Resistentiae

In the pathogenesis of retinal detachment in eyes with coloboma of the choroid, one has to understand the contribution of breaks in the retina, breaks in the ICM and the sites of communication between the subretinal and sub-ICM space. The breaks in the retina can be similar to any other case of retinal detachment in the form of lattice with holes or tractional related tears in the periphery. Breaks in the ICM can be located along the border of the coloboma margin or in the central part of the coloboma.[5,6] These breaks are difficult to identify due to the lack of contrast. They can be multiple and can sometimes involve the anatomical macula if it is involved in the coloboma. Breaks in the Locus minoris resistentiae indicate the presence of sites of communication between subretinal space and sub-ICM space. These are not clinically identifiable but may be identified on carefully done OCT.[7]

Characteristics of the Retinal Detachment

Careful examination of the margin of the coloboma will show whether the retinal detachment is extending into the coloboma or not (i.e. the retinal detachment is continuing as ICM detachment). If ICM detachment is definitely excluded, the retinal detachment is only due to a peripheral break and can be handled like any other case of retinal detachment, ignoring the coloboma. If however ICM detachment is present, the coloboma is partly or totally responsible for the retinal detachment. Most cases of coloboma related retinal detachments start as ICM detachments and spill over into the normal retina, once a communication is established between the sub-ICM space and subretinal space through a break in the Locus minoris resistentiae.

Management

If one is sure of the absence of the ICM detachment and a peripheral break is clearly identified and if the retinal detachment is fresh, one can perform a scleral buckling. If ICM detachment is noted (even if it is a small rim), it is best to perform vitreoretinal surgery since the contribution of coloboma to the retinal detachment can be confirmed during the surgery and the management appropriately tailored.

Steps of Surgical Procedure

The sclerotomy position depends on the degree of microphthalmos. In small eyes, correspondingly the sclerotomies may have to be made anteriorly. Lensectomy is not needed as a routine. During vitrectomy, one assesses the presence or absence of posterior vitreous detachment (PVD). If PVD is absent, one can use intravitreal triamcinolone acetonide to guide the induction and complete removal of the posterior vitreous. Detaching the vitreous from the posterior pole could be sometimes difficult and can actually induce breaks in the Locus minoris resistentiae. Once the peripheral vitreous is trimmed, fluid air exchange is performed. This step is the most important and the behavior of the retina guides the further steps of the surgery. During fluid air exchange when one keeps the extrusion needle on the bed of the coloboma, the following observations can be made.

The retina balloons around the coloboma with no extension of retinal detachment into the coloboma. This confirms the lack of ICM detachment and one should look for a peripheral break as a cause of the retinal detachment and the coloboma in such case is only incidental.

The retina balloons around the coloboma but extends into the coloboma as ICM detachment. This indicates the presence of communication between the subretinal space and sub-ICM space through breaks in the Locus minoris resistentiae, but ICM does not have breaks and hence the subretinal fluid is unable to find its way into the vitreous space.

The retina flattens totally without having to deliberately suck the subretinal fluid (i.e. there is no need for any drainage retinotomy). This is possible only if there is communication between the subretinal and sub-ICM space and the presence of breaks in the ICM. Peripheral retinal breaks can coexist.

If there is no ICM break and the peripheral break is too peripheral to permit endodrainage, one may have to make a retinotomy to settle the retina.

Once the retina is flattened laser photocoagulation is performed. The peripheral retinal breaks if any are treated. Then the coloboma border is treated if the retinal detachment is associated with ICM detachment. The coloboma border is ideally treated with diode laser so that the risk of nerve fiber layer damage is minimized. This becomes especially important in cases where the disc is involved within the coloboma. Heavy burns with green laser around the disc coloboma could potentially result in loss of vision due to nerve fiber layer damage and hence diode laser is preferred with the deeper burns sparing the nerve fiber layer.

No attempt is made to treat the visible ICM breaks. The treatment around the coloboma border is carried on along the ora serrata. Usually silicone tamponade is preferred (Fig. 36.2).

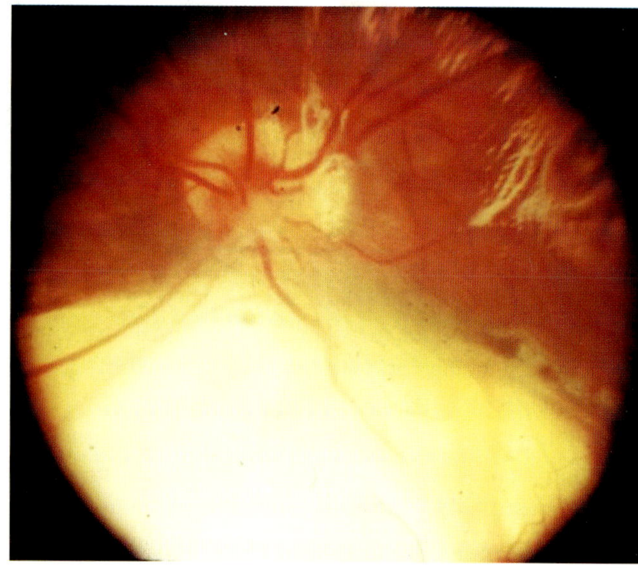

▲ **Figure 36.2**

Posterior pole of an eye with coloboma of the choroid not involving the disc.

Note: The silicone oil reflexes, attached retina and photocoagulation marks along the margin of the coloboma

▶ Causes of Failure of Surgery

- Failure to detach the vitreous.
- Failure to treat the coloboma margin properly and break the communication between the sub-ICM space and the subretinal space.
- Failure to identify the peripheral dialysis and treat the same properly.
- A relatively rigid ICM with traction on the retina beyond the coloboma border. A relatively broad area of laser treatment can protect the retina in such cases. On occasion one may have to cut the ICM to relieve the traction on the coloboma border.[8] However one must be conscious of the fact that major blood vessels may be traversing the ICM before entering the normal retina. Failure to recognize this fact can result in inducing retinal arteriolar occlusion in functional retina.
- Proliferative vitreoretinopathy.

Results

Prior to vitrectomy the success rate of surgery for retinal detachment in these cases was very low. In a series published by us, 81.2% had anatomical success and 69.4% recovered equal or better than 10/200 vision.[8] Pal et al.[9] reported an anatomical success rate of 88.1% with 10/200 or better vision seen in 78.4%.

References

1. Forrester JV, Dick AD, McMenarmin PG, Lee WR. The eye: Basic sciences in practice, 2nd edition. Edinburgh: WB Saunders; 2002. pp. 99-129.
2. Jesberg DO, Schepens CL. Retinal detachment associated with coloboma of choroid. Arch opthalmol. 1961;65:163-73.
3. Schubert HD. Schisis like rhegmatogenous retinal detachment associated with choroidal colobomas. Graefes Arch Clin Exp Ophthalmol. 1995;233:74-9.
4. Gopal L, Badrinath SS, Kumar KS, et al. Optic disc in fundal coloboma. Ophthalmology. 1996;103:2120-6.
5. Gopal L, Badrinath SS, Sharma T, et al. Surgical management of retinal detachments related to coloboma of the choroid. Ophthalmology. 1998;105:804-9.
6. Gopal L, Badrinath SS, Sharma T, et al. Pattern of retinal breaks and retinal detachments in eyes with choroidal coloboma. Ophthalmology. 1995;102:1212-7.
7. Gopal L, Khan B, Jain S, et al. A clinical and optical coherence tomography study of the margins of the choroidal colobomas. Ophthalmology. 2007;114:571-80.
8. Gopal L, Kinin MM, Badrinath SS, et al. Management of retinal detachment with choroidal coloboma. Ophthalmology. 1991;98:1622-7.
9. Pal N, Azad RV, Sharma YR. Long term anatomical and visual outcome of vitreous surgery for retinal detachment with choroidal coloboma. Indian J Ophthalmol. 2006;54:85-8.

SECTION 11

Oncology

37 Eye-conserving Surgical Treatment Methods in Intraocular Tumors

Kaan Gündüz

Introduction

Eye-conserving surgical treatment methods used in the management of some commonly seen intraocular tumors are discussed here.

Laser Photocoagulation

Laser photocoagulation raises the tissue temperature above 60° C and causes coagulation of the proteins and immediate cell death. Laser photocoagulation has been used in the treatment of choroidal melanoma, retinoblastoma, circumscribed choroidal hemangioma and retinal capillary hemangioma.

▶ Choroidal Melanoma

Surface laser photocoagulation using green or red wavelengths has been used in the treatment of selected small choroidal melanomas in the past.[1] Long exposure (0.5 seconds) burns are used. Photocoagulation is first applied around the tumor margins to induce choroidal atrophy. Next, the entire tumor surface is treated with heavy burns to induce retinal and choroidal atrophy. Laser photocoagulation is associated with high recurrence rates in the treatment of choroidal melanoma, reaching 64% in one study.[2] Today, laser photocoagulation is used for the treatment of proliferative radiation retinopathy after brachytherapy or teletherapy of choroidal melanoma and not as primary treatment.

▶ Retinoblastoma

In retinoblastoma, the objective of treatment is to surround the tumor and close off all feeder tumor vessels. Laser photocoagulation was used as primary treatment for retinoblastoma less than 3 mm in base diameter and less than 2 mm in thickness. Surface photocoagulation in retinoblastoma may be dangerous as it may lead to rupture of the internal limiting membrane and spread of the tumor cells into the vitreous cavity.[3] Laser photocoagulation is rarely used for retinoblastoma today.

▶ Circumscribed Choroidal Hemangioma

The goal of laser photocoagulation in circumscribed choroidal hemangioma (CCH) is to induce adhesions between the retina and retinal pigment epithelium (RPE) (Fig. 37.1). Surface laser photocoagulation has been reported to be successful in inducing resolution of subretinal fluid (Fig. 37.1).[4] Unfortunately, in these cases the subretinal fluid has a tendency to recur and as many as 40% of patients require additional laser treatments.[5] The major limitations of laser photocoagulation in CCH are failure to induce tumor regression and the need for repeated treatments. Laser photocoagulation is rarely used today in the treatment of CCH and has largely been superseded by photodynamic therapy (PDT), discussed later in this chapter.

▶ Retinal Capillary Hemangioma-Retinal Hemangioblastoma

Laser photocoagulation is usually targeted either directly at the tumor, to feeder vessels, or both in retinal capillary

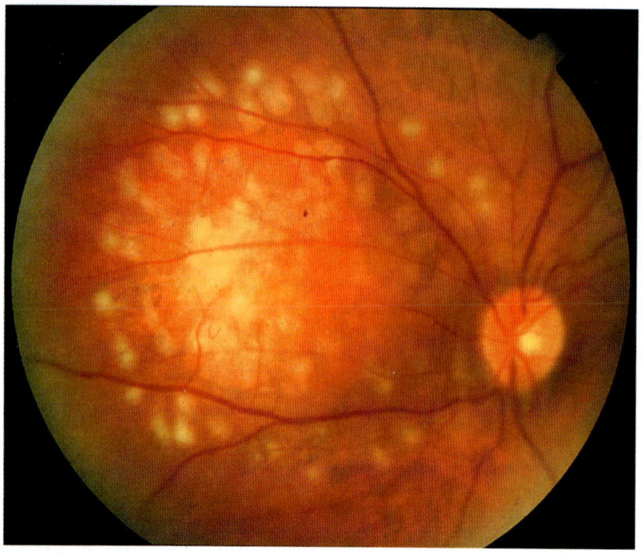

▲ **Figure 37.1**

Laser spots over a choroidal hemangioma located temporal to the optic disc. This tumor was treated with surface laser photocoagulation using green argon (514 nm) laser (Dr Jerry and Carol Shields)

hemangioma (RCH). This treatment has been successful in treating RCHs that are up to 4.5 mm in size, but is particularly effective for tumors that are 1.5 mm or smaller.[6] Repeated treatment sessions usually spaced 1–2 weeks apart may be necessary to achieve tumor regression, resolution of retinal exudates and subretinal fluid.

Transpupillary Thermotherapy

Transpupillary thermotherapy (TTT) is a laser treatment that uses infrared radiation (810 nm) to increase tissue temperature to 42–60°C, at which temperature range DNA damage and cytolytic changes occur.[7] Tumor regression starts within weeks and continues for months, resulting in a regressed tumor or an atrophic chorioretinal scar at the site of the tumor. TTT has a number of advantages, including lower cost than plaque radiotherapy, avoidance of invasive surgery and of radiation complications and convenience of outpatient treatment, which uses a widely available infrared diode laser system.[8] TTT has been used for the treatment of a number of intraocular tumors including choroidal melanoma, retinoblastoma and CCH.

▶ Choroidal Melanoma

Transpupillary thermotherapy was initially developed as an adjunctive treatment to plaque radiotherapy in choroidal melanomas by Oosterhuis et al.[9] Experimental studies showed that thermal penetration of the tumor reaches a maximum depth of 4 mm, thereby making TTT a potentially ideal treatment for small choroidal melanomas.[10] Primary TTT has recently gained popularity as an outpatient procedure for the treatment of small choroidal melanomas, especially for tumors near the critical visual areas, where radiation would potentially result in vision loss.[11,12] Primary TTT has generally been used in choroidal melanomas less than 4 mm in thickness and less than 10 mm in base diameter (Figs 37.2A to D).

Despite the initial enthusiasm for TTT, analyses of long-term patient data showed that primary TTT was associated with high rates of complications and recurrence in the treatment of choroidal melanoma.[8,13-16] About 30–50% of the eyes develop complications, and these complications need to be followed carefully, as they can lead to vision loss and even globe loss.[8,13-16] TTT may be associated with complications, including macular pucker and retinal traction, refractory cystoid macular edema, branch retinal vein and artery occlusions, focal iris atrophy, increased sensory retinal detachment and pigment dispersion into the vitreous cavity.[8,13-16]

About 25% of the eyes fail TTT and develop recurrence by 5 year follow-up.[8,15] In one study, the recurrence rate was higher when the tumor abutted the optic nerve or when more than three sessions of TTT were required for tumor control. Amelanotic melanomas responded poorly to TTT owing to decreased heat uptake in the tumor.[8] Another study found that tumor diameter more than 10 mm, tumor thickness more than 3 mm, and high-risk characteristics (including subretinal fluid, orange pigment and thickness > 2 mm) were significant predictors of failure.[15] Recurrences can be intraocular or extraocular.

Although TTT may be useful in the treatment of small choroidal melanocytic lesions, the high complication and recurrence rates warrant close monitoring of patients after primary TTT. Patients treated with TTT should be followed with both clinical examination and ultrasonography to detect intraocular and extraocular tumor growth, even when a flat chorioretinal scar has been achieved.

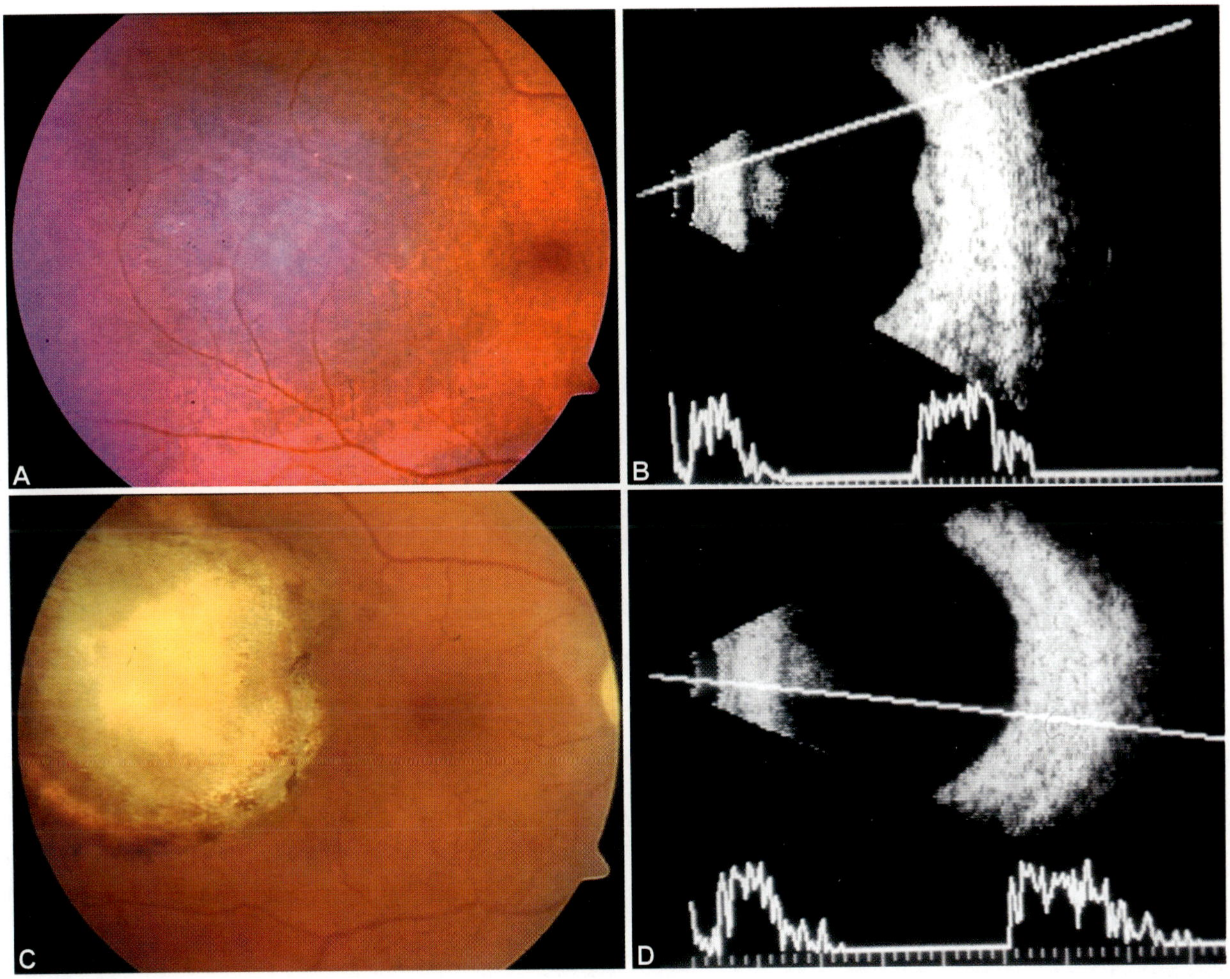

▲ **Figures 37.2A to D**

(A) Pigmented choroidal melanoma measuring 6.0 x 6.0 mm in base diameter located temporal to the fovea; (B) B-mode ultrasonogram shows a 2.5 mm-thick choroidal melanoma with acoustic solidity at baseline. The vitreous appears clear, and there is no extraocular extension; (C) Complete regression of the melanoma into a flat chorioretinal scar after 3 sessions of TTT; (D) B-mode ultrasonogram after three sessions of TTT demonstrates complete regression of choroidal melanoma. Source: Gündüz K, Karslioglu MZ, Köse K. Primary transpupillary thermotherapy of choroidal melanocytic lesions. Middle East Afr J Ophthalmol.2011;18:183-8.

▶ Retinoblastoma

Transpupillary thermotherapy is an effective treatment for small retinoblastoma located posterior to the equator of the eye and has been widely used. As primary treatment, TTT is mainly used for retinoblastoma less than 3 mm in base diameter and less than 2 in thickness.[17,18] TTT can also be used to treat residual tumor in larger retinoblastomas treated with chemoreduction. When used in conjunction with chemoreduction, TTT is usually performed on the same or the next day after chemoreduction (Figs 37.3A and B). The uptake of TTT by retinoblastoma is variable and recurrent tumors on a white background (such as atrophic scar or calcified tissue) often demonstrate poor uptake. TTT can also be used for more anteriorly located tumors with scleral depression; however, cryotherapy is usually preferred for tumors in this location.

A special application of TTT in retinoblastoma is thermo-chemotherapy.[19] The rationale for this treatment is based on the finding that cytotoxicity of carboplatin is enhanced by hyperthermia of 6–9° C. Chemothermotherapy is done by administering carboplatin intravenously and delivering diode laser (810 nm) within a couple of hours.

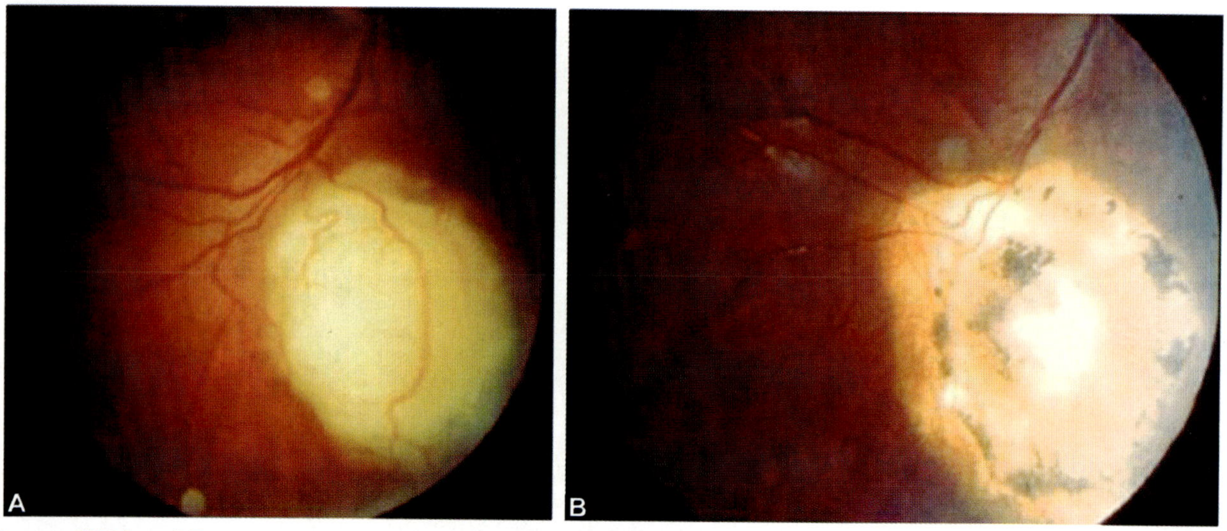

▲ **Figures 37.3A and B**

(A) Inferiorly located retinoblastoma in the right eye measuring 6.0 x 6.0 mm in base diameter and 3.0 mm in thickness; (B) After 6 chemoreduction and 2 sessions of TTT the tumor is completely atrophic. Source: Gündüz K, Günalp I, Yalcindag NY, et al. Causes of chemoreduction failure in retinoblastoma and analysis of associated factors leading to eventual treatment with external beam radiotherapy and enucleation. Ophthalmology. 2004;111:1917-24.

Circumscribed Choroidal Hemangioma

Transpupillary thermotherapy is an effective treatment for symptomatic CCH not associated with significant retinal detachment. In a review of 38 patients with CCH treated with TTT, 95% showed complete or partial tumor regression with resolution of subretinal fluid and corresponding improvement in visual acuity (Figs 37.4A to D).[20] Reported complications of TTT in CCH included cystoid macular edema, preretinal fibrosis and retinal vascular occlusion. TTT may not be the best treatment option for CCH located in subfoveal, juxtafoveal, or juxtapapillary regions. PDT provides better visual results for CCHs in these locations, as dissussed later.

Transpupillary thermotherapy has been preferred over PDT in the treatment of CCH in many parts of the world, especially the developing countries because of cost reasons.[20] In general, tumor regression is usually evident within 3 months after TTT. Additional treatment sessions may be offered after a 3 month period if subretinal fluid persists.

Photodynamic Therapy

Circumscribed Choroidal Hemangioma

Photodynamic therapy with verteporfin may be the most ideal treatment for symptomatic CCH without extensive retinal detachment because it offers the possibility of tumor destruction with sparing of the overlying retina and performing this treatment in an outpatient setting (Figs 37.5A to D). The principal effect of PDT is a selective occlusion of the choriocapillaris layer with relative sparing of photoreceptors and retinal pigment epithelium.[21] This mode of action may explain the disappearance in subretinal fluid after PDT as the reduced blood flow in choriocapillaris results in less fluid transudation through the RPE. Mechanisms that have been shown to be involved in the tumoricidal effect of PDT include direct cytotoxicity to tumor cells and selective occlusion of the tumor vasculature, thus starving the tumor of oxygen or nutrients.[22,23]

Different PDT parameters including verteporfin injection parameters (bolus vs. injection over 10 minutes), light dose settings (50–100 J/cm^2), and duration of exposure (83–166 seconds) have been used by different investigators.[24-26] However, a standard fluence PDT (light dose of 50 J/cm^2 and duration of 83 seconds) with infusion of verteporfin over 10 minutes followed by laser 5 minutes after completion of the infusion is generally used. Multiple overlapping spots may be used to cover the entire tumor surface. In general, tumor regression is most dramatic following the first session following photodynamic therapy and is usually evident within 3 months.[25] If the tumor fails to respond and the subretinal fluid does not regress after standard fluence PDT, a higher

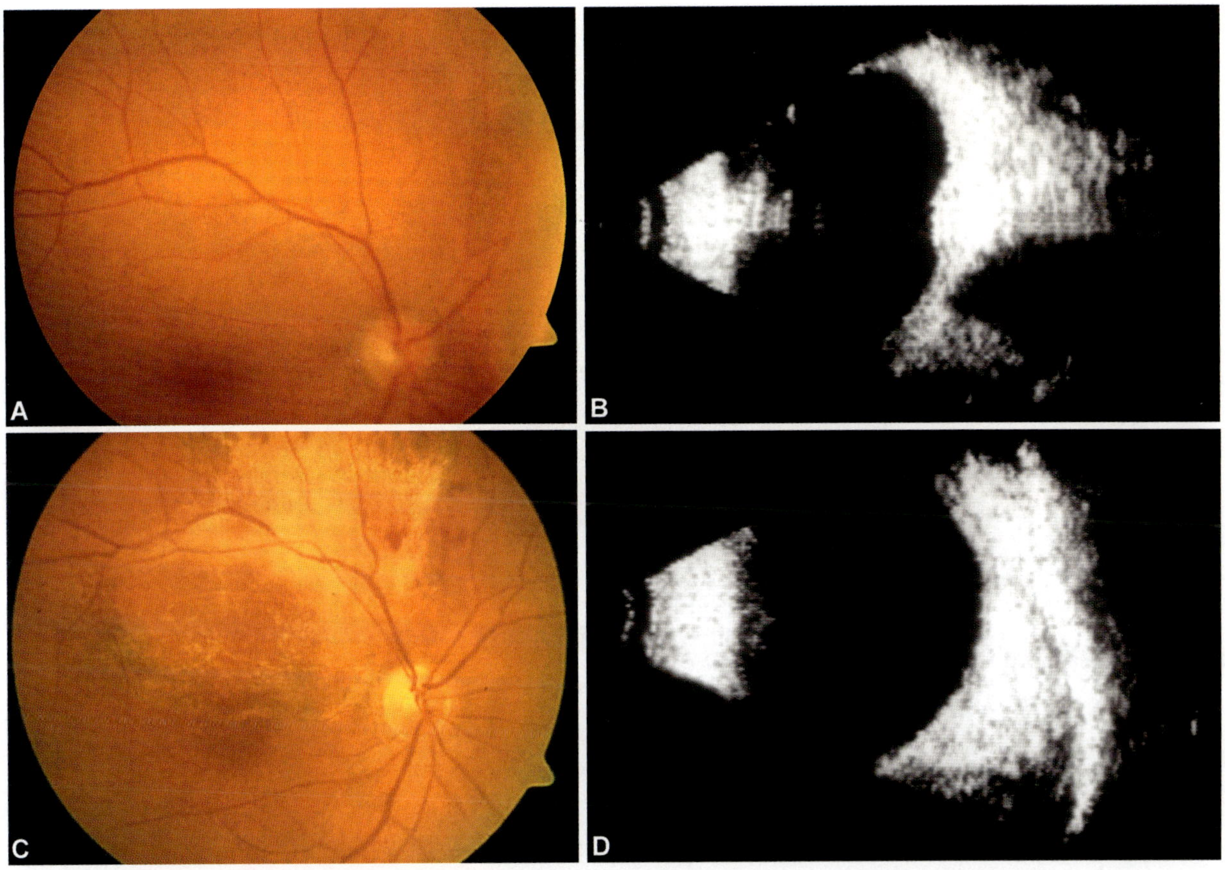

▲ **Figures 37.4A to D**

(A) Circumscribed choroidal hemangioma measuring 6.0 x 6.0 mm in base diameter located superotemporal to the optic disc; (B) B-mode ultrasonogram demonstrates 2.0 mm thick choroidal hemangioma with acoustic solidity; (C) Complete regression of the CCH 3 months after a single session of TTT; (D) B-mode ultrasonogram demonstrates complete disappearance of the choroidal hemangioma 3 months after a single session of TTT. Source: Reproduced from Gündüz K. Transpupillary thermotherapy in the management of circumscribed choroidal hemangioma. Surv Ophthalmol. 2004;49:316-27.

light dose (100 J/cm^2) may be tried at the second attempt. However, repeated treatments and over-treatment may result in delayed choroidal atrophy adversely affecting final visual acuity outcomes.[26]

▶ Diffuse Choroidal Hemangioma

Low-dose (20 Gy) external beam radiotherapy is generally used in the treatment of symptomatic diffuse choroidal hemangioma (DCH), especially if it is associated with bullous retinal detachment.[27] Recently, PDT has also been reported with good short-term results in the treatment of DCH with little or no overlying subretinal fluid.[28,29] Multiple spots are necessary to cover the epicenter of the tumor. Tumor regression and resolution of exudative retinal detachment with visual acuity improvement have been reported.

▶ Choroidal Nevus

Photodynamic therapy has also been used for the treatment of symptomatic choroidal nevi located near the fovea with subretinal fluid extending under the fovea (Figs 37.6A to E).[30] The mechanism of action is similar to that for CCH. Because of light absorption characteristics, the regressive effect appears to be more marked in amelanotic choroidal nevi compared to heavily pigmented lesions. The potential advantage of PDT for lesions close to the macula is a greater potential for preservation of visual acuity.

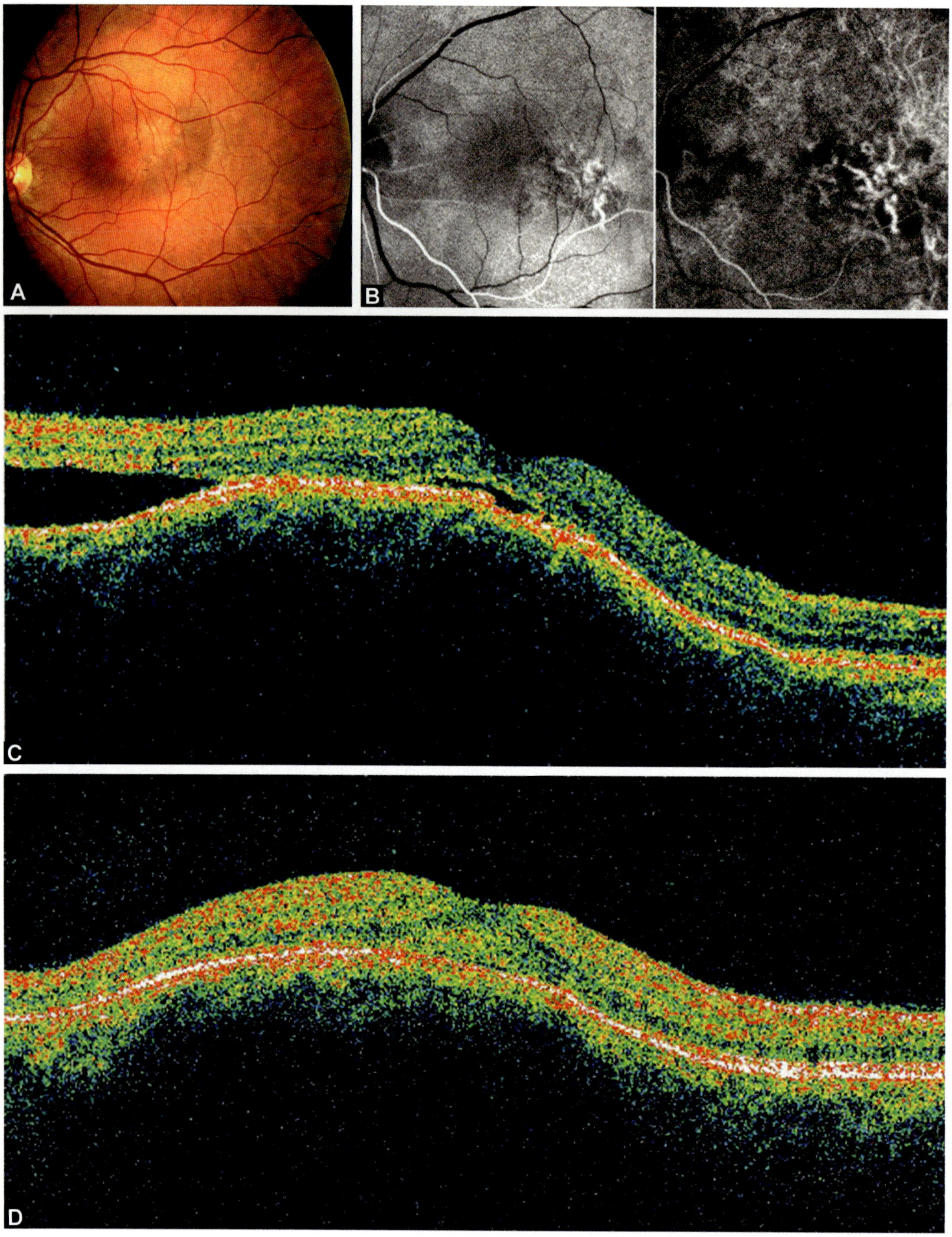

▲ **Figures 37.5A to D**

(A) Small orange color circumscribed choroidal hemangioma (CCH) located temporal to the fovea producing visual loss to 20/60. The tumor thickness is 1.9 mm; (B) Fluorescein (right of the composite picture) and indocyanine green (left of the composite picture) angiograms show intralesional hyperfluorescence in the arterial phase of the fluorescein angiogram and the early phase of indocyanine angiogram consistent with the diagnosis of CCH; (C) Vertical OCT (time-domain) cut through the fovea demonstrates the choroidal elevation from the CCH and subretinal fluid over the tumor that involves the fovea; (D) The patient underwent standard fluence PDT. One year later, vertical OCT (time-domain) cut through the fovea shows complete resolution of the subretinal fluid. There was only a slight regression in the CCH to a thickness of 1.6 mm. The visual acuity one year later is 20/30. Source: Patient from Mayo Clinic, Rochester, MN

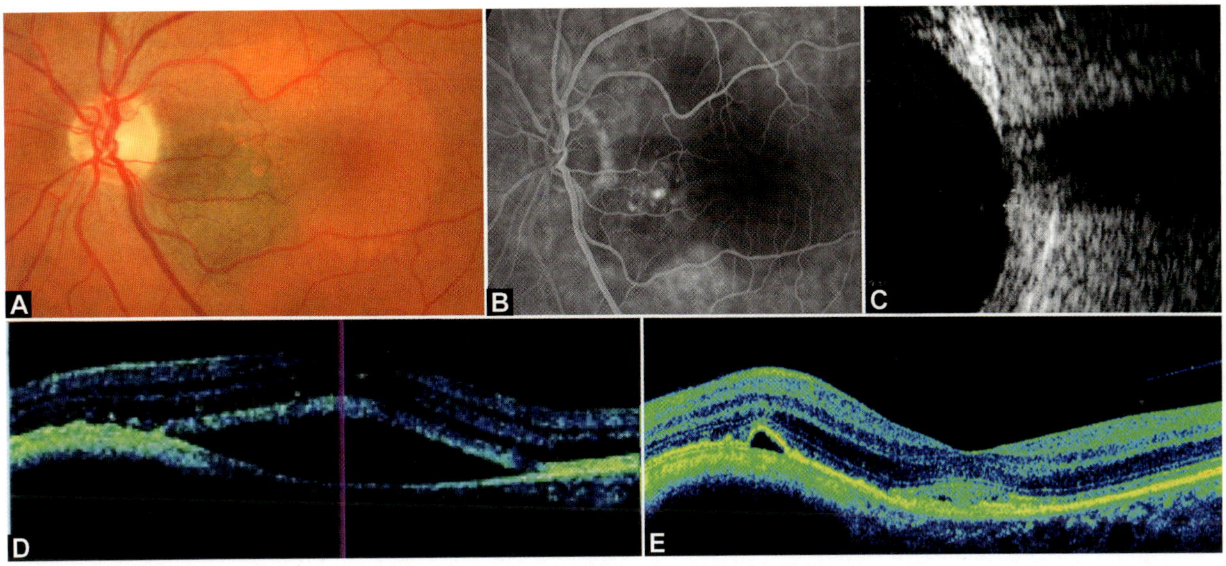

▲ **Figures 37.6A to E**

(A) Juxtapapillary choroidal nevus with orange pigment on the lesion surface and subretinal fluid extending to the fovea; (B) Mid-phase fluorescein angiogram demonstrates patchy hyperfluorescence in the lesion; (C) B-mode ultrasonogram shows a 0.7 mm acoustically solid lesion; (D) Spectral domain OCT showing the subfoveal fluid; (E) Spectral domain OCT 3 months after a single session of PDT shows marked resolution of the subretinal fluid. Source: Garcia-Arumi J, Amselem L, Gunduz K, et al. Photodynamic therapy for symptomatic subretinal fluid related to choroidal nevus. Retina (in press)

Vascular Retinal Tumors

Photodynamic therapy has been reported to induce the occlusion of both juxtapapillary and peripheral RCHs.[31] For juxtapapillary RCH, PDT probably provides the best treatment approach (Figs 37.7A and B). PDT leads to resolution of exudates and subretinal fluid with variable regression of the main tumor mass in retinal vasoproliferative tumors.[32] A standard light dose setting (50 J/cm^2) can be used although the higher light dose setting of 100 J/cm^2 has been used by several investigators.[31,32]

Choroidal Osteoma

There is insufficient information in the literature about the effects of PDT on choroidal osteomas. PDT has been used in one case of extrafoveal choroidal osteoma to induce decalcification and prevent growth of the tumor to the fovea.[33] However, this encouraging result should not be extrapolated to subfoveal osteomas because PDT may induce decalcification of subfoveal choroidal osteoma which can result in vision decrease due to RPE loss. PDT should probably be undertaken in subfoveal osteomas only if there is choroidal neovascularization.

Acquired Retinal Astrocytoma and Astrocytic Hamartomas

There are few reports in the literature about PDT of aggressive acquired astrocytomas and astrocytic hamartomas.[34,35] Astrocytic hamartomas can be seen in association with tuberous sclerosis. PDT has been found to be effective in resolution of macular exudation and edema with variable regression of the tumor (complete disappearance of the tumor in a case of astrocytic hamartoma[35] vs. no change in tumor in a case of acquired astrocytoma[34]).

Cryotherapy

Retinoblastoma

Cryotherapy is usually done transconjunctivally. However, in selected cases, if there is difficulty in reaching the tumor, a snip incision can be made in the conjunctiva and the cryoprobe inserted through the incision to reach the more posteriorly located tumors. Cryotherapy is usually used for retinoblastoma less than 4 mm in base diameter and less than

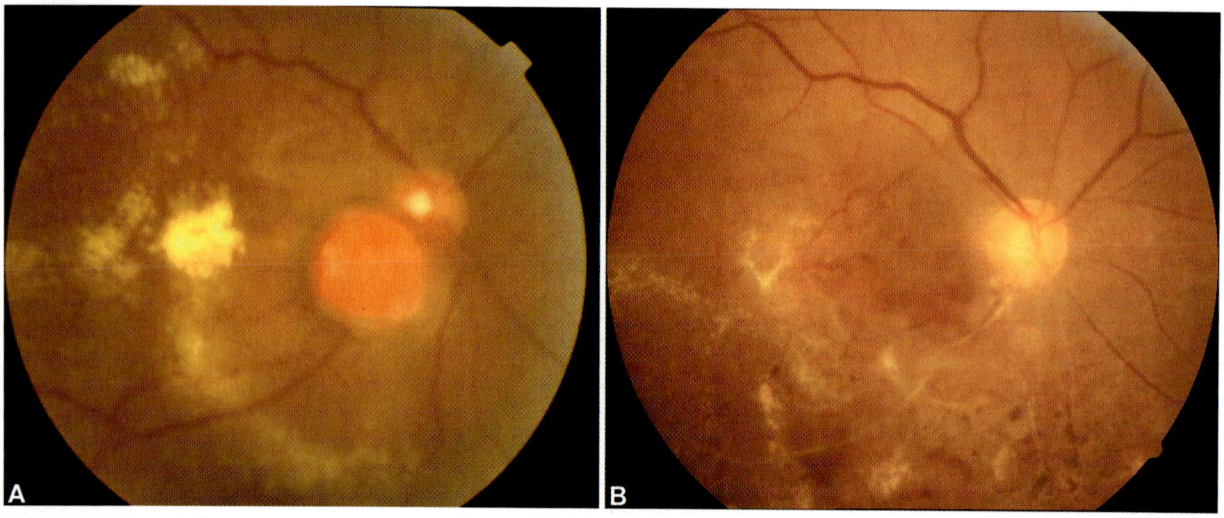

▲ **Figures 37.7A and B**

(A) Juxtapapillary retinal capillary hemangioma associated with subretinal fluid and macular exudation. The lesion was treated with multiple surface laser photocoagulation sessions but failed to regress; (B) Disappearance of the tumor with resolution of subretinal fluid and macular exudates 6 months after a single session of standard fluence PDT. Source: Yaman A, Saatci AO, Arikan G, Gündüz K, et al. Involution of endophytic optic disc hemangioma with a single session of photodynamic treatment. Ann Ophthalmol. 2007;39:63-6.

3 mm thick without vitreous seeds located anterior to the equator of the eye (Fig. 37.8).[36] Cryotherapy can be used either singly or in combination with chemoreduction. A triple freeze-thaw techique is used to ensure effective tumor destruction.

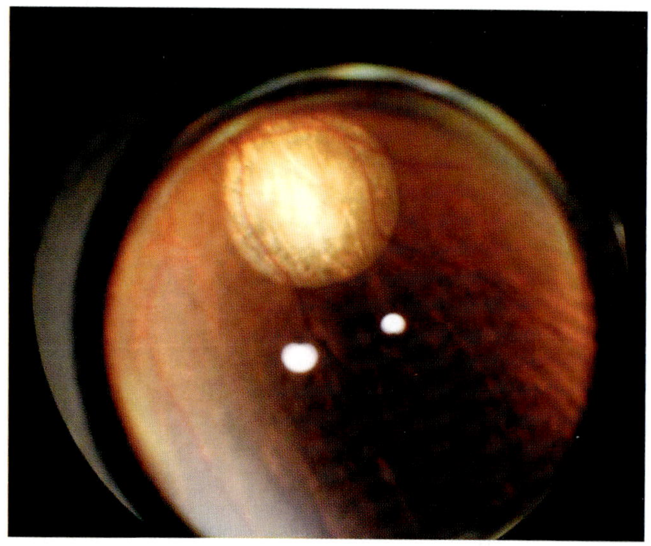

▲ **Figure 37.8**

Flat atrophic chorioretinal scar tissue resulting from cryotherapy of a small peripheral retinoblastoma. Note that the tumor is completely gone

Vascular Retinal Tumors

Cryotherapy has also been used in peripheral retinal vasoproliferative tumor and RCH. Triple freeze-thaw transconjunctival cryotherapy has been reported to be successful in a small number of retinal vasoproliferative tumor cases; however repeated treatment sessions may be required (Figs 37.9A and B).[37] Cryotherapy may be preferable to photocoagulation in RCHs where tumors are anteriorly located, associated with a moderate degree of subretinal fluid, or are more than 3.0 mm in base diameter.[38] The best therapeutic result is obtained if the tumor is less than 1.5 mm in base diameter. Both triple and double freeze-thaw techniques have been used in benign vascular retinal tumors.

Episcleral Plaque Radiotherapy (Brachytherapy)

Plaque radiotherapy requires two surgical operations, one to insert the plaque and the other to remove the plaque. The plaque usually stays on the eye for about 3–6 days, the duration of treatment is dependent on the type of tumor being treated (i.e. the apex dose required), tumor thickness and the radioactivity of the plaque. The radiation calculations are made by the help of a Plaque Simulator program.

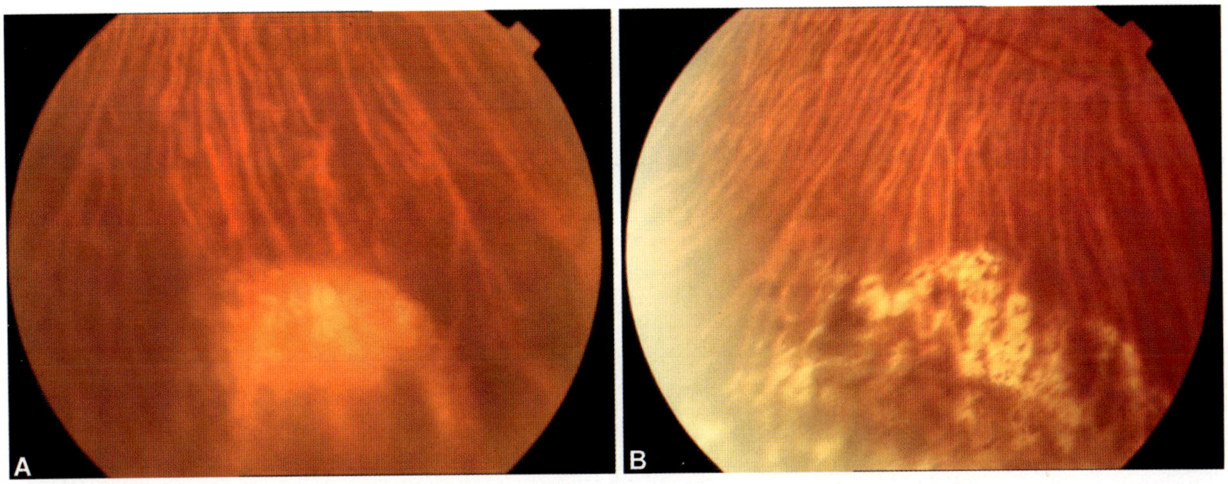

▲ **Figures 37.9A and B**

(A) Inferiorly located retinal vasoproliferative tumor 3.0 x 3.0 in base diameter and 2.0 mm in thickness associated with localized subretinal fluid over and surrounding the tumor; (B) Complete regression of the vasoproliferative tumor with resolution of the subretinal fluid following 2 sessions of triple-freeze thaw cryotherapy 1 month apart

Choroidal and Ciliary Body Melanoma

Episcleral plaque radiotherapy is probably the most common method used currently in developed countries for the treatment of choroidal melanoma. Different radioisotopes have been used, including cobalt-60 (60Co), ruthenium-106 (106Ru), iodine-125 (125I), palladium-103 (103Pd) and iridium-192 (192Ir).[39,40] Currently, the most popular ones are ruthenium-106 and iodine-125. Notched plaques are available to treat juxtapapillary tumors. Radiation cytotoxicity develops from radiation-induced DNA damage in the tumor cells and the vascular system. Iodine-125 emits gamma-rays and is useful in the treatment of tumors up to 10 mm thick, although the use of episcleral plaque brachytherapy for thicker tumors is associated with a higher enucleation risk in the long run because of the associated radiation complications. The largest tumor-base diameter suitable for treatment with plaque brachytherapy is considered to be approximately 16 mm, although in rare cases plaque brachytherapy has been used for larger tumors. The current practice is to deliver a dose of 80–100 Gy to the tumor apex. Ruthenium-106 emits beta-rays and is useful in the treatment of tumors up to 5 mm thick. However, it can be used melanomas up to 8 mm in thickness, delivering 120 Gy to a 5 mm tumor depth (Figs 37.10A to D). The tumor apex receives less than 85 Gy radiation dose in these circumstances, which is the normally recommended dose for uveal melanoma. The rationale for this application may be to close tumor vessels by delivering high-dose radiotherapy to the tumor base. The half-life of Ruthenium-106 is 369 days, and this allows the plaque to be used successively on a number of patients, reducing cost and making it affordable in many developing countries. Because Iodine-125 has a half-life of only 60 days, it is available for use in a smaller number of patients than the longer-lived Ru-106.

Following brachytherapy, the tumor begins to regress within 3 months of treatment. The rate of tumor regression is faster with 106Ru plaques than with 125I plaques, presumably because of the higher radiation dose delivered to the tumor base. A slow regression pattern is desired because tumors that undergo rapid and complete regression are thought to have a malignant cell type and are thus associated with a poorer prognosis (Figs 37.11A and B).[41] This is because more malignant, rapidly cycling tumors grow faster and respond to radiation-induced DNA damage with more rapid shrinkage.

Radiation complications of episcleral plaque radiotherapy include dry eye, cataract, neovascular glaucoma, optic neuropathy and retinopathy.[42] Although choroidal melanoma with extraocular extension is usually treated with enucleation, plaque radiotherapy can also be used in tumors with limited extraocular extension less than 3 mm thick. The area of extraocular extension should be left untouched in these circumstances to avoid dissemination of melanoma cells.[43]

There are three main situations in which TTT may be combined with episcleral plaque brachytherapy (the so-called

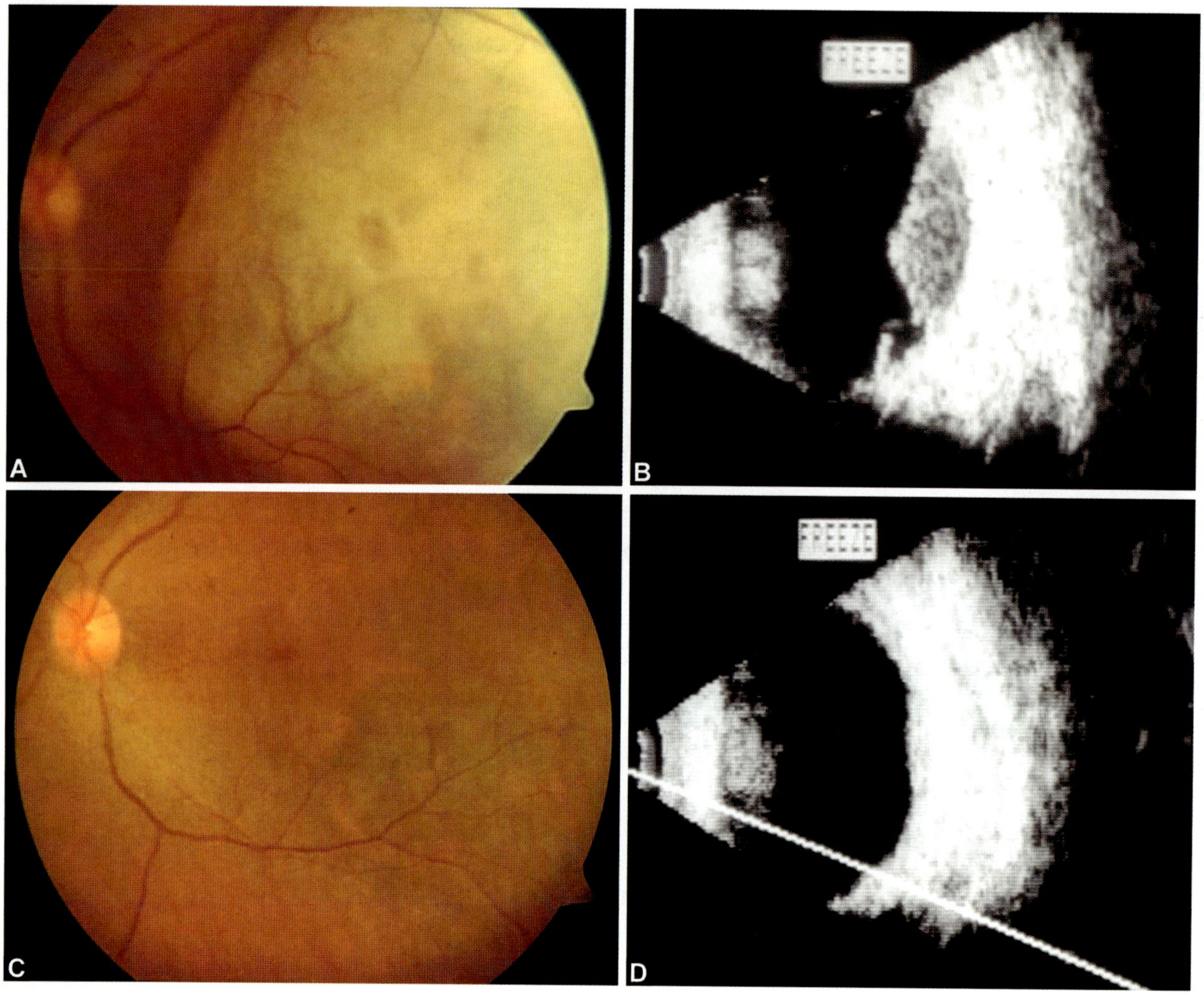

▲ **Figures 37.10A to D**

(A) Amelanotic macular choroidal melanoma measuring 12.0 x 10.0 mm in base diameter in the left eye; (B) The tumor measures 6.0 mm in thickness and shows medium acoustic solidity and retinal detachment on B-mode ultrasonogram; (C) 9 months after Ruthenium-106 plaque radiotherapy, the tumor has demonstrated marked regression; (D) On B-mode ultrasonogram, the residual tumor has a thickness of only about 0.5 mm

sandwich therapy).[7] First, TTT is used to treat the posterior tumor margin in juxtapapillary melanomas, which may not be well covered with the plaque because of difficulties in plaque placement in this position (Figs 37.12A and B). Second, TTT may be used to augment the effect of 106Ru plaque brachytherapy in tumors 5–8 mm thick. Third, TTT can be used to treat central or marginal recurrence of choroidal melanoma after plaque radiotherapy.

▶ Retinoblastoma

The indications for tumor thickness, base and choice of radioactive isotopes discussed above for melanomas also apply to plaque radiotherapy of retinoblastoma. Minimal retinoblastoma vitreous seeds overlying the tumor can also be treated with plaque radiotherapy. However, extensive vitreous and subretinal seeds are difficult to control with this method. The recommended apex dose is 40 Gy.[44]

▶ Circumscribed Choroidal Hemangioma

Plaque radiotherapy causes tumor regression in addition to resolution of exudative retinal detachment and improvement in visual acuity in the majority of cases with CCH (Figs 37.13A and B). There have been several papers on the use of different radioisotopes in plaque radiotherapy including

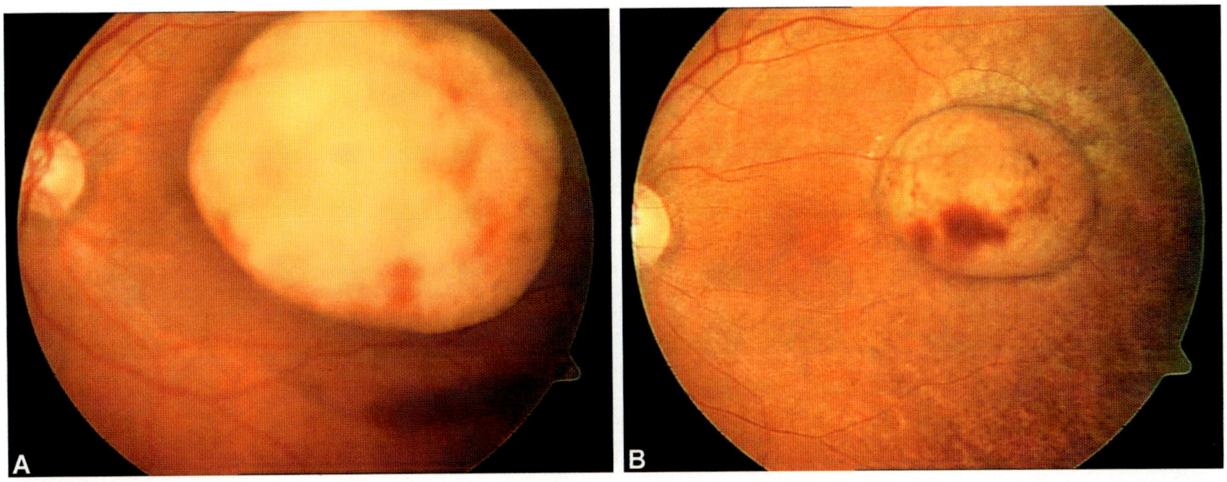

▲ **Figures 37.11A and B**

(A) Amelanotic choroidal melanoma with a mushroom (collar-button) shape occupying the macular area in the left eye. The tumor features retinal hemorrhages on the surface resulting from break through the Bruch's membrane. The tumor measures 9.0 x 8.0 mm in base diameter and 5.5 mm in thickness; (B) One year after Iodine-125 plaque radiotherapy, the tumor has shown a nice slow regression to a thickness of 2.8 mm

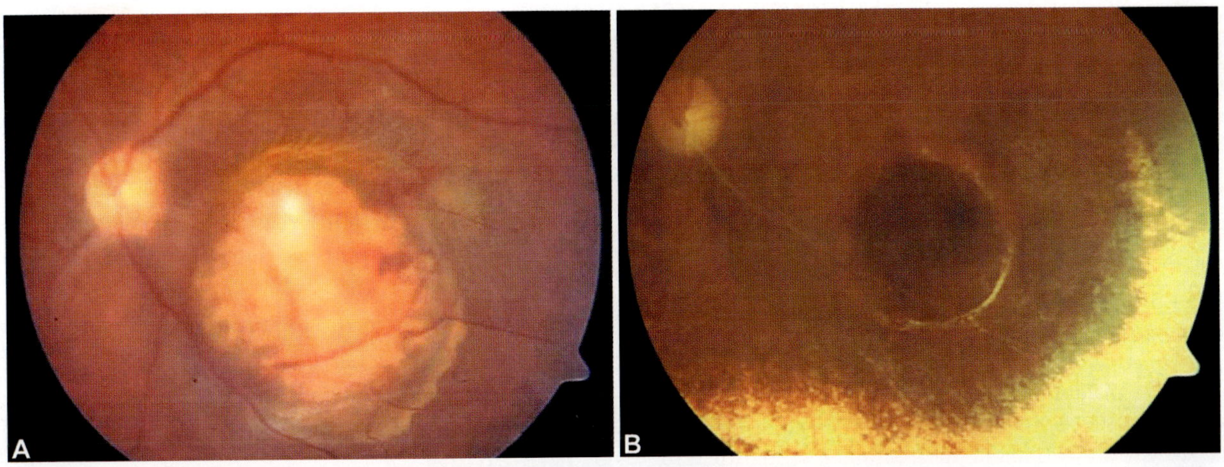

▲ **Figures 37.12A and B**

(A) Mushroom-shaped amelanotic choroidal melanoma with break through Bruch's membrane and retinal hemorrhages on the tumor surface. The tumor measures 6.0 x 6.0 mm in base diameter and 4.0 mm in thickness. The tumor is located in the macular area near the optic disc, a location where accurate plaque placement is difficult; (B) 15 months after Ruthenium-106 plaque radiotherapy and 3 sessions of TTT, the tumor is markedly regressed to a thickness of 2.1 mm. Note the widespread retinal pigment epithelial atrophy resulting from plaque radiotherapy surrounding the tumor. The tumor has a brownish color from the accumulation of dead melanophagic pigment on the tumor surface after TTT

iodine-125, cobalt-60, and ruthenium-106.[45,46] The apex doses that have been used for CCH ranged from 25–60 Gy but probably a 20 Gy dose is sufficient for the treatment of this condition.

▶ Vascular Retinal Tumors

Plaque radiotherapy has also been used in selected cases of retinal vasoproliferative tumors and RCH. Both iodine-125 and ruthenium-106 brachytherapy have been used to treat

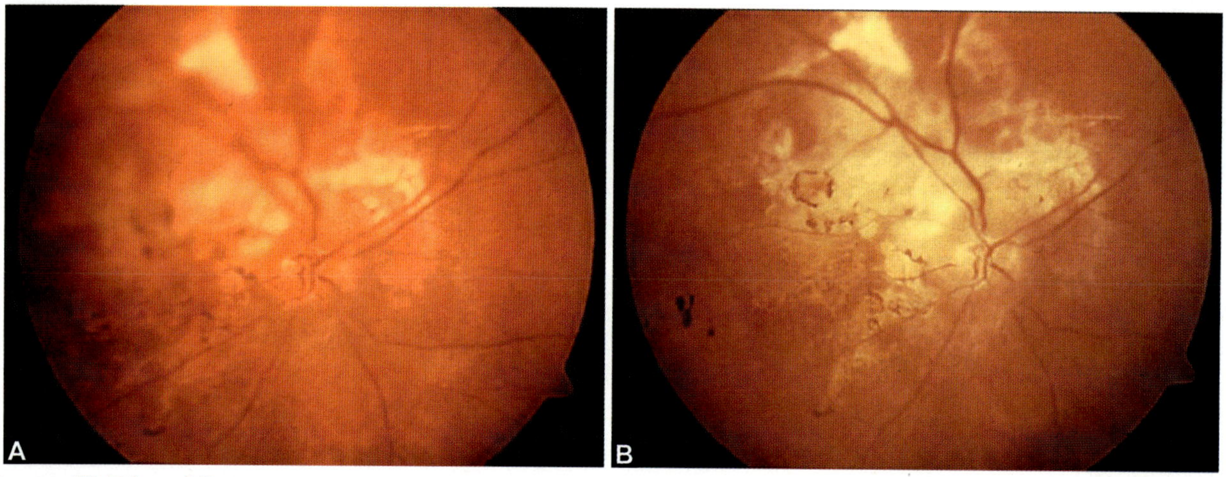

▲ **Figures 37.13A and B**

(A) CCH located above the optic disc associated with marked subretinal fibrosis and subretinal fluid. The tumor has a thickness of 4.0 mm on B-mode ultrasonography; (B) One year after Ruthenium-106 plaque radiotherapy, the tumor is markedly regressed to a thickness of 1.5 mm with complete resolution of the subretinal fluid. Note that the vessels over the tumor are now clearly visible

vasoproliferative tumors.[47,48] In a series of 30 eyes with retinal vasoproliferative tumor treated with iodine I-125 brachytherapy, tumor regression was observed in 97%, exudative retinal detachment resolved in 65% and visual acuity improved or remained stable in 73%.[47]

For RCH less than 5.0 mm in base diameter or those that have been resistant to either prior photocoagulation or cryotherapy, plaque radiotherapy has been used successfully. However, visual results are better in eyes with no preoperative exudative retinal detachment.[49]

Surgical Resection

Parallel to the development of treatment modalities for choroidal melanomas utilizing ionizing radiation either by brachytherapy discussed above or teletherapy (proton beam irradiation), eye retaining surgical excision of these tumors was developed either by means of "exo or transscleral resection" or by means of pars plana vitrectomy described as "endoresection".

The indications for surgical removal of uveal tumors are numerous. Removal is indicated for iris and iridociliary tumors of indeterminate pathology that present suspicious features, such as pigment seeding, prominent vascularity and increased thickness and size.[50,51] It may not be possible to perform fine-needle aspiration biopsy (FNAB) of these tumors, especially if they are located in the iridocorneal angle. Moreover, different portions of the tumor may harbor different pathologies, so small FNAB samples may be misleading. Second, iris or iridociliary tumors with documented growth, such as leiomyoma and melanocytoma, need to be surgically excised to restore intraocular structure and prevent complications such as lens subluxation and cataract.[52] Growing necrotic iris or iridociliary melanocytomas can cause increase in intraocular pressure (IOP); thus, removal is also necessary to achieve control of IOP and intraocular inflammation.[53] Third, thick ciliary body and choroidal melanomas require high radiation doses to the tumor and surrounding tissues, resulting in severe radiation complications. Surgical resection is believed to be safer under these circumstances.[54]

Iridectomy

Iris tumors involving less than 3 clock hours of the iris without angle involvement are treated via iridectomy done through a limbal incision (Figs 37.14A and B). It is best to preserve the pupillary rim if possible. If the tumor involves the angle on gonioscopy and extends into the ciliary body, it is necessary to perform a iridogoniectomy or iridogoniocyclectomy via a partial lamellar sclerouvectomy approach.

Partial Lamellar Sclerouvectomy or Exoresection

In partial lamellar sclerouvectomy (PLSU), a scleral flap (80–90% of scleral thickness) is dissected and the ciliary

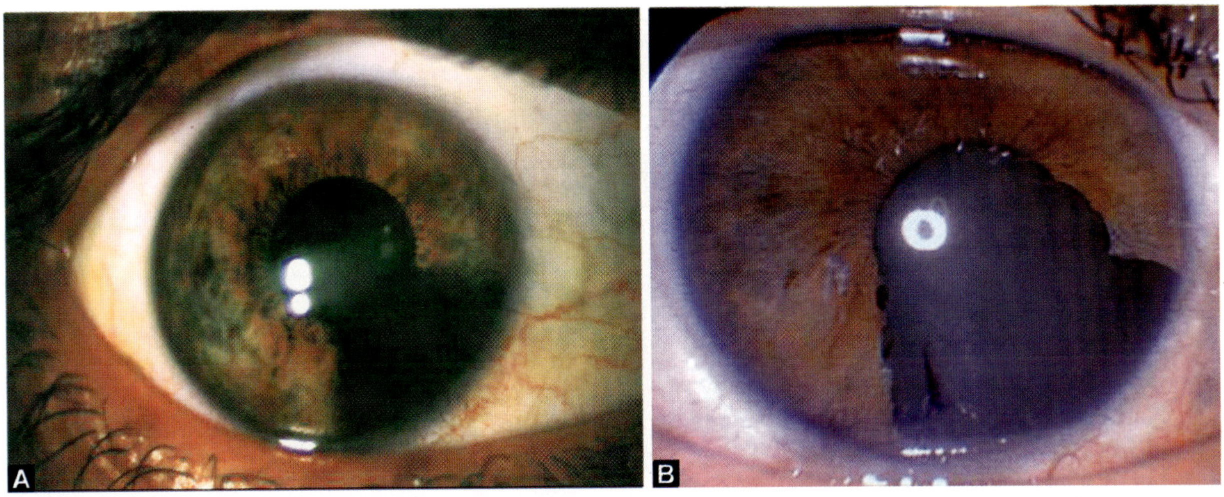

▲ Figures 37.14A and B

(A) Iris melanoma extending for 3 clock hours with no angle involvement; (B) Sectoral iris defect 1 year after total iridectomy surgery for the iris melanoma

body tumor with possible iris and/or choroidal extensions is excised intact with the overlying scleral fibers. The surgical technique has previously been described in detail.[54,55] The margins of the tumor on the sclera are marked with a marking pencil around the tumor shadow. Subsequently, the margins of the anteriorly hinged scleral flap positioned 3–4 mm outside this mark are marked on the sclera. The shape of the scleral flap is usually rectangular to allow easier scleral suturing after the cyclectomy. With a #57 beaver blade, a groove is created to an approximately 80–90% thickness of the sclera and the scleral flap is then developed and carried anteriorly to the corneoscleral limbus. If the blue color of the underlying choroid is not visible, the plane of dissection is gently deepened until it could be seen. Any bleeding from emissary vessels is controlled with bipolar cautery.

When the scleral flap is fully developed, a small circumferential incision using a 15° microsurgical knife is then made on the inner scleral fibers about 3 mm outside the margins of the tumor. Then, Vannas scissors are used to complete the scleral incision until the uveal tract is exposed. The uveal tract is cauterized using bipolar cautery until blanching and a gray color change of the uveal tissue is achieved.

In uveal tumors involving the iris, a 15° microsurgical knife is used to create a paracentesis port in the limbus approximately 90° from the area of the main incision and viscoelastic is injected into the anterior chamber. The anterior chamber is then entered using a 15° microsurgical knife at the center of the flap area, and the corneoscleral incision is carried laterally with Westcott scissors. For uveal tumors not involving the iris, the anterior chamber is not entered. In most cases of ciliary body and choroidal melanomas, a limited pars plana vitrectomy (20- or 23-gauge) without infusion is advised to reduce the possibility of uveal, retinal, and vitreous prolapse during the excision procedure. Vitreous aspiration with a 22-gauge needle should probably be avoided. Subsequently, the uveal tumor is excised using blunt Vannas scissors. The choroidal or ciliary part of the tumor is excised first, followed by excision of the iris part if the tumor has an iris component. The pupillary rim is spared, if possible. Care is taken to leave the underlying retina or, in the case of ciliary tumors, the nonpigmented ciliary pigment epithelium intact. The uveal tumor together with the overlying scleral fibers is carefully lifted off the surgical field using a "no-touch technique" to avoid spilling tumor cells into the surgical field. If vitreous loss occurs, vitreous is removed with a vitrectomy instrument. Before doing vitrectomy, three to five 9-0 nylon sutures may be placed at the corners and the free margin of the rectangular scleral flap, if possible. Vitrectomy is subsequently done at the margins of the flap to prevent vitreous wick in the wound area. Following completion of the vitrectomy, the scleral flap is sutured to its original position with more 9-0 nylon sutures. Any previously detached rectus muscle is sutured to its original position/insertion and the conjunctiva is reapproximated to the limbus with 7/0 vicryl sutures.

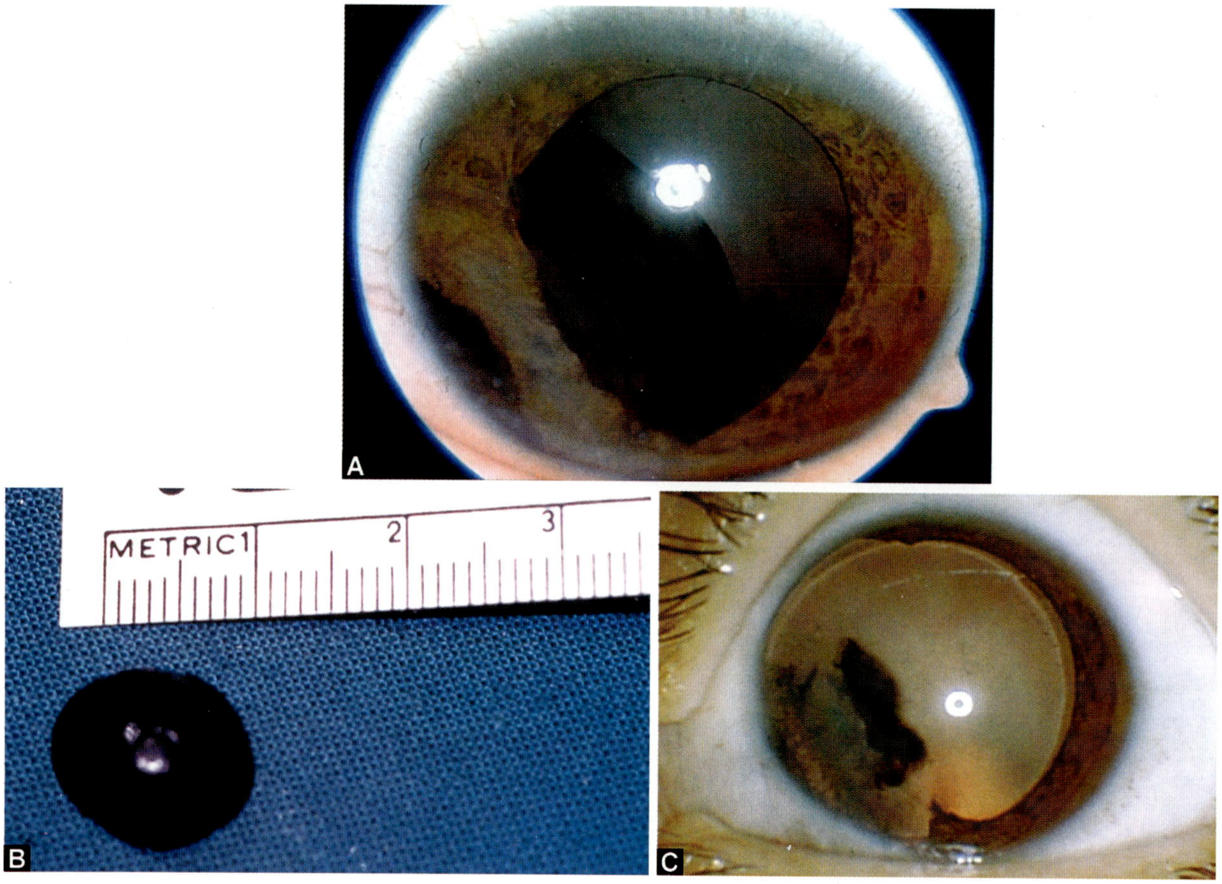

▲ **Figures 37.15A to C**

(A) Massive iridociliochoroidal melanoma producing corneal touch; (B) Gross photograph of the excised tumor showing a greater than 10 mm diameter uveal melanoma; (C) Anterior segment view 1 month after PLSU showing the absence of the iris from 7–11 o'clock after pupillary dilation. The corneal pigment was left untreated. Source: Kurt RA, Gündüz K. Exoresection via a partial lamellar sclerouvectomy approach: A successful performance by a novice surgeon. Clin Ophthalmol. 2010;4:59-65.

The largest tumor-base diameter suitable for this surgery is generally considered to be approximately 15 mm (Figs 37.15A to C).[55] This is a difficult surgical procedure carried out under hypotensive anesthesia with a significant learning curve. Since uveal melanoma cells can demonstrate intrascleral extension, plaque radiotherapy can be used postoperatively to eradicate any possible remaining melanoma cells.[56] A 100 Gy dose is given to a 1 mm depth from the inner surface of the sclera. Adjunctive plaque radiotherapy is usually done in ciliary melanomas with iris and/or choroidal involvement but not in iridociliary or iridocorneal melanomas where the epicenter of the tumor is in the iris with limited involvement of the adjacent ciliary body.

The indications for exoresection have evolved over the past years. Today, many surgeons reserve exoresection for anteriorly located tumors with ciliary body involvement. In tumors extending posterior to the ora serrata into the choroid, separation of the retina from the tumor can be difficult and is more frequently associated with intraoperative complications the closer, the posterior tumor margin is located to posterior pole. It is generally believed that iridociliary tumors occupying less than 3 clock hours of pars plicata and choroidal melanomas less than 15 mm in base diameter are eligible for surgical exoresection.[54,55,57]

Certain inherent difficulties of exoresection via PLSU can result in intraoperative, early (occurring < 8 weeks after surgery) and late complications (> 8 weeks after surgery). One of the major intraoperative problems is the failure to dissect a scleral flap of desired thickness.[55,57,58] The second major intraoperative challenge is to open the choroidal slit and dissect the uveal tissue without damaging the underlying retina or the nonpigmented ciliary epithelium.[58] Early postoperative complications include vitreous hemorrhage, hyphema, subretinal hemorrhage, transient blepharoptosis, cataract, retinal detachment, choroidal detachment, corneal edema and elevated IOP.[55,58] The most common early complication after PLSU surgery is vitreous hemorrhage.[55] Transient vitreous hemorrhage can occur in up to 30% of patients and generally develops from inadequately cauterized choroidal or ciliary body blood vessels.[53] In general, vitreous hemorrhage resolves spontaneously; however, when it persists beyond 8 weeks, pars plana vitrectomy can be performed. Persistent vitreous hemorrhage was seen in only 2 of 22 (9%) patients in one series.[58]

Late postoperative complications include cataract, subretinal fibrosis, posterior synechiae, rhegmatogenous retinal detachment with or without proliferative vitreoretinopathy, cystoid macular edema, elevated IOP, scleral thinning and rarely iris neovascularization.[55,57,58] Iatrogenic lens damage will lead to cataract formation during or after surgery. However, often, there is a slow and progressive cataract development many months after surgery, occurring as a late complication. It is believed that if the retrolenticular vitreous is not disturbed, the risk of cataract decreases.

Tumor recurrence after exoresection may follow incomplete removal of malignant tumors with positive surgical margins. One study found that lack of adjuvant radiotherapy, larger basal tumor diameter, older age and preoperative retinal detachment increased the incidence of tumor recurrence.[59] There is no statistically significant difference in the survival rate of patients treated with PLSU versus those treated with plaque radiotherapy.[60,61]

Endoresection

Endoresection of choroidal melanomas is an alternative surgical resection technique where the tumor is excised by a vitreous cutter during pars plana vitrectomy, providing access to tumors located posteriorly near the optic disc and/or macula.[62-64] This treatment is particularly useful in large uveal melanomas with more than 7 mm thickness because of the frequent radiogenic side effects of both brachy- and teletherapy (Figs 37.16A to D).

In phakic patients it is advisable to perform phacoemulsification with IOL implantation before starting pars plana vitrectomy in order to get better access to the vitreous base during the vitrectomy procedure. Following phacoemulsification, a 20- or 23- gauge 3 port pars plana vitrectomy is performed by inducing a complete posterior vitreous detachment by suction with the vitreous cutter, care being taken to also detach the posterior hyaloid from the anterior tumor margin. It is advisable to use a fourth port for an additional endoilluminating device such as chandelier endoillumination to facilitate bimanual manipulations during endoresection. After endodiathermy of the retinal vessels over the tumor base, the subretinal fluid is drained through a peripheral retinectomy after application of 1–2 cc perfluorocarbon liquid to the posterior pole. This is followed by transretinal endoresection with increased IOP (up to 85 mm Hg) and low systolic blood pressure ($\leq$ 90 mm Hg) to minimize bleeding from tumor vessels. The tumor is excised up to the sclera accompanied by endodiathermy and/or endolaser of individual scleral ciliary arteries and choroidal vessels. After flattening the retina by further perfluorocarbon injection, the retinectomy and choroidectomy edges are coagulated by an endolaser in continuous-wave mode and by cryocoagulation for the anterior endoresection and retinectomy borders. Flat tumor residues still remaining at the bare sclera are subjected to hyperthermia using 810 nm diode endolaser with low energy and continuous wave settings. Perfluorocarbon liquid is then directly exchanged for 5000 centistokes (cSt) silicone.[64,65]

A potential problem with endoresection is the intraoperative dissemination of vital tumor cells that can lead to recurrences. Aiming to reduce the incidence of tumor cell dissemination during endoresection a combined approach has been developed, including preoperative irradiation of the tumor (with proton beam irradiation or other stereotactic radiosurgical techniques)with subsequent endoresection.[65] The reasoning of tumor resection after tumoricidal irradiation to the tumor can be described as addressing the issue of the so called "toxic tumor syndrome", namely the removal of already necrotic or potentially necrotic tumor tissue that produces or is expected to produce in the future hypoxia and necrosis induced cytokines, inducing further radiation related retinal and optic nerve toxiciy. By removing or debulking the irradiated tumor and reattaching the detached retina, long-term ocular morbidity could be reduced significantly especially in large uveal melanomas that have undergone irradiation.[66]

In endoresection there is no limitation with regard to tumor thickness, but with largest tumor base exceeding 15 mm the intra- and postoperative complications increase. In addition, endoresection should be considered for tumors that do not infiltrate the ciliary body (due to the difficulty of

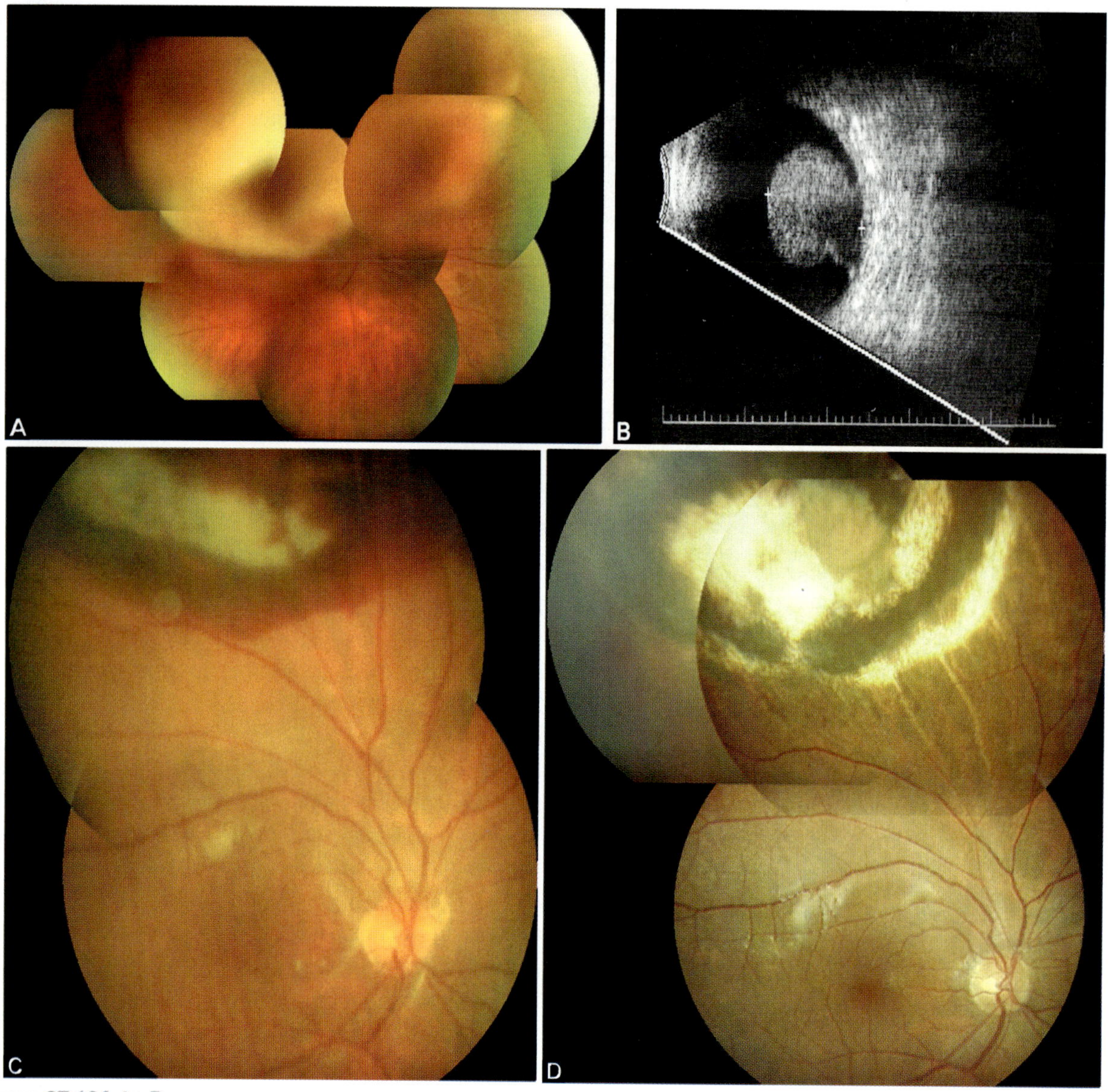

▲ **Figures 37.16A to D**

(A) Large choroidal melanoma obscuring funduscopic view to the posterior pole. Visual acuity is 20/100; (B) B-scan ultrasound of the tumor depicted in 37.4A showing a 11.9 mm thick mushroom-shaped choroidal melanoma; (C) Early postoperative view of the fundus of the eye depicted in (A) 2 days after endoresection. Visual acuity is 20/200; (D) Late postoperative view of the fundus of the eye depicted in (B) 18 months after endoresection. Visual acuity is 20/25. Source: Reproduced from Gündüz K, Bechrakis NE. Exoresection and endoresection for uveal melanoma. Middle East Afr J Ophthalmol. 2010;17:210-6

visualizing this area during vitrectomy) and ideally there should be at least one disc diameter distance from the posterior tumor margin to the optic disc and fovea.

Surgical resection by either exo- or endoresection provides histopathological and cytogenetic information of the tumor, which helps in prognostic predictions.

Other Vitreoretinal Procedures

Primary Vitreoretinal Lymphoma

Primary vitreoretinal lymphoma, a diffuse large B-cell lymphoma, is a subset of primary central nervous system

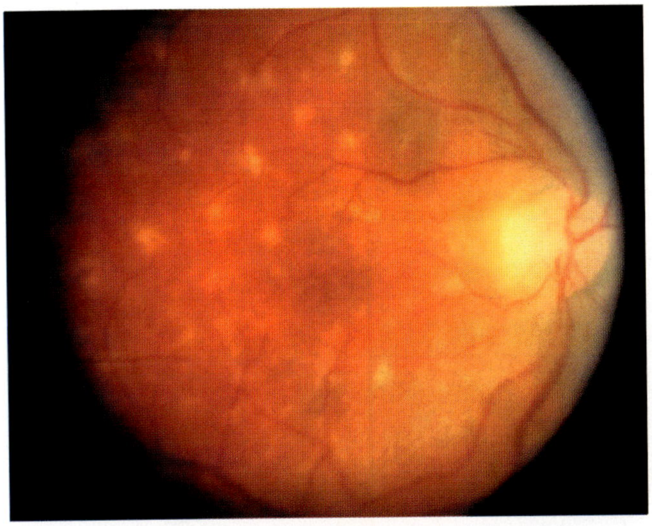

▲ Figure 37.17

Primary vitreoretinal lymphoma (subset of primary central nervous system lymphoma and formerly called primary intraocular lymphoma) characterized by whitish sub-retinal pigment epithelium infiltrates

lymphoma. Primary vitreoretinal lymphoma was previously called primary intraocular lymphoma. However, this term does not distinguish between uveal lymphoma which can also be primary and vitreoretinal lymphoma. Hence, the use of the new term primary vitreoretinal lymphoma should be endorsed. Primary vitreoretinal lymphoma is characterized by subretinal pigment epithelium infiltrates in addition to vitreous infiltration by the lymphoma cells (Fig. 37.17). Pars plana vitrectomy is required in many cases of primary vitreoretinal lymphoma to establish the diagnosis by providing material for cytopathology and improve vision by removing the cellular clumps and debris in the vitreous cavity.[67] The vitreous material should be transported to the cytology unit immediately to ensure a better diagnostic yield.

▶ Retinal Capillary Hemangioma

Pars plana vitrectomy, retinal detachment repair with or without a scleral buckle and other related procedures are occasionally required for large retinal vasoproliferative tumors and RCHs that have produced complications of tractional or rhegmatogenous retinal detachment. An endoresection type of procedure has also been used to excise mainly indolent RCHs by some surgeons.[68] However, the indications for this type of procedure are tentative and the risks of surgery should potentially be weighed against the advantages of other less invasive surgical methods including cryotherapy and PDT.

▶ Choroidal Melanoma

Vitreous hemorrhage resulting from radiation-induced changes (either brachytherapy or teletherapy) in choroidal melanomas can also be treated with vitrectomy methods to remove the vitreous blood. These cases may also benefit from additional endoresection to remove the dead tumor and relieve the toxic tumor syndrome.[69]

Intravitreal Injections

▶ Primary Vitreoretinal Lymphoma

Intravitreal injections of methotrexate (400 micrograms/0.1 ml) and rituximab (1 mg/0.1 ml), either separately or in combination, have been used in primary vitreoretinal lymphoma.[70,71] Rituximab is a monoclonal antibody targeting CD20(+) B-cell surface marker and methotrexate inhibits folate metabolism and DNA synthesis. Therefore, the use of combination chemotherapy and immunotherapy may be the way to go in the treatment of primary vitreoretinal lymphoma.

Although the frequency of injections may vary depending on the severity of the disease, biweekly injections of methotrexate and rituximab may be used for more severe forms of primary vitreoretinal lymphoma. Monthly injections may be more appropriate for less severe forms of the disease. Intravitreal injections are continued until regression of the intraocular disease is achieved. It has been suggested that a lower dose of methotrexate (200 micrograms/0.05 ml) can be used in the combination treatment with rituximab.[70] The common complications of intravitreal methotrexate included cataract (73%), corneal epitheliopathy (58%), maculopathy (42%), vitreous hemorrhage (8%), optic atrophy (4%) and sterile endophthalmitis (4%) in one series where twice weekly injections were given followed for weekly injections and then monthly injections.[71] Combination therapy with rituximab may help to decrease the complications associated with more frequent injections of methotrexate.

A patient with primary vitreoretinal lymphoma may or may not present with central nervous system involvement. For concomitant primary central nervous system lymphoma

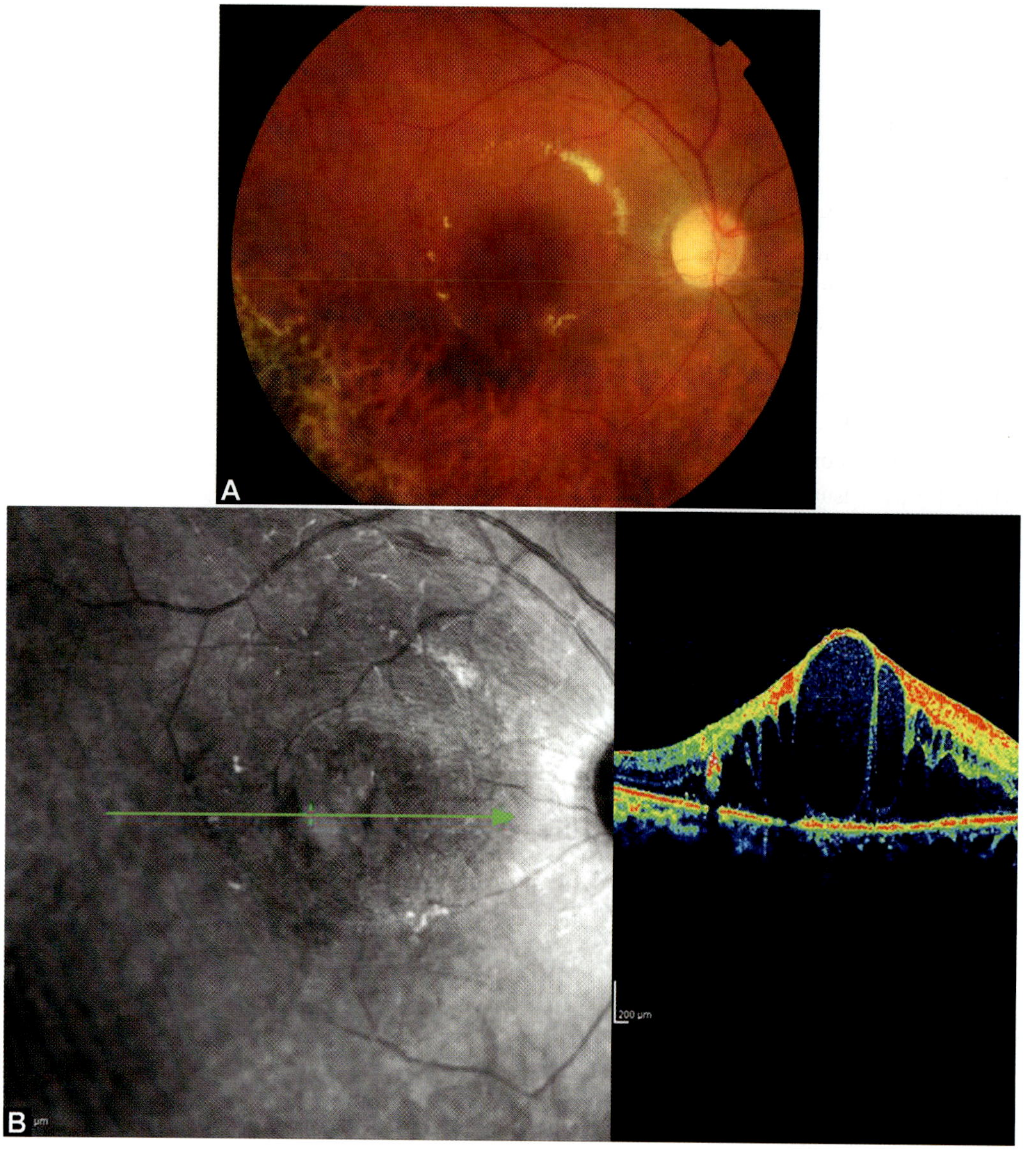

▲ **Figures 37.18A and B**

(A) Radiation maculopathy with circinate macular exudates developing 2 years after Ruthenium-106 plaque radiotherapy. The margin of the tumor is visible inferotemporally in the color photograph. Vision in this eye is 0.05; (B) Spectral domain OCT shows extensive intraretinal fluid accumulation almost simulating a serous retinal detachment in the macular area. The macular edema in this patient showed very litte response to intravitreal bevacizumab in terms of central foveal thickness reduction. However, vision remained stable at 0.05. After 5 intravitreal injections of bevacizumab given 4–6 weeks apart, the injections were halted on the grounds that there was no significant response

(PCNSL), high dose systemic chemotherapy with methotrexate and cytarabine with or without intrathecal methotrexate or rituximab are usually used. Cranial external beam radiotherapy is usually reserved for resistant or recurrent cases. However, there is concern about the efficacy of systemic chemotherapy as the sole therapy in patients with primary vitreoretinal lymphoma. In one report, all patients with primary vitreoretinal lymphoma treated with systemic chemotherapy suffered intraocular recurrence.[72] Therefore, adjunctive intraocular chemotherapy and immunotherapy should be considered in patients with primary vitreoretinal lymphoma.

Intravitreal Injections of Vascular Targeting Agents

Intravitreal injection of anti-VEGF (vascular endothelial growth factor) agents including bevacizumab and ranibizumab as well as triamcinolone acetonide have been used to treat radiation maculopathy and radiation papillopathy in choroidal melanoma (Figs 37.18A and B) and macular edema and exudation in retinal vascular tumors.[73-75] Radiation maculopathy may respond to bevacizumab with regression of macular edema and slight vision improvement in the early term.[73] Visual acuity increase usually does not occur in eyes with macular ischemia from radiation treatment. Intravitreal triamcinolone does not significantly improve the visual acuity in radiation papillopathy but may hasten the resolution of optic disc changes.[74] Intravitreal bevacizumab with or without PDT has been used in RCH and has been found to be useful in resolving the macular edema in a small number of patients.[75]

The role of intravitreal anti-VEGF agents as primary treatment for intraocular tumors is still unclear. A single case of retinal vasoproliferative tumor treated successfully with bevacizumab was reported. This patient experienced a 35% reduction in tumor thickness as well as resolution of macular edema at a short follow-up of 3 weeks.[76]

References

1. Eide N. Primary laser photocoagulation of "small" choroidal melanomas. Acta Ophthalmol Scand. 1999;77:351-4.
2. Shields JA, Glazer LC, Mieler WF. Comparison of xenon arc and argon laser photocoagulation in the treatment of choroidal melanomas. Am J Ophthalmol. 1990;109:647-55.
3. Shields CL, Shields JA, Kiratli H, et al. Treatment of retinoblastoma with indirect ophthalmoscope laser photocoagulation. J Pediatr Ophthalmol Strabismus. 1995;32:317-22.
4. Shields CL, Honavar S, Shields JA, et al. Circumscribed choroidal hemangioma: clinical manifestations and factors predictive of visual outcome in 200 consecutive cases. Ophthalmology. 2001;108:2237-48.
5. Anand R, Augsburger JJ, Shields JA. Circumscribed choroidal hemangiomas. Arch Ophthalmol. 1989;107:1338-42.
6. Schmidt D, Natt E, Neumann HP. Long-term results of laser treatment for retinal angiomatosis in von Hippel-Lindau disease. Eur J Med Res. 2000;5:47-58.
7. Bartlema YM, Oosterhius JA, Journee-De Korver JG, et al. Combined plaque radiotherapy and transpupillary thermotherapy in choroidal melanoma: 5 years' experience. Br J Ophthalmol. 2003;87:1370-3.
8. Shields CL, Shields JA, Perez N, et al. Primary transpupillary thermotherapy for small choroidal melanoma in 256 consecutive cases. Ophthalmology. 2002;109:225-34.
9. Oosterhuis JA, Journee-de Korver HG, Kakebeeke-Kemme HM, et al. Arch Ophthalmol. 1995;113:315-21.
10. Journee-de-Korver JG, Oosterhius JA, de Wolff-Rouendall D, et al. Histopathological findings in human choroidal melanomas after transpupillary thermotherapy. Br J Ophthalmol. 1997;81:234-9.
11. Shields CL, Shields JA, Cater J, et al. Transpupillary thermotherapy for choroidal melanoma. Tumor control and visual results in 100 consecutive cases. Ophthalmology. 1998;105: 581-90.
12. Godfrey DG, Waldron RG, Capone A. Transpupillary thermotherapy for small choroidal melanoma. Am J Ophthalmol. 1999;128:88-93.
13. Win PH, Robertson DM, Buttner H, et al. Extended follow-up of small melanocytic choroidal tumors treated with transpupillary thermotherapy. Arch Ophthalmol. 2006;124:503-6.
14. Pan Y, Diddie K, Lim JI. Primary transpupillary thermotherapy for small choroidal melanomas. Br J Ophthalmol. 2008;92:747-50.
15. Aaberg TM, Bergstrom CS, Hickner ZJ, et al. Long-term results of primary transpupillary thermal therapy for the treatment of choroidal malignant melanoma. Br J Ophthalmol. 2008;92:741-6.
16. Spire M, Devouassoux MSB, Kodjikian L, et al. Primary transpupillary thermotherapy for 18 small posterior pole uveal melanomas. Am J Ophthalmol. 2006;141:840-9.
17. Shields CL, Santos MC, Diniz W, et al. Thermotherapy for retinoblastoma. Arch Ophthalmol. 1999;117:885-93.
18. Abramson DH, Schefler AC. Transpupillary thermotherapy as initial treatment for small intraocular retinoblastoma: technique and predictors of success. Ophthalmology. 2004;111:984-91.
19. Murphree AL, Villablanca JG, Deegan WF, et al. Chemotherapy plus local treatment in the management of intraocular retinoblastoma. Arch Ophthalmol. 1996;114:1348-56.
20. Gündüz K. Transpupillary thermotherapy in the management of circumscribed choroidal hemangioma. Surv Ophthalmol. 2004;49:316-27.
21. Schmidt-Erfurth U, Laqua H, Schlotzer-Schrehard U, et al. Histopathological changes following photodynamic therapy in human eyes. Arch Ophthalmol. 2002;120:835-44.
22. Murphree AL, Cote M, Gomer CJ. The evolution of photodynamic therapy techniques in the treatment of intraocular tumors. Photochem Photobiol. 1987;46:919-23.
23. Schmidt-Erfurth U, Birngruber R, Hasan T. Photodynamic therapy in ocular vascular disease. Laser Physics. 1998;8:191-8.

24. Singh AD, Kaiser PK. Uveal vascular tumors. In: Singh AD, Damato BE, Pe'er J (Eds). Clinical Ophthalmic Oncology. Philadelphia (PA): Saunders-Elsevier; 2007. pp. 289-99.
25. Madreperla SA. Choroidal hemangioma treated with photodynamic therapy using verteporfin. Arch Ophthalmol. 2001;119:1606-10.
26. Jurklies B, Anastassiou G, Ortmans S, et al. Photodynamic therapy using verteporfin in circumscribed choroidal haemangioma. Br J Ophthalmol. 2003;87:84-9.
27. Scott TA, Augsburger JJ, Brady LW, et al. Low dose ocular irradiation for diffuse choroidal hemangiomas associated with bullous nonrhegmatogenous retinal detachment. Retina. 1991;11:389-93.
28. Singh AD, Rundle PA, Vardy SJ, et al. Photodynamic therapy of choroidal hemangioma associated with Sturge-Weber syndrome. Eye. 2004;19:365-7.
29. Bains HS, Cirino AC, Ticho BH, et al. Photodynamic therapy using verteporfin for a diffuse choroidal hemangioma in Sturge-Weber syndrome. Retina. 2004;24:152-5.
30. Rundle P, Rennie I. Management of symptomatic choroidal naevi with photodynamic therapy. Eye. 2007;21:1531-33.
31. Schmidt-Erfurth UM, Kusserow C, Barbazetto IA, et al. Benefits and complications of photodynamic therapy of papillary capillary hemangiomas. Ophthalmology. 2002;109: 1256-66.
32. Blasi MA, Scupola A, Tiberti AC, et al. Photodynamic therapy for vasoproliferative retinal tumors.Retina. 2006;26:404-9.
33. Shields CL, Materin MA, Mehta S, et al. Regression of extrafoveal choroidal osteoma following photodynamic therapy. Arch Ophthalmol. 2008;126:135-7.
34. Shields CL, Materin MA, Marr BP, et al. Resolution of exudative retinal detachment from retinal astrocytoma following photodynamic therapy. Arch Ophthalmol. 2008;126:273-4.
35. Mennel S, Hausmann N, Meyer CH, et al. Photodynamic therapy for exudative hamartoma in tuberous sclerosis. Arch Ophthalmol. 2006;124:597-9.
36. Shields CL, Shields JA. Recent developments in the management of retinoblastoma. J Pediatr Ophthalmol Strabismus. 1999;36:8-18.
37. Shields CL, Shields JA, Barrett J, et al. Vasoproliferative tumors of the ocular fundus. Classification and clinical manifestations in 103 patients. Arch Ophthalmol. 1995;113:615-23.
38. Singh AD, Nouri M, Shields CL, et al. Treatment of retinal capillary hemangioma. Ophthalmology. 2002;109:1799-806.
39. Gündüz K, Shields CL, Shields JA, et al. Plaque radiotherapy of uveal melanoma with predominant ciliary body involvement. Arch Ophthalmol. 1999;117:170-7.
40. Lommatzsch PK, Werschnik C, Schuster E. Long-term follow-up of Ru-106/Rh-106 brachytherapy for posterior uveal melanoma. Graefes Arch Clin Exp Ophthalmol. 2000;238:129-37.
41. Augsburger JJ, Gamel JW, Shields JA, et al. Post-irradiation regression of choroidal melanomas as a risk factor for death from metastatic disease. Ophthalmology. 1987;94:1173-7.
42. Gündüz K, Shields CL, Shields JA, et al. Radiation retinopathy following plaque radiotherapy for posterior uveal melanoma. Arch Ophthalmol. 1999;117:609-14.
43. Gündüz K, Shields CL, Shields JA, et al. Plaque radiotherapy for management of ciliary body and choroidal melanoma with extraocular extension. Am J Ophthalmol. 2000;130:97-102.
44. Shields CL, Shields JA, Cater J, et al. Plaque radiotherapy for retinoblastoma: long-term tumor control and treatment complications in 208 tumors. Ophthalmology. 2001;108:2116-21.
45. Madreperla SA, Hungerford JL, Plowman PN, et al. Choroidal hemangiomas: visual and anatomic results of treatment by photocoagulation or radiation therapy. Ophthalmology. 1997;104:1773-8.
46. Zografos L, Bercher L, Chamot L, et al. Cobalt-60 treatment of choroidal hemangiomas. Am J Ophthalmol. 1996;121:190-9.
47. Cohen VM, Shields CL, Demirci H, et al. Iodine I 125 plaque radiotherapy for vasoproliferative tumors of the retina in 30 eyes. Arch Ophthalmol. 2008;126:1245-51.
48. Anastassiou G, Bornfeld N, Schueler AO, et al. Ruthenium-106 plaque brachytherapy for symptomatic vasoproliferative tumours of the retina. Br J Ophthalmol. 2006;90:447-50.
49. Kreusel KM, Bornfeld N, Lommatzsch A, et al. Ruthenium-106 brachytherapy for peripheral retinal capillary hemangiomas. Ophthalmology. 1998;105:1386-92.
50. Shields CL, Manquez ME, Ehya H, et al. Fine-needle aspiration biopsy of iris tumors in 100 consecutive cases: technique and complications. Ophthalmology. 2006;113:2080-6.
51. Marigo FA, Finger PT. Anterior segment tumors: current concepts and innovations. Surv Ophthalmol. 2003;48:569-93.
52. Biswas J, Kumar SK, Gopal L, et al. Leiomyoma of the ciliary body extending to the anterior chamber: clinicopathologic and ultrasound biomicroscopic correlation. Surv Ophthalmol. 2000;44:336-42.
53. Fineman MS, Eagle RC, Shields J, et al. Melanocytomalytic glaucoma in eyes with necrotic iris melanocytoma. Ophthalmology. 1998;105:492-6.
54. Damato B, Woulds WS. Indications for trans-scleral local resection of uveal melanoma. Br J Ophthalmol. 1996;80:1029-30.
55. Shields JA, Shields CL, Shah P, et al. Partial lamellar sclerouvectomy for ciliary body and choroidal tumors. Ophthalmology. 1991;98:971-83.
56. Damato B. Adjunctive plaque radiotherapy after local resection of uveal melanoma. Front Radiat Ther Oncol. 1997;30:123-32.
57. Damato BE, Paul J, Foulds WS. Risk factors for residual and recurrent uveal melanoma after trans-scleral local resection. Br J Ophthalmol. 1996;80:102-8.
58. Kurt RA, Gündüz K. Exoresection via a partial lamellar sclerouvectomy approach: A successful performance by a novice surgeon. Clin Ophthalmol. 2010;4:59-65.
59. Bechrakis NE, Petousis VE, Willerding G, et al. Ten year results transcleral resection of large uveal melanomas: Local

tumour control and metastatic rate. Br J Ophthalmol. 2010;94:460-6.
60. Bechrakis NE, Bornfeld N, Zöller I, et al. Iodine 125 plaque brachytherapy versus transscleral tumor resection in the treatment of large uveal melanomas. Ophthalmology. 2002;109:1855-61.
61. Augsburger JJ, Lauritzen K, Gamel JW, et al. Matched group study of surgical resection versus cobalt-60 plaque radiotherapy for primary choroidal or ciliary body melanoma. Ophthalmic Surg. 1990;21:682-8.
62. Peyman GA, Cheema RA, Lagouros PA. Endoresection of a ciliochoroidal melanoma. Can J Ophthalmol. 2001;36:411-4.
63. Damato B, Groenewald C, McGalliard J, et al. Endoresection of choroidal melanoma. Br J Ophthalmol. 1998;82:213-8.
64. Garcia-Arumi J, Zapata MA, Balaguer O, et al. Endoresection in high posterior choroidal melanomas: long-term outcome. Br J Ophthalmol. 2008;92:1040-5.
65. Bechrakis NE, Foerster MH. Neoadjuvant proton beam radiotherapy combined with subsequent endoresection of choroidal melanomas. Int Ophthalmol Clin. 2006;46:95-107.
66. Bechrakis NE, Blatsios G, Schmid E, et al. Surgical resection techniques of large uveal melanomas. Spektrum Augenheilkd. 2010;24:17-22.
67. Yeh S, Weichel ED, Faia LJ, et al. 25-Gauge transconjunctival sutureless vitrectomy for the diagnosis of intraocular lymphoma. Br J Ophthalmol. 2010;94:633-8.
68. Kreusel KM, Bechrakis NE, Neumann HP, et al. Pars plana vitrectomy for juxtapapillary capillary retinal angioma. Am J Ophthalmol. 2006;141:587-9.
69. Ferreyra HA, Goldbaum MH, Weinreb RN. Endoresection of irradiated choroidal melanoma as a treatment for intractable vitreous hemorrhage and secondary blood-induced glaucoma. Semin Ophthalmol. 2008;23:135-8.
70. Kitzmann AS, Pulido JS, Mohney BG, et al. Intraocular use of rituximab. Eye. 2007;21:1524-7.
71. Smith JR, Rosenbaum JT, Wilson DJ, et al. Role of intravitreal methotrexate in the management of primary central nervous system lymphoma with ocular involvement. Ophthalmology. 2002;109:1709-16.
72. Velez G, Yuan P, Sung C, et al. Pharmacokinetics and toxicity of intravitreal chemotherapy for primary intraocular lymphoma. Arch Ophthalmol. 2001;119:1518-24.
73. Mason JO, Albert MA, Persaud TO, et al. Intravitreal bevacizumab treatment for radiation macular edema after plaque radiotherapy for choroidal melanoma. Retina. 2007;27:903-7.
74. Shields CL, Demirci H, Dai V, et al. Intravitreal triamcinolone acetonide for radiation maculopathy after plaque radiotherapy for choroidal melanoma. Retina. 2005;25:868-74.
75. Mennel S, Meyer CH, Callizo J. Combined intravitreal anti-vascular endothelial growth factor (Avastin) and photodynamic therapy to treat retinal juxtapapillary capillary haemangioma. Acta Ophthalmol. 2009 Feb 12. [Epub ahead of print]
76. Kenawy N, Groenwald C, Damato B. Treatment of a vasoproliferative tumour with intravitreal bevacizumab (Avastin). Eye. 2007;21:893-4.

Index

Page numbers with *f* and *t* indicate figure and table, respectively.

A

B

C

D

M

N

Q

R

S

T

U

V

W

X

Y